Nutrition and Metabolism

NUTRITION AND HEALTH

Adrianne Bendich, PhD, FACN, Series Editor

For other titles published in this series, go to
www.springer.com/series/7659

NUTRITION AND METABOLISM

Underlying Mechanisms and Clinical Consequences

Editor

Christos S. Mantzoros, MD, DSc
Division of Endocrinology, Diabetes and Metabolism,
Beth Israel Deaconess Medical Center, Harvard Medical School,
Boston, MA, USA

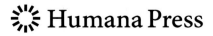

Humana Press

Editor
Christos S. Mantzoros, MD, DSc
Division of Endocrinology
Diabetes and Metabolism
Beth Israel Deaconess Medical Center
Harvard Medical School
Boston, MA
USA

Series Editor
Adrianne Bendich, PhD, FACN
GlaxoSmithKline Consumer Healthcare
Parsippany, NJ
USA

ISBN: 978-1-60327-452-4   e-ISBN: 978-1-60327-453-1
DOI: 10.1007/978-1-60327-453-1

Library of Congress Control Number: 2009922619

Dedication

To my parents, whose lifelong service to their suffering fellow human beings became a true inspiration and enlightened guidance for my professional and personal life

Series Preface

The Nutrition and Health™ series of books have, as an overriding mission, to provide health professionals with texts that are considered essential because each includes: (1) a synthesis of the state of the science, (2) timely, in-depth reviews by the leading researchers in their respective fields, (3) extensive, up-to-date fully annotated reference lists, (4) a detailed index, (5) relevant tables and figures, (6) identification of paradigm shifts and the consequences, (7) virtually no overlap of information between chapters, but targeted, inter-chapter referrals, (8) suggestions of areas for future research, and (9) balanced, data-driven answers to patient/health professionals questions which are based upon the totality of evidence rather than the findings of any single study.

The series volumes are developed to provide valuable in-depth information to nutrition health professionals and health providers interested in practical guidelines. Each editor has the potential to examine a chosen area with a broad perspective, both in subject matter as well as in the choice of chapter authors. The international perspective, especially with regard to public health initiatives, is emphasized where appropriate. The editors, whose trainings are both research and practice oriented, have the opportunity to develop a primary objective for their book, define the scope and focus, and then invite the leading authorities from around the world to be part of their initiative. The authors are encouraged to provide an overview of the field, discuss their own research, and relate the research findings to potential human health consequences. Because each book is developed de novo, the chapters are coordinated so that the resulting volume imparts greater knowledge than the sum of the information contained in the individual chapters.

Nutrition and Metabolism: Underlying Mechanisms and Clinical Consequences, edited by Christos S. Mantzoros, MD is a very welcome addition to the Nutrition and Health Series and fully exemplifies the Series' goals. This volume is especially timely since the obesity epidemic continues to increase around the world and the comorbidities, such as the metabolic syndrome, type II diabetes, hypertension, and hyperlipidemia are seen even in very young children. The editor reminds us that, for most people, their weight remains relatively stable despite wide variations in the types of foods we consume each day, differences in caloric content, and differences in daily physical activity. It is only recently that physicians, scientists, and health providers have begun to think about the complexities of excess body weight. This volume contains informative chapters that look at the genetics associated with obesity, the role of the nervous system and the endocrine system, the gastrointestinal tract and of great importance, adipose tissue, as more than a fat storage site. The last decade has seen an explosion of identification and characterization of the many bioactive molecules that are synthesized and secreted by adipose cells (adipokines). The adipokines and other molecules synthesized in the stomach, intestines, pancreas, and other gastrointestinal organs have been associated with the development of obesity and its comorbidities as well as many, often thought of as unrelated, consequences including insulin resistance, cardiovascular complications, lipid disorders, hypertension, and hormonal imbalances as examples. Thus, the relevance of obesity-related pathophysiology to the clinical setting is of great interest to not only academic researchers, but also healthcare providers. This text is the first to synthesize the knowledge base concerning obesity and its comorbidities including metabolic syndrome, diabetes, hypertension, and hyperlipidemia, and relate these to the mechanisms behind the alterations in metabolism that increase chronic disease risk. This unique volume also contains practice guidelines and tools for obesity management to help the practicing health professional as well as those professionals who have an interest in the latest, up-to-date information on obesity treatments and their implications for improving human health and reducing obesity-related diseases.

This volume serves the dual purposes of providing current clinical assessment and management guidelines as well as relevant background information on the genetics and pathophysiology associated with the consequences of obesity. The chapters include an historic perspective as well as suggestions for future research opportunities. Dr. Mantzoros is an internationally recognized leader in the field of obesity research as well as clinical outcomes. He and his authors are excellent communicators and he has worked tirelessly to develop a book that is destined to be the benchmark in the field because of its extensive, in-depth chapters covering the most important aspects of the complex interactions between cellular functions, diet and obesity, and its impact on disease states. The editor has chosen 32 of the most well-recognized and respected authors from around the world to contribute the 18 informative chapters in the volume. Hallmarks of all of the chapters include complete definitions of terms with the abbreviations fully defined for the reader and consistent use of terms between chapters. Key features of this comprehensive volume include the informative key points and keywords that are at the beginning of each chapter, appendices that include detailed tables of major nutrient recommendations for weight reduction in the obese as well as for those with diabetes; detailed descriptions of the Dietary Approaches to Stop Hypertension (DASH) diet protocol; an extensive list of foods and their glycemic index and many other practical guidelines to help in patient management. The volume also contains more than 80 detailed tables and informative figures, an extensive, detailed index, and more than 2,000 up-to-date references that provide the reader with excellent sources of worthwhile information about the role of diet, exercise, food intake, physiology and pathophysiology of obesity, the metabolic syndrome, types I and II diabetes, and other obesity-related comorbidities.

Dr. Mantzoros has coauthored many of the chapters and he has chosen chapter authors who are internationally distinguished researchers, clinicians, and epidemiologists who provide a comprehensive foundation for understanding the role of weight control in the maintenance of human health as well as its role in obesity and related co-morbidities. The book is organized into logical sections that provide the reader with an overview of the complexities of weight control. There is an extensive discussion of the genetics of obesity and the involvement of at least 11 human genes in the control of food intake and metabolism. Genetically linked obesity syndromes are described including Prader–Willi syndrome. This chapter includes new information on the genetics of metabolic syndrome, types I and II diabetes and reviews the findings that link these diseases genetically. The interaction between the central and peripheral nervous systems, the endocrine system, and molecules synthesized during digestion are discussed in the next chapter that introduces the reader to the concepts of metabolic signals, orosensory stimuli, GI tract peptides and adipokines from fat tissue. Explanations are provided for the role of leptin, insulin, peptide YY, ghrelin, visfatin, cholecystokinin, and many other important modulators in human metabolism. An important chapter is devoted to the description of the central nervous system with detailed explanations of the importance of the hypothalamus and the brain stem. We learn that control of appetite resides in the arcuate nucleus area of the hypothalamus, whereas the paraventricular nucleus is involved with energy homeostasis. This chapter reviews the importance of orexigenic and anorexigenic neuropeptides as well as the effects of thyroid hormones, adrenergic receptors, and thermogenic tissues. The final chapter in the section on genetics and pathophysiology looks at insulin resistance and its consequences. The concept of adipose tissue inflammation is introduced and there is discussion about body fat distribution including the effects of visceral vs. subcutaneous fat.

Childhood obesity is a major public health concern as the percentage of young children that are obese or overweight continues to grow globally. There is an extensive review of the published studies that have attempted to control weight gain in children and adolescents most of which do not use pharmacological agents. Certainly, more research is needed in this area as long-term successful strategies have not been developed and well-accepted guidelines for clinical practice are not currently available. Two chapters review recommendations for diet and physical activity for healthy adults in one chapter and for the prevention and management of diabetes in the other chapter. These chapters discuss the importance of reducing trans fats, total fat, refined grains, and sugar-sweetened beverages. The authors review the data on the importance of physical activity to help control lipid levels and improve energy balance. The final chapter in this section examines the association of obesity and cancer risk. Poor dietary habits account for about 35% of incident cancers and smoking accounts for 30%; obesity accounts for 15%. About 16–20% of cancer deaths in US women and 14% in US men can be attributed to obesity. The chapter includes an analysis of the dietary habits around the globe that can result in a sevenfold difference in the rates of breast and prostate cancers between Western type diets and the rates seen in Japan.

Many nations have developed nutrition recommendations for the general population as well as for those individuals who suffer from the co-morbidities associated with obesity including diabetes and cardiovascular disease. This section of the volume considers the guidance that has been provided, reviews the history of the development of US national dietary guidelines and the most recent Food Guide Pyramid, and follows with a provocative chapter by Drs. Willett and Stampfer that questions the scientific basis for some of the more general national recommendations given in the Pyramid. Nutrition recommendation for those with cardiovascular disease includes reduction of salt, saturated and trans fats and increases in dietary fiber, antioxidants, B vitamins, omega-3 fatty acids, mono-unsaturated fatty acids, calcium, and potassium. Examples of food-based intervention studies that have reduced cardiovascular disease (CVD) risk factors including the prudent diet, DASH diet, Mediterranean diet and the guidelines from the American Heart

Association and the European Society of Cardiology are discussed in detail. Details are also provided for the assessment of cardiovascular disease including the biochemical markers currently used to stage the patient. This chapter also discussed the role of dietary supplements in CVD management. In the past 20 years, a new field of patient care has emerged called medical nutrition therapy (MNT). MNT has been particularly important in the management of patients with types I and II diabetes. Practice guidelines have been developed for children, adolescents, and adults and have been of value in the control of blood glucose levels as well as glycosylated hemoglobin. Diets are recommended that contain levels of essential micronutrients important to the diabetic. This chapter and the additional information in the related appendices provide practical information for the health provider. There is also a separate chapter that describes the Mediterranean diet and the clinical studies, including survey data, case–control and intervention studies that have examined the potential for this diet to reduce obesity and CVD.

The final section includes in-depth chapters on the clinical assessment and management of obesity and its co-morbidities. There is a comprehensive chapter on lifestyle and pharmacological treatments for obesity. It is of interest that even today that hyper-cholesterolemia remains undiagnosed in 50% of the US population and 95% remain undertreated. This chapter explains the effects of hypertension, often seen in the obese, on carotid medial intimal thickness and the clinical studies that have included treatments. A comprehensive review of statin use is also included. Accurate diagnosis tools for obesity and diabetes are provided in the next chapter and also include management tools for gestational diabetes. Another informative chapter describes the use of bariatric surgery and the critical importance of the preoperation evaluation. We are reminded that to date weight loss surgery is the only effective treatment for severe, medically complicated, and refractory obesity. Guidelines for patient inclusion, types of operations, and importantly, postoperation care are provided in detail. The final chapter reviews the major co-morbidities associated with obesity and weight loss due to bariatric surgery that have not been included in other chapters. These areas include the increased risk of osteoporosis and fracture following bariatric surgery and the increased risk of gallstones that also occurs after this surgery. On the other hand, there appears to be a significant decrease in mortality as well as a decrease in sleep apnea and osteoarthritis. The literature on the increased risk of certain cancers with obesity is also included. Each of the chapter authors has integrated the newest research findings so the reader can better understand the complex interactions that can result from excess weight gain as well as loss of excess weight.

Given the growing concern with the increase in adult as well as childhood obesity, it is not surprising to find that all chapters in this valuable book are devoted to the clinical aspects of obesity, weight control, diabetes, and other chronic diseases associated with obesity. Moreover, both the cultural aspects of weight gain and the emotional triggers of eating are reviewed. Emphasis is also given to the growing awareness that obesity is associated with a low-grade inflammatory state. The editor and authors have integrated the information within these chapters so that the healthcare practitioner can provide guidance to the patient about the potential consequences of chronic obesity. The inclusion of both the earlier chapters on the complexity of human physiology and the chapters that contain clinical discussions helps the reader to have a broader basis of understanding of obesity and the attendant co-morbidities.

In conclusion, *Nutrition and Metabolism: Underlying Mechanisms and Clinical Consequences*, edited by Christos S. Mantzoros, MD provides health professionals in many areas of research and practice with the most up-to-date, well-referenced volume on the importance of maintaining normal weight so that obesity and the obesity-related chronic diseases that can adversely affect human health are avoided. This volume will serve the reader as the benchmark in this complex area of interrelationships between body weight, the central nervous system, endocrine organs, the GI tract, the biochemical reactions in fat cells, inflammation of adipose tissue, and the functioning of all other organ systems in the human body. Moreover, the interactions between obesity, genetic factors, and the numerous co-morbidities are clearly delineated so that students as well as practitioners can better understand the complexities of these interactions. Dr. Mantzoros is applauded for his efforts to develop the most authoritative resource in the field to date and this excellent text is a very welcome addition to the Nutrition and Health series.

Adrianne Bendich, PhD, FACN
Parsippany, NJ

Preface

Research on obesity spans a wide range of disciplines, from molecular biology to physiology to epidemiology and translational research to clinical medicine. This book attempts to review comprehensively, for practicing clinicians and scientists alike, our current understanding of how nutrition interacts with the genetic substrate as well as environmental-exogenous factors, including physical activity or the lack thereof, to result in insulin resistance and the metabolic syndrome. Furthermore, the causation, epidemiology, clinical presentation, prevention, and treatment of the most common manifestations of disease states associated with the metabolic syndrome are reviewed. After presenting the Scope of the Problem, the first major part of the book is devoted to Genetics and Pathophysiology, the second part of the book presents the Public Health Perspective of the most prevalent problems associated with nutrition and the metabolic syndrome, whereas the third major part of the book focuses on Clinical Assessment and Management of the main disease states associated with inappropriate nutrition and the metabolic syndrome. Finally, general information useful for both clinicians and researchers alike is presented in the Appendix.

Covering the entire field of nutrition or metabolism would have been a daunting task, far beyond the scope of a single volume book. Thus, *Nutrition and Metabolism: Underlying Mechanisms and Clinical Consequences* offers only an up-to-date and authoritative review of the major scientific and clinical aspects of the overlapping areas between nutrition and metabolism. I am indebted to all my colleagues, most of them scientists and distinguished professors at Harvard University, for their valuable contributions. I thank the staff at Humana Press for their hard work in putting together this book in close collaboration with staff in my group, especially Lauren Kuhn and Jess Fargnoli. We also wish to express our gratitude to Dr. Adrianne Bendich, the Series Editor, for her thoughtful suggestions.

I certainly hope that the efforts of all of us will not only provide much needed information to our practicing colleagues but also serve as a stimulus for further research in this scientific topic of utmost importance for the developed world in the twenty-first century. Our mission will be eventually accomplished if, through higher quality research, superior teaching, and consequently improved health services, the quality of our prevention programs as well as the quality of health care we provide to our suffering fellow human beings is ultimately enhanced.

Christos S. Mantzoros
Boston, MA

Contents

Contributors

CAROLINE APOVIAN, MD • *Division of Endocrinology, Diabetes, and Nutrition, Boston University School of Medicine and Boston Medical Center, Boston, MA, USA*

EIRINI BATHRELLOU, MSc • *Department of Nutrition and Dietetics, Harokopio University, Athens, Greece*

GEORGE L. BLACKBURN, PhD, MD • *Division of Nutrition, Beth Israel Deaconess Medical Center, Harvard Medical School, Boston, MA, USA*

SUSANN BLÜHER, MD • *Hospital for Children and Adolescents, University of Leipzig, Leipzig, Germany and Division of Endocrinology, Diabetes & Metabolism, Beth Israel Deaconess Medical Center, Boston, MA, USA*

AOIFE BRENNAN, MD • *Division of Endocrinology, Diabetes & Metabolism, Beth Israel Deaconess Medical Center, Harvard Medical School, Boston, MA, USA*

JEAN L. CHAN, MD • *Division of Endocrinology, Diabetes & Metabolism, Beth Israel Deaconess Medical Center, Harvard Medical School, Boston, MA, USA*

THOMAS DANNE, MD • *Diabetes Center for Children and Adolescents, Childrens' Hospital at the Bult, Hannover, Germany*

KRISTINA DAY, RD • *Division of Surgery, Beth Israel Deaconess Medical Center, Harvard Medical School, Boston, MA, USA*

CARA B. EBBELING, PhD • *Children's Hospital Boston, Harvard Medical School, Boston, MA, USA*

EVAGGELIA FAPPA, MSc • *Department of Nutrition and Dietetics, Harokopio University, Athens, Greece*

JESSICA FARGNOLI, BS • *Division of Endocrinology, Diabetes & Metabolism, Beth Israel Deaconess Medical Center, Harvard Medical School, Boston, MA, USA*

FRANK B. HU, PhD, MD • *Department of Nutrition, Harvard School of PublicHealth, Boston, MA, USA*

JANICE JIN HWANG, MD • *Division of Endocrinology, Diabetes & Metabolism, Beth Israel Deaconess Medical Center, Harvard Medical School, Boston, MA, USA*

DANIEL B. JONES MD, MS • *Section of Minimally Invasive Surgery, Beth Israel Deaconess Medical Center, Harvard Medical School, Boston, MA, USA*

IOSIF KELESIDIS, MD • *Division of Endocrinology, Diabetes & Metabolism, Beth Israel Deaconess Medical Center, Harvard Medical School, Boston, MA, USA*

THEODORE KELESIDIS, MD • *Division of Endocrinology, Diabetes & Metabolism, Beth Israel Deaconess Medical Center, Harvard Medical School, Boston, MA, USA*

YOON KIM, MD • *Division of Endocrinology, Diabetes & Metabolism, Beth Israel Deaconess Medical Center, Harvard Medical School, Boston, MA, USA*

MEROPI KONTOGIANNI, MD • *Department of Nutrition and Dietetics, Harokopio University, Athens, Greece*

OLGA KORDONOURI, MD • *Diabetes Center for Children and Adolescents, Childrens' Hospital at the Bult, Hannover, Germany*

LAUREN KUHN, BS • *Division of Endocrinology, Diabetes & Metabolism, Beth Israel Deaconess Medical Center, Harvard Medical School, Boston, MA, USA*

CHRISTOS S. MANTZOROS, MD, DSc • *Division of Endocrinology, Diabetes & Metabolism, Beth Israel Deaconess Medical Center, Harvard Medical School, Boston, MA, USA*

J. PETER OETTGEN, MD • *Division of Cardiology, Beth Israel Deaconess Medical Center, Harvard Medical School, Boston, MA, USA*

TORSTEN OLBERS, MD, PhD • *Department of Surgery and Gastro Research, Sahlgrenska University Hospital, Goteborg, Sweden*

DEANNA OLENCZUK, BS • *Division of Endocrinology, Diabetes & Metabolism, Beth Israel Deaconess Medical Center, Harvard Medical School, Boston, MA, USA*

VIVIAN M. SANCHEZ, MD • *Section of Minimally Invasive Surgery, Beth Israel Deaconess Medical Center, Harvard Medical School, Boston, MA, USA*

DESPINA SANOUDOU, PhD • *Division of Molecular Biology, Foundation for Biomedical Research of the Academy of Athens, Athens, Greece*

BENJAMIN E. SCHNEIDER, MD • *Section of Minimally Invasive Surgery, Beth Israel Deaconess Medical Center, Harvard Medical School, Boston, MA, USA*

SUNALI SHAH, BS • *Division of Endocrinology, Diabetes & Metabolism, Beth Israel Deaconess Medical Center, Harvard Medical School, Boston, MA, USA*

MEIR STAMPFER, MD • *Departments of Nutrition and Epidemiology, Harvard School of Public Health, Boston, MA, USA*

ELIZABETH VAFIADAKI, PhD • *Division of Molecular Biology, Foundation for Biomedical Research of the Academy of Athens, Athens, Greece*

WALTER WILLETT, MD • *Department of Nutrition, Harvard School of Public Health, Boston, MA, USA*

ALICJA WOLK, DMSc • *Institute of Environmental Medicine, Karolinska Institutet, Stockholm, Sweden*

MARY YANNAKOULIA, PhD • *Department of Nutrition and Dietetics, Harokopio University, Athens, Greece*

I SCOPE OF THE PROBLEM

1 Nutrition and the Metabolic Syndrome: A Twenty-First-Century Epidemic of Obesity and Eating Disorders

Christos S. Mantzoros

Lack of sufficient nutrition is the main problem of billions of persons in the underdeveloped world, while excessive caloric intake leading to obesity is becoming more and more prevalent in Western societies of affluence. As a result, obesity, which leads to the metabolic syndrome and is thus closely associated with significant morbidity and mortality from diabetes, cardiovascular diseases, and cancers, to mention a few, is considered the epidemic of our century in Western societies.

Positive energy balance, as reflected by increasing BMI, is not a recent phenomenon. BMI has been increasing for many decades, but until the mid or late 1970s, it was rather associated with improved health and increased longevity. In the past few decades, however, the risk-to-benefit ratio has been shifting in such a way that the continued increase in body fatness is increasingly being recognized as underlying several chronic disease states. This phenomenon is slowing or even reversing gains made in terms of life expectancy in the past. More than 30% of Americans are currently overweight and another 30% are obese, defined as a body mass index (BMI) between 25.0 and 29.9 kg m^{-2} and higher than 30.0 kg m^{-2} respectively. Moreover, if the current trends continue, it is expected that by the year 2020 more than 50% of Americans will be obese, possibly making obesity the "norm" and leanness the "exception." In children, use of the term overweight is usually preferred, to avoid potential stigmatization, and thus the definition of obesity in children is based on exceeding the 95th percentile of BMI-for-age using the 2000 Centers for Disease Control charts.

From: *Nutrition and Health: Nutrition and Metabolism*
Edited by: C.S. Mantzoros, DOI: 10.1007/978-1-60327-453-1_1,
© Humana Press, a part of Springer Science+Business Media, LLC 2009

Obesity is currently considered as being responsible for increasing morbidity as well as mortality, i.e., for the deaths of several hundreds of thousands of persons every year in Western societies. This fact makes obesity the second important potentially preventable cause of death after smoking. In addition to leading to illness, obesity can reduce significantly functional capacity and can increase disability. Realization of the above has prompted a heightened research interest in the factors influencing energy balance, and intensified research efforts on the links between obesity and its complications. It has also created an increasing demand for the study of new methods to diagnose, prevent, or treat obesity and associated comorbidities.

Negative energy balance, either due to lack of availability of appropriate nutrition leading to starvation in underdeveloped nations, or due to voluntary (dieting for weight loss) or involuntary caloric restriction (anorexia nervosa, exercise-induced or hypothalamic amenorrhea) in developed nations, is also of increasing prevalence. Immune dysfunction as well as certain well-defined neuroendocrine abnormalities leading to important adverse health consequences such as osteoporosis and infertility are the end result of energy deprivation. Research efforts to identify missing links between energy deficiency and these pathophysiological abnormalities have also been intensified over the past several years. In the area of epidemiology of obesity, the good news is that increasing rates of obesity appear to be reaching a plateau either because public health campaigns and interventions have started working and/or because almost all people with the genetic potential to develop obesity upon exposure to adverse environmental and dietary factors have already developed obesity. The bad news is that the prevalence of obesity continues to rise around the world and that this rising prevalence of obesity is associated with increasing rates of disability, morbidity, and mortality.

1. CAN WE DISCERN HOPEFUL SIGNS IN THE MIDDLE OF THE CURRENT DIFFICULTIES CREATED BY THESE DISEASE STATES?

Several discoveries over the past 10 years have created opportunities for prevention and/or treatment, including discoveries of new genes, molecules, and regulatory pathways. Central, in my opinion, may prove to be developments in the field encompassed by the question: How does negative energy balance lead to neuroendocrine abnormalities? Recent work, mainly from our laboratory, has demonstrated that levels of an adipocyte-secreted hormone, circulating levels of which reflect the amount of energy stored in fat, i.e. leptin, fall in response to negative energy balance and this fall can lead to the neuroendocrine dysfunction that has traditionally been associated with energy, and thus leptin, deficiency states, such as anorexia nervosa and exercise-induced or hypothalamic amenorrhea. Importantly, exogenous administration of leptin, in replacement doses, can correct these neuroendocrine abnormalities in these leptin deficiency states. These novel advances, discussed in the relevant chapters of this book, open new and exciting avenues for diagnosing and treating these conditions in the future. Whether additional factors may also play a role or modify the effects of leptin administration remains to be seen. It also remains to be seen whether falling leptin levels in response to caloric/energy deprivation in obese persons who diet to lose weight may also be responsible for their neuroendocrine changes, which, in turn, tend to defend the original body weight and to make the obese person regain any weight lost in response to dieting.

2. EPIDEMIOLOGY TRENDS IN CHILDREN AND ADULTS

The prevalence of obesity has been increasing steadily over the past several years. This has been documented in both genders and in every ethnic group and socioeconomic status in Western societies of affluence. Importantly, the increasing prevalence of obesity is not confined to adults; children and adolescents are becoming increasingly overweight and obese. This phenomenon has resulted in increasing prevalence of type 2 diabetes among adolescents and is expected to shift the age of diagnosis of obesity-associated comorbidities, including cardiovascular diseases and cancers, earlier in life. The potential financial, psychological, and public health implications of these changes are enormous, and have not yet been fully appreciated.

Recent evidence indicates that in addition to long-recognized genetic and environmental factors, including nutrition and exercise, social networks are closely associated with and may play an important role in the spread of obesity. What are the links between significant interpersonal relationships, human behavior, and the pathogenesis of obesity and its complications? What is their impact on obesity prevention and treatment in societies of affluence, as well as in developing societies? Also, how does inappropriate nutrition lead to obesity and how is obesity linked to morbidity and mortality? A considerable amount of work is currently underway to identify and characterize the environmental, social, genetic, cognitive, sensory, metabolic, hormonal, and neural factors leading to obesity and associated comorbidities. The end result is the significant growth of specific clusters of knowledge in each one of the above specific scientific areas; over the past 15 years, none is currently emerging, unfortunately, as developed enough to explain a meaningful proportion of the problem and/or to allow meaningful predictions of future developments in the areas of prevention or treatment (see below). This not only underlines the multifactorial pathogenesis of the problem but is also considered by many as the last step before major breakthroughs occur on the basis of this accumulating knowledge. Significant progress is being made in the scientific area of hormonal and other factors linking excessive amounts of energy stored in adipose tissue with insulin resistance, the metabolic syndrome, and related complications. All these are outlined in detail in the respective chapters of this book.

3. ENVIRONMENTAL AND EXOGENOUS INFLUENCES AS OPPORTUNITIES FOR PUBLIC HEALTH INTERVENTIONS

Our current environment is distinctly different from the one our ancestors encountered several centuries or even just a century ago. One would thus argue that obesity may be, in part, the result of several factors set in motion by changes in the environment we live in, including the immediate availability of food at the expense of a lower cost and less physical labor, less physical activity, and possibly potential hormonal and epigenetic effects. Questions related to these notions are not only what the best interventions, including diet and exercise, should be, but also how could one help people adhere to an appropriate intervention program for the long term?

Two commonly attacked environmental factors are food marketing practices and institutionally and technologically driven reductions in physical activity. Yet, many have argued that, despite emerging data from controlled interventional studies, available data supporting the above are largely circumstantial and observational in nature. We all realize, however, that if we are to make pervasive and enduring changes to the prevalence of obesity and associated comorbidities, it is likely that we will need to make pervasive and enduring changes to the ways we live across our entire lifespan and these changes are admittedly difficult to implement.

4. MECHANISMS UNDERLYING THE LINK BETWEEN NUTRITION, METABOLISM, AND DISEASE STATES AS OPPORTUNITIES FOR MEDICAL INTERVENTIONS

Although we realize that obesity is associated with adverse health outcomes, we do not fully understand the mechanisms underlying these associations. New genes linked to obesity have been discovered and novel neuroendocrine mechanisms have been proposed. Although scientific developments in basic and translational research over the past decade have greatly advanced our understanding of the mechanisms underlying the development of the metabolic syndrome and associated abnormalities, as discussed in detail herein, much more needs to be done in the not so distant future.

5. HOW EFFECTIVE ARE WE IN ACHIEVING OUR GOALS?

Assuming that weight loss is desirable, can we really achieve it? Behavioral modifications such as diet and exercise, while first-line recommendations, remain ultimately largely ineffective at maintaining long-term weight loss at desirable levels. Despite intensive research efforts in the field, it remains to be fully elucidated which diet or dietary pattern, if any, is the most beneficial in terms of reducing weight loss or improving metabolic profile. This is related, in part, to the difficulty in reproducing in an experimental setting the real life dietary patterns of populations, let alone to perform long-term clinical trials utilizing these specific diets or dietary patterns. Thus, although data from interventional studies have started to emerge, current dietary recommendations are based mainly on expert opinion, based, to a large extent, on observational studies (which do not prove causality), expected outcomes and risk–benefit estimations.

We discuss herein the effects of different treatment modalities, including behavioral modifications such as diet and exercise, pharmacotherapy, and bariatric surgery, on obesity and its comorbidities, including cardiovascular risk factors, risk for malignancy, bone disease, biliary disease, and overall quality of life. Pertinent randomized controlled clinical trial and meta-analysis data are discussed and when these are not available, or do not fully elucidate relevant questions, data from observational studies and case series are reported in the relevant chapters of this book.

6. WHERE WOULD WE LIKE TO BE IN THE NOT SO DISTANT FUTURE?

In energy deficiency states we clearly need to advance further our understanding of the role of leptin (and other hormones) to improve and/or correct the neuroendocrine abnormalities of women with hypothalamic amenorrhea and anorexia nervosa as well as those of obese subjects dieting to lose weight and/or having had surgery for obesity. We also need conclusive evidence from randomized trials on whether leptin and/or other treatment options could also improve the osteoporosis of subjects with anorexia nervosa or hypothalamic amenorrhea. Importantly, we need to learn whether the effect of leptin in improving neuroendocrine function could facilitate weight maintenance of obese subjects who strive to lose weight. Much needed investigations are underway in this area.

With obesity affecting greater numbers of people each year and with currently available methods having only modest success to reduce the increasing prevalence of obesity, there is an urgent need to develop better weight loss and weight maintenance programs. We also need to clearly identify the many genetic and environmental components that are involved in the pathogenesis of the problem and to carefully study the underlying molecular, cellular, and hormonal mechanisms. On the basis of elucidating these factors, effective diagnostic tools and pharmaceuticals could hopefully be designed, appropriate behavioral modification programs could be investigated, and well-informed public health recommendations could be formulated to direct and implement pervasive, effective, and enduring changes to the ways we live our lives.

7. WHAT CAN WE RECOMMEND TODAY?

Diet and exercise are the cornerstones of prevention and treatment of obesity and related disorders. Although dietary recommendations have been changing over the past few years, it is hoped that, as we learn more from both observational and interventional studies, our recommendations will continue to be refined and will hopefully prove to be more and more effective. It is also hoped that diagnostic and therapeutic methods will continue to improve significantly. New medications and new surgical methods are continually tested, developed, and applied. We present herein our current understanding of underlying scientific principles and current recommendations with the explicit understanding that medical approaches should not only be characterized by continuous quality improvements but need to also be individualized and guided by the responsible treating physician.

Each chapter in this book provides an authoritative review of the current status of research and knowledge in each one of the most important clusters of current work in the Nutrition and Metabolism field. Text and graphs of several chapters appeared in their original form in the textbook "Nutrition and Metabolism", C. Mantzoros (editor), published by the Aristides Daskalopoulos Foundation in Athens, Greece, 2007. Material from these chapters is reproduced herein with permission granted by the Aristides Daskalopoulos Foundation. The chapters in this book are relatively brief, analytical, based on scientific evidence, and are written in an accessible style. We all hope that putting together cutting-edge research and reviewing critically current knowledge in all these fields will result in a sum that will be greater than its individual components. We also hope that ongoing work will lead, in the not so distant future, to a better understanding of the problems we are facing and to a more efficient creation of novel solutions that would allow us to effectively combat and hopefully eliminate this epidemic of the twenty-first century.

II   GENETICS AND PATHOPHYSIOLOGY

2 Genes and Gene–Environment Interactions in the Pathogenesis of Obesity and the Metabolic Syndrome

Despina Sanoudou, Elizabeth Vafiadaki, and Christos S. Mantzoros

KEY POINTS

- In recent years, the prevalence of obesity has risen sharply, becoming a major public health problem, especially in western countries.
- According to the World Health Organization (http://www.who.int), an estimated 1 billion adults are overweight (body mass index > 25 kg/m^2), and 300 million of these are considered clinically obese (body mass index > 30 kg/m^2).
- In part as a result of the rising prevalence of obesity, the incidence of the metabolic syndrome and type 2 diabetes are also reaching the levels of an epidemic.
- Although our genetic make-up has not changed significantly over the last 50 years, our diet and lifestyle have. This has unveiled how genetic predisposition can affect our response to environmental factors such as nutrition and exercise.
- In the present chapter we discuss how our genes, alone and in combination with the environment, can give rise to obesity, the metabolic syndrome and diabetes.

Key Words: Mutations, Polymorphisms, Chromosomal loci, Animal models

1. OBESITY

Obesity is a complex trait with multifactorial etiology, including environmental, behavioral, and genetic factors. The genetic contribution to human body weight has been established through family studies, investigations of parent–offspring relationships, and the study of twins and adopted children *(1,2)*. The estimated heritability for body weight is 40–70% *(3)*. Although obesity was first considered to be a disease that obeys Mendelian inheritance, the application of continuously evolving molecular biology technologies

From: *Nutrition and Health: Nutrition and Metabolism*
Edited by: C.S. Mantzoros, DOI: 10.1007/978-1-60327-453-1_2,
© Humana Press, a part of Springer Science+Business Media, LLC 2009

has revealed a far more complex picture for this metabolic disease and has led to fascinating new developments.

The contribution of genetic factors to obesity can be either a single, dysfunctional gene (monogenic obesity) or, as in the case of common (polygenic) obesity, numerous genes that make up minor contributions in determining the phenotype.

In general, the two methods used for the study of genetic factors in complex diseases include the candidate gene approach and the genome-wide scan approach. The candidate gene approach examines the association of a given allele and the presence of the disease, while the genome-wide scan, or linkage analysis, locates genes through their genomic position and is based on the rationale that family members sharing a specific phenotype will also share chromosomal regions surrounding the gene involved. Linkage and linkage disequilibrium analysis in specific rely on the fact that genes with similar chromosome positions will only rarely be separated during genetic recombination, so susceptibility to causative genes can be localized by searching for genetic markers that cosegregate.

In addition to genetic studies in human families, the existence of naturally or genetically modified animal models has provided valuable information on our understanding of the pathophysiology of disease. The mouse represents the most frequently used species for the creation of transgenic or gene knockout animals, allowing the analysis of the effects of gene overexpression, modification, or deletion. Rats are also used for transgenic studies, but this animal model has practical and technical disadvantages over the mouse model and hence is less frequently used. Transgenic animal models provide critical tools for in vivo functional characterization of single genes and for the search of unknown genes implicated in disease manifestation. Nevertheless, there are also limitations that call for great care in interpreting results from transgenic animal models and in translating them to humans. For example, loss or overexpression of individual proteins may produce compensatory mechanisms that could mask the resulting phenotype. Most important however, the phenotypic or pathophysiological consequences of genetic manipulation in animal models may not always match the human disease *(4)*.

1.1. Monogenic Obesity

Initial knowledge on the genetic involvement in monogenic obesity was derived from large-scale linkage analysis in obese mice carrying naturally occurring mutations. These analyses have pointed to disease-related loci and have identified the majority of gene mutations leading to monogenic obesity in mice *(3)*. In particular, the genetic characterization of naturally occurring obese animal models, such as *ob/ob*, *db/db*, *fat* and *tubby* mice, led to the discovery of recessive mutations in the genes encoding leptin (Lep or ob), leptin receptor (Lepr or db), carboxypeptidase E (Cpe, or fat), and tubby (Tub) *(5,6)*. Furthermore, the latest murine obesity gene map identified 248 genes that, when mutated or expressed as transgenes in the mouse, result in phenotypes affecting body weight and adiposity *(7)*. Transfer of this knowledge to clinical cases has confirmed the role of the above genes in human monogenic obesity and uncovered the critical role of the leptin/melanocortin pathway in the regulation of energy homeostasis *(8)*. Briefly, this hypothalamic pathway is activated following the systemic release of leptin and its subsequent interaction with the leptin receptor located on the surface of neurons of the arcuate nucleus of the hypothalamus. The downstream signals that regulate energy homeostasis are then propagated via proopiomelanocorin (POMC), cocaine- and amphitamine-related transcript (CART) and the melanocortin system *(9,10)*. While POMC/CART neurons synthesize the anorectic peptide α-melanocyte-stimulating hormone (α-MSH), a separate group of neurons express the orexigenic neuropeptide Y (NPY) and the agouti-related protein, which acts as a potent inhibitor of melanocortin 3 receptor (MC3R) and melanocortin 4 receptor (MC4R).

To date, mutations in 11 different genes (Table 1), including *LEP, LEPR, POMC,* and proconvertase 1 *(PC1)*, have been linked to obesity, in nearly 200 patients *(7,30)*. Patients with monogenic obesity have extremely severe phenotypes that present in childhood and are often associated with additional behavioral, developmental, and endocrine disorders *(31)*. MC4R-linked obesity represents the most prevalent form of

Table 1
Genes Implicated in Monogenic Obesity

Gene	Gene symbol	Locus	Mode of transmission	Obesity	Reference
Leptin	*LEP*	7q31.3	Recessive	Severe, from first days of life	11–13
Leptin receptor	*LEPR*	1q31	Recessive	Severe, from first days of life	14, 15
Proopiomelano-cortin	*POMC*	2p23.3	Recessive	Severe, from first month of life	16, 17
Proconvertase 1	*PC1*	5q15–q21	Recessive	Considerable, from first month of life	18
Melanocortin-4-receptor	*MC4R*	18q22	Dominant	Variable severity, early onset	19–22
Single-minded homolog 1	*SIM1*	6q16.3–q21	Dominant	Severe, from childhood	23
Neurotropic tyrosine kinase receptor type 2	*NTRK2*	9q22.1	Dominant	Severe, from first months of life	24
Corticotropin-releasing hormone receptor 1	*CRHR1*	17q12–q22	Dominant	Severe, early onset	25
Corticotropin-releasing hormone receptor 2	*CRHR2*	7p14.3	Not known	Not known	25
G-protein-coupled receptor 24	*GPR24*	22q13.3	Dominant	Severe, early onset	26
Melanocortin-3-receptor	*MC3R*	20q13.2	Dominant	Severe, early onset	27–29

monogenic obesity identified to date, representing ~2–3% of childhood and adult obesity *(30,32,33)*. MC4R is a G-protein-coupled receptor with seven transmembrane domains that plays an important role in controlling weight homeostasis *(10)*. MC4R knockout mice develop morbid obesity and increased linear growth, whereas heterozygous mice are also obese but with a varying degree of severity *(34)*. Investigations in the molecular mechanisms by which loss of function mutations in *MC4R* cause obesity have suggested a number of functional anomalies, including abnormal MC4R membrane expression, a defect in agonist response, and disruption in the intracellular transport of the protein *(35)*. Other single gene mutations leading to obesity involve single-minded homolog 1 (*SIM1*), melanocortin receptor 3 (*MC3R*), and neurotrophic tyrosine kinase receptor type 2 (*TRKB/NTRK2*) *(23,24,27)*.

The major goal of the extensive ongoing research is the development of therapies targeting monogenic obesity, in order to ameliorate the metabolic status of obese individuals. Leptin therapy, by subcutaneous injection of leptin in children and adults deficient in this adipokine, markedly reduced their body weight, having a major effect on reducing food intake and on other dysfunctions, including immunity *(36)*. Although treatments are not available yet for cases of LEPR, POMC-, PC1-, SIM1-, MC4R-, and TRKB-linked obesity, preliminary studies suggest that targeted therapies could be possible to develop *(37)*.

1.2. Syndromic Obesity

In addition to the monogenic forms of obesity, this phenotype is also associated with many genetic syndromes. Syndromic obesity was initially thought of as monogenic; however, the contribution of multiple genetic factors in a syndrome is significantly more challenging than localizing the single gene involved in monogenic disorders.

There are currently 20–30 Mendelian disorders in which, in addition to mental retardation, dysmorphic features, and organ-specific developmental abnormalities, patients are also clinically obese *(30,31)*. Such cases are referred to as syndromic obesity. These syndromes arise from discrete genetic defects or chromosomal abnormalities and can be either autosomal or X-linked disorders. The most common disorders known are Prader–Willi syndrome (PWS), Bardet-Biedl syndrome (BBS), and Alström syndrome *(38)*.

PWS, the most frequent of these syndromes (1 in 25,000 births), is characterized by obesity, hyperphagia, diminished fetal activity, mental retardation, and hypogonadism. PWS is caused by the absence of the paternal segment 15q11.2–q12, through chromosomal loss *(39–41)*. Several candidate genes in this chromosomal region have been studied; however, the genetic basis of polyphagia remains undefined because none of the PWS mouse models have an obese phenotype *(42)*. One genetic candidate that may disrupt the control of food intake is the gastric hormone ghrelin, which could act through the regulation of hunger and stimulation of growth hormone *(43)*.

BBS is characterized by early onset obesity, retinal dystrophy, morphological finger abnormalities, mental disabilities, and kidney diseases *(44,45)*. To date, BBS has been associated with at least 12 distinct chromosomal locations, with several mutations identified so far *(46–57)*. Although the precise function of the BBS proteins is yet to be determined, current data support a role in cilia function and intraflagellar transport *(58–60)*.

Alström syndrome is a very rare disorder, which in addition to obesity, is associated with congenital retinal cone dystrophy, cardiomyopathy, and type 2 diabetes *(61,62)*. Family studies have identified several mutations in the Alström syndrome 1 gene *(ALMS1)*, the majority of which are nonsense and frameshift (insertion or deletion) mutations predicted to lead to premature protein termination *(63–65)*. ALMS1 is a ubiquitously expressed protein with recently proposed functional involvement in cilia formation *(66,67)*.

As the above genetic syndromes involving obesity are rare, their underlying genetic involvement has been difficult to decipher. Furthermore, even in the cases where the responsible genes have been identified, the pathophysiological link between the protein products and the development of the disease has not yet been fully elucidated.

1.3. Polygenic Obesity

Polygenic, or common, obesity arises when an individual's genetic makeup is susceptible to an environment that promotes energy intake over energy expenditure. Specifically, environments in most westernized societies favor weight gain rather than loss because of food abundance and lack of physical activity, thus rendering common obesity as a major epidemic currently challenging the medical and financial resources in these societies *(37)*.

A range of polygenic mouse models have been generated through inbreeding of mouse lines or repeated selections of noninbred mice, and have enabled the identification of >408 quantitative trait loci (QTL) associated with obesity (http://obesitygene. pbrc.edu). A recent meta-analysis of ~280 QTL, from 34 mouse cross-breeding experiments involving >14,500 mice, revealed 58 QTL regions associated with body weight and adiposity (http://www.obesitygenes.org) *(68)*. Different QTL have been associated with the age of onset and gender in obesity, while certain loci may only contribute to obesity by interacting with other loci *(69)*.

In humans, studies of polygenic obesity are based on the analysis of single nucleotide polymorphisms (SNPs) or repetition of bases (polyCAs or microsatellites) located within or near a candidate gene. These studies are carried out in family members (family study) or unrelated individuals (case–control study), and their objective is to determine a potential association between a gene's allelic variant and obesity-related traits *(70)*. However, unlike monogenic obesity, many genes and chromosomal regions contribute to the common obese phenotype *(7,71)*. For this purpose, large DNA banks have been established from different populations throughout the world and are used for the extensive investigation of large number of genes and chromosomal regions. The findings of these genetic studies are reported every year by the Human Obesity Gene Map consortium. According to their latest report, 253 QTL have been identified, in 61 genome-wide scans *(7)*. All chromosomes, except the Y chromosome, have been found linked with an obesity-related phenotype, such as fat mass, distribution of adipose tissue, resting energy expenditure, or levels of circulating leptin and insulin. Genes associated with obesity include solute carrier family 6 (neurotransmitter transporter) member 14 *(SLC6A14)*, glutamate decarboxylase 2 *(GAD2)*, and ectonucleotide pyrophosphatase/ phosphodiesterase I *(ENPPI) (72–74)*. These genes have been implicated in a variety of biological functions such as the regulation of food intake, energy expenditure, lipid and glucose metabolism, adipose tissue development, and inflammatory processes. Recent genome-wide association studies have identified genetic variants (SNPs) associated with obesity-related traits in both children and adults, in the fat mass and obesity associated (*FTO*) gene *(75–77, 272)*. It has been proposed that through its catalytic activity, FTO may regulate the transcription of genes involved in metabolism *(78)*.

In contrast to genetically identical mice, whose environments can be controlled, the genetic and environmental diversity in humans has proved problematic for data replication. To date, only 22 obesity-related genes are supported by at least five positive studies *(7,37)*. The reasons for the lack of replication in association and linkage studies include lack of statistical power to detect modest effect, lack of control over type I error rate, and overinterpretation of marginal data *(79)*. Thus, the use of novel approaches may provide the means to circumvent classical statistical obstacles in identifying new candidate genes and possible gene–environment interactions (see Sect. 4).

The immense ongoing research on the identification of new molecular targets for antiobesity drugs and the significance of the generated findings is reflected by the rapidly increasing number of patent applications. Specifically, a total of 173 US patents were issued between January 2001 and March 2004, with the word "obesity" included in the abstract *(80,81)*. Among the molecular targets with the highest number of new patents are the serotonin receptor ligands (24 patents), neuropeptide Y receptor ligands (20 patents), and adrenergic receptor ligands (20 patents).

2. THE METABOLIC SYNDROME AND TYPE 2 DIABETES

2.1. The Metabolic Syndrome

The term metabolic syndrome (occasionally called insulin resistance syndrome) refers to a constellation of clinical findings including obesity, hypertension, hyperlipidemia, and insulin resistance, with increased risk for type 2 diabetes and cardiovascular disease. It has also been linked with chronic kidney disease, liver disease with steatosis, fibrosis, and cirrhosis, and cognitive decline and dementia. Despite recent controversy regarding the concept of a metabolic syndrome, the International Diabetes Federation (IDF) developed a new unifying worldwide definition building upon the World Health Organization (WHO) and ATP III definitions, as will be discussed in later chapters *(82)*.

On the basis of the IDF definition, almost 40% of US adults are classified as having the metabolic syndrome *(83)*. Although environmental factors such as smoking, low economic status, high intake of carbohydrates, no alcohol consumption, and physical inactivity can play a role in the development of the metabolic syndrome, a series of evidence indicates that there is also a genetic component involved. Specifically the metabolic syndrome has different prevalence between men and women, and among ethnic groups, as well as different concordance rates between monozygotic twins. Furthermore, there is increased incidence in individuals with a parental history of metabolic syndrome, and a general familial clustering of the metabolic syndrome and its components *(83–91)*.

Ongoing work on spontaneous and engineered animal models has revealed that several genetic loci are associated with metabolic syndrome components in different rodent models *(92)*. Examples of metabolic syndrome rodent models include the spontaneous hypertensive rat (SHR), the transgenic SHR overexpressing a dominant-positive form of the human sterol regulatory element binding transcription factor 1 (*SREBP-1*), the SHR/

NDmcr-cp rat, the polydactylous rat strain (PD/cub), the obese Zucker rats (OZR), the New Zealand obese (NZO), the Wistar Ottawa Karlsburg W rats, as well as congenic, consomic, and double-introgressed strains *(93–100)*.

Linkage analyses in patients with the metabolic syndrome have aimed at identifying loci with pleiotropic effects on multiple aspects of the syndrome. Several different linkage analysis approaches have been applied in the study of the metabolic syndrome, such as principal components or principal factor analysis, multivariate analysis, metabolic syndrome score from combined residuals and the structural equation model *(101)*. One of the most consistent findings was the linkage to chromosome 1q, while multiple phenotypes linked to this region indicate that it likely harbors a gene with pleiotropic effects on measure of glucose, lipids, hypertension, and adipocity, or multiple genes that contribute to each one of these features *(102–106)*. Other consistent loci implicated in the development of the metabolic syndrome include chromosomes 2p, 2q, 3p, 6q, 7q, 9q, and 15q *(103,106–111)*.

Many of these loci have also been linked to individual components of the metabolic syndrome. For example, chromosome 2p has been linked to serum triglycerides, systolic blood pressure, obesity, body fat percentage, and HDL *(111–113)*, while chromosome 7q has been linked to systolic blood pressure, triglyceride–HDL-C ratio, fasting glucose, insulin, and insulin resistance *(114–116)*.

Despite the wide use and important findings that have emerged from linkage analysis, this method presents with a number of limitations that need to be carefully considered and addressed in the interpretation of current findings and the design of future studies. Some of the common obstacles in this type of studies are the inadequate statistical power, the multiple hypothesis testing, the population stratification, the publication bias and phenotypic variation *(117)*. The identification of true genetic associations in common multifactorial conditions, such as the metabolic syndrome, requires large studies consisting of thousands of subjects. This need is further accentuated by the large number of implicated genetic loci and their potentially small contribution to the phenotype when individually considered.

In parallel to linkage and association studies, several studies have evaluated the contribution of specific candidate genes to the metabolic syndrome pathogenesis. These candidate genes have been selected based on their biological function and/or previous associations to any of the phenotypic aspects of the syndrome. However, the large number of metabolic pathways implicated in the pathogenesis of the metabolic syndrome (including insulin signaling, glucose homeostasis, lipoprotein metabolism, adipogenesis, inflammation, coagulation, etc.) renders this search a highly challenging task that has yielded a relatively limited success. There are many examples of genes directly or indirectly implicated in the development of the metabolic syndrome or specific clinical features related to it, but an equal number of negative studies have also been published *(118)*.

The peroxisome proliferator-activated receptor γ (*PPARγ*) is one of the strong candidates for conferring susceptibility to the metabolic syndrome because of its involvement in adipocyte differentiation, fatty acid metabolism, insulin sensitivity, and glucose homeostasis *(119–121)*. Despite some inconsistencies in the PPARγ association studies, the overall evidence seems to suggest that *PPARγ* polymorphisms can increase the risk for developing the metabolic syndrome *(122–124)*. Direct correlations to the metabolic syndrome have also been described for genetic variants of the β_3-adrenergic receptor (*ADRβ-3*), nitric oxide synthase 3 (*NOS3*), angiotensin I converting enzyme (*ACE*), beacon (*BEACON*), lamin A/C (*LMNA*), interleukin-6 (*IL-6*), interleukin-β (*IL1-β*), and protein tyrosine phosphatase nonreceptor type 1 (*PTPN1*) genes *(122,125–131)*. Interestingly, *PPARγ* and *IL1-β* polymorphisms have been implicated in gene–environment interactions (see Sect. 4).

Fatty acid binding protein 2 (*FABP2*) and apolipoprotein C-III (*APOC3*) polymorphisms have been directly associated with increased risk for dyslipidemia and the metabolic syndrome in Asian-Indians *(132)*. Other examples include a number of lipid-sensitive transcription factors (nuclear receptor subfamily 1, member 4 (*FXR*), nuclear receptor subfamily 1, member 3 (*LXR-α*), retinoid X receptor α (*RXR-α*), *PPAR-α*, *PPAR-δ*, peroxisome proliferator-activated receptor (*PGC1-α*), *PCG1-β*, sterol regulatory element binding transcription factor 1 (*SREBP-1c*)) that have been implicated in the development of dyslipidemia, one of the very early features of the metabolic syndrome *(124)*. Since lipoprotein metabolism plays a central role in the metabolic syndrome, several genes related to the former are also good candidates for the latter. These include variants of scavenger receptor class B, member 1 (*SCARB1*), ATP-binding cassette subfamily A, member 1 (*ABCA1*), cholesteryl ester transfer protein (*CETP*), lipoprotein lipase (*LPL*), lipase (*LIPG*), pancreatic lipase (*PNLIP*), apolipoprotein A-V (*APOA5*), and the apolipoprotein gene clusters *ApoA1/C3/A4/A5* and *ApoE/C1/C2* that affect HDL-cholesterol and triaglyceride metabolism *(133–138)*.

2.2. Hypertension

Hypertension is one of the components of the metabolic syndrome and a major risk factor for cardiovascular disease. Similar to obesity and the metabolic syndrome, hypertension seems to be the outcome of combined genetic and environmental etiologies *(139)*. Mutations in eight genes have been identified to cause severe but rare forms of monogenic hypertension *(140)*. Interestingly, all of these genes participate in the same physiological pathway in the kidney, altering net renal salt reabsorption. However, the genetic factors behind the common, less severe forms of hypertension, collectively termed essential hypertension (i.e., hypertension with unknown cause), are poorly understood. A large number of candidate gene, linkage, and association studies have sporadically implicated a range of different genetic loci in hypertension development. Polymorphisms in the angiotensinogen (*AGT*), the natriuretic peptide receptor A (*NRP1*), and *ACE* are prime examples of the most consistent findings in the literature *(141–144)*. Nonetheless, genome-wide linkage analyses have not consistently implicated specific chromosomal loci, suggesting a model in which there may be many loci, each imparting small effects on hypertension in the general population *(145–148)*. Similar to other multifactorial diseases, the study of hypertension in humans will require the consistent replication of results in large and rigorously characterized populations that are well suited for detecting alleles imparting small effects. Such populations would include cohorts of unrelated individuals as well as family-based linkage disequilibrium studies. These latter tests minimize the chance of false-positive associations arising from population admixture of individuals of different genetic backgrounds *(149)*. Meta-analysis of the combined results from multiple different studies/populations can also greatly contribute towards this end, as for example in the case of a methylenetetrahydrofolate reductase (*MTHFR*) polymorphism that appears to be significantly associated with hypertension in multiple populations *(150)*.

In parallel to human studies, a series of spontaneous and engineered animal models of hypertension have been extensively studied. For example, inbred rat strains that display hypertension as an inherited trait have long been used as a means for identifying genes that can give rise to essential hypertension. Examples of these strains include SHRs, Dahl salt-sensitive rats, Sabra hypertensive-prone rats, Molan, Lyon, fawn-hooded and Prague hypertensive rats *(151)*. Importantly, some of the findings in these animal models have later been translated to humans, such as in the case of brain and muscle Arnt-like protein-1 (*Bmal1*) polymorphisms which are associated with susceptibility to hypertension and type 2 diabetes *(152)*. Congenic and consomic rat strains have also been used to identify QTL for hypertension, in an effort to eliminate the variability arising from the often heterogeneous genetic background of these animals *(151,153–157)*. In support of the notion that hypertension is a polygenic condition, at least one blood-pressure-related QTL has been identified on almost all rat chromosomes *(151)*. Genetically engineering mouse models with increased or decreased expression of targeted genes has also provided useful insights *(158)*. For example, deletions of various genes (including the bradykinin B2 receptor, D1A and D3 dopamine receptors, atrial natriuretic peptide, endothelial nitric oxide synthase, and others) have resulted in elevated blood pressure, while in other cases, gene mutations have had little or no effect *(159–163)*. Furthermore, mouse models have enabled the confirmation of various observations in humans, and the more detailed characterization of the disease physiology *(158)*.

2.3. Type 2 Diabetes

Diabetes mellitus represents a group of metabolic disorders characterized by hyperglycemia resulting from defects in insulin secretion, insulin action, or both. The pathogenic processes involved in the development of diabetes range from autoimmune destruction of the pancreatic β cells with consequent insulin deficiency to abnormalities that result in resistance to insulin action *(164)*. There are two main etiopathogenetic categories of diabetes: (1) type 1 diabetes, which is caused by deficiency of insulin secretion and rises independently of obesity or the metabolic syndrome (will be covered in Sect. 3), and (2) type 2 diabetes, which is caused by a combination of resistance to insulin action and inadequate compensatory insulin secretion. Type 2 diabetes, or noninsulin-dependent diabetes mellitus, is the most frequent form of diabetes, accounting for 90% of the disease prevalence, with an estimated 150 million affected people worldwide *(165,166)*. Overall, type 2 diabetes is characterized by impairment of insulin secretion and decrease in insulin sensitivity. Initial studies in families with rare monogenic forms of diabetes pointed towards a genetic component of type 2 diabetes *(167)*. However, it has become evident that the incidence of the disease is also affected by environmental influences, such as lifestyle and diet.

On the basis of the role of genetic factors, type 2 diabetes may be divided into monogenic and polygenic forms, where monogenic forms are the consequence of rare mutations in a single gene whereas polygenic forms are the result of the interaction between the environment and genetic contribution of many different genes *(168,169)*.

2.3.1. Polygenic Type 2 Diabetes

Polygenic, or the common form, type 2 diabetes is a complex and heterogeneous disorder that is influenced by the contribution/impact of multiple genes and various environmental factors that can affect disease predisposition. In many cases obesity and the metabolic syndrome precede the development of type 2 diabetes. Owing to its complexity, with both gene–gene and gene–environment interactions, the genetic influences on this form of type 2 diabetes have been difficult to elucidate and the identification of genes has not been easily achieved (Fig. 1).

Animal models for type 2 diabetes have enabled the study of the molecular pathways involved in disease pathophysiology, providing useful information on the molecular etiology of type 2 diabetes and pointing towards potential therapeutic interventions. The numerous spontaneous animal models for type 2 diabetes have facilitated our understanding of disease physiology and have aided towards the identification of underlying genetic factors. Examples of such models include the Nagoya-Shibata-Yasuda (NSY) mouse model, which spontaneously develops diabetes in an age-dependent manner, the diabetic db/db mice and the KK mouse strain, which shows inherently glucose intolerance and insulin resistance *(170–172)*. Additional spontaneous animal models presenting insulin resistance and impaired insulin secretion include the Goto Kakizaki rat, the Otsuka Long-Evans Tokushima fatty (OLETF) rat and the Zucker Diabetic Fatty rat model *(173–175)*. Genome-wide linkage scans in OLETF rats have identified susceptibility loci on chromosomes 1, 7, 14, and the X chromosome, while a sequence variation in the hepatocyte nuclear factor 1β (*Hnf1β*), a gene implicated in human MODY (maturity-onset diabetes of the young) disease, was identified in the NSY mouse model *(176–178)*.

In addition to spontaneous animal models, an increasing number of genetically engineered models have been generated for type 2 diabetes. In an attempt to recreate the human disease in animals, investigations have focused on the understanding of β-cell dysfunction or insulin resistance pathways. Depending on the targeted protein and its importance on insulin signaling, various degrees of insulin resistance can be created. Insulin-receptor (IRS)-deficient mice were among the first knockout mice to be generated with affected proteins in the insulin signaling cascade. Heterozygous mice exhibit normal glucose tolerance and only 10% of adult animals develop diabetes, while homozygous

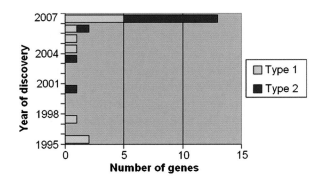

Fig. 1. Progress in the identification of susceptibility genes for type 1 and type 2 diabetes over the past decade.

IRS-deficient mice rapidly develop diabetes and die within 3–7 days after birth, thus demonstrating the essential role of IRS in the control of glucose metabolism *(179,180)*. Deficiency of the insulin receptor substrate 1 protein (IRS-1) in mice results in postnatal growth retardation with only mild insulin resistance and no diabetes, whereas deletion of IRS-2 causes impaired insulin signaling and β-cell function, resulting in progressive deterioration of glucose metabolism *(181,182)*. On the other hand, IRS-3 and IRS-4 knockout mice show respectively either mild glucose intolerance or have no phenotype, therefore suggesting that they are unlikely to play a major role in glucose homeostasis *(183,184)*.

In an attempt to resemble the polygenic nature of type 2 diabetes, polygenic animal models containing combined gene disruptions have been created. Double heterozygous mice for IRS and IRS-1 exhibit a synergistic impairment on insulin action, presenting a phenotype that is much stronger than individual gene deficiency *(185)*. In contrast to their respective individual gene deficiency models, double knockout mice for IRS-1 and β-cell glucokinase (*Gck*) develop overt diabetes, demonstrating that combination of minor mutations in genes involved in either insulin action alone or insulin secretion and action can cause diabetes *(186)*. Overall, polygenic mouse models have demonstrated that, when combined, minor defects in insulin secretion and action can lead to diabetes, therefore emphasizing the interaction between different genetic loci in diabetes.

Animal models with tissue-specific inactivation of insulin receptor genes have also been generated, in order to assess insulin action in individual tissues. These include the muscle-specific insulin receptor knockout mice, the liver insulin receptor knockout mice, and the β-cell insulin receptor knockout mice *(187–189)*. Such tissue-specific models have helped in dissecting the contribution of individual insulin-responsive organs to glucose metabolism.

In humans, candidate gene analyses towards the identification of type-2–diabetes-related genes have focused on genes implicated in insulin resistance and particularly in β-cell development, insulin signaling, or hypothalamic regulation. This has included genes such as the *PPARγ*, the ATP-binding cassette subfamily C member 8 (*ABCC8*) and potassium-inward rectifier 6.2 (*KCJN11*), and *IRS-1 (119,190)*. The best-characterized and most robust variant is the highly prevalent Pro21Ala polymorphism in *PPARγ*. Two meta-analyses have shown that the proline allele, which is the most frequent allele, is associated with a moderate increase in risk for type 2 diabetes. Furthermore, a 21–27% risk reduction was shown for the presence of the alanine allele, hence suggesting that the alanine genotype results in greater insulin sensitivity *(191–193)*. Other meta-analyses studies have determined that in the *KCJN11* gene, which encodes the ATP-sensitive potassium channel subunit Kir6.2, the frequent variant E23K shows association with a slightly increased susceptibility to type 2 diabetes in some populations, with the risk for the disease increasing by about 15% in the presence of the K allele *(190,194)*. However, in many cases the initial associations have not been replicated in subsequent studies. For example, a meta-analysis of ~9,000 individuals initially determined that the G971R variant in *IRS-1* had a significant effect on diabetes risk; however, two subsequent studies failed to confirm this association *(195–197)*.

To date, more that 50 linkage studies have been conducted in a variety of populations. Although initially the regions of linkage determined by the different studies were inconsistent (because of differences in study design, family configuration, ethnic heterogeneity), the completion of additional scans revealed that some chromosomal regions, and in particular chromosomes 1q21–24, 1q31–q42, 9q21, 10q23, 11p15, 12q12, 19q13, and 20q11–q13, are showing positive association with the disease in more than one study *(198)*. Calpain 10 *(CAPN10)* was the first polygenic diabetes gene to be cloned *(199)* and it encodes for a ubiquitously expressed cysteine protease. Although widespread acceptance of *CAPN10* as a type-2-diabetes-predisposing gene was not initially achieved, recent studies have provided further evidence for the biological importance of *CAPN10* variation in susceptibility for the disease. A meta-analysis of more than 7,500 patients of diverse ethnic origin has determined a significant association for the presence of a *CAPN10* variant (SNP-44; CAPN10-g4841 T → C) and the disease *(200)*. It has been proposed that genetic variants of *CAPN10* might affect insulin sensitivity, insulin secretion, or the relation between the two *(201–203)*. Other genes associated with the common form of type 2 diabetes include transcription factor 7-like 2 gene *(TCF7L2)* *(204,205)*, *FTO (77,206,273)*, and ectonucleotide pyrophosphatase/phosphodiesterase 1 *(ENPP1)*, genetic variants of which impair insulin binding to its receptor in muscle and brain, hence leading to fat deposition *(207)*.

The shape of genetic association studies for type 2 diabetes is set to be transformed in the next few years, with the advent of truly genome-wide association scans. The availability of array-based platforms that will allow the performance of massive parallel genotyping (between 250,000 and 1 million SNPs per assay), combined with the information provided by the International HapMap Consortium, will provide powerful means for a global view of genetic associations in type 2 diabetes *(208)*. Indeed, through the simultaneous analysis of thousands of genetic variants (SNPs) in large diabetes patient cohorts, genome-wide association studies have recently identified the solute carrier family 30 member 8 *(SLC30A8)*, the insulin degrading enzyme *(IDE)*, and hematopoetically expressed homeodomain *HHEX (HHEX/IDE)* genes, as well as the cyclin-dependent kinase 5 *(CDK5)* regulatory subunit associated protein-1-like 1 *(CDKAL1)* melatonin receptor 1B *(MTNR1B) (274)*, the insulin-like growth factor 2 mRNA binding protein *(IGF2BP2)*, and the cyclin-dependent kinase inhibitor 2A *(CDKN2A)* genes as type 2 diabetes susceptibility genes *(204,206, 209, 210)*. However, as these loci explain a small proportion of the observed familial cases of the disease, it is expected that additional loci will be revealed in the near future by further systematic screens *(211)*.

Our understanding of the molecular pathways involved in the pathogenesis of the disease could also be enhanced by the utilization of novel technologies. For example, the microarray technology has been used to identify differential mRNA expression patterns in muscle tissue of type 2 diabetes patients and normal controls *(212)*. The application of metabolomics, which is defined as the measurement of all metabolites present within a cell, tissue, or organism following genetic medication or physiological stimulus, will also contribute valuable insights into the understanding of the pathophysiology of the disease as it provides the potential of globally profiling the metabolome of an organism *(213,214)*. Although few studies of metabolomics have focused on diabetes, a recent application of the technology to type 2 diabetes has identified characteristic alterations in the plasma phospholipids profile, therefore enabling the identification of patients from control individuals *(215,216)*.

2.3.2. Monogenic Type 2 Diabetes

The monogenic form of type 2 diabetes constitutes a small group accounting for ~5% of the disease and is characterized by high phenotypic penetrance, early disease onset, and often a severe clinical picture *(69,168,169)*. The most frequent monogenic type 2 diabetes form is the autosomal dominant MODY, a term that was first used by Tattersall and Fajans in 1975 *(217)*. So far, six genes responsible for MODY have been described, and they include hepatocyte nuclear factor-4α, -1α, -1β (*HNF-4α, -1α, -1β*), *GCK*, insulin promoter factor 1α (*IPF-1α*), and neurogenic differentiation 1 (*NEUROD1*) *(218–223)*. All of the MODY genes are expressed in the pancreatic β-cells, and, with the exception of *GCK*, all code for transcription factors with a role in β-cell development and function *(224)*. Moreover, these MODY genes are functionally related, forming part of an integrated transcriptional network. However, as in 16–45% of MODY families, termed MODY X, there have been no mutations detected in any of the known MODY genes, it has been proposed that additional MODY genes could exist *(225,226)*. In addition to the established MODY genes, mutations in familial diabetes have been implicated in two other genes, mitogen-activated protein kinase 8 interacting protein 1 (*MAPK8IP1*), which codes for another β-cell transcription factor, and *ABCC8*, the gene that codes for SUR1 *(227,228)*.

Another monogenic form of type 2 diabetes, with distinct molecular involvement, is the maternally inherited diabetes. This is a very rare form of the disease that is caused by mutations in mitochondrial DNA, most often by mutations in the tRNA for leucine *(229)*. Maternally inherited diabetes is associated with deafness (maternally inherited diabetes with deafness) or mitochondrial encephalopathy, lactic acidosis, and stroke-like episodes syndrome (MELAS) *(230,231)*. Mitochondrial mutations could perturb glucose homeostasis/metabolism through impairment of the glucosensory function of the β cells and their decreased ability for insulin production *(232)*.

3. TYPE 1 DIABETES

Insulin-dependent diabetes mellitus (IDDM), or type 1 diabetes, is characterized by autoimmune destruction of insulin-producing β cells in the pancreas and severe insulin deficiency *(233)*. Type 1 diabetes accounts for around 10% of all cases of diabetes, occurs more frequently in people of European descent, and affects 2 million people in Europe and North America *(234)*. Currently, there is a 3% global increase in incidence per year, but this is predicted to increase considerably within the next few years *(235)*.

Type 1 diabetes is a complex trait, the etiology of which has only been partially characterized. It is generally recognized though that the disease has both genetic (Fig. 1) and environmental influences. The advances in our understanding of the pathophysiology and the genetic factors underlying type 1 diabetes have benefited immensely from studies on spontaneous or genetically manipulated animal models of the disease. Autoimmune diabetes in such models shares many molecular and genetic characteristics to human type 1 diabetes. Animal models have therefore provided valuable information that can be applied on studies of human type-1-diabetes-associated molecular and cellular pathways. The nonobese diabetic (NOD) mouse represents the most studied animal model for type 1 diabetes and has been utilized for the determination of over 20 non-HLA regions (known as insulin-dependent diabetes, *Idd*) associated with disease risk in this diabetic mouse strain *(236)*. By narrowing down genetic intervals in animal models, a small number of candidate genes have been highlighted for association testing in human patients. An example of this is illustrated by the IL-2 pathway, which was considered as a candidate for the *Idd3* locus in the nonobese diabetic mouse. Following extensive investigation, its involvement in human disease was revealed. Analysis of its orthologue gene in humans confirmed its association in type 1 diabetes, therefore providing an example where genes discovered in animal models can be considered as primary candidates for investigation in humans *(236)*. Other widely used animal models include the BioBreeding diabetes-prone rat and the Komeda diabetes-prone rat *(237)*. In addition to the naturally occurring animal models, a range of transgenic animals have been generated for a long series of different genes, including major histocompatibility molecules (e.g., *D57, HLA-DRα, HLA-DQ6*), cytokines (*Il2, Tnfα, Tgfβ1*), autoantigens (proinsulin, *HSP60, GAD*), costimulatory molecules (*Cd152, Cd80*), and T-cell receptors (*BDC2.5, 8.3*) *(69)*.

Through association studies and linkage analysis in humans, an increasing number – 19 to date – of IDDM susceptibility loci have been identified (named by the abbreviation IDDM and a number reflecting the order with which they were reported, e.g., *IDDM1*, *IDDM2*, etc.) *(69,238,239)*. The human leukocyte antigen (HLA) locus on chromosome 6p21 was the first to be associated with the disease and is thought to contribute for around 50% of the familial basis of type 1 diabetes *(234,240–242)*. It has been shown that the HLA-DR$_4$-DQ$_8$ and HLA-DR$_3$-DQ$_2$ haplotypes are present in 90% of children with type 1 diabetes, whereas HLA-DR$_{15}$-DQ$_6$ is found in only 1% of affected children but more than 20% in the general population, therefore suggesting that it is protective *(243)*. The genotype combining the two susceptibility haplotypes (DR$_4$-DQ$_8$/DR$_3$-DQ$_2$) contributes the greatest risk for the disease. Despite extensive research, the specific details as to how genes in this region modulate type 1 diabetes risk have still not been fully elucidated.

The insulin gene, or IDDM2 locus, on chromosome 11p15.5 was the second locus to be identified and is the second most common factor, contributing to 10% of the genetic susceptibility of type 1 diabetes *(244)*. Susceptibility in the insulin gene has been primarily mapped to a variable number of tandem repeats located in the promoter region of the gene. Shorter forms of these repeats are associated with susceptibility to the diseases whereas longer repeats are associated with protection *(245)*.

Other genes associated with type 1 diabetes include cytotoxic T-lymphocyte antigen 4 (*CTLA4*), protein tyrosine phosphatase, nonreceptor type 22 (*PTPN22*), small ubiquitin-like modifier 4 (*SUMO4*), and the α-chain of interleukin-2 receptor gene (*IL2R*) *(246–248,275,276,277)*. The KIAA0350 gene, encoding for a protein with predicted sugar binding properties, was the latest one identified *(249)*. Overall, a number of whole genome scans using families and affected sibling pairs performed over the past decade have provided evidence for the existence of many additional loci associated with type 1 diabetes, including but not limited to the IDDM loci *(211,250–254,278)*.

In a coordinated effort on the analysis of existing type 1 diabetes families for the elucidation of the genetic etiology of the disease, the type 1 Diabetes Genetics Consortium (T1DGC) (http://www.t1dgc.org) has been established. The T1DGC represents a worldwide collaboration on the study of a large collection of patients and their families from around the world. The first report from this consortium was published in 2005, and it included a combined linkage analysis of four datasets, three previously published genome scans, and a new dataset of 254 families *(252)*. The T1DGC analysis included 1,435 families with 1,636 affected sibling pairs from the UK, the USA, and Scandinavia, representing one of the largest linkage studies performed so far. In addition to HLA, this large study determined evidence for linkage to ten other chromosomal regions. In particular chromosomes 2q31–q33, 6q21, 10p14–q11, and 16q22–24 showed genome-wide significance, therefore indicating a strong non-HLA genetic contribution to type 1 diabetes *(252)*.

The T1Dbase database (http://T1DBase.org) represents a powerful resource, which combines and organizes data for type 1 diabetes, focusing on the molecular genetics and biology of disease susceptibility and pathogenesis *(255)*. This public database allows scientists to search across different data sources/types, and thus find new relationships among factors contributing to the complex pathogenesis of type 1 diabetes *(256)*.

In addition to the genetic contributions of type 1 diabetes, it is becoming evident that additional factors, such as environmental influences, are also involved in the development of the disease. Such factors include viruses, such as enteroviruses, rotavirus, and rubella *(257,258)*. Nevertheless, even though Finland has effectively eradicated rubella through vaccination, it has one of the highest incidences of type 1 diabetes. This therefore supports the hygiene hypothesis, which proposes that environmental exposure to microbes early in life promotes innate immune responses that suppress atopy and autoimmunity. To address the role of environmental factors in type 1 diabetes, large-scale studies are required. For this purpose, the international consortium Environmental Determinants of Diabetes in the Young (TEDDY; http://www.niddk.nih.gov/patient/TEDDY/TEDDY.htm) has been established so as to follow large number of babies with high-risk HLA genotypes during early life and thus identify infectious agents, dietary factors, or other environmental factors that could trigger autoimmunity in susceptible populations *(234)*.

3.1. Evidence for Genetic Overlap between Type 1 and Type 2 Diabetes

Even though, as described above, type 1 and type 2 diabetes represent two different disease entities, the clinical and etiological distinction between them is becoming more difficult as there is increasing evidence of a significant overlap between the two disease states. Clinical studies have reported that even within the same family both type 1 and type 2 diabetes may co-occur and patients with such double genetic predisposition have intermediate phenotype *(259)*. As an example of common genetic predisposition, a variable number of tandem repeats polymorphism in the insulin gene promoter region has been associated with both type 1 and type 2 diabetes *(259)*.

The "accelerator hypothesis" suggests that both type 1 and type 2 diabetes are the same disorder of insulin resistance set against different genetic background *(260)*. According to this hypothesis, type 1 and type 2 diabetes are one and the same entity, distinguished only by the rate of β cell loss. Instead of overlap between the two types of diabetes, the hypothesis envisages overlay between the two types, with one disease representing a subset of the other.

4. GENE–ENVIRONMENT INTERACTION

All evidence so far appears to support a shared genetic and environmental (with diet and exercise being among the most important) contribution to disease predisposition, including obesity, metabolic syndrome, and type 2 diabetes (Fig. 2). Nevertheless, the relative contribution of each of these two main parameters and the extent of their interaction are difficult to determine, and varies for each condition. It is noteworthy, that although the human genome has not changed significantly over the last few decades, the prevalence of obesity, metabolic syndrome, and type 2 diabetes are increasing exponentially. Although the genetic and environmental factors have long been studied independently, an increasing effort is now placed on deciphering the gene–environment interaction. Obesity, metabolic syndrome, and type 2 diabetes are classic examples of such gene–environment interactions *(261–263)*. For example, in a cohort of 287 monozygotic and 189 dizygotic young adult male twin pairs, it was shown that sedentary twins were more likely to develop high waist circumference if they were genetically susceptible to obesity than if they were not *(264)*. The complexity, however, of these multifactorial diseases has emphasized the need for development of more sophisticated statistical methods that would enable more accurate assessment of the interplay between complex combinations of multiple gene variants and environmental factors *(265)*.

A large set of common genetic variants are currently under study in the European programs Nutrient–Gene Interactions in Human Obesity (NUGENOB) (http://www.nugenob.com) and Diet, Obesity and Genes (DIOGENES) (http://www.diogenes-eu.org). Such programs comprising both academic and industrial partners, aim to study gene–environment interactions and thus identify genetic determinants susceptible to environmental stimuli that are capable of influencing obesity development. Within these programs, the use of comprehensive platforms (i.e., genetics, transcriptomics, peptidomics, and metabolomics) coupled with clinical data will have a predominant role in elucidating the perturbed functions leading to obesity, and ultimately in developing better targeted therapies.

In the context of the metabolic syndrome development, a study of 303 elderly twin pairs recently showed that glucose intolerance, obesity, and low HDL-cholesterol concentrations are significantly higher among monozygotic twins than among dizygotic twins,

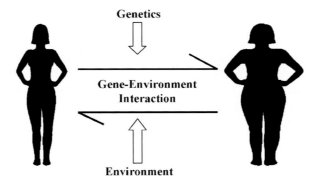

Fig. 2. Genetic polymorphisms can affect predisposition to mutlifactorial diseases, such as obesity, on their own or in response to environmental factors, such as nutrition and exercise.

indicating a genetic influence on the development of these phenotypes. In contrast, the heritability estimates for hyperinsulinemia, hypertension, and hypertriacylglycerolemia are low, indicating a more important environmental influence on these components of the metabolic syndrome *(266)*. Nevertheless, gene–environment interactions are slowly emerging for them too. For example, polymorphisms in endothelin 1 (*EDN1*) are associated with increased risk for hypertension in low-fit, but not in high-fit, white individuals *(267)*.

Similar observations are emerging for the other multifactorial conditions described in this chapter, and they are likely to play a key role in addressing and reversing the current epidemic of obesity, metabolic syndrome, and type 2 diabetes.

4.1. Nutrigenomics

One of the rapidly expanding scientific fields that address the way genes and bioactive food components interact is nutrigenomics. It specifically focuses on understanding how diet (1) affects the genome, directly (e.g. via methylation) or indirectly (e.g. at the gene expression level); (2) may compensate for or accentuate the effect of genetic polymorphisms; and (3) can alter the risk for disease development by interfering with the molecular processes involved in disease onset, incidence, progression, and/or severity. The ultimate goal is the in-depth understanding of the genome–nutrient interaction, which will lead to carefully targeted dietary intervention strategies for restoring health and fitness and for preventing diet-related disease. Many studies are beginning to address the interplay between genome and nutrition, such as in the case of type 2 diabetes *(268)*. A characteristic example of the importance of nutrigenomic studies lies in the discovery of a polymorphism in the angiotensinogen gene, which alters the effect of dietary fiber on human blood pressure. Specifically, individuals with the angiotensinogen TT genotype have decreased blood pressure, when provided with high insoluble fiber diets. In contrast, individuals with the TM or MM genotype do not experience a significant effect on their blood pressure in response to dietary fiber *(269)*. Similarly, in individuals with a specific polymorphism in PPARgamma (Pro12Ala), a low polyunsaturated-to-saturated fat ratio is associated with an increase in body mass index and fasting insulin concentrations, suggesting that when the dietary polyunsaturated-to-saturated fat ratio is low, the body mass index in Ala carriers is greater than that in Pro homozygotes *(270)*. When the dietary ratio is high, the opposite is seen. Analysis of 1,120 white subjects in the context of the Genetics of Lipid Lowering Drugs and Diet Network (GOLDN) Study demonstrated that common genetic variants at the *IL1β* locus were associated with risk of metabolic syndrome and related phenotypes. Importantly, a significant interaction was identified between dietary polyunsaturated fatty acids, and specifically docosahexaenoic acids and eicosapentaenoic acids, intake and the *IL1β* 6054G>A polymorphism, with AA subjects having significantly lower risk of metabolic syndrome. This suggests that the increasing genetic predisposition towards the development of metabolic syndrome in these individuals, could be reduced by a diet rich in polyunsaturated fatty acids, supporting the notion that more tailored dietary recommendations could be successfully used to prevent chronic diseases *(131)*. Furthermore, the Framingham Heart Study, involving 2,148 participants, identified an *APOA5* polymorphism that was associated with polyunsaturated fatty acid intake in a dose-dependent manner thus determining fasting triglyceride levels *(271)*.

5. FUTURE DIRECTIONS

Current technological advances are enabling an unprecedented width and speed of scientific discovery, thus increasing rapidly our understanding of the genetic etiology of obesity, metabolic syndrome, and diabetes. Although the number of disease-associated genes has recently risen sharply, many more yet-to-be-discovered genes are believed to be implicated in the above-mentioned complex diseases. Better designed, large-scale, multipopulation meta-analyses are starting to provide the necessary statistical power and biological breadth to uncover new genetic players in disease development. In parallel to causative gene mutations and single nucleotide polymorphisms (SNPs – the most common form of polymorphisms associated with obesity, metabolic syndrome, and diabetes), new forms of genome variation such as DNA copy number variants or novel mechanisms of genome/transcriptome regulation, such as microRNAs, are introducing an additional level of complexity that needs to be considered. Advanced technological tools, together with cumulative biological knowledge, will allow us to answer the many open questions in disease pathophysiology such as, for example, the effect of type 1 diabetes genetic variants in immune response and tolerance or their role on insulin action and β-cell function in type 2 diabetes. Meanwhile, the long-suspected gene–environment interplay will be molecularly deciphered through rapidly evolving disciplines such as nutrigenomics. All this wealth of knowledge should translate in presymptomatic genetic diagnosis and effective preventive approaches, as well as improved clinical management when disease development is inevitable. Therapies will be better targeted to specific molecular pathways and therefore likely to be more efficient and effective. Ultimately, the advent of pharmacogenomics will allow the promise of personalized medicine to be fulfilled.

REFERENCES

1. Sorensen TI. The genetics of obesity. Metabolism 1995; 44:4–6.
2. Maes HH, Neale MC, Eaves LJ. Genetic and environmental factors in relative body weight and human adiposity. Behav. Genet. 1997; 27:325–351.
3. Barsh GS, Farooqi IS, O'Rahilly S. Genetics of body-weight regulation. Nature 2000; 404:644–651.
4. Bluher M. Transgenic animal models for the study of adipose tissue biology. Best Pract. Res. Clin. Endocrinol. Metabol. 2005; 19:605–623.
5. Leibel RL, Chung WK, Chua SCJ. The molecular genetics of rodent single gene obesities. J. Biol. Chem 1997; 275:31937–31940.
6. Chagnon YC, Bouchard C. Genetics of obesity: advances from rodent studies. Trends Genet. 1996; 12:441–444.
7. Rankinen T, Zuberi A, Chagnon YC, et al. The human obesity map: the 2005 update. Obesity 2006; 14:529–644.
8. Coll AP, Farooqi IS, Challis BG, Yeo S, O'Rahilly S. Proopiomelanocortin and energy balance: insights from human and murine genetics. J. Endocrinol. Metab. 2004; 89:2557–2562.
9. Clement K. Genetics of human obesity. Proc. Nutr. Soc. 2005; 64:133–142.
10. Harrold JA, Williams G. Melanocortin-4 receptors, beta-MSH and leptin: key elements in the satiety pathway. Peptides 2006; 27:365–371.
11. Strobel A, Issad T, Camoin L, Ozata M, Strosberg AD. A leptin missense mutation associated with hypogonadism and morbid obesity. Nat. Genet. 1998; 18:213–215.
12. Montague CT, Farooqi IS, Whitehead JP, et al. Congenital leptin deficiency is associated with severe early-onset obesity in humans. Nature 1997; 387:903–90.
13. Ozata M, Ozdemir IC, Licinio J. Human leptin deficiency caused by a missense mutation: multiple

endocrine defects, decreased sympathetic tone, and immune system dysfunction indicate new targets for leptin action, greater central than peripheral resistance to the effects of leptin, and spontaneous correction of leptin-mediated defects. J. Clin. Endocrinol. Metab. 1999; 84:3686–3695.

14. Clement K, Vaisse C, Lahlou N, et al. A mutation in the human leptin receptor gene causes obesity and pituitary dysfunction. Nature 1998; 392:398–401.

15. Farooqi IS, Wangensteen T, Collins S, et al. Clinical and molecular genetic spectrum of congenital deficiency of the leptin receptor. N. Engl. J. Med. 2007; 356:237–247.

16. Challis BG, Pritchard LE, Creemers JW, et al. A missense mutation disrupting a dibasic prohormone processing site in pro-opiomelanocortin (POMC) increases susceptibility to early-onset obesity through a novel molecular mechanism. Hum. Mol. Genet. 2002; 11:1997–2004.

17. Krude H, Biebermann H, Luck W, Horn R, Brabant G, Gruters A. Severe early-onset obesity, adrenal insufficiency and red hair pigmentation caused by POMC mutations in humans. Nat. Genet. 1998; 19:155–157.

18. Jackson RS, Creemers JW, Ohagi S, et al. Obesity and impaired prohormone processing associated with mutations in the human prohormone convertase 1 gene. Nat. Genet. 1997; 16:303–306.

19. Yeo GS, Farooqi IS, Aminian S, Halsall DJ, Stanhope RG, O'Rahilly S. A frameshift mutation in MC4R associated with dominantly inherited human obesity. Nat. Genet. 1998; 20:111–112.

20. Vaisse C, Clement K, Guy-Grand B, Froguel P. A frameshift mutation in human MC4R is associated with a dominant form of obesity. Nat. Genet. 1998; 20:113–114.

21. Hinney A, Schmidt A, Nottebom K, et al. Several mutations in the melanocortin-4 receptor gene including a nonsense and a frameshift mutation associated with dominantly inherited obesity in humans. J. Clin. Endocrinol. Metab. 1999; 84:1483–1486.

22. Gu W, Tu Z, Kleyn PW, et al. Identification and functional analysis of novel human melanocortin-4 receptor variants. Diabetes 1999; 48:635–639.

23. Holder JL, Butte NF, Zinn AR. Profound obesity associated with a balanced translocation that disrupts the SIM1 gene. Hum. Mol. Genet. 2000; 9:101–108.

24. Yeo GS, Connie Hung CC, Rochford J, et al. A de novo mutation affecting human TrkB associated with severe obesity and developmental delay. Nat. Neurosci. 2004; 7:1187–1189.

25. Challis BG, Luan J, Keogh J, Wareham NJ, Farooqi IS, O'Rahilly S. Genetic variation in the corticotrophin-releasing factor receptors: identification of single-nucleotide polymorphisms and association studies with obesity in UK Caucasians. Int. J. Obes. Relat. Metab. Disord. 2004; 28:442–446.

26. Gibson WT, Pissios P, Trombly DJ, et al. Melanin-concentrating hormone receptor mutations and human obesity: functional analysis. Obes. Res. 2004; 12:743–749.

27. Tao YX. Molecular mechanisms of the neural melanocortin receptor dysfunction in severe early onset obesity. Mol. Cell. Endocrinol. 2005; 239:1–14.

28. Lee YS, Poh LK, Loke KY. A novel melanocortin 3 receptor gene (MC3R) mutation associated with severe obesity. J. Clin. Endocrinol. Metab. 2002; 87:1423–1326.

29. Rached M, Buronfosse A, Begeot M, Penhoat A. Inactivation and intracellular retention of the human I183N mutated melanocortin 3 receptor associated with obesity. Biochim. Biophys. Acta. 2004; 1689:229–234.

30. Bell CG, Walley AJ, Froguel P. The genetics of human obesity. Nat. Rev. Genet. 2005; 6:221–234.

31. Farooqi IS, O'Rahilly S. Monogenic obesity in humans. Ann. Rev. Med. 2005; 56:443–458.

32. Hinney A, Bettecken T, Tarnow P, et al. Prevalence, spectrum, and functional characterization of melanocortin-4 receptor gene mutations in a representative population-based sample and obese adults from Germany. J. Clin. Endocrinol. Metab. 2006; 91:1761–1769.

33. Lubrano-Berthelier C, Cavazos M, Dubern B, et al. Molecular genetics of human obesity-associated MC4R mutations. Ann. N.Y. Acad. Sci. 2003; 994:49–57.

34. Huszar D, Lynch CA, Fairchild-Huntress V, et al. Targeted disruption of the melanocortin-4 receptor results in obesity in mice. Cell 1997; 88:131–141.

35. Ho G, MacKenzie RG. Functional characterization of mutations in melanocortin-4 receptor associated with human obesity. J. Biol. Chem. 1999; 274:35816–35822.

36. Farooqi IS, Matarese G, Lord GM, et al. Beneficial effects of leptin on obesity, T cell hyporesponsiveness and neuroendocrine/metabolic dysfunction of human congenital leptin deficiency. J. Clin. Invest. 2002; 110:1093–1103.

37. Mutch DM, Clement K. Unraveling the genetics of human obesity. PLoS Genet. 2006; 2:1956–1963.

38. Chung WK, Leibel RL. Molecular physiology of syndromic obesities in humans. Trends Endocrinol. Metab. 2005; 16:267–272.

39. Gilhuis HJ, van Ravenswaaij CM, Hamel BJ, Gabreels FJ. Interstitial 6q deletion with a Prader–Willi-like phenotype: a new case and review of the literature. Eur. J. Paediatr. Neurol. 2000; 4:39–43.

40. Stein CK, Stred SE, Thomson LL, Smith FC, Hoo JJ. Interstitial 6q deletion and Prader–Willi-like phenotype. Clin. Genet. 1996; 49:306–310.

41. Smith A. The diagnosis of Prader–Willi syndrome. J. Paediatr. Child Health 1999; 35:335–337.

42. Goldstone AP. Prader–Willi syndrome: advances in genetics and pathophysiology and treatment. Trends Endocrinol. Metab. 2004; 15:12–20.

43. Cummings DE, Clement K, Purnell JQ, et al. Elevated plasma ghrelin levels in Prader–Willi syndrome. Nat. Med. 2002; 8:643–644.

44. Green JS, Parfrey PS, Harnett JD, et al. The cardinal manifestations of Bardet-Biedl syndrome, a form of Laurence-Moon-Biedl syndrome. New Eng. J. Med. 1989; 321:1002–1009.

45. Beales PL, Elcioglu N, Woolf AS, Parker D, Flinter FA. New criteria for improved diagnosis of Bardet-Biedl syndrome: results of a population survey. J. Med. Genet. 1999; 36:437–446.

46. Fan Y, Esmail MA, Ansley SJ, et al. Mutations in a member of the Ras superfamily of small GTP-binding proteins causes Bardet-Biedl syndrome. Nat. Genet. 2004; 36:989–993.

47. Mykytyn K, Braun T, Carmi R, et al. Identification of the gene that, when mutated, causes the human obesity syndrome BBS4. Nat. Genet. 2001; 28:188–191.

48. Mykytyn K, Nishimura DY, Searby CC, et al. Identification of the gene (BBS1) most commonly involved in Bardet-Biedl syndrome, a complex human obesity syndrome. Nat. Genet. 2002; 31:435–438.

49. Nishimura DY, Searby CC, Carmi R, et al. Positional cloning of a novel gene on chromosome 16q causing Bardet-Biedl syndrome (BBS2). Hum. Mol. Genet. 2001; 10:865–874.

50. Li JB, Gerdes JM, Haycraft CJ, et al. Comparative genomics identifies a flagellar and basal body proteome that includes the BBS5 human disease gene. Cell 2004; 117:541–552.

51. Katsanis N, Beales PL, Woods MO, et al. Mutations in MKKS cause obesity, retinal dystrophy and renal malformations associated with Bardet-Biedl syndrome. Nat. Genet. 2000; 26:67–70.

52. Nishimura DY, Swiderski RE, Searby CC, et al. Comparative genomics and gene expression analysis identifies BBS9, a new Bardet-Biedl syndrome gene. Am. J. Hum. Genet. 2005; 77:1021–1033.

53. Badano JL, Ansley SJ, Leitch CC, Lewis RA, Lupski JR, Katsanis N. Identification of a novel Bardet-Biedl syndrome protein, BBS7, that shares structural features with BBS1 and BBS2. Am. J. Hum. Genet. 2003; 72:650–658.

54. Ansley SJ, Badano JL, Blacque OE, et al. Basal body dysfunction is a likely cause of pleiotropic Bardet-Biedl syndrome. Nature 2003; 425:628–633.

55. Chiang AP, Beck JS, Yen HJ, et al. Homozygosity mapping with SNP arrays identifies TRIM32, an E3 ubiquitin ligase, as a Bardet-Biedl syndrome gene (BBS11). Proc. Natl. Acad. Sci. USA 2006; 103:6287–6292.

56. Stoetzel C, Laurier V, Davis EE, et al. BBS10 encodes a vertebrate-specific chaperonin-like protein and is a major BBS locus. Nat. Genet. 2006; 38:521–524.

57. Stoetzel C, Muller J, Laurier V, et al. Identification of a novel BBS gene (BBS12) highlights the major role of a vertebrate-specific branch of chaperonin-related proteins in Bardet-Biedl syndrome. Am. J. Hum. Genet. 2007; 80:1–11.

58. Katsanis N. The oligogenic properties of Bardet-Biedl syndrome. Hum. Mol. Genet. 2004; 13(Spec. No. 1):R65–R71.

59. Yen HJ, Tayeh MK, Mullins RF, Stone EM, Sheffield VC, Slusarski DC. Bardet-Biedl syndrome genes are important in retrograde intracellular trafficking and Kupffer's vesicle cilia function. Hum. Mol. Genet. 2006; 15:667–677.

60. Nachury MV, Loktev AV, Zhang Q, et al. A core complex of BBS proteins cooperates with the GTPase Rab8 to promote ciliary membrane biogenesis. Cell 2007; 129:1201–1213.

61. Russell-Eggitt IM, Clayton PT, Coffey R, Kriss A, Taylor DS, Taylor JF. Alstrom syndrome. Report of 22 cases and literature review. Ophthalmology 1998; 105:1274–1280.

62. Marshall JD, Bronson RT, Collin GB, et al. New Alstrom syndrome phenotypes based on the evaluation of 182 cases. Arch. Intern. Med. 2005; 165:675–683.

63. Hearn T, Renforth GL, Spalluto C, et al. Mutation of ALMS1, a large gene with a tandem repeat encoding 47 amino acids, causes Alstrom syndrome. Nat. Genet. 2002; 31:79–83.

64. Collin GB, Marshall JD, Ikeda A, et al. Mutations in ALMS1 cause obesity, type 2 diabetes and neurosensory degeneration in Alstrom syndrome. Nat. Genet. 2002; 31:74–78.
65. Marshall JD, Hinman EG, Collin GB, et al. Spectrum of ALMS1 variants and evaluation of genotype–phenotype correlations in Alstrom syndrome. Hum. Mutat. 2007; 28:1114–1123.
66. Hearn T, Spalluto C, Phillips VJ, et al. Subcellular localization of ALMS1 supports involvement of centrosome and basal body dysfunction in the pathogenesis of obesity, insulin resistance, and type 2 diabetes. Diabetes 2005; 54:1581–1587.
67. Li G, Vega R, Nelms K, et al. A role for Alstrom syndrome protein, alms1, in kidney ciliogenesis and cellular quiescence. PLoS Genet. 2007; 3:e8.
68. Wuschke S, Dahm S, Schmidt C, Joost HG, Al-Hasani H. A meta-analysis of quantitative trait loci associated with body weight and adiposity in mice. Int. J. Obes. (Lond.) 2007; 31:829–841.
69. Sanoudou D, Mantzoros C. Genetics of obesity and diabetes. In: Mantzoros C, ed. Obesity and Diabetes. Totowa: Humana, 2006; 39–67.
70. Hebebrand J, Friedel S, Schauble N, Geller F, Hinney A. Perspectives: molecular genetic research in human obesity. Obesity Rev. 2003; 4:139–146.
71. Glazier AM, Nadeau JH, Aitman TJ. Finding genes that underlie complex traits. Science 2002; 298:2345–2349.
72. Abate N, Chandalia M, Satija P, et al. ENPPI/PC-I K121Q polymorphism and genetic susceptibility to type 2 diabetes. Diabetes 2005; 54:1207–1213.
73. Boutin P, Dina C, Vasseur F, et al. GAD2 on chromosome 10p12 is a candidate gene for human obesity. PLoS Biol. 2003; 1:361–371.
74. Durand E, Boutin P, Meyre D, et al. Polymorphisms in the amino acid transporter solute carrier family 6 (neurotransmitter transporter) member 14 gene contribute to polygenic obesity in French Caucasians. Diabetes 2004; 53:2483–2486.
75. Dina C, Meyre D, Gallina S, et al. Variation in FTO contributes to childhood obesity and severe adult obesity. Nat. Genet. 2007; 39:724–726.
76. Scuteri A, Sanna S, Chen WM, et al. Genome-wide association scan shows genetic variants in the FTO gene are associated with obesity-related traits. PLoS Genet. 2007; 3:e115.
77. Frayling TM, Timpson NJ, Weedon MN, et al. A common variant in the FTO gene is associated with body mass index and predisposes to childhood and adult obesity. Science 2007; 316:889–894.
78. Gerken T, Girard CA, Tung YC, et al. The obesity-associated FTO gene encodes a 2-oxoglutarate-dependent nucleic acid demethylase. Science 2007; 318:1469–1472.
79. Mutch DM, Clement K. Genetics of human obesity. Best. Pract. Res. Clin. Endocrinol. Metab. 2006; 20:647–664.
80. Jandacek RJ, Woods SC. Pharmaceutical approaches to the treatment of obesity. Drug Discov. Today 2004; 15:874–880.
81. Wasan KM, Looije NA. Emerging pharmacological approaches to the treatment of obesity. J. Pharmaceut. Sci. 2005; 8:259–271.
82. Federation ID. International Diabetes Federation consensus worldwide definition of the metabolic syndrome. International Diabetes Federation, 2005.
83. Ford ES, Ajani UA, Mokdad AH. The metabolic syndrome and concentrations of C-reactive protein among U.S. youth. Diabetes Care 2005; 28:878–881.
84. Cameron AJ, Shaw JE, Zimmet PZ. The metabolic syndrome: prevalence in worldwide populations. Endocrinol. Metab. Clin. North Am. 2004; 33:351–375; table of contents.
85. Edwards KL, Newman B, Mayer E, Selby JV, Krauss RM, Austin MA. Heritability of factors of the insulin resistance syndrome in women twins. Genet. Epidemiol. 1997; 14:241–253.
86. Carmelli D, Cardon LR, Fabsitz R. Clustering of hypertension, diabetes, and obesity in adult male twins: same genes or same environments? Am. J. Hum. Genet. 1994; 55:566–573.
87. Chen W, Srinivasan SR, Elkasabany A, Berenson GS. The association of cardiovascular risk factor clustering related to insulin resistance syndrome (Syndrome X) between young parents and their offspring: the Bogalusa Heart Study. Atherosclerosis 1999; 145:197–205.
88. Hong Y, Rice T, Gagnon J, et al. Familial clustering of insulin and abdominal visceral fat: the HERITAGE Family Study. J. Clin. Endocrinol. Metab. 1998; 83:4239–4245.
89. Liese AD, Mayer-Davis EJ, Tyroler HA, et al. Familial components of the multiple metabolic syndrome: the ARIC study. Diabetologia 1997; 40:963–970.

90. Mayer EJ, Newman B, Austin MA, et al. Genetic and environmental influences on insulin levels and the insulin resistance syndrome: an analysis of women twins. Am. J .Epidemiol. 1996; 143:323–332.

91. Sweeney L, Brennan A, Mantzoros C. Metabolic syndrome. In: Regensteiner J, Reusc J, Stewart J, Veves A, eds. Diabetes and Exercise. Totowa: Humana, 2007.

92. Russell JC, Proctor SD. Small animal models of cardiovascular disease: tools for the study of the roles of metabolic syndrome, dyslipidemia, and atherosclerosis. Cardiovasc. Pathol. 2006; 15:318–330.

93. Freedman BD, Lee EJ, Park Y, Jameson JL. A dominant negative peroxisome proliferator-activated receptor-gamma knock-in mouse exhibits features of the metabolic syndrome. J. Biol. Chem. 2005; 280:17118–17125.

94. Ortlepp JR, Kluge R, Giesen K, et al. A metabolic syndrome of hypertension, hyperinsulinaemia and hypercholesterolaemia in the New Zealand obese mouse. Eur. J. Clin. Invest. 2000; 30:195–202.

95. Yamaguchi Y, Yoshikawa N, Kagota S, Nakamura K, Haginaka J, Kunitomo M. Elevated circulating levels of markers of oxidative-nitrative stress and inflammation in a genetic rat model of metabolic syndrome. Nitric Oxide 2006; 15:380–386.

96. Qi NR, Wang J, Zidek V, et al. A new transgenic rat model of hepatic steatosis and the metabolic syndrome. Hypertension 2005; 45:1004–1011.

97. Seda O, Liska F, Krenova D, et al. Dynamic genetic architecture of metabolic syndrome attributes in the rat. Physiol. Genomics 2005; 21:243–252.

98. van den Brandt J, Kovacs P, Kloting I. Features of the metabolic syndrome in the spontaneously hypertrig-lyceridemic Wistar Ottawa Karlsburg W (RT1u Haplotype) rat. Metabolism 2000; 49:1140–1144.

99. Kloting I, Kovacs P, van den Brandt J. Sex-specific and sex-independent quantitative trait loci for facets of the metabolic syndrome in WOKW rats. Biochem. Biophys. Res. Commun. 2001; 284:150–156.

100. Strahorn P, Graham D, Charchar FJ, Sattar N, McBride MW, Dominiczak AF. Genetic determinants of metabolic syndrome components in the stroke-prone spontaneously hypertensive rat. J. Hypertens. 2005; 23:2179–2186.

101. Sale MM, Woods J, Freedman BI. Genetic determinants of the metabolic syndrome. Curr. Hypertens. Rep. 2006; 8:16–22.

102. McQueen MB, Bertram L, Rimm EB, Blacker D, Santangelo SL. A QTL genome scan of the metabolic syndrome and its component traits. BMC Genet. 2003; 4 (Suppl. 1):S96.

103. Arya R, Blangero J, Williams K, et al. Factors of insulin resistance syndrome-related phenotypes are linked to genetic locations on chromosomes 6 and 7 in nondiabetic Mexican-Americans. Diabetes 2002; 51:841–847.

104. Langefeld CD, Wagenknecht LE, Rotter JI, et al. Linkage of the metabolic syndrome to 1q23–q31 in Hispanic families: the Insulin Resistance Atherosclerosis Study Family Study. Diabetes 2004; 53:1170–1174.

105. Hamet P, Merlo E, Seda O, et al. Quantitative founder-effect analysis of French Canadian families identifies specific loci contributing to metabolic phenotypes of hypertension. Am. J. Hum. Genet. 2005; 76:815–832.

106. Loos RJ, Katzmarzyk PT, Rao DC, et al. Genome-wide linkage scan for the metabolic syndrome in the HERITAGE Family Study. J. Clin. Endocrinol. Metab. 2003; 88:5935–5943.

107. Stein CM, Song Y, Elston RC, Jun G, Tiwari HK, Iyengar SK. Structural equation model-based genome scan for the metabolic syndrome. BMC Genet. 2003; 4 (Suppl. 1):S99.

108. Olswold C, de Andrade M. Localization of genes involved in the metabolic syndrome using multivariate linkage analysis. BMC Genet. 2003; 4 (Suppl. 1):S57.

109. Ng MC, So WY, Lam VK, et al. Genome-wide scan for metabolic syndrome and related quantitative traits in Hong Kong Chinese and confirmation of a susceptibility locus on chromosome 1q21–q25. Diabetes 2004; 53:2676–2683.

110. Cai G, Cole SA, Freeland-Graves JH, MacCluer JW, Blangero J, Comuzzie AG. Principal component for metabolic syndrome risk maps to chromosome 4p in Mexican Americans: the San Antonio Family Heart Study. Hum. Biol. 2004; 76:651–665.

111. Tang W, Miller MB, Rich SS, et al. Linkage analysis of a composite factor for the multiple metabolic syndrome: the National Heart, Lung, and Blood Institute Family Heart Study. Diabetes 2003; 52:2840–2847.

112. Imperatore G, Knowler WC, Pettitt DJ, et al. A locus influencing total serum cholesterol on chromosome 19p: results from an autosomal genomic scan of serum lipid concentrations in Pima Indians. Arterioscler. Thromb. Vasc. Biol. 2000; 20:2651–2656.

113. Krushkal J, Ferrell R, Mockrin SC, Turner ST, Sing CF, Boerwinkle E. Genome-wide linkage analyses of systolic blood pressure using highly discordant siblings. Circulation 1999; 99:1407–1410.

114. Cheng LS, Davis RC, Raffel LJ, et al. Coincident linkage of fasting plasma insulin and blood pressure to chromosome 7q in hypertensive Hispanic families. Circulation 2001; 104:1255–1260.

115. An P, Freedman BI, Hanis CL, et al. Genome-wide linkage scans for fasting glucose, insulin, and insulin resistance in the National Heart, Lung, and Blood Institute Family Blood Pressure Program: evidence of linkages to chromosome 7q36 and 19q13 from meta-analysis. Diabetes 2005; 54:909–914.

116. Shearman AM, Ordovas JM, Cupples LA, et al. Evidence for a gene influencing the TG/HDL-C ratio on chromosome 7q32.3-qter: a genome-wide scan in the Framingham study. Hum. Mol. Genet. 2000; 9:1315–1320.

117. Hirschhorn JN, Lohmueller K, Byrne E, Hirschhorn K. A comprehensive review of genetic association studies. Genet. Med. 2002; 4:45–61.

118. Pollex RL, Hegele RA. Genetic determinants of the metabolic syndrome. Nat. Clin. Pract. Cardiovasc. Med. 2006; 3:482–489.

119. Barroso I, Gurnell M, Crowley VE, et al. Dominant negative mutations in human PPARgamma associated with severe insulin resistance, diabetes mellitus and hypertension. Nature 1999; 402:880–883.

120. Barak Y, Nelson MC, Ong ES, et al. PPAR gamma is required for placental, cardiac, and adipose tissue development. Mol. Cell 1999; 4:585–595.

121. Gurnell M. PPARgamma and metabolism: insights from the study of human genetic variants. Clin. Endocrinol. (Oxf.) 2003; 59:267–277.

122. Frederiksen L, Brodbaek K, Fenger M, et al. Comment: studies of the Pro12Ala polymorphism of the PPAR-gamma gene in the Danish MONICA cohort: homozygosity of the Ala allele confers a decreased risk of the insulin resistance syndrome. J. Clin. Endocrinol. Metab. 2002; 87:3989–3992.

123. Meirhaeghe A, Cottel D, Amouyel P, Dallongeville J. Association between peroxisome proliferator-activated receptor gamma haplotypes and the metabolic syndrome in French men and women. Diabetes 2005; 54:3043–3048.

124. Phillips C, Lopez-Miranda J, Perez-Jimenez F, McManus R, Roche HM. Genetic and nutrient determinants of the metabolic syndrome. Curr. Opin. Cardiol. 2006; 21:185–193.

125. Dallongeville J, Helbecque N, Cottel D, Amouyel P, Meirhaeghe A. The Gly16 Arg16 and Gln27 Glu27 polymorphisms of beta2-adrenergic receptor are associated with metabolic syndrome in men. J. Clin. Endocrinol. Metab. 2003; 88:4862–4866.

126. Fernandez ML, Ruiz R, Gonzalez MA, et al. Association of NOS3 gene with metabolic syndrome in hypertensive patients. Thromb. Haemost. 2004; 92:413–418.

127. Lee YJ, Tsai JC. ACE gene insertion/deletion polymorphism associated with 1998 World Health Organization definition of metabolic syndrome in Chinese type 2 diabetic patients. Diabetes Care 2002; 25:1002–1008.

128. Jowett JB, Elliott KS, Curran JE, et al. Genetic variation in BEACON influences quantitative variation in metabolic syndrome-related phenotypes. Diabetes 2004; 53:2467–2472.

129. Steinle NI, Kazlauskaite R, Imumorin IG, et al. Variation in the lamin A/C gene: associations with metabolic syndrome. Arterioscler. Thromb. Vasc. Biol. 2004; 24:1708–1713.

130. Hamid YH, Rose CS, Urhammer SA, et al. Variations of the interleukin-6 promoter are associated with features of the metabolic syndrome in Caucasian Danes. Diabetologia 2005; 48:251–260.

131. Shen J, Arnett DK, Peacock JM, et al. Interleukin1beta genetic polymorphisms interact with polyunsaturated fatty acids to modulate risk of the metabolic syndrome. J. Nutr. 2007; 137:1846–1851.

132. Guettier JM, Georgopoulos A, Tsai MY, et al. Polymorphisms in the fatty acid-binding protein 2 and apolipoprotein C-III genes are associated with the metabolic syndrome and dyslipidemia in a South Indian population. J. Clin. Endocrinol. Metab. 2005; 90:1705–1711.

133. Acton S, Osgood D, Donoghue M, et al. Association of polymorphisms at the SR-BI gene locus with plasma lipid levels and body mass index in a white population. Arterioscler. Thromb. Vasc. Biol. 1999; 19:1734–1743.

134. Borggreve SE, Hillege HL, Wolffenbuttel BH, et al. The effect of cholesteryl ester transfer protein -629C A promoter polymorphism on high-density lipoprotein cholesterol is dependent on serum triglycerides. J. Clin. Endocrinol. Metab. 2005; 90:4198–4204.

135. Hutter CM, Austin MA, Farin FM, et al. Association of endothelial lipase gene (LIPG) haplotypes with high-density lipoprotein cholesterol subfractions and apolipoprotein AI plasma levels in Japanese Americans. Atherosclerosis 2006; 185:78–86.

136. Deeb SS, Zambon A, Carr MC, Ayyobi AF, Brunzell JD. Hepatic lipase and dyslipidemia: interactions among genetic variants, obesity, gender, and diet. J. Lipid. Res. 2003; 44:1279–1286.

137. Srinivasan SR, Li S, Chen W, Boerwinkle E, Berenson GS. R219K polymorphism of the ABCA1 gene and its modulation of the variations in serum high-density lipoprotein cholesterol and triglycerides related to age and adiposity in white versus black young adults. The Bogalusa Heart Study. Metabolism 2003; 52:930–934.

138. Lai CQ, Demissie S, Cupples LA, et al. Influence of the APOA5 locus on plasma triglyceride, lipoprotein subclasses, and CVD risk in the Framingham Heart Study. J. Lipid Res. 2004; 45:2096–2105.

139. Lifton RP, Gharavi AG, Geller DS. Molecular mechanisms of human hypertension. Cell 2001; 104:545–556.

140. Lang F, Capasso G, Schwab M, Waldegger S. Renal tubular transport and the genetic basis of hypertensive disease. Clin. Exp. Nephrol. 2005; 9:91–99.

141. Jeunemaitre X, Soubrier F, Kotelevtsev YV, et al. Molecular basis of human hypertension: role of angiotensinogen. Cell 1992; 71:169–180.

142. Nakayama T, Soma M, Takahashi Y, Rehemudula D, Kanmatsuse K, Furuya K. Functional deletion mutation of the 5¢-flanking region of type A human natriuretic peptide receptor gene and its association with essential hypertension and left ventricular hypertrophy in the Japanese. Circ. Res. 2000; 86:841–845.

143. Fornage M, Amos CI, Kardia S, Sing CF, Turner ST, Boerwinkle E. Variation in the region of the angiotensin-converting enzyme gene influences interindividual differences in blood pressure levels in young white males. Circulation 1998; 97:1773–1779.

144. O'Donnell CJ, Lindpaintner K, Larson MG, et al. Evidence for association and genetic linkage of the angiotensin-converting enzyme locus with hypertension and blood pressure in men but not women in the Framingham Heart Study. Circulation 1998; 97:1766–1772.

145. Hsueh WC, Mitchell BD, Schneider JL, et al. QTL influencing blood pressure maps to the region of PPH1 on chromosome 2q31–34 in Old Order Amish. Circulation 2000; 101:2810–2816.

146. Izawa H, Yamada Y, Okada T, Tanaka M, Hirayama H, Yokota M. Prediction of genetic risk for hypertension. Hypertension 2003; 41:1035–1040.

147. Yatsu K, Mizuki N, Hirawa N, et al. High-resolution mapping for essential hypertension using microsatellite markers. Hypertension 2007; 49:446–452.

148. Chang YP, Liu X, Kim JD, et al. Multiple genes for essential-hypertension susceptibility on chromosome 1q. Am. J. Hum. Genet. 2007; 80:253–264.

149. Spielman RS, Ewens WJ. The TDT and other family-based tests for linkage disequilibrium and association. Am. J. Hum. Genet. 1996; 59:983–989.

150. Qian X, Lu Z, Tan M, Liu H, Lu D. A meta-analysis of association between C677T polymorphism in the methylenetetrahydrofolate reductase gene and hypertension. Eur. J. Hum. Genet. 2007; 15:1239–1245.

151. Rapp JP. Genetic analysis of inherited hypertension in the rat. Physiol. Rev. 2000; 80:135–172.

152. Woon PY, Kaisaki PJ, Braganca J, et al. Aryl hydrocarbon receptor nuclear translocator-like (BMAL1) is associated with susceptibility to hypertension and type 2 diabetes. Proc. Natl. Acad. Sci. USA 2007; 104:14412–14417.

153. Printz MP, Jirout M, Jaworski R, Alemayehu A, Kren V. Genetic models in applied physiology. HXB/BXH rat recombinant inbred strain platform: a newly enhanced tool for cardiovascular, behavioral, and developmental genetics and genomics. J. Appl .Physiol. 2003; 94:2510–2522.

154. Kreutz R, Hubner N. Congenic rat strains are important tools for the genetic dissection of essential hypertension. Semin. Nephrol. 2002; 22:135–147.

155. Kwitek-Black AE, Jacob HJ. The use of designer rats in the genetic dissection of hypertension. Curr. Hypertens. Rep. 2001; 3:12–18.

156. Nabika T, Kobayashi Y, Yamori Y. Congenic rats for hypertension: how useful are they for the hunting of hypertension genes? Clin. Exp. Pharmacol. Physiol. 2000; 27:251–256.

157. Dominiczak AF, Negrin DC, Clark JS, Brosnan MJ, McBride MW, Alexander MY. Genes and hypertension: from gene mapping in experimental models to vascular gene transfer strategies. Hypertension 2000; 35:164–172.

158. Takahashi N, Smithies O. Gene targeting approaches to analyzing hypertension. J. Am. Soc. Nephrol. 1999; 10:1598–1605.

159. Kurihara Y, Kurihara H, Suzuki H, et al. Elevated blood pressure and craniofacial abnormalities in mice deficient in endothelin-1. Nature 1994; 368:703–710.

160. Huang PL, Huang Z, Mashimo H, et al. Hypertension in mice lacking the gene for endothelial nitric oxide synthase. Nature 1995; 377:239–242.

161. Ohuchi T, Kuwaki T, Ling GY, et al. Elevation of blood pressure by genetic and pharmacological disruption of the ETB receptor in mice. Am. J. Physiol. 1999; 276:R1071–R1077.

162. Cvetkovic B, Sigmund CD. Understanding hypertension through genetic manipulation in mice. Kidney Int. 2000; 57:863–874.

163. Rohrer DK, Desai KH, Jasper JR, et al. Targeted disruption of the mouse beta1-adrenergic receptor gene: developmental and cardiovascular effects. Proc. Natl. Acad. Sci. USA 1996; 93:7375–7380.

164. Association AD. Diagnosis and classification of diabetes mellitus. Diabetes Care 2006; 29:S43–S48.

165. Freeman H, Cox RD. Type-2 diabetes: a cocktail of genetic discovery. Hum. Mol. Genet. 2006; 15:R202–R209.

166. Zimmet P, Alberti KG, Shaw J. Global and societal implications of the diabetes epidemic. Nature 2001; 414:782–787.

167. Gottlieb GS. Diabetes in offspring and siblings of juvenile- and maturity-onset-type diabetes. J. Chronic. Dis. 1980; 33:331–339.

168. McCarthy MI. Susceptibility gene discovery for common metabolic and endocrine traits. J. Mol. Endocrinol. 2002; 28:1–17.

169. McCarthy MI, Froguel P. Genetic approaches to the molecular understanding of type 2 diabetes. Am.J. Physiol. Endocrinol. Metab. 2002; 283:E217–E225.

170. Ueda H, Ikegami H, Yamato E, et al. The NSY mouse: a new animal model of spontaneous NIDDM with moderate obesity. Diabetologia 1995; 38:503–508.

171. Coleman DL. Lessons from studies with genetic forms of diabetes in the mouse. Metabolism 1983; 32:162–164.

172. Ikeda H. KK mouse. Diabetes. Res. Clin. Pract. 1994; 24:S313–S316.

173. Kawano K, Hirashima T, Mori S, Saitoh Y, Kurosumi M, Natori T. Spontaneous long-term hyperglycemic rat with diabetic complications. Otsuka Long-Evans Tokushima Fatty (OLETF) strain. Diabetes 1992; 41:1422–1428.

174. Goto Y, Kakizaki M. The spontaneous-diabetes rat: a model of noninsulin-dependent diabetes mellitus. Proc. Jpn Acad. 1981; 57:381–384.

175. Peterson RG, Shaw WN, Neel M, Little LA, Eichberg J. Zucker diabetic fatty rat as a model for non-insulin-dependent diabetes mellitus. ILAR J.1990; 32:16–19.

176. Kose H, Moralejo DH, Ogino T, Mizuno A, Yamada T, Matsumoto K. Examination of OLETF-derived non-insulin-dependent diabetes mellitus QTL by construction of a series of congenic rats. Mamm. Genome 2002; 13:558–562.

177. Moralejo DH, Wei S, Wei K, Yamada T, Matsumoto K. X-linked locus is responsible for non-insulin-dependent diabetes mellitus in the OLETF rat. J. Vet. Med. Sci. 1998; 60:373–375.

178. Ueda H, Ikegami H, Kawaguchi Y, et al. Genetic analysis of late-onset type 2 diabetes in a mouse model of human complex trait. Diabetes 1999; 48:1168–1174.

179. Accili D, Drago J, Lee EJ, et al. Early neonatal death in mice homozygous for a null allele of the insulin receptor gene. Nat. Genet. 1996; 12:106–109.

180. Joshi RL, Lamothe B, Cordonnier N, et al. Targeted disruption of the insulin receptor gene in the mouse results in neonatal lethality. EMBO J. 1996; 15:1542–1547.

181. Araki E, Lipes MA, Patti ME, et al. Alternative pathway of insulin signalling in mice with targeted disruption of the IRS-1 gene. Nature 1994; 372:186–190.

182. Withers DJ, Gutierrez JS, Towery H, et al. Disruption of IRS-2 causes type 2 diabetes in mice. Nature 1998; 391:900–904.

183. Liu SC, Wang Q, Lienhard GE, Keller SR. Insulin receptor substrate 3 is not essential for growth or glucose metabolism. J. Biol. Chem. 1999; 274:18093–18099.

184. Fantin VR, Wang Q, Lienhard GE, Keller SR. Mice lacking insulin receptor substrate 4 exhibit mild defects in growth, reproduction and glucose metabolism. Am. J. Physiol. Endocrinol. Metab. 2000; 278: E127–E133.

185. Brunning JC, Winnay J, Bonner-Weir S, Taylor SI, Accili D, Kahn CR. Development of a novel poly-genic model of NIDDM in mice heterozygous for IR and IRS-1 null alleles. Cell 1997; 88:561–572.

186. Terauchi Y, Iwamoto K, Tamemoto H, et al. Development of non-insulin-dependent diabetes mellitus in the double knockout mice with disruption of insulin receptor substrate-1 and beta cell glucokinase genes. Genetic reconstitution of diabetes as a polygenic disease. J. Clin. Invest. 1997; 99:861–866.

187. Bruning JC, Michael MD, Winnay JN, et al. A muscle specific insulin receptor knockout exhibits features of the metabolic syndrome of NIDDM without altering glucose tolerance. Mol. Cell 1998; 2:559–569.

188. Michael MD, Kulkarni RN, Postic C, Previs SF, Shulman GI, Magnuson MA. Loss of insulin signal-ling in hepatocytes leads to severe insulin resistance and progressive hepatic dysfunction. Mol. Cell 2000; 6:87–97.

189. Kulkarni RN, Bruning JC, Winnay JN, Postic C, Magnuson MA, Kahn CR. Tissue-specific knockout of the insulin receptor in pancreatic beta cells creates an insulin secretory defect similar to that in type 2 diabetes. Cell 1999; 96:329–339.

190. Gloyn AL, Weedon MN, Owen KR, et al. Large-scale association studies of variants in genes encod-ing the pancreatic beta-cell KATP channel subunits Kir6.2 (KCNJ11) and SUR1 (ABCC8) confirm that the KCNJ11 E23K variant is associated with type 2 diabetes. Diabetes 2003; 52:568–572.

191. Lohmueller KE, Pearce CL, Pike M, Lander ES, Hirschhorn JN. Meta-analysis of genetic association studies supports a contribution of common variants to susceptibility to common disease. Nat. Genet. 2003; 33:177–182.

192. Memisoglu A, Hu FB, Hankinson SE, et al. Prospective study of the association between the proline to alanine codon 12 polymorphism in the PPARgamma gene and type 2 diabetes. Diabetes Care 2003; 26:2915–2917.

193. Deeb SS, Fajas L, Nemoto M, et al. A Pro12Ala substitution in PPARg2 associated with decreased recep-tor activity, lower body mass index and improved insulin sensitivity. Nat. Genet. 1998; 20:284–287.

194. Hani EH, Boutin P, Durand E, et al. Missense mutations in the pancreatic islet beta cell inwardly rectifying K⁺ channel gene (KIR6.2/BIR): a meta-analysis suggests a role in the polygenic basis of type II diabetes mellitus in Caucasians. Diabetologia 1998; 41:1511–1515.

195. Jellema A, Zeegers MP, Feskents EJ, Dagnelie PC, Mensink RP. Gly972Arg variant in the insulin receptor substrate-1 gene and association with type 2 diabetes: a meta-analysis of 27 studies. Diabe-tologia 2003; 46:990–995.

196. Zeggini E, Parkinson JR, Halford S, et al. Association studies of insulin receptor substrate 1 gene (IRS1) variants in type 2 diabetes samples enriched for family history and early age of onset. Diabetes 2004; 53:3319–3322.

197. Florez JC, Sjogren M, Burtt N, et al. Association testing in 9,000 people fails to confirm the associa-tion of the insulin receptor substrate-1 G972R polymorphism with type 2 diabetes. Diabetes 2004; 53:3313–3318.

198. Rhodes CJ, White MF. Molecular insights into insulin action and secretion. Eur. J. Clin. Invest. 2002; 32:3–13.

199. Horikawa Y, Oda N, Cox NJ, et al. Genetic variation in the gene encoding calpain-10 is associated with type 2 diabetes mellitus. Nat. Genet. 2000; 26:163–175.

200. Weedon MN, Schwarz PEH, Horikawa Y, et al. Meta-analysis confirms the role of calpain-10 variation in type 2 diabetes susceptibility. Am. J. Hum. Genet. 2003; 73:1208–1212.

201. Baier LJ, Permana PA, Yang X, et al. A calpain-10 gene polymorphism is associated with reduced muscle mRNA levels and insulin resistance. J. Clin. Invest. 2000; 106:R69–R73.

202. Sreenan SK, Zhou YP, Otani K, et al. Calpains play a role in insulin secretion and action. Diabetes 2001; 50:2013–2020.

203. Tripathy D, Eriksson KF, Orho-Melander M, Fredriksson J, Ahlqvist G, Groop L. Parallel manifestation of insulin resistance and beta cell decompensation is compatible with a common defect in type 2 diabetes. Diabetologia 2004; 47:782–793.

204. Sladek R, Rocheleau G, Rung J, et al. A genome-wide association study identifies novel risk loci for type 2 diabetes. Nature 2007; 445:881–885.

205. Grant SF, Thorleifsson G, Reynisdottir I, et al. Variant of transcription factor 7-like 2 (TCF7L2) gene confers risk of type 2 diabetes. Nat. Genet. 2006; 38:320–323.

206. Scott LJ, Mohlke KL, Bonnycastle LL, et al. A genome-wide association study of type 2 diabetes in Finns detects multiple susceptibility variants. Science 2007; 316:1341–1345.

207. Meyre D, Lecoeur C, Delplanque J, et al. Variants of ENPP1 are associated with childhood and adult obesity and increase the risk of glucose intolerance and type 2 diabetes. Nat. Genet. 2005; 37:863–867.

208. McCarthy MI, Zeggini E. Genetics of type 2 diabetes. Curr. Diabetes Rep. 2006; 6:147–154.

209. Zeggini E, Weedon MN, Lindgren CM, et al. Replication of genome-wide association signals in UK samples reveals risk loci for type 2 diabetes. Science 2007; 316:1336–1341.

210. Diabetes Genetics Initiative of Broad Institute of Harvard and MIT, LU and NIoBR: Saxena R, Voight BF, et al. Genome-wide association analysis identifies loci for type 2 diabetes and triglyceride levels. Science 2007; 316:1331–1336.

211. Frayling TM, McCarthy MI. Genetic studies of diabetes following the advent of the genome-wide association study: where do we go from here? Diabetologia 2007; 50:2229–2233.

212. Mootha VK, Lindgren CM, Eriksson KF, et al. PGC-1alpha-responsive genes involved in oxidative phosphorylation are coordinately downregulated in human diabetes. Nat. Genet. 2003; 34:267–273.

213. Bino RJ, Hall RD, Fiehn O, et al. Potential of metabolomics as a functional genomics tool. Trends Plant Sci. 2004; 9:418–425.

214. Griffin JL, Nicholls AW. Metabolomics as a functional genomics tool for understanding lipid dysfunction in diabetes, obesity and related disorders. Pharmacogenomics 2006; 7:1095–1107.

215. Wang C, Kong H, Guan Y, et al. Plasma phospholipid metabolic profiling and biomarkers of type 2 diabetes mellitus based on high-performance liquid chromatography/electrospray mass spectrometry and multivariate statistical analysis. Anal. Chem. 2005; 77:4108–4116.

216. Yang J, Xu G, Hong Q, et al. Discrimination of type 2 diabetic patients from healthy controls by using metabonomics method based on their serum fatty acid profiles. J. Chromatogr. B. Anal. Technol. Biomed. Life. Sci. 2004; 813:53–58.

217. Tattersall RB, Fajans SS. A difference between the inheritance of classical juvenile-onset and maturity onset type of diabetes in young people. Diabetes 1975; 24:44–53.

218. Yamagata K, Furuta H, Oda N, et al. Mutations in the hepatocyte nuclear factor-4a gene in the maturity-onset diabetes of the young (MODY1). Nature 1996; 384:458–460.

219. Yamagata K, Oda N, Kaisaki PJ, et al. Mutations in the hepatocyte nuclear factor-1a gene in maturity-onset diabetes of the young (MODY3). Nature 1996; 384:455–458.

220. Vionnet N, Stoffel M, Takeda J, et al. Nonsense mutation in the glucokinase gene causes early-onset non-insulin-dependent diabetes mellitus. Nature 1992; 356:721–722.

221. Stoffers DA, Ferrer J, Clarke WL, Habener JF. Early onset type-II diabetes mellitus (MODY4) linked to IPF1. Nat. Genet. 1997; 17:138–139.

222. Malecki MT, Jhala US, Antonellis A, et al. Mutations in NEUROD1 gene are associated with the development of type 2 diabetes mellitus. Nat Genet. 1999; 23:323–328.

223. Horikawa Y, Iwasaki N, Hara M, et al. Mutation in hepatocyte nuclear factor-1 beta gene (TCF2) associated with MODY. Nat. Genet. 1997; 17:384–385.

224. Barroso I. Genetics of type 2 diabetes. Diabetes 2005; 22:517–535.

225. Shih D, Stoffel M. Molecular etiologies of MODY and other early-onset forms of diabetes. Curr. Diabetes. Rep. 2002; 2:125–134.

226. Velho G, Robert JJ. Maturity-onset diabetes of the young (MODY): genetic and clinical characteristics. Horm. Res. 2002; 57:29–33.

227. Shimomura H, Sanke T, Hanabusa T, Tsunoda K, Furuta H, Nanjo K. Nonsense mutation of islet-1 gene (Q310X) found in a type 2 diabetic patient with strong family history. Diabetes 2000; 49:1597–1600.

228. Huopio H, Otonkoski T, Vauhkonen I, Reimann F, Ashcroft FM, Laakso M. A new subtype of autosomal dominant diabetes attributable to a mutation in the gene for sulfonylurea receptor 1. Lancet 2003; 361:301–307.

229. van den Ouweland JM, Lemkes HH, Ruitenbeek W, et al. Mutation in mitochondrial tRNA(Leu) (UUR) gene in a large pedigree with maternally transmitted type II diabetes mellitus and deafness. Nat. Genet. 1992; 1:368–371.

230. Maassen JA, Kadowaki T. Maternally inherited diabetes and deafness: a new diabetes subtype. Diabetologia 1996; 39:375–382.

231. Goto Y, Nonaka I, Horai S. A mutation in the tRNA(-Leu)(UUR) gene associated with the MELAS subgroup of mitochondrial encephalomyopathies. Nature 1990; 348:651–653.

232. Malecki MT. Genetics of type 2 diabetes mellitus. Diabetes. Res. Clin. Pract. 2005; 68 (Suppl. 1):S10–S21.

233. Genuth S, Alberti KG, Bennett P, et al. Follow-up report on the diagnosis of diabetes mellitus. Diabetes Care 2003; 26:3160–3167.

234. Gillespie KM. Type 1 diabetes: pathogenesis and prevention. CMAJ 2006; 175:165–170.

235. Onkamo P, Vaananen S, Karnoven M, Tuomilehto J. Worldwide increase in incidence of type I diabetes – the analysis of the data on published incidence trends. Diabetologia 1999; 42:1395–1403.

236. Maier LM, Smyth DJ, Vella A, et al. Construction and analysis of tag single nucleotide polymorphism maps for six human-mouse orthologous candidate genes in type 1 diabetes. BMC Genet. 2005; 6:9.

237. Eisenbarth GS. Animal models of type 1 diabetes: genetics and immunological function. In: Eisenbarth GS, ed. Type 1 Diabetes: Molecular, Cellular and Clinical Immunology. New York: Kluwer, 2004, pp. 91–108.

238. Pugliese A, Eisenbarth GS. Type 1 diabetes mellitus of man: genetic susceptibility and resistance. Adv. Exp. Med. Biol. 2004; 552:170–203.

239. Smyth DJ, Cooper JD, Bailey R, et al. A genome-wide association study of nonsynonymous SNPs identifies a type 1 diabetes locus in the interferon-induced helicase (IFIH1) region. Nat. Genet. 2006; 38:617–619.

240. Nerup J, Platz P, Andersen OO, et al. HLA antigens and diabetes mellitus. Lancet 1974; 2:864–866.

241. Cudworth AG, Woodworth JC. HLA system and diabetes mellitus. Diabetes 1975; 24:345–349.

242. Nejentsev S, Howson JM, Walker NM, et al. Localization of type 1 diabetes susceptibility to the MHC class I genes HLA-B and HLA-A. Nature 2007; 450:887–892.

243. Eisenbarth GS, Gottlieb PA. Autoimmune polyendocrine syndromes. N. Engl. J. Med. 2004; 350:2068–2079.

244. Bell GI, Horita S, Karam JH. A polymorphic locus near the insulin gene is associated with insulin-dependent diabetes mellitus. Diabetes 1984; 33:176–183.

245. Bennett ST, Lucassen AM, Gough SCL, et al. Susceptibility to human type 1 diabetes at IDDM2 is determined by tandem repeat variation at the insulin gene minisatellite locus. Nat. Genet. 1995; 9:284–292.

246. Bottini N, Musumeci L, Alonso A, et al. A functional variant of lymphoid tyrosine phosphatase is associated with type I diabetes. Nat. Genet. 2004; 36:337–338.

247. Vella A, Cooper JD, Lowe CE, et al. Localization of a type 1 diabetes locus in the IL2RA/CD25 region by use of tag single-nucleotide polymorphisms. Am. J. Hum. Genet. 2005; 76:773–779.

248. Ueda H, Howson JM, Esposito L, et al. Association of the T-cell regulatory gene CTLA4 with susceptibility to autoimmune disease. Nature 2003; 423:506–511.

249. Hakonarson H, Grant SF, Bradfield JP, et al. A genome-wide association study identifies KIAA0350 as a type 1 diabetes gene. Nature 2007; 448:591–594.

250. Wicker LS, Miller BJ, Coker LZ, et al. Genetic control of diabetes and insulitis in the nonobese diabetic (NOD) mouse. J. Exp. Med. 1987; 165:1639–1654.

251. Mein CA, Esposito L, Dunn MG, et al. A search for type 1 diabetes susceptibility genes in families from the United Kingdom. Nat. Genet. 1998; 19:297–300.

252. Concannon P, Erlich HA, Julier C, et al. Evidence for susceptibility loci from four genomic-wide linkage scans in 1,435 multiplex families. Diabetes 2005; 54:2995–3001.

253. Concannon P, Gogolin-Ewens KJ, Hinds DA, et al. A second-generation screen of the human genome for susceptibility to insulin-dependent diabetes mellitus. Nat. Genet. 1998; 19:292–296.

254. Todd JA, Walker NM, Cooper JD, et al. Robust associations of four new chromosome regions from genome-wide analyses of type 1 diabetes. Nat. Genet. 2007; 39:857–864.

255. Smink LJ, Helton EM, Healy BC, et al. T1DBase, a community Web-based resource for type 1 diabetes research. Nucleic Acids Res. 2005; 33:D544–D549.

256. Hulbert EM, Smink LJ, Adlem EC, et al. T1DBase: integration and presentation of complex data for type 1 diabetes research. Nucleic Acid Res. 2007; 35(Database issue):D742–D746.

257. Hyoty H. Enterovirus infections and type I diabetes. Ann. Med. 2002; 34:138–147.

258. Honeyman MC, Coulson BS, Stone NL, et al. Association between rotavirus infection and pancreatic islet autoimmunity in children at risk of developing type 1 diabetes. Diabetes 2000; 49:1319–1324.

259. Tuomi T. Type 1 and type 2 diabetes: what do they have in common? Diabetes 2005; 54:S40–S45.

260. Wilkin TJ. The accelerator hypothesis: weight gain as the missing link between type I and type II diabetes. Diabetologia 2001; 44:914–922.

261. Hill JO. Understanding and addressing the epidemic of obesity: an energy balance perspective. Endocr. Rev. 2006; 27:750–761.

262. Sharma V, McNeill JH. The etiology of hypertension in the metabolic syndrome part two: the gene–environment interaction. Curr. Vasc. Pharmacol. 2006; 4:305–320.

263. Wareham NJ, Franks PW, Harding AH. Establishing the role of gene–environment interactions in the etiology of type 2 diabetes. Endocrinol. Metab. Clin. North. Am. 2002; 31:553–566.

264. Karnehed N, Tynelius P, Heitmann BL, Rasmussen F. Physical activity, diet and gene–environment interactions in relation to body mass index and waist circumference: the Swedish young male twins study. Public Health Nutr. 2006; 9:851–858.

265. Grarup N, Andersen G. Gene–environment interactions in the pathogenesis of type 2 diabetes and metabolism. Curr. Opin. Clin. Nutr Metab. Care 2007; 10:420–426.

266. Poulsen P, Vaag A, Kyvik K, Beck-Nielsen H. Genetic versus environmental aetiology of the metabolic syndrome among male and female twins. Diabetologia 2001; 44:537–543.

267. Rankinen T, Church T, Rice T, et al. Effect of endothelin 1 genotype on blood pressure is dependent on physical activity or fitness levels. Hypertension 2007; 50:1120–1125.

268. Kaput J, Dawson K. Complexity of type 2 diabetes mellitus data sets emerging from nutrigenomic research: a case for dimensionality reduction? Mutat. Res. 2007; 622:19–32.

269. Hegele RA, Harris SB, Hanley AJ, Sun F, Connelly PW, Zinman B. Angiotensinogen gene variation associated with variation in blood pressure in aboriginal Canadians. Hypertension 1997; 29:1073–1077.

270. Luan J, Browne PO, Harding AH, et al. Evidence for gene–nutrient interaction at the PPARgamma locus. Diabetes 2001; 50:686–689.

271. Lai CQ, Corella D, Demissie S, et al. Dietary intake of n-6 fatty acids modulates effect of apolipoprotein A5 gene on plasma fasting triglycerides, remnant lipoprotein concentrations, and lipoprotein particle size: the Framingham Heart Study. Circulation 2006; 113:2062–2070.

272. Meyre D, Delplanque J, Chèvre JC, Lecoeur C, et al. Genome-wide association study for early-onset and morbid adult obesity identifies three new risk loci in European populations. Nat. Genet. 2009; 41:157–159.

273. Willer CJ, Speliotes EK, Loos RJ, et al. Six new loci associated with body mass index highlight a neuronal influence on body weight regulation. Nat. Genet. 2009; 41:25–34.

274. Lyssenko V, Nagorny CL, Erdos MR, et al. Common variant in MTNR1B associated with increased risk of type 2 diabetes and impaired early insulin secretion. Nat. Genet. 2009; 41(1):82–88.

275. Lowe CE, Cooper JD, Brusko T, et al. Large-scale genetic fine mapping and genotype-phenotype associations implicate polymorphism in the IL2RA region in type 1 diabetes. Nat. Genet. 2007; 39:1074–1082.

276. Wang CY, Podolsky R, She JX. Genetic and functional evidence supporting SUMO4 as a type 1 diabetes susceptibility gene. Ann. N. Y. Acad. Sci. 2006; 1079:257–267.

277. Guo D, Li M, Zhang Y, et al. A functional variant of SUMO4, a new I kappa B alpha modifier, is associated with type 1 diabetes. Nat. Genet. 2004; 36:837–841.

278. Concannon P, Chen WM, Julier C, et al. Genome-wide scan for linkage to type 1 diabetes in 2,496 multiplex families from the Type 1 Diabetes Genetics Consortium. Diabetes 2009; Jan 9. [Epub ahead of print]

3

Environmental Inputs, Intake of Nutrients, and Endogenous Molecules Contributing to the Regulation of Energy Homeostasis

Theodore Kelesidis, Iosif Kelesidis, and Christos S. Mantzoros

KEY POINTS

- In the last 20 years the rapid increase in obesity and associated pathologies in developed countries has been accompanied by intensification of research efforts and subsequently a substantial increase in the knowledge of the physiological and molecular mechanisms regulating body mass.
- These efforts have resulted in the recent discovery of new peripheral hormonal signals as well as new neuropeptides, involved in body-weight homeostasis.
- This review summarizes new research findings in the area of energy balance regulation, starting from the original classical hypotheses proposing metabolite sensing, through peripheral tissue–brain interactions, and coming full circle to the recently discovered pathways regulating energy homeostasis.
- Understanding these molecular mechanisms will provide new pharmacological targets for the treatment of obesity and eating disorders and associated comorbidities.

Key Words: Body-weight homeostasis, Energy balance regulation, Obesity, Eating disorders

1. INTRODUCTION

The incidences of both obesity and type 2 diabetes mellitus are rising at epidemic proportions and have emerged as a major threat to human health in the late twentieth and early twenty-first century. Growing evidence suggests that nutrient and hormonal

From: *Nutrition and Health: Nutrition and Metabolism*
Edited by: C.S. Mantzoros (ed.), DOI: 10.1007/978-1-60327-453-1_3,
© Humana Press, a part of Springer Science+Business Media, LLC 2009

signals converge and act directly on brain centers, leading to changes in fuel metabolism. Many newly discovered molecules that are proposed to play an active role in the physiology and pathophysiology of energy homeostasis have changed our understanding of obesity and metabolism and have attracted the attention of many researchers who strive to investigate and characterize the mechanisms underlying energy homeostasis. The purpose of this chapter is to summarize our current understanding of peripheral pathways regulating energy homeostasis and to outline new targets for the treatment of obesity, metabolic disorders, and associated comorbidities.

2. INPUTS IMPORTANT IN THE REGULATION OF ENERGY HOMEOSTASIS

Afferent signals to the brain convey information via exogenous and/or environmental factors influencing energy homeostasis, nutrients or metabolic factors, and finally hormonal signals regarding long- or short-term energy availability. These inputs can be classified into three distinct types, namely, neural environmental, nutrient/metabolic, and endocrine signals.

2.1. Exogenous Inputs–Environmental Signals

In modern societies of affluence, high palatability and orosensory properties of certain foods, in combination with environmental influences that promote a sedentary way of life, promote a positive energy balance and development of obesity. Mood and other signals that affect "emotional eating" and are being processed by complex neural circuits have a significant effect on these environmental signals and also regulate energy homeostasis.

2.2. Metabolic Signals

Sensors expressed in hypothalamic neurons such as ion channels [1,2] and surface enzymes [3] act as direct sensors of nutrients such as carbohydrates and lipids and activate intracellular second messenger pathways to regulate energy homeostasis. The role of nutrients and metabolic signals to regulate energy homeostasis is discussed in detail below.

2.3. Endocrine Signals

Hormones are released from peripheral endocrine organs, including the white adipose tissue (leptin), pancreas (insulin, amylin), stomach (ghrelin), and intestine (cholecystokinin, CCK). Hormonal signals such as the adipose-tissue-secreted hormone leptin and the pancreatic hormone insulin regulate the long-term metabolic status and body's energy stores whereas other signals such as gastrointestinal hormones convey information on the amount or composition of the food entering the gastrointestinal tract.

2.4. Neural Signals

Short-term regulation of feeding is also regulated by neural afferent signals from the periphery which are activated by a combination of mechanical stimuli (distension, contraction) [4], chemical stimuli (presence of nutrients in the gut lumen), and neurohumoral stimuli (gut hormones, neurotransmitters) [5] and are mainly conveyed via the vagus nerve to important CNS target centers such as the hypothalamus and the brain stem. The central integration of exogenous, environmental metabolic and peripherally secreted molecules by the CNS is discussed in detail in the subsequent chapter.

3. ENVIRONMENTAL INPUTS

The rapidly changing environment and the associated lifestyle changes are increasingly recognised as one of the primary causes of obesity in western nations *(6)*. The impact of the environment on energy balance seems to be unidirectional; modern lifestyle promotes sedentary rather than physically active pursuits and thus positive rather than negative energy balance *(7–9)*. Variations in the specific set of susceptibility genes of individuals determine the physiological impact of particular factors by which lifestyle and the environment influence energy balance *(10)* and subsequently individual susceptibility to obesity and the metabolic syndrome. Hill et al. *(11)* proposed that susceptibility to developing obesity could be due to metabolic susceptibility (e.g., tendency to store rather than burn excess body fat, differences in skeletal muscle composition), and/or to behavioral susceptibility (tendency to overeat or to be sedentary). The fact that obesity rates have been gradually increasing might also suggest that people with a high metabolic susceptibility are experiencing weight gain first as the environment becomes more obesigenic (i.e., increased food availability, high energy dense food supply, decreased need for physical activity).

How are exogenous–environmental inputs contributing to the regulation of energy homeostasis? It is important to recognize the existence of at least two influential systems. First a central neural network stretching from the hypothalamus to the caudal medulla, responsive to leptin and other peripherally secreted signals conveying information on energy and metabolic status, has been identified as the homeostatic control system for the regulation of food intake and energy balance. This system acts as an integrative metabolic sensor generating output signals to control energy intake and expenditure in a coordinated fashion (see subsequent chapter on central regulation of energy homeostasis). While this system is remarkably powerful in defending the lower limits of adiposity, it is apparently very weak in curbing appetite in a world of affluence.

Alongside the above-mentioned homeostatic neural system operates another neural non-homeostatic, "hedonic" system that processes appetite, sensory inputs, and rewarding aspects of food intake, ultimately resulting in increased energy intake in genetically predisposed individuals. Food palatability may have an independent effect and/or interact with a number of neurotransmitter systems (including dopamine *(12)*, serotonin *(13)*, and endorphins *(12,14,15)*) that contribute to appetite, reward, and mood regulation. Although it is not well understood how the reward value of pleasurable taste and flavor guides ingestive behavior, psychological components that translate reward into learning, liking, and wanting more food play a very important role in the pathogenesis of obesity and have been outlined in recent reports *(16)*.

A further question is whether these systems operate independently of each other or whether they may interact. Recent finding suggest a role for nucleus accumbens–hypothalamic pathways in the interaction between the "cognitive" and "emotional" brain and the "metabolic" brain and thus between non-homeostatic and homeostatic factors that control food intake *(17–21)*; however, more studies are clearly needed to elucidate these mechanisms.

3.1. Orosensory Properties of Food

The orosensory properties of food, mainly mediated by palatability, play a significant role in regulating eating. On a moment-to-moment basis, eating is controlled predominantly by the orosensory effects of food such as taste, flavor, aroma, and texture of food that provide positive feedback, and the postingestive effects that provide negative feedback. The effects of entry of palatable food in the mouth are stimulatory, while the entry of food into the stomach is inhibitory *(22)*. Thus, heightened responsiveness to hedonic factors, including increased palatability, is often cited as a major factor in the development of obesity, but more needs to be learned in this field and this area is currently the focus of intensive research efforts *(23)*.

3.2. Emotional Eating

Both appetite and food preferences are altered across a range of mood states; preference for "junk food" and increased caloric intake is enhanced during negative mood states whereas preference for healthier foods is increased during positive mood states *(24)*. Numerous associations between mood states and emotional eating have been reported *(25)*, and stress-associated eating (i.e., emotional eating) is more common in those who are overweight or obese. Various psychological theories of emotional eating have been proposed *(26,27)*, most of which conclude that emotional eating fails to produce any lasting benefit to psychological and mood states.

In summary, eating behavior links the internal world of molecules and physiological processes with the external world of physical and cultural systems. The extent to which human eating patterns are a function of physiological or environmental pressure is not always clear. Understanding the pathways responsible for the neural control of feeding and how the integration of diverse signaling systems could be translated into the expression of behavior and the accompanying subjective feelings is deemed to be important for the development of behavioral strategies and pharmacological therapies against obesity.

4. NUTRIENTS

Development of obesity and type 2 diabetes could ensue from alteration in the balance in the nutrient-activated mechanisms/nutrient-sensing pathways *(28)*. It has been proposed that circulating factors, e.g., lipids, glucose, or protein products, that are generated in proportion to body fat stores and/or nutritional status act as signals to the brain, eliciting changes in energy intake and expenditure *(29)*. A prolonged period of excessive food intake has been proposed to lead to weight gain and insulin resistance by activating nutrient-sensing pathways which process the signal for the availability of nutrients at central sites (hypothalamus) as well as directly in peripheral tissues (muscle and fat). All these pathways may either act independently or converge to decrease expression of proliferator-activated receptor coactivator 1 (PGC-1) α and β, key coactivators of PPAR α, γ, and δ, leading to mitochondrial dysfunction and reduced energy expenditure, all of which enhance the risk for obesity and insulin resistance *(30)*.

We will further discuss the role of fatty acid metabolism in regulation of energy homeostasis, since very recent modalities for treating obesity are based on this metabolic pathway. We will then review the role of dietary fat and dietary carbohydrates in regulating body weight, since diet, including low fat or low carbohydrate diets, still remain the most important therapeutic modality for weight loss.

4.1. The Role of Fatty Acid Metabolism in Regulation of Energy Homeostasis

A potential role in the regulation of energy balance for fatty acid metabolism acting in the brain or in the periphery has been considered only recently. Several studies indicate that inhibition of FAS, the enzyme that catalyzes the synthesis of long-chain fatty acids, using either cerulenin, a natural FAS inhibitor, or synthetic FAS inhibitors, reduces food intake and causes profound and reversible weight loss *(31–38)*. Through central, peripheral, or combined central and peripheral mechanisms, these compounds increase energy consumption to augment weight loss *(39)*. Centrally, these compounds reduce the expression of orexigenic peptides *(40)*. In vitro and in vivo studies indicate that, at least in part, C75's effect is mediated by modulation of adenosine-monophosphate-activated protein kinase (AMPK), a member of an energy-sensing kinase family *(41,42)*. These compounds, with chronic treatment, also alter gene expression peripherally to favor a state of enhanced energy consumption *(36,37)*. While the question of the physiological role of fatty acid metabolism remains to be fully elucidated, these effects raise the possibility that pharmacological alterations targeting molecules important in fatty acid synthesis/degradation may prove to be useful targets for obesity therapeutics.

4.2. The Role of Dietary Fat in the Regulation of Energy Homeostasis

Dietary fat is the most energy-dense macronutrient in the diet *(43)*. Short-term feeding studies have indicated that dietary fat might be used more efficiently than carbohydrates and thus it accumulates as body fat *(44)*. When these short-term feeding studies are extended to 4 days, however, no difference in stored energy is observed *(44,45)*. It has thus been suggested that carbohydrate intake, unlike fat intake, is regulated *(46)*. The rationale underlying the promotion of low-fat diets is largely based on the belief that dietary fat is positively associated with body fat through the high energy density of fat and enhanced palatability of high-fat foods *(43)*. However, traditional recommendations of fat restriction have been shown to have a negligible effect on long-term weight loss *(43)* whereas low-fat diets may also not offer any benefit in terms of reducing the risk of cardiovascular disease *(47)*. Thus, further studies are needed to clarify the role of dietary fat in regulation of energy homeostasis.

4.3. The Role of Dietary Carbohydrates in Regulation of Energy Homeostasis

Recent studies indicate that low-carbohydrate diets might be more effective for short-term weight loss than low-fat diets, although this has not been verified by longer-term studies *(48)*. Weight loss while following a low-carbohydrate diet is thought to result from a combination of factors: the satiating effect of protein *(49)*, increased energy expenditure *(50,51)*, appetite suppression from ketosis, as well as restriction of food choice *(52–60)*. More research is needed to fully define the exact role of low carbohydrate diet in the long-term regulation of body weight, and to elucidate the underlying mechanisms.

5. HORMONES

Hormonal systems serve as peripheral signals to CNS to provide information regarding energy storage and metabolic state. These hormones deriving mainly from the adipose tissue, the gastrointestinal tract, and the pancreas contribute to the homeostatic control system for the regulation of food intake and energy balance.

5.1. Adipose Tissue – Adipokines

Adipocytes are active endocrine cells that secrete numerous proteins and bioactive peptides known as adipokines, which act at both the local (paracrine/autocrine) and systemic (endocrine) level. The adipose tissue is therefore considered today as a true endocrine organ (see Table 1 and Fig. 1) *(61)*. The most intensively studied and cur-

Table 1

The Adipose Tissue as an Endocrine Organ: Molecules Secreted by Adipose Tissue

Category	Molecules
Hormones	Leptin, adiponectin, resistin, estrogens, angiotensinogen, retinol binding protein 4, visfatin, apelin
Cytokines	IL-6, TNF-α
Complement factors	Adipsin (complement factor D), complement C3, complement factor B, ASP
Extracellular matrix proteins	Type I, II, IV, VI collagen, fibronectin, osteonectin, laminin, entactin, matrix metalloproteinases 2 and 9
Other immune-related proteins	MCP-1
Proteins of the RAS	Renin, AGT, AT1, AT2, ACE
Acute phase response proteins	α1-acid glycoprotein, haptoglobin
Proteins involved in the fibrinolytic system	PAI-1, tissue factor
Enzymes and transporters involved in Lipid metabolism	LPL, CETP Apolipoprotein E, Adipocyte fatty acid binding protein, CD36.
Enzymes and transporters involved in glucose metabolism	Insulin receptor substrate 1,2, Phosphatidylinositol 3-kinase, protein kinase B (Akt), GLUT4, protein kinase λ/ζ
Enzymes involved in steroid metabolism	Cytochome-P450-dependent aromatase, 17βHSD, 11βHSD1
Receptors of peptides and glycoproteins	Insulin, glucagon, thyroid-stimulating hormone, growth hormone, angiotensin-II, gastrin/cholecystokinin B, adiponectin
Receptors of cytokines	IL-6, TNF-α, leptin
Nuclear receptors	PPARγ, glucocorticoid, estrogen, progesterone, androgen, thyroid, vitamin D, nuclear factor-kB
Other	Prostacyclin, FFAs

Il-6 interleukin 6, *TNF* tumor necrosis factor, *MCP-1* monocyte chemoatractant protein 1, *ASP* acylation stimulating protein, *11βHSD-1* 11β-hydroxysteroid dehydrogenase type 1, *17βHSD* 17β-hydroxysteroid dehydrogenase, *LPL* lipoprotein lipase, *CETP* cholesterol ester transfer protein, *AGT* angiotensinogen, *AT1 and 2* angiotensin receptor type 1 and 2, *ACE* angiotensin-converting enzyme, *PAI-1* plasminogen activator inhibitor, *FFAs* free fatty acids, *PPARγ* peroxisome proliferator-activated receptor gamma

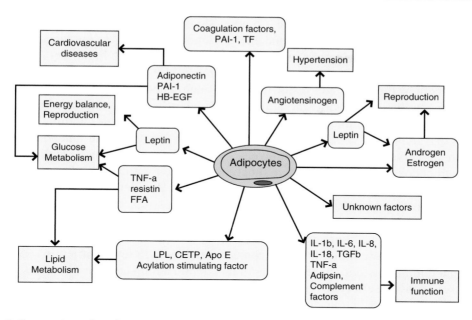

Fig. 1. Integration of environmental and peripheral signals by the central nervous system.

rently considered most important molecules secreted by the adipose tissue are leptin, adiponectin, and interleukin-6 (IL-6), which are discussed below.

5.1.1. LEPTIN

Leptin, a 16-kDa protein, is the product of the *ob* (leptin) gene. Its discovery has changed the concept of white adipose tissue from that of an inert tissue to that of an active endocrine organ. Leptin is expressed predominantly in adipocytes *(62)* but has also been found in the hypothalamus, pituitary, placenta, skeletal muscle, and the gastrointestinal tract *(63)*. Leptin circulates in the blood stream in a free and a bound form, and mediates its metabolic effects by binding to and activating the long isoform of a specific receptor known as ObRb *(64)*. Signaling pathways downstream of leptin include the JAK STAT pathway, MAP kinase, and PI3 kinase *(65)*. Leptin levels decrease in response to caloric restriction *(66)* and they increase in response to overfeeding irrespective of adipose tissue mass. Leptin secretion is also increased by insulin, glucocorticoids, tumor necrosis factor alpha, and estrogens, and is decreased in response to starvation *(67)*, β_3-adrenergic activity *(68)*, free fatty acids, growth hormone, androgens, and PPARγ agonists, as reviewed in detail elsewhere *(69)*.

The discovery of leptin not only led to the realization that leptin per se plays a pivotal role in the regulation of energy homeostasis but also opened the black box of energy homeostasis regulation. Leptin is thought to act as a lipostat: as the amount of fat stored in adipocytes rises, leptin is released into the blood and signals to the brain information on adequacy of energy stores. Recent studies in mice underline the important role of leptin in the development of hypothalamic circuits regulating energy homeostasis *(70)* since leptin may affect the synaptic plasticity of hypothalamic neurons *(71)* and may also act as a neurotrophic factor during hypothalamic development *(72)*.

Although the role of leptin appears to be of significance in both ends of the energy homeostasis spectrum, i.e., obesity and energy-deficient states *(73)*, our work has demonstrated that in humans leptin's role appears to be of much more important in states of energy deprivation *(74–76)*. Our group has also recently shown that falling leptin levels below a certain threshold can result in several neuroendocrine changes and immune abnormalities that occur with starvation *(75,77)* whereas no alterations of these neuroendocrine axes and immune response occur when leptin fluctuates within the normal range *(78)*. Importantly, extremely thin women with hypothalamic amenorrhea and/ or anorexia nervosa have low leptin levels *(79,80)*, whereas exogenous leptin normalizes neuroendocrine and reproductive function in women with relative hypoleptinemia *(76)*. The role of leptin in human obesity is intriguing. In rodents diet-induced obesity has been correlated with the development of leptin resistance *(81,82)*. Mutations in *ob* gene (leptin gene), as well as the leptin receptor gene, result in morbid obesity and diabetes in rodents and humans *(62,83–85)*; however, these cases are extremely rare. The majority of obese individuals are characterized by high levels of leptin *(86)*, suggesting leptin insensitivity or resistance; in fact, leptin administration to obese subjects has only a moderate effect on body weight *(87)*. Importantly, negative regulators of both leptin and insulin signal transduction, such as inhibitors of protein tyrosine phosphatase 1B, may provide opportunities for the treatment of both obesity and insulin resistance by improving these hormone resistance syndromes *(69,88)*. Finally, the prospect that leptin administration in replacement doses might prove clinically useful to maintain weight loss and the resulting relative hypoleptinemia that has been achieved by more traditional means *(89,90)* is an exciting possibility. Further testing of this concept in humans is the focus of many research efforts. The complex role of leptin in regulation of energy homeostasis and neuroendocrine function is summarized in Figs. 2 and 3a and in Tables 2 and 3.

5.1.2. ADIPONECTIN

Adiponectin, a 247-amino-acid protein produced exclusively by adipocytes, circulates in trimers and higher order oligomers *(91–94)* (Figs. 3b and 4). Different adiponectin isoforms, bind and activate at least two adiponectin receptors, which in turn alter the phosphorylation state of 5′-AMP kinase and possibly other downstream molecules *(94,95)*. Adiponectin receptor 1 (AdipoR1), which is expressed ubiquitously, but most abundantly in skeletal muscle, has a high affinity for globular adiponectin and a very low affinity for full-length adiponectin, whereas adiponectin receptor 2 (AdipoR2), which is found predominantly in the liver, has an intermediate affinity for both forms *(96)*.

Adiponectin is currently considered to regulate not only insulin resistance but also possibly energy homeostasis *(91)*. It decreases with increasing overall and central adiposity *(92,97–99)*, and increases with long-term weight reduction *(100)*. Adiponectin is increased after food restriction in rodents *(101)*. Its levels are regulated in rodents by ageing and high fat diet *(102)*, and in humans by certain genetic polymorphisms *(103)*, Mediterranean diet *(104)*, glycemic load *(105)*, and exercise *(106)*. Studies in rodents have revealed that peripheral adiponectin administration reduces body weight and visceral adiposity without affecting food intake *(107,108)*, increases insulin sensitivity, and decreases lipid levels in rodents *(109–111)*. These effects are proposed to occur mainly by regulating energy expenditure, increasing glucose uptake, free fatty

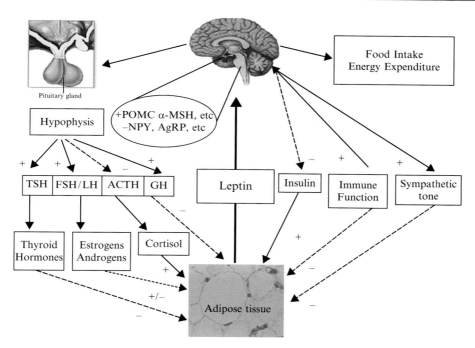

Fig. 2. Leptin's role in energy homeostasis and neuroendocrine regulation. States of energy excess are associated with increased leptin levels but both neuroendocrine function and energy homeostasis are resistant to the effects of increased leptin. Energy deficiency results in decreasing leptin levels and reduced leptin receptor activation in the arcuate nucleus of the hypothalamus. This leads to activation of a complex neural circuitry comprising orexigenic and anorexigenic signals. The main anorexigenic peptides are proopiomelanocortin and cocaine and amphetamine regulated transcript; these are stimulated by leptin. The main orexigenic peptides downstream of leptin are neuropeptide Y and agouti-related protein; both potently stimulate food intake and reduce energy expenditure, thereby promoting weight gain in response to reducing leptin levels. In the figure the response to anorexigenic stimuli (activated in states of energy excess) is shown. "+" indicates stimulatory effects; "–" inhibitory effects. In states of energy deficiency the exact reverse pathways are activated.

acid oxidation, and oxygen consumption in the periphery *(95,108,109)*. This effect on energy expenditure appears to be mediated by the hypothalamic melanocortin system *(111)*. Adiponectin knockout mice have severe diet-induced insulin resistance *(112)*. Importantly, accumulating evidence indicates that the primary role for adiponectin is to regulate insulin sensitivity *(96,110,113–115)*.

Circulating adiponectin levels correlate negatively with insulin resistance *(98)*, and low adiponectin levels predict increased risk for developing insulin resistance, diabetes, cardiovascular disease and may represent a link between obesity and certain malignancies *(116)*. On the other hand, adiponectin levels are higher in states of improved insulin sensitivity, such as after weight reduction or treatment with insulin-sensitizing drugs, e.g. thiazolidinediones *(94)*. In addition to its insulin-sensitizing effects, adiponectin can decrease lipid levels *(111)* and has potent anti-inflammatory *(117)* and atheroprotective effects *(118–120)*. Although metabolic pathways that are involved in regulation of food intake, gluconeogenesis, and lipogenesis *(121)* mediate some of the actions of adiponectin,

Table 2
Actions of Leptin That Can Regulate Energy Homeostasis and Metabolism by Organ and System

Action of leptin	Type of action of leptin
Energy intake	Binding to and activation of leptin receptors found in hypothalamic nuclei (mainly, but not exclusively, in arcuate and paraventricular nucleus of the hypothalamus) and brainstem, triggers circuits inhibiting appetite (mainly through upregulation of α-MSH (POMC)) and inhibits circuits stimulating appetite (mainly by suppressing neuropeptide Y and agouti-related peptide (AgRP) expression in hypothalamic nuclei) (300).
Energy expenditure	Experimental evidence points to both acute and chronic effects of leptin to increase energy expenditure, both via activation of BAT and increases in SNS firing per se (301,302). Acute effects of leptin include increased catecholamine turnover in BAT (301), increased SNS firing in numerous thermogenic tissues (302), and lipolysis (303). The acute effects of leptin may be important for body weight regulation because leptin may prevent the decrease in energy expenditure that normally accompanies decreased food intake in mice (304) and humans (89). Leptin administration has not been shown to alter SNS activity in healthy humans in the short term (305) but may alter SNS activity in long-term weight-loss-induced hypoleptinemia in humans (89). In any case, leptin's effect on energy expenditure in both weight-loss-induced and congenital hypoleptinemia appears to be relatively small (85).
Autonomic nervous system axis	Activation of leptin receptors in the ventromedial hypothalamus and arcuate nucleus results in modulation of autonomic nervous system activity. Acute leptin injections (i.v., intracerebroventricular – ICV, or intrahypothalamic into the VMH) increase sympathetic nerve activity in mice (306–308). Through activation of sympathetic nerves, leptin stimulates free fatty acid oxidation and thermogenesis in brown adipose tissue in rodents (309). No similar effects have been demonstrated to date in humans (305).
Peripheral tissues	Leptin increases glucose uptake in several tissues, including muscle and brown adipose tissue, and thus seems to play a role in modulating peripheral insulin sensitivity (310). The latter is likely to also involve activation of central melanocortin neurons but more research is needed for underlying mechanisms to be fully elucidated. Leptin administration has been shown to improve insulin resistance in humans with congenital (311) or relative acquired leptin deficiency (310). Other important actions of leptin include regulation of immune function, hematopoiesis in mice (312) and humans (313,314), angiogenesis (73) and finally bone metabolism (73).

BAT brown adipose tissue, *MSH* a-melanocyte-stimulating hormone, *POMC* proopiomelanocortin, *SNS* sympathetic nervous system

Table 3
The Role of Leptin in Energy Homeostasis

The role of leptin in states of energy excess

- Children with leptin deficiency due to a leptin or leptin receptor *(85)* gene mutation are normal at birth but develop morbid obesity in early childhood, which is responsive to leptin treatment *(315–317)*. Although monogenic obesity syndromes due to mutations in the leptin or leptin receptor genes remain an uncommon cause of obesity, their existence underlines the importance of the leptin system in the control of energy homeostasis in humans.
- Most obese humans and almost all mouse models of obesity (except ob/ob) have elevated levels of leptin in serum *(318)*. Administration of leptin to diet-induced obese mice, a model of human obesity, resulted in only minimal weight loss *(304)*, demonstrating that these hyperleptinemic mice are leptin-resistant, probably because of receptor or postreceptor defects *(318)*.
- Common human obesity is a leptin-resistant state with high circulating levels of leptin in obese subjects and relative tolerance or deficiency in the actions of leptin *(86,317,318)*.
- Although defective leptin transport through the blood–brain barrier to the hypothalamus, induction of leptin signaling inhibitors, or intracellular signaling defects in leptin-responsive hypothalamic neurons have been designated as potential defects accountable for leptin resistance *(319–321)*, the exact mechanism of leptin tolerance or resistance to its actions remains to be elucidated in humans.
- In view of the fact that leptin treatment depletes body fat specifically *(304)* the notion of leptin tolerance or resistance to its actions was supported by clinical trials in which only modest weight loss occurred in response to recombinant leptin (r-metHuLeptin) administration *(87)*.
- Although rare patients with partial leptin deficiency may respond to exogenous leptin treatment *(322)*, larger, prospective, double-blinded and placebo-controlled clinical trials in obese patients have shown only modest, dose-dependent weight loss in obese patients, along with a high degree of variability in response *(87)*.
- A possible role for falling leptin levels in the plateau phenomenon and the return to baseline body weight in response to weight loss has been raised in a recent small and uncontrolled study where leptin administration to maintain levels equal to those prior to weight loss reversed changes observed with weight loss *(89)*.

The role of leptin in states of energy deficiency

- Accumulating evidence suggests that leptin is physiologically more important as a signal of energy deficiency than as a signal of energy excess.
- In contrast to the observation that leptin levels increase gradually over time as fat mass increases, leptin levels are very sensitive to acute energy deprivation *(77)* and fall rapidly in response to complete fasting, before and/or out of proportion to changes in fat mass *(77,323,324)*.
- Starvation also elicits physiological adaptations of several neuroendocrine axes that can be considered protective, from a teleological point of view, since they may divert energy away from processes that are not essential for immediate survival during acute starvation. We have shown that several neuroendocrine changes that occur with starvation are the result of falling leptin levels in mice *(67)* and in humans *(67,77)*.
- Exogenous leptin administration to normalize falling leptin levels in response to starvation restores neuroendocrine function in normal men *(77)*, but has only minimal effect when leptin fluctuates within the normal range *(75)*.
- Extremely thin women with hypothalamic amenorrhea and/or anorexia nervosa have low leptin levels *(79,80,325,326)*. Leptin treatment of strenuously exercising women normalizes neuroendocrine and reproductive functions, as well as bone formation markers in women with relative hypoleptinemia *(76)*.

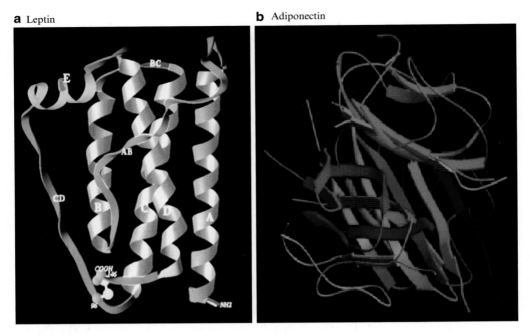

Fig. 3. Tertiary structure of leptin (**a**) and adiponectin (**b**).

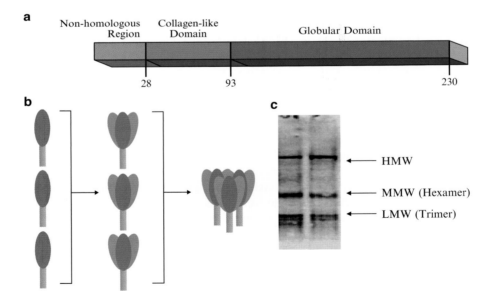

Fig. 4. (**a**) Primary structure of adiponectin. (**b**) Multimeric structure of adiponectin. (**c**) Multimers of adiponectin in an SDS gel (Western blot). *HMW* high molecular weight, *MMW* middle molecular weight, *LMW* low molecular weight adiponectin.

the mechanism by which this adipokine improves insulin resistance, glucose metabolism, and attenuation of weight gain remains to be fully elucidated. Further studies are needed to fully elucidate the role of adiponectin in regulation of energy homeostasis.

5.1.3. Interleukin-6 and Interleukin-1

IL-6 is a multifunctional immune-modulating cytokine that circulates at high levels in the blood stream. It has been suggested to have important functions in glucose and lipid metabolism. IL-6 is secreted from adipose tissue into the circulation, and its expression is positively correlated with BMI and total fat tissue mass. IL-6-knockout mice develop obesity, which can partly be reversed by IL-6 replacement, suggesting a role for IL-6 in the long-term regulation of adipose tissue mass *(122)*. Furthermore, central administration of a low dose of IL-6 decreases feeding and increases energy expenditure in rats, suggesting a central site of action for IL-6 *(122)*. Importantly, obesity can be associated with relative deficiency of IL-6 centrally, since IL-6 levels in the CNS correlate inversely with subcutaneous and total body fat in overweight and obese humans *(123)*. Serum levels and tissue expression of IL-6 decrease in response to diet-induced weight loss and increase with increasing adiposity *(124)*. Increased production of IL-6 by the adipose tissue, especially visceral adipose tissue *(125)*, of obese subjects may represent a compensatory mechanism attempting to limit obesity. Plasma concentrations of IL-6 can predict the development of type 2 diabetes and cardiovascular disease *(61)* since increased IL-6 levels result in a proinflammatory state, as well as insulin signaling defects and thus insulin resistance *(125,126)*.

Other interleukins, including IL-18 and IL-1, are also involved in body-weight homeostasis. IL-1 type I receptor knockout mice display an obese and insulin-resistant phenotype. This obese phenotype is characterised by a decrease in leptin sensitivity, fat utilization, and locomotor activity *(127)*. The emerging role of interleukins in energy homeostasis and insulin resistance has been recently reviewed extensively elsewhere.

5.1.4. Resistin

Resistin, a recently identified 114-amino-acid protein, is almost exclusively expressed in white-adipose tissue. Its concentrations have been reported to be higher in insulin-resistant states as well as in visceral vs. subcutaneous adipose tissue *(128)*. Circulating resistin is increased in obese rodents *(128)* and humans *(129)* and falls after weight loss in humans *(130)*. Whether resistin influences obesity or insulin resistance either directly or by altering glucose and insulin levels and/or whether resistin may play a direct or indirect role in inflammation associated with obesity *(131)* warrants further investigation. Studies have shown contradictory results *(128,132–139)*. Further studies are clearly needed to elucidate the role of resistin in regulation of energy homeostasis *(140)*.

5.1.5. Apelin

Apelin, a hormone with considerable sequence similarity with the angiotensin receptor type 1 (AT-1) gene, was discovered many years ago *(141)* but its production in adipose tissue and its potential modulating effect on obesity were recognized only very recently *(142)*. Apelin, similar to leptin and insulin, is an adipocyte-generated signal circulating in proportion to body fat stores that may be acting to reduce food intake. In addition, similar to leptin, upregulation of apelin gene expression has been observed in certain mouse models of obesity while insulin regulates apelin expression in adipose tissue *(142,143)*. Thus except for the previously described beneficial effects of apelin on cardiovascular physiology and insulin sensitivity *(143)*, apelin may also play a protective role in obesity-associated disease states. However, more experimental evidence on the proposed roles of apelin is needed since available data remain controversial *(142,144–146)*.

5.1.6. VISFATIN

Pre-B-cell colony-enhancing factor, a growth factor for early B lymphocytes previously known to be synthesized in bone marrow, liver, and skeletal muscle, was recently found to be highly expressed in human visceral fat *(147,148)* and was referred to as "visfatin" since plasma visfatin concentration was found to correlate strongly with the amount of visceral fat *(147)*. Plasma visfatin levels were found to be almost twofold higher in mice made obese by a high-fat diet in comparison to lean animals *(147)*. In humans, plasma visfatin has also been reported to correlate significantly with visfatin mRNA level in visceral adipose tissue, percent body fat, and body mass index *(148)*. Experimental data also suggest that endogenous visfatin is involved in the regulation of glucose homeostasis *(147)* and plasma visfatin levels are also higher in patients with type 2 diabetes mellitus than in normoglycemic controls *(149,150)*, although this has not been confirmed by all studies *(151)*. Future studies are needed to clearly establish the exact role of visfatin in the development of obesity and diabetes.

5.1.7. OTHER HORMONES PRODUCED BY ADIPOSE TISSUE

Adipocytes produce other cytokines also, including tumor necrosis factor alpha *(152)* and proteins such as macrophages and monocyte chemoatractant protein 1, plasminogen activator inhibitor 1, and acylation stimulating protein (ASP), all of which have also been studied in the context of regulation of obesity, metabolism, and the insulin resistance syndrome *(61)*. These and other adipocyte-secreted molecules (see Table 1) are the focus of intensive research efforts and their study is expected to contribute significantly to our understanding of the mechanisms regulating nutrition, metabolism, and energy homeostasis.

5.2. Pancreas/Pancreatic Hormones

5.2.1. INSULIN

Insulin, a 51-amino-acid hormone, appears to be one of the most important hormones regulating energy homeostasis. It is secreted from pancreatic beta cells and acts by binding to and activating a glycoprotein insulin receptor expressed on the plasma membrane of almost all cells. Subsequent tyrosine phosphorylation of the insulin receptor and initiation of intracellular signaling lead to regulation of key cellular activities, including gene expression, glucose uptake and oxidation, and synthesis of glycogen, triglycerides, and protein *(153)*.

Key areas responsible for controlling food intake, such as the arcuate nucleus in the hypothalamus, express insulin binding sites *(154)*, and intracerebroventricular infusion of insulin dramatically decreases food intake and body weight in animals *(155)*. In contrast, neuron-specific insulin receptor knockout mice demonstrate increased food intake, body weight, and adiposity, suggesting that insulin, similar to leptin, plays a key role in regulating energy balance *(156,157)*. Animal models of diet-induced obesity and leptin resistance are also characterized by insulin resistance and reduced insulin transport into the brain and thus weight gain and increased food intake may be due to decreased central insulin levels in addition to defective leptin transport and leptin resistance *(158)*. Although both the melanocortin and neuropeptide Y (NPY) systems are important downstream mediators of insulin's actions on food intake and body weight, the pathways mediating insulin's effects on food intake remain to be fully elucidated *(159–161)*.

In humans, insulin, similar to leptin, circulates in levels proportional to the degree of adiposity *(162)* which may serve to overcome impaired insulin-mediated intracellular signaling or to increase insulin levels centrally *(153)*. Negative regulators of both leptin and insulin signal transduction, such as inhibitors of protein tyrosine phosphatase 1B, may provide opportunities for the treatment of both obesity and insulin resistance *(88)*. Several compounds are currently in preclinical development by several pharmaceutical companies and are anticipated with great interest as potential new treatment options for obesity and diabetes.

5.2.2. PANCREATIC POLYPEPTIDE

Pancreatic polypeptide (PP) is primarily produced by cells of the islets of Langerhans *(163)*. It may modulate expression of other gut hormones such as ghrelin *(164)* and/or regulate other hypothalamic neuropeptides such as NPY and orexin *(164)* and convey anorectic signals via brain stem pathways *(165)*. Thus even though PP could be unable to cross the blood–brain barrier, it is possible that it could still regulate appetite. Although less data are available on the interaction between PP and other adipokines such as leptin, it has been shown that PP administration in leptin-deficient *ob/ob* mice decreases body weight *(164)*. We did not find any leptin-induced alterations in PP levels in a recent interventional study in humans *(166)*.

Transgenic mice overexpressing PP are leaner than controls *(167)*, and chronic peripheral administration of PP to mice reduces body weight *(168)*. The actions of PP on food intake seem to depend on the route of administration. In obese rodents, peripheral PP administration decreases food intake, reduces energy expenditure and body weight, and improves insulin resistance and dyslipidemia *(164,169)*. In humans, PP may reduce food intake in normal-weight human volunteers *(170)* and in patients with Prader–Willi syndrome *(171)*. In contrast to the peripheral actions of PP, central administration of PP into the third ventricle increases food intake *(172)* but the mechanisms involved remain to be fully elucidated. Plasma PP concentrations have been inversely associated with adiposity and subjects with anorexia have elevated levels of this peptide *(173,174)*, while reduced levels of plasma PP *(175,176)* have been linked to hyperphagia and obesity in obese subjects *(177,178)*. However, other studies show no difference in plasma PP concentrations in response to weight loss in obese subjects *(179)*, or between lean and obese subjects *(180)*, with the exception of Prader–Willi syndrome. Although observational studies of PP levels in humans are conflicting *(176,181)*, intravenous infusion of PP in normal-weight subjects has been shown to reduce 24-h energy intake *(170)*. Longitudinal prospective evaluation of Pima Indians over 5 years indicate that PP's role in regulating energy balance may be complex, since higher fasting PP levels were associated with greater risk of weight gain, but higher postprandial PP levels were associated with decreased risk of weight gain *(182)*. Thus, the efficacy of PP infusion in obesity remains to be further studied.

5.2 3. AMYLIN

Amylin, produced by the beta cells of the pancreas, is secreted along with insulin in response to food ingestion. Its best known functions are to reduce food intake and gastric emptying, and to inhibit pancreatic glucagon secretion and pancreatic and gastric enzyme secretion *(183)*. Importantly, amylin is deficient in patients with type 1 diabetes, who are also deficient in insulin *(183)*. In rats, amylin decreases food intake, body weight, and fat mass, while inhibition of amylin signaling has the opposite effect *(184,185)*.

Finally, there is evidence that amylin functions as an adiposity signal controlling body weight *(183,186)*, but the magnitude of its effects appears to be relatively small. Amylin may interact with other signals controlling energy homeostasis at the level of the hypothalamus and probably elsewhere, enhances the action of other satiety signals at the level of the hindbrain, and can lead to reduction of meal size *(185,187,188)*. In rats, amylin has a synergistic effect with leptin to induce weight loss *(189)*, specifically decreasing fat mass *(190)*, and a recent clinical trial in humans involving administration of amylin and leptin suggests a similar synergy (http://www.amylin.com). Using an interventional study design in healthy normal-weight humans, we have recently demonstrated that amylin levels are decreased during short-term complete fasting, but this effect is not mediated by leptin; we have also shown that amylin levels are not altered by chronic energy deficit or normalizing leptin levels for up to 3 months *(166)*. Thus, any potential synergistic effect of amylin and leptin to mediate weight loss is likely not due to alterations of amylin levels by leptin, but may be related to central mechanisms and/or synergies in enhancing intracellular signaling.

The synthetic amylin analog pramlintide is marketed for diabetes treatment, but its administration for at least 16 weeks in humans also causes mild progressive weight loss *(191,192)* and can induce weight loss in individuals with *(193)* and without diabetes *(194)*. More studies are needed to fully quantitate amylin's weight reducing capacity, its potential synergistic effects with other peptides, and to carefully study potential side effects.

5.3. Gastrointestinal Tract Hormones

The gastrointestinal tract is also an endocrine organ and an important source of peptide hormones which regulate energy balance. Gastrointestinal hormones have been proposed to contribute to short-term regulation of energy homeostasis in contrast to adipose-tissue-secreted or pancreas-derived hormones which have been proposed to provide long-term signals that regulate energy homeostasis,. Therefore, gut hormone signaling systems represent important pharmaceutical targets for potential antiobesity therapies that would have a short acting role. Of the several gastrointestinal-tract-generated molecules we will focus herein on those considered to be the most important, such as ghrelin, peptide YY (PYY), glucagon-like peptide 1 (GLP-1) and oxyntomodulin, cholecystokinin (CCK), and bombesin-like peptides.

5.3.1. Ghrelin

Ghrelin, a 28-amino-acid peptide, is mainly expressed in enterochromaffin cells of the stomach fundus *(195)* but may also be expressed centrally in the hypothalamus *(196)*. Its action is thought to be mediated via the growth hormone secretagogue receptor (GHS-R) type 1a expressed in numerous tissues, including hypothalamus, pituitary, liver, and the gastrointestinal tract *(195)*. Plasma ghrelin levels are regulated both by food intake and by endogenous diurnal rhythms *(197)*. In normal humans, ghrelin levels rise before meals *(197)* and in response to diet-induced weight loss *(198)* whereas they fall acutely after feeding. The rise in preprandial ghrelin correlates with hunger scores in human subjects eating spontaneously *(199)*. Interestingly, the levels of ghrelin are correlated with adiposity in humans, with an inverse relationship between plasma ghrelin levels and BMI *(200)*. Obese human subjects show reduced levels of plasma ghrelin, which rise to normal after diet-induced weight loss *(198)*. Moreover, in obese individuals the postprandial regulation of ghrelin seems to be altered, which may be related to continuous food intake and/ or obesity *(201)*. Obese patients have also decreased ghrelin levels after gastric bypass surgery, which may contribute to maintaining decreased weight after surgery *(198)*. Furthermore, recent data in humans have demonstrated an inverse correlation between ghrelin and leptin, but we have shown no direct regulation of ghrelin by leptin administration over the short term (period of a few hours to a few days) *(202)*. Peripheral and central administration of ghrelin to rodents induces positive energy balance by decreasing feeding, as well as fat mass, and reduces fat utilization *(203,204)*. Ghrelin is unique because it is the only known gut hormone stimulating food intake. Intravenous administration of ghrelin to healthy volunteers increases food intake *(205)*.

A potentially important application of ghrelin is that ghrelin antagonists could possibly be developed as antiobesity drugs. It has been shown that GHS-R knockout mice are resistant to diet-induced obesity *(206,207)* and favor fat as a metabolic substrate when on a high-fat diet *(208)*. In another study, ghrelin and GHS-R knockout mice were found not to have profoundly altered food intake or body weight on a normal diet *(209,210)*. GHS-R antagonists may therefore have beneficial effects in obese humans on high-fat diet, but more experiments are needed to establish this hypothesis.

Knockout models have also provided further evidence for the role of ghrelin in glucose homeostasis. Diabetic ghrelin knockout mice show less dramatic hyperphagia than do controls *(211)*, and ablating ghrelin attenuates diabetes in the ob/ob mouse models of obesity *(212)*. Moreover, ghrelin administration has been demonstrated to increase food intake in certain patient groups such as in cancer *(213)* and dialysis patients *(214)* and thus reduced ghrelin levels may be responsible in part for the loss of appetite and weight often observed in these patients *(213,214)*. Whether ghrelin plays an important role in regulating energy homeostasis in humans remains to be seen through future interventional studies involving new ghrelin analogs and antagonists currently in development by pharmaceutical companies.

5.3.2. PEPTIDE YY

PYY, a 36-amino-acid peptide *(215)*, is secreted from the L cells of the small and large bowel *(216)*. There are two main forms of PYY in the circulation: PYY1–36 and PYY3–36 *(217)*. PYY levels decrease with fasting and increase rapidly after a meal *(218)*. PYY inhibits food intake through a gut–hypothalamic pathway that involves inhibition of NPY via Y2 receptors in the arcuate nucleus and the dorsal motor nucleus of the vagus nerve *(219)*. Peripheral administration of PYY delays gastric emptying and gastric secretion, inhibits food intake, and reduces weight gain in animals and humans *(220–225)*. However, centrally administered PYY increases food intake in rodents *(226,227)*. In humans, endogenous levels of PYY may be lower in obese subjects, and PYY reduces appetite and food intake when administered to obese or normal-weight subjects, suggesting that a relative PYY deficiency may contribute to the development of obesity *(228)*. We have shown in humans that PYY increases after meal ingestion and decreases after fasting in a manner consistent with a meal-related signal of energy homeostasis but circulating levels of this gut-secreted molecule are independent of regulation by leptin over the short term *(229)*.We have also recently found that PYY levels are higher in obese patients after gastric bypass surgery, a fact that may contribute to the increased efficiency of this procedure in decreasing body weight *(230)*. In a short phase Ic trial of 37 obese participants a PYY nasal spray yielded somewhat promising results causing 1.3 lb of weight loss in 6 days whereas an injectable PYY analog (AC-162352) has been tested in phase I studies, with limited success due to nausea *(231)*. Ongoing clinical trials involving PYY administration are awaited with great anticipation to further elucidate the role of this peptide in the treatment of obesity in humans.

5.3.3. INCRETINS: GLUCAGON-LIKE PEPTIDES (GLP-1,2) AND GLUCOSE-DEPENDENT INSULINOTROPIC PEPTIDE

Incretins such as glucose-dependent insulinotropic polypeptide (GIP) and the glucagon-like peptides (mostly GLP-1 but also GLP-2) are intestinal hormones that are released in response to ingestion of nutrients, especially carbohydrate *(232)*. They have a number of important biological effects, which include release of insulin, inhibition of postprandial glucagon release, maintenance of β-cell mass, delay of gastric emptying, and inhibition of feeding which result in negative energy balance *(232)*. These properties allow them to be potentially suitable agents for the treatment of type 2 diabetes.

Exogenous GLP-1 (central or peripheral administration) has been found to reduce food and caloric intake *(233,234)*, and to decrease weight gain *(235)*, body weight, and adiposity in rodents, whereas immunoblockade of central GLP-1 with antibodies results in increased energy intake *(236,237)*. Moreover, mice deficient in dipeptidyl peptidase IV (DPP-IV), an inhibitor of GLP-1 degradation, are resistant to diet-induced obesity and insulin resistance. Regardless of the anorectic actions of GLP-1 reported in rodents, GLP-1 receptor knockout mice have normal feeding behavior *(238,239)*. The anorectic effect of GLP-1 is also present in humans *(240,241)*. Preprandial subcutaneous GLP-1 injections reduce caloric intake by 15% and result in 0.5 kg of weight loss over 5 days in obese individuals *(242)*. Therefore, low circulating GLP-1 could likely contribute to the pathogenesis and maintenance of obesity, and GLP-1 replacement could restore satiety. The actions of both GLP-1 on feeding may be mediated via the GLP-1 receptor, which is expressed in the hypothalamus, brainstem, and periphery *(243)*. Although GLP-1 is presumed to produce its anorectic effect by acting centrally, the exact mechanism of its action and its potential efficacy in humans need to be further studied *(232)*.

The role of GLP-2 has not been fully established; however, central administration reduces feeding, probably via GLP-1 receptor *(244)*. No effect of GLP-2 on feeding has been reported in man *(245)*.

GIP, a peptide secreted by the duodenum upon absorption of fat or glucose, is a potent insulin secretagogue *(246)*. It has been suggested that GIP may be implicated in a peripheral decrease of energy expenditure and fat oxidation and is oversecreted in the diet-induced mouse model of obesity. GIP receptor knockout mice are protected from obesity and insulin resistance *(246)*, but the role of GIP in humans is currently thought to be less important than that of GLP-1.

In clinical trials, incretin mimetics and GLP-1 agonists such as exenatide and liraglutide reduced fasting and postprandial glucose concentrations, with improvements in HbA1c and modest weight loss when added to existing metformin and/or sulfonylurea therapy in patients with type 2 diabetes *(247–250)*. The modest weight loss caused by incretin mimetics underlines the important role of incretins in regulation of body weight and energy homeostasis. However, side effects, including nausea and vomiting, limit the development of stronger, more efficacious, incretins that could lead to new potential medications for treatment of obesity. Another important category of agents that target the incretin axis include DPP-IV inhibitors, which act by suppressing the degradation of a variety of bioactive peptides, including GLP-1, thereby extending their duration of action *(251)*. Sitagliptin was recently approved for the treatment of type 2 diabetes whereas vildagliptin is furthest along in late-stage clinical development among other DPP-IV inhibitors *(251,252)*. Significant improvement of glycemic control in patients with type 2 diabetes has been observed with sitagliptin *(253–256)* and vildagliptin *(257–259)* treatment in several clinical trials. Long-term clinical studies are needed to determine the benefits of targeting the incretin axis (alone or in combination with other medications) for the treatment of type 2 diabetes.

5.3.4. OXYNTOMODULIN

Oxyntomodulin (OXM) is released from the small intestine in proportion to caloric intake *(260)*. Both central and peripheral OXM administration acutely reduces food intake in rodents *(261,262)*, and repeated administration reduces body weight gain and adiposity *(262)* possibly through an effect on the thyroid axis and via increased energy expenditure *(262)*. Studies in humans *(263)* have shown that OXM reduces hunger and food intake *(263,264)* and may also result in increased energy expenditure *(265)*. Long-term trials are needed to establish OXM as an antiobesity drug and whether it may be the first therapy to suppress appetite and to concurrently increase spontaneous activity.

5.3.5. CHOLECYSTOKININ

CCK is a peptide that is released by the duodenum and jejunum in response to nutrient ingestion (protein and fatty acid) *(266)*, and by acting via specific receptors, it slows gastric emptying and stimulates gastric distension, intestinal motility, gall bladder contraction, and pancreatic enzyme secretion *(267,268)*. Antagonists of these receptors increase food and energy intake in rodents *(269)* and in human subjects *(270)*.

Although peripheral administration of CCK reduces food intake acutely in animals and humans *(267)*, it may also lead to a compensatory increase in daily meal number and thus results in little weight loss. Thus, despite its anorectic actions, repeated administration of CCK does not influence body weight, and CCK is mostly involved in the short-term control of food intake *(271)*. Chronic administration of CCK antagonists or anti-CCK antibodies increases weight gain in rodents, but without a significant change in food intake *(272,273)*. The long-term effect of CCK on body weight may be the result of interaction with other signals of adiposity such as leptin, which enhances the satiating effect of CCK *(274)*. The evidence for a role of CCK in long-term body weight regulation, and hence as a potential therapy for obesity, remains to be fully elucidated.

5.3.6. BOMBESIN-LIKE PEPTIDES

Bombesin and bombesin-like peptides such as gastrin-releasing peptide and neuromedin B are released from the gastrointestinal tract in response to food intake. These peptides result in decreased food intake *(275)* and duration of feeding *(276,277)* and act through specific G-protein-coupled receptors *(278)* which are widely expressed both in the gastrointestinal tract and centrally *(275,279)* and signal to the brain information on energy intake. Peripheral or central injections of bombesin reduce food intake *(280,281)* independently of CCK in rodents *(282)*. Bombesin receptor 3 (BRS-3) knockout mice display hyperphagia, mild obesity, diabetes, and hypertension *(283)* New compounds targeting this pathway are currently under preclinical development and are expected to soon shed light on the role of these molecules in humans.

5.3.7. Apo A-IV

Apolipoprotein (apo) A-IV is a circulating glycoprotein secreted by the small intestine in humans. It has been considered a key peptide involved in the processing of ingested fat by the body *(284)*. One site of action of the anorexic effect of apo A-IV appears to be within the brain since apo A-IV is synthesized in the ventrobasal hypothalamus *(285)*, a general area in which other important feeding-related neuropeptides are also produced, and hypothalamic apo A-IV mRNA levels fluctuate with metabolic state as well as with time of day *(286–288)*. Apo A-IV is also present in the cerebrospinal fluid, and its cerebrospinal levels increase when fat is absorbed *(289)*. Moreover, administration of exogenous apo A-IV in the third ventricle reduces food intake *(290)*. Because both intestinal and hypothalamic apo A-IV are regulated by absorption of lipids, but not carbohydrates, this peptide may be an important link between short- and long-term regulation of body fat *(286–288)*. A possible signaling role of apo A-IV in energy homeostasis is suggested by the fact that systemic administration of exogenous apo A-IV decreases dose dependently food intake of rats *(286–289)* and that administration of apo A-IV antiserum increases food intake and body weight *(290)*. All of these findings suggest that apo A-IV likely interacts with other signals involved in the regulation of energy homeostasis, but more studies are clearly needed to fully elucidate its role.

5.3.8. Enterostatin

Enterostatin is the aminoterminal pentapeptide of procolipase and is released from pancreatic procolipase by proteolytic activity in the small intestine after the ingestion of dietary fat *(291)*. Enterostatin is expressed in both the gastrointestinal tract and the CNS since both procolipase and enterostatin have been localized to the gastric mucosa and to certain brain regions (amygdala, hypothalamus, cortex) *(292)*. Enterostatin when administrated centrally or peripherally to overnight fasted rats induces satiation since it suppresses intake of a high-fat diet, but not a high-carbohydrate diet *(293,294)*. Finally, a role for endogenously produced enterostatin in feeding behavior is suggested by its ability to increase intake of high-fat diets by the enterostatin antagonist β-casomorphin$_{1-7}$ *(295)*. Further studies are needed to fully elucidate the role of this peptide in regulation of food intake and energy homeostasis.

5.3.9. Obestatin

It has recently been reported that obestatin, a new peptide derived from the ghrelin gene, inhibits food intake by acting through the orphan receptor GPR39 *(296,297)*. Despite this evidence there are some discrepancies in relation to the anorectic effect of obestatin *(298)* as well as its binding to GPR39 *(299)*. If the anorectic effect is confirmed, this finding could provide a new drug target for the treatment of obesity.

6. CONCLUSION

In summary, regulation of energy homeostasis is extremely complex. Signals from the environment and the periphery are integrated by the CNS to regulate both energy intake and energy expenditure. As the secrets of the systems responsible for the energy homeostasis regulation continue to be decoded, promising prospects emerge for the development of novel antiobesity medications which should produce more substantial weight loss than is currently achieved with nonsurgical interventions. This will hopefully provide in the not so distant future substantial benefits to the increasing percentage of the population striving to control their body weight.

REFERENCES

1. Akabayashi A, Zaia CT, Silva I, Chae HJ, Leibowitz SF. Neuropeptide Y in the arcuate nucleus is modulated by alterations in glucose utilization. Brain Res 1993; 621(2):343–348.
2. Muroya S, Yada T, Shioda S, Takigawa M. Glucose-sensitive neurons in the rat arcuate nucleus contain neuropeptide Y. Neurosci Lett 1999; 264(1–3):113–116.
3. Lynch RM, Tompkins LS, Brooks HL, Dunn-Meynell AA, Levin BE. Localization of glucokinase gene expression in the rat brain. Diabetes 2000; 49(5):693–700.
4. Burdyga G, Spiller D, Morris R, Lal S, Thompson DG, Saeed S et al. Expression of the leptin receptor in rat and human nodose ganglion neurones. Neuroscience 2002; 109(2):339–347.
5. Moriarty P, Dimaline R, Thompson DG, Dockray GJ. Characterization of cholecystokininA and cholecystokininB receptors expressed by vagal afferent neurons. Neuroscience 1997; 79(3):905–913.
6. Peters JC, Wyatt HR, Donahoo WT, Hill JO. From instinct to intellect: the challenge of maintaining healthy weight in the modern world. Obes Rev 2002; 3(2):69–74.
7. Brownell K. Public policy and the prevention of obesity. In: Fairburn CG, Brownell K, editors. Eating disorders and obesity. New York: The Guilford, 2001: 619–624.
8. Hill JO, Peters JC. Environmental contributions to the obesity epidemic. Science 1998; 280(5368):1371–1374.
9. Hill JO, Wyatt HR, Reed GW, Peters JC. Obesity and the environment: where do we go from here. Science 2003; 299(5608):853–855.
10. Boutin P, Froguel P. Genetics of human obesity. Best Pract Res Clin Endocrinol Metab 2001; 15(3):391–404.
11. Hill J, Pagliassotti M, Peters J. Nongenetic determinants of obesity and fat topography. In: Bouchard C, editor. Genetic determinants of obesity. Boca Raton, FL: CRC, 1994: 35–48.
12. Lingford-Hughes A, Nutt D. Neurobiology of addiction and implications for treatment. Br J Psychiatry 2003; 182:97–100.
13. Rogers PJ, Smit HJ. Food craving and food "addiction": a critical review of the evidence from a biopsychosocial perspective. Pharmacol Biochem Behav 2000; 66(1):3–14.
14. Gulati K, Ray A, Sharma KK. Role of diurnal variation and receptor specificity in the opioidergic regulation of food intake in free-fed and food-deprived rats. Physiol Behav 1991; 49(6):1065–1071.
15. Triscari J, Nelson D, Vincent GP, Li CH. Effect of centrally and peripherally administered beta-endorphin on food intake in rats. Int J Pept Protein Res 1989; 34(5):358–362.
16. Berridge KC, Robinson TE. Parsing reward. Trends Neurosci 2003; 26(9):507–513.
17. Mogenson GJ, Jones DL, Yim CY. From motivation to action: functional interface between the limbic system and the motor system. Prog Neurobiol 1980; 14(2–3):69–97.
18. Zahm DS. An integrative neuroanatomical perspective on some subcortical substrates of adaptive responding with emphasis on the nucleus accumbens. Neurosci Biobehav Rev 2000; 24(1):85–105.
19. Otake K, Nakamura Y. Possible pathways through which neurons of the shell of the nucleus accumbens influence the outflow of the core of the nucleus accumbens. Brain Dev 2000; 22(Suppl 1):S17–S26.
20. Usuda I, Tanaka K, Chiba T. Efferent projections of the nucleus accumbens in the rat with special reference to subdivision of the nucleus: biotinylated dextran amine study. Brain Res 1998; 797(1):73–93.

21. Berthoud HR. Homeostatic and non-homeostatic pathways involved in the control of food intake and energy balance. Obesity (Silver Spring) 2006; 14(Suppl 5):197S–200S.

22. Yeomans MR. Palatability and the micro-structure of feeding in humans: the appetizer effect. Appetite 1996; 27(2):119–133.

23. Drewnowski A, Greenwood MR. Cream and sugar: human preferences for high-fat foods. Physiol Behav 1983; 30(4):629–633.

24. Lyman B. The nutritional values and food group characteristics of foods preferred during various emotions. J Psychol 1982; 112(1st Half):121–127.

25. Taylor GJ, Parker JD, Bagby RM, Bourke MP. Relationships between alexithymia and psychological characteristics associated with eating disorders. J Psychosom Res 1996; 41(6):561–568.

26. Parker G, Parker I, Brotchie H. Mood state effects of chocolate. J Affect Disord 2006; 92(2–3):149–159.

27. Heatherton TF, Herman CP, Polivy J. Effects of distress on eating: the importance of ego-involvement. J Pers Soc Psychol 1992; 62(5):801–803.

28. Obici S, Rossetti L. Minireview: nutrient sensing and the regulation of insulin action and energy balance. Endocrinology 2003; 144(12):5172–5178.

29. Campfield LA, Smith FJ, Burn P. The OB protein (leptin) pathway – a link between adipose tissue mass and central neural networks. Horm Metab Res 1996; 28(12):619–632.

30. Patti ME, Kahn BB. Nutrient sensor links obesity with diabetes risk. Nat Med 2004; 10(10):1049–1050.

31. Loftus TM, Jaworsky DE, Frehywot GL, Townsend CA, Ronnett GV, Lane MD et al. Reduced food intake and body weight in mice treated with fatty acid synthase inhibitors. Science 2000; 288(5475):2379–2381.

32. Makimura H, Mizuno TM, Yang XJ, Silverstein J, Beasley J, Mobbs CV. Cerulenin mimics effects of leptin on metabolic rate, food intake, and body weight independent of the melanocortin system, but unlike leptin, cerulenin fails to block neuroendocrine effects of fasting. Diabetes 2001; 50(4):733–739.

33. Kumar MV, Shimokawa T, Nagy TR, Lane MD. Differential effects of a centrally acting fatty acid synthase inhibitor in lean and obese mice. Proc Natl Acad Sci USA 2002; 99(4):1921–1925.

34. Mobbs CV, Makimura H. Block the FAS, lose the fat. Nat Med 2002; 8(4):335–336.

35. Shimokawa T, Kumar MV, Lane MD. Effect of a fatty acid synthase inhibitor on food intake and expression of hypothalamic neuropeptides. Proc Natl Acad Sci USA 2002; 99(1):66–71.

36. Thupari JN, Landree LE, Ronnett GV, Kuhajda FP. C75 increases peripheral energy utilization and fatty acid oxidation in diet-induced obesity. Proc Natl Acad Sci USA 2002; 99(14):9498–9502.

37. Tu Y, Thupari JN, Kim EK, Pinn ML, Moran TH, Ronnett GV et al. C75 alters central and peripheral gene expression to reduce food intake and increase energy expenditure. Endocrinology 2005; 146(1):486–493.

38. Clegg DJ, Benoit SC, Air EL, Jackman A, Tso P, D'Alessio D et al. Increased dietary fat attenuates the anorexic effects of intracerebroventricular injections of MTII. Endocrinology 2003; 144(7):2941–2946.

39. Ronnett GV, Kleman AM, Kim EK, Landree LE, Tu Y. Fatty acid metabolism, the central nervous system, and feeding. Obesity (Silver Spring) 2006; 14(Suppl 5):201S–207S.

40. Kim EK, Miller I, Landree LE, Borisy-Rudin FF, Brown P, Tihan T et al. Expression of FAS within hypothalamic neurons: a model for decreased food intake after C75 treatment. Am J Physiol Endocrinol Metab 2002; 283(5):E867–E879.

41. Kim EK, Miller I, Aja S, Landree LE, Pinn M, McFadden J et al. C75, a fatty acid synthase inhibitor, reduces food intake via hypothalamic AMP-activated protein kinase. J Biol Chem 2004; 279(19):19970–19976.

42. Landree LE, Hanlon AL, Strong DW, Rumbaugh G, Miller IM, Thupari JN et al. C75, a fatty acid synthase inhibitor, modulates AMP-activated protein kinase to alter neuronal energy metabolism. J Biol Chem 2004; 279(5):3817–3827.

43. Willett WC. Dietary fat plays a major role in obesity: no. Obes Rev 2002; 3(2):59–68.

44. Astrup A. Dietary composition, substrate balances and body fat in subjects with a predisposition to obesity. Int J Obes Relat Metab Disord 1993; 17(Suppl 3):S32–S36.

45. McDevitt RM, Poppitt SD, Murgatroyd PR, Prentice AM. Macronutrient disposal during controlled overfeeding with glucose, fructose, sucrose, or fat in lean and obese women. Am J Clin Nutr 2000; 72(2):369–377.

46. Flatt J. Energetics of intermediary metabolism. In: Garrow JS, Halliday D, editors. Substrate and energy metabolism in man. London: John Libbey, 1985: 58–69.

47. Malik VS, Hu FB. Popular weight-loss diets: from evidence to practice. Nat Clin Pract Cardiovasc Med 2007; 4(1):34–41.

48. Nordmann AJ, Nordmann A, Briel M, Keller U, Yancy WS, Jr, Brehm BJ et al. Effects of low-carbohydrate vs low-fat diets on weight loss and cardiovascular risk factors: a meta-analysis of randomized controlled trials. Arch Intern Med 2006; 166(3):285–293.

49. Halton TL, Hu FB. The effects of high protein diets on thermogenesis, satiety and weight loss: a critical review. J Am Coll Nutr 2004; 23(5):373–385.

50. Feinman RD, Fine EJ. Thermodynamics and metabolic advantage of weight loss diets. Metab Syndr Relat Disord 2003; 1:209–219.

51. Segal-Isaacson CJ, Johnson S, Tomuta V, Cowell B, Stein DT. A randomized trial comparing low-fat and low-carbohydrate diets matched for energy and protein. Obes Res 2004; 12(Suppl 2):130S–140S.

52. Astrup A, Meinert LT, Harper A. Atkins and other low-carbohydrate diets: hoax or an effective tool for weight loss. Lancet 2004; 364(9437):897–899.

53. Buchholz AC, Schoeller DA. Is a calorie a calorie. Am J Clin Nutr 2004; 79(5):899S–906S.

54. Brehm BJ, Seeley RJ, Daniels SR, D'Alessio DA. A randomized trial comparing a very low carbohydrate diet and a calorie-restricted low fat diet on body weight and cardiovascular risk factors in healthy women. J Clin Endocrinol Metab 2003; 88(4):1617–1623.

55. Erlanson-Albertsson C, Mei J. The effect of low carbohydrate on energy metabolism. Int J Obes (Lond) 2005; 29(Suppl 2):S26–S30.

56. Adam-Perrot A, Clifton P, Brouns F. Low-carbohydrate diets: nutritional and physiological aspects. Obes Rev 2006; 7(1):49–58.

57. Haymond MW, Karl IE, Clarke WL, Pagliara AS, Santiago JV. Differences in circulating gluconeogenic substrates during short-term fasting in men, women, and children. Metabolism 1982; 31(1):33–42.

58. Denke MA. Metabolic effects of high-protein, low-carbohydrate diets. Am J Cardiol 2001; 88(1):59–61.

59. Schoeller DA, Buchholz AC. Energetics of obesity and weight control: does diet composition matter? J Am Diet Assoc 2005; 105(5 Suppl 1):S24–S28.

60. Dansinger ML, Gleason JA, Griffith JL, Selker HP, Schaefer EJ. Comparison of the Atkins, Ornish, Weight Watchers, and Zone diets for weight loss and heart disease risk reduction: a randomized trial. JAMA 2005; 293(1):43–53.

61. Kershaw EE, Flier JS. Adipose tissue as an endocrine organ. J Clin Endocrinol Metab 2004; 89(6):2548–2556.

62. Zhang Y, Proenca R, Maffei M, Barone M, Leopold L, Friedman JM. Positional cloning of the mouse obese gene and its human homologue. Nature 1994; 372(6505):425–432.

63. Moschos S, Chan JL, Mantzoros CS. Leptin and reproduction: a review. Fertil Steril 2002; 77(3):433–444.

64. Auwerx J, Staels B. Leptin. Lancet 1998; 351(9104):737–742.

65. Flier JS. Obesity wars: molecular progress confronts an expanding epidemic. Cell 2004; 116(2):337–350.

66. Mantzoros CS, Flier JS. Editorial: leptin as a therapeutic agent – trials and tribulations. J Clin Endocrinol Metab 2000; 85(11):4000–4002.

67. Ahima RS, Prabakaran D, Mantzoros C, Qu D, Lowell B, Maratos-Flier E et al. Role of leptin in the neuroendocrine response to fasting. Nature 1996; 382(6588):250–252.

68. Mantzoros CS, Qu D, Frederich RC, Susulic VS, Lowell BB, Maratos-Flier E et al. Activation of beta(3) adrenergic receptors suppresses leptin expression and mediates a leptin-independent inhibition of food intake in mice. Diabetes 1996; 45(7):909–914.

69. Brennan AM, Mantzoros CS. Drug insight: the role of leptin in human physiology and pathophysiology – emerging clinical applications. Nat Clin Pract Endocrinol Metab 2006; 2(6):318–327.

70. Matochik JA, London ED, Yildiz BO, Ozata M, Caglayan S, DePaoli AM et al. Effect of leptin replacement on brain structure in genetically leptin-deficient adults. J Clin Endocrinol Metab 2005; 90(5):2851–2854.

71. Pinto S, Roseberry AG, Liu H, Diano S, Shanabrough M, Cai X et al. Rapid rewiring of arcuate nucleus feeding circuits by leptin. Science 2004; 304(5667):110–115.

72. Bouret SG, Draper SJ, Simerly RB. Trophic action of leptin on hypothalamic neurons that regulate feeding. Science 2004; 304(5667):108–110.

73. Kelesidis T, Mantzoros CS. The emerging role of leptin in humans. Pediatr Endocrinol Rev 2006; 3(3):239–248.
74. Chan JL, Mantzoros CS. Role of leptin in energy-deprivation states: normal human physiology and clinical implications for hypothalamic amenorrhoea and anorexia nervosa. Lancet 2005; 366(9479):74–85.
75. Chan JL, Matarese G, Shetty GK, Raciti P, Kelesidis I, Aufiero D et al. Differential regulation of metabolic, neuroendocrine, and immune function by leptin in humans. Proc Natl Acad Sci USA 2006; 103(22):8481–8486.
76. Welt CK, Chan JL, Bullen J, Murphy R, Smith P, DePaoli AM et al. Recombinant human leptin in women with hypothalamic amenorrhea. N Engl J Med 2004; 351(10):987–997.
77. Chan JL, Heist K, DePaoli AM, Veldhuis JD, Mantzoros CS. The role of falling leptin levels in the neuroendocrine and metabolic adaptation to short-term starvation in healthy men. J Clin Invest 2003; 111(9):1409–1421.
78. Chan JL, Matarese G, Shetty GK, Raciti P, Kelesidis I, Aufiero D et al. Differential regulation of metabolic, neuroendocrine, and immune function by leptin in humans. Proc Natl Acad Sci USA 2006; 103(22):8481–8486.
79. Miller KK, Parulekar MS, Schoenfeld E, Anderson E, Hubbard J, Klibanski A et al. Decreased leptin levels in normal weight women with hypothalamic amenorrhea: the effects of body composition and nutritional intake. J Clin Endocrinol Metab 1998; 83(7):2309–2312.
80. Laughlin GA, Yen SS. Hypoleptinemia in women athletes: absence of a diurnal rhythm with amenorrhea. J Clin Endocrinol Metab 1997; 82(1):318–321.
81. Van Heek M, Compton DS, France CF, Tedesco RP, Fawzi AB, Graziano MP et al. Diet-induced obese mice develop peripheral, but not central, resistance to leptin. J Clin Invest 1997; 99(3):385–390.
82. Levin BE, Dunn-Meynell AA. Reduced central leptin sensitivity in rats with diet-induced obesity. Am J Physiol Regul Integr Comp Physiol 2002; 283(4):R941–R948.
83. Coleman DL. Obese and diabetes: two mutant genes causing diabetes-obesity syndromes in mice. Diabetologia 1978; 14(3):141–148.
84. Friedman JM, Leibel RL. Tackling a weighty problem. Cell 1992; 69(2):217–220.
85. Farooqi IS, Wangensteen T, Collins S, Kimber W, Matarese G, Keogh JM et al. Clinical and molecular genetic spectrum of congenital deficiency of the leptin receptor. N Engl J Med 2007; 356(3):237–247.
86. Considine RV, Sinha MK, Heiman ML, Kriauciunas A, Stephens TW, Nyce MR et al. Serum immunoreactive-leptin concentrations in normal-weight and obese humans. N Engl J Med 1996; 334(5):292–295.
87. Heymsfield SB, Greenberg AS, Fujioka K, Dixon RM, Kushner R, Hunt T et al. Recombinant leptin for weight loss in obese and lean adults: a randomized, controlled, dose-escalation trial. JAMA 1999; 282(16):1568–1575.
88. Dadke S, Chernoff J. Protein-tyrosine phosphatase 1B as a potential drug target for obesity. Curr Drug Targets Immune Endocr Metabol Disord 2003; 3(4):299–304.
89. Rosenbaum M, Goldsmith R, Bloomfield D, Magnano A, Weimer L, Heymsfield S et al. Low-dose leptin reverses skeletal muscle, autonomic, and neuroendocrine adaptations to maintenance of reduced weight. J Clin Invest 2005; 115(12):3579–3586.
90. Boozer CN, Leibel RL, Love RJ, Cha MC, Aronne LJ. Synergy of sibutramine and low-dose leptin in treatment of diet-induced obesity in rats. Metabolism 2001; 50(8):889–893.
91. Scherer PE, Williams S, Fogliano M, Baldini G, Lodish HF. A novel serum protein similar to C1q, produced exclusively in adipocytes. J Biol Chem 1995; 270(45):26746–26749.
92. Arita Y, Kihara S, Ouchi N, Takahashi M, Maeda K, Miyagawa J et al. Paradoxical decrease of an adipose-specific protein, adiponectin, in obesity. Biochem Biophys Res Commun 1999; 257(1):79–83.
93. Wang GJ, Volkow ND, Fowler JS. The role of dopamine in motivation for food in humans: implications for obesity. Expert Opin Ther Targets 2002; 6(5):601–609.
94. Chandran M, Phillips SA, Ciaraldi T, Henry RR. Adiponectin: more than just another fat cell hormone? Diabetes Care 2003; 26(8):2442–2450.
95. Yamauchi T, Kamon J, Ito Y, Tsuchida A, Yokomizo T, Kita S et al. Cloning of adiponectin receptors that mediate antidiabetic metabolic effects. Nature 2003; 423(6941):762–769.
96. Kubota N, Terauchi Y, Yamauchi T, Kubota T, Moroi M, Matsui J et al. Disruption of adiponectin causes insulin resistance and neointimal formation. J Biol Chem 2002; 277(29):25863–25866.

97. Hu E, Liang P, Spiegelman BM. AdipoQ is a novel adipose-specific gene dysregulated in obesity. J Biol Chem 1996; 271(18):10697–10703.

98. Hotta K, Funahashi T, Bodkin NL, Ortmeyer HK, Arita Y, Hansen BC et al. Circulating concentrations of the adipocyte protein adiponectin are decreased in parallel with reduced insulin sensitivity during the progression to type 2 diabetes in rhesus monkeys. Diabetes 2001; 50(5):1126–1133.

99. Gavrila A, Chan JL, Yiannakouris N, Kontogianni M, Miller LC, Orlova C et al. Serum adiponectin levels are inversely associated with overall and central fat distribution but are not directly regulated by acute fasting or leptin administration in humans: cross-sectional and interventional studies. J Clin Endocrinol Metab 2003; 88(10):4823–4831.

100. Yang WS, Lee WJ, Funahashi T, Tanaka S, Matsuzawa Y, Chao CL et al. Weight reduction increases plasma levels of an adipose-derived anti-inflammatory protein, adiponectin. J Clin Endocrinol Metab 2001; 86(8):3815–3819.

101. Berg AH, Combs TP, Scherer PE. ACRP30/adiponectin: an adipokine regulating glucose and lipid metabolism. Trends Endocrinol Metab 2002; 13(2):84–89.

102. Bullen JW, Jr, Bluher S, Kelesidis T, Mantzoros CS. Regulation of adiponectin and its receptors in response to development of diet induced obesity in mice. Am J Physiol Endocrinol Metab 2007; 292(4):E1079–E1086.

103. Qi L, Doria A, Manson JE, Meigs JB, Hunter D, Mantzoros CS et al. Adiponectin genetic variability, plasma adiponectin, and cardiovascular risk in patients with type 2 diabetes. Diabetes 2006; 55(5):1512–1516.

104. Mantzoros CS, Williams CJ, Manson JE, Meigs JB, Hu FB. Adherence to the Mediterranean dietary pattern is positively associated with plasma adiponectin concentrations in diabetic women. Am J Clin Nutr 2006; 84(2):328–335.

105. Qi L, Rimm E, Liu S, Rifai N, Hu FB. Dietary glycemic index, glycemic load, cereal fiber, and plasma adiponectin concentration in diabetic men. Diabetes Care 2005; 28(5):1022–1028.

106. Bluher M, Bullen JW, Jr, Lee JH, Kralisch S, Fasshauer M, Kloting N et al. Circulating adiponectin and expression of adiponectin receptors in human skeletal muscle: associations with metabolic parameters and insulin resistance and regulation by physical training. J Clin Endocrinol Metab 2006; 91(6):2310–2316.

107. Masaki T, Chiba S, Yasuda T, Tsubone T, Kakuma T, Shimomura I et al. Peripheral, but not central, administration of adiponectin reduces visceral adiposity and upregulates the expression of uncoupling protein in agouti yellow (Ay/a) obese mice. Diabetes 2003; 52(9):2266–2273.

108. Fruebis J, Tsao TS, Javorschi S, Ebbets-Reed D, Erickson MR, Yen FT et al. Proteolytic cleavage product of 30-kDa adipocyte complement-related protein increases fatty acid oxidation in muscle and causes weight loss in mice. Proc Natl Acad Sci USA 2001; 98(4):2005–2010.

109. Berg AH, Combs TP, Du X, Brownlee M, Scherer PE. The adipocyte-secreted protein Acrp30 enhances hepatic insulin action. Nat Med 2001; 7(8):947–953.

110. Yamauchi T, Kamon J, Waki H, Terauchi Y, Kubota N, Hara K et al. The fat-derived hormone adiponectin reverses insulin resistance associated with both lipoatrophy and obesity. Nat Med 2001; 7(8):941–946.

111. Qi Y, Takahashi N, Hileman SM, Patel HR, Berg AH, Pajvani UB et al. Adiponectin acts in the brain to decrease body weight. Nat Med 2004; 10(5):524–529.

112. Maeda N, Shimomura I, Kishida K, Nishizawa H, Matsuda M, Nagaretani H et al. Diet-induced insulin resistance in mice lacking adiponectin/ACRP30. Nat Med 2002; 8(7):731–737.

113. Bluher M, Michael MD, Peroni OD, Ueki K, Carter N, Kahn BB et al. Adipose tissue selective insulin receptor knockout protects against obesity and obesity-related glucose intolerance. Dev Cell 2002; 3(1):25–38.

114. Stefan N, Vozarova B, Funahashi T, Matsuzawa Y, Weyer C, Lindsay RS et al. Plasma adiponectin concentration is associated with skeletal muscle insulin receptor tyrosine phosphorylation, and low plasma concentration precedes a decrease in whole-body insulin sensitivity in humans. Diabetes 2002; 51(6):1884–1888.

115. Lindsay RS, Funahashi T, Hanson RL, Matsuzawa Y, Tanaka S, Tataranni PA et al. Adiponectin and development of type 2 diabetes in the Pima Indian population. Lancet 2002; 360(9326):57–58.

116. Kelesidis I, Kelesidis T, Mantzoros CS. Adiponectin and cancer: a systematic review. Br J Cancer 2006; 94(9):1221–1225.

117. Yokota T, Oritani K, Takahashi I, Ishikawa J, Matsuyama A, Ouchi N et al. Adiponectin, a new member of the family of soluble defense collagens, negatively regulates the growth of myelomonocytic progenitors and the functions of macrophages. Blood 2000; 96(5):1723–1732.

118. Ouchi N, Kihara S, Arita Y, Maeda K, Kuriyama H, Okamoto Y et al. Novel modulator for endothelial adhesion molecules: adipocyte-derived plasma protein adiponectin. Circulation 1999; 100(25):2473–2476.

119. Ouchi N, Kihara S, Arita Y, Nishida M, Matsuyama A, Okamoto Y et al. Adipocyte-derived plasma protein, adiponectin, suppresses lipid accumulation and class A scavenger receptor expression in human monocyte-derived macrophages. Circulation 2001; 103(8):1057–1063.

120. Mantzoros CS, Li T, Manson JE, Meigs JB, Hu FB. Circulating adiponectin levels are associated with better glycemic control, more favorable lipid profile, and reduced inflammation in women with type 2 diabetes. J Clin Endocrinol Metab 2005; 90(8):4542–4548.

121. Shklyaev S, Aslanidi G, Tennant M, Prima V, Kohlbrenner E, Kroutov V et al. Sustained peripheral expression of transgene adiponectin offsets the development of diet-induced obesity in rats. Proc Natl Acad Sci USA 2003; 100(24):14217–14222.

122. Wallenius K, Wallenius V, Sunter D, Dickson SL, Jansson JO. Intracerebroventricular interleukin-6 treatment decreases body fat in rats. Biochem Biophys Res Commun 2002; 293(1):560–565.

123. Stenlof K, Wernstedt I, Fjallman T, Wallenius V, Wallenius K, Jansson JO. Interleukin-6 levels in the central nervous system are negatively correlated with fat mass in overweight/obese subjects. J Clin Endocrinol Metab 2003; 88(9):4379–4383.

124. Bastard JP, Jardel C, Bruckert E, Blondy P, Capeau J, Laville M et al. Elevated levels of interleukin 6 are reduced in serum and subcutaneous adipose tissue of obese women after weight loss. J Clin Endocrinol Metab 2000; 85(9):3338–3342.

125. Fried SK, Bunkin DA, Greenberg AS. Omental and subcutaneous adipose tissues of obese subjects release interleukin-6: depot difference and regulation by glucocorticoid. J Clin Endocrinol Metab 1998; 83(3):847–850.

126. Hotamisligil GS, Arner P, Caro JF, Atkinson RL, Spiegelman BM. Increased adipose tissue expression of tumor necrosis factor-alpha in human obesity and insulin resistance. J Clin Invest 1995; 95(5):2409–2415.

127. Garcia MC, Wernstedt I, Berndtsson A, Enge M, Bell M, Hultgren O et al. Mature-onset obesity in interleukin-1 receptor I knockout mice. Diabetes 2006; 55(5):1205–1213.

128. Steppan CM, Bailey ST, Bhat S, Brown EJ, Banerjee RR, Wright CM et al. The hormone resistin links obesity to diabetes. Nature 2001; 409(6818):307–312.

129. Savage DB, Sewter CP, Klenk ES, Segal DG, Vidal-Puig A, Considine RV et al. Resistin/Fizz3 expression in relation to obesity and peroxisome proliferator-activated receptor-gamma action in humans. Diabetes 2001; 50(10):2199–2202.

130. Valsamakis G, McTernan PG, Chetty R, Al Daghri N, Field A, Hanif W et al. Modest weight loss and reduction in waist circumference after medical treatment are associated with favorable changes in serum adipocytokines. Metabolism 2004; 53(4):430–434.

131. Holcomb IN, Kabakoff RC, Chan B, Baker TW, Gurney A, Henzel W et al. FIZZ1, a novel cysteine-rich secreted protein associated with pulmonary inflammation, defines a new gene family. EMBO J 2000; 19(15):4046–4055.

132. McTernan PG, Fisher FM, Valsamakis G, Chetty R, Harte A, McTernan CL et al. Resistin and type 2 diabetes: regulation of resistin expression by insulin and rosiglitazone and the effects of recombinant resistin on lipid and glucose metabolism in human differentiated adipocytes. J Clin Endocrinol Metab 2003; 88(12):6098–6106.

133. Steppan CM, Lazar MA. Resistin and obesity-associated insulin resistance. Trends Endocrinol Metab 2002; 13(1):18–23.

134. Way JM, Gorgun CZ, Tong Q, Uysal KT, Brown KK, Harrington WW et al. Adipose tissue resistin expression is severely suppressed in obesity and stimulated by peroxisome proliferator-activated receptor gamma agonists. J Biol Chem 2001; 276(28):25651–25653.

135. Lee JH, Chan JL, Yiannakouris N, Kontogianni M, Estrada E, Seip R et al. Circulating resistin levels are not associated with obesity or insulin resistance in humans and are not regulated by fasting or leptin administration: cross-sectional and interventional studies in normal, insulin-resistant, and diabetic subjects. J Clin Endocrinol Metab 2003; 88(10):4848–4856.

136. Silha JV, Krsek M, Hana V, Marek J, Jezkova J, Weiss V et al. Perturbations in adiponectin, leptin and resistin levels in acromegaly: lack of correlation with insulin resistance. Clin Endocrinol (Oxf) 2003; 58(6):736–742.

137. Banerjee RR, Rangwala SM, Shapiro JS, Rich AS, Rhoades B, Qi Y et al. Regulation of fasted blood glucose by resistin. Science 2004; 303(5661):1195–1198.

138. Lee JH, Bullen JW, Jr, Stoyneva VL, Mantzoros CS. Circulating resistin in lean, obese, and insulin-resistant mouse models: lack of association with insulinemia and glycemia. Am J Physiol Endocrinol Metab 2005; 288(3):E625–E632.

139. Barb D, Pazaitou-Panayiotou K, Mantzoros CS. Adiponectin: a link between obesity and cancer. Expert Opin Invest Drugs 2006; 15(8):917–931.

140. Tovar S, Nogueiras R, Tung LY, Castaneda TR, Vazquez MJ, Morris A et al. Central administration of resistin promotes short-term satiety in rats. Eur J Endocrinol 2005; 153(3):R1–R5.

141. O'Dowd BF, Heiber M, Chan A, Heng HH, Tsui LC, Kennedy JL et al. A human gene that shows identity with the gene encoding the angiotensin receptor is located on chromosome 11. Gene 1993; 136(1–2):355–360.

142. Boucher J, Masri B, Daviaud D, Gesta S, Guigne C, Mazzucotelli A et al. Apelin, a newly identified adipokine up-regulated by insulin and obesity. Endocrinology 2005; 146(4):1764–1771.

143. Beltowski J. Apelin and visfatin: unique "beneficial" adipokines upregulated in obesity? Med Sci Monit 2006; 12(6):RA112–RA119.

144. Taheri S, Murphy K, Cohen M, Sujkovic E, Kennedy A, Dhillo W et al. The effects of centrally administered apelin-13 on food intake, water intake and pituitary hormone release in rats. Biochem Biophys Res Commun 2002; 291(5):1208–1212.

145. Sunter D, Hewson AK, Dickson SL. Intracerebroventricular injection of apelin-13 reduces food intake in the rat. Neurosci Lett 2003; 353(1):1–4.

146. O'Shea M, Hansen MJ, Tatemoto K, Morris MJ. Inhibitory effect of apelin-12 on nocturnal food intake in the rat. Nutr Neurosci 2003; 6(3):163–167.

147. Fukuhara A, Matsuda M, Nishizawa M, Segawa K, Tanaka M, Kishimoto K et al. Visfatin: a protein secreted by visceral fat that mimics the effects of insulin. Science 2005; 307(5708):426–430.

148. Berndt J, Kloting N, Kralisch S, Kovacs P, Fasshauer M, Schon MR et al. Plasma visfatin concentrations and fat depot-specific mRNA expression in humans. Diabetes 2005; 54(10):2911–2916.

149. Chen MP, Chung FM, Chang DM, Tsai JC, Huang HF, Shin SJ et al. Elevated plasma level of visfatin/pre-B cell colony-enhancing factor in patients with type 2 diabetes mellitus. J Clin Endocrinol Metab 2006; 91(1):295–299.

150. Hammarstedt A, Pihlajamaki J, Rotter SV, Gogg S, Jansson PA, Laakso M et al. Visfatin is an adipokine, but it is not regulated by thiazolidinediones. J Clin Endocrinol Metab 2006; 91(3):1181–1184.

151. Pagano C, Pilon C, Olivieri M, Mason P, Fabris R, Serra R et al. Reduced plasma visfatin/pre-B cell colony-enhancing factor in obesity is not related to insulin resistance in humans. J Clin Endocrinol Metab 2006; 91(8):3165–3170.

152. Warne JP. Tumour necrosis factor alpha: a key regulator of adipose tissue mass. J Endocrinol 2003; 177(3):351–355.

153. Niswender KD, Schwartz MW. Insulin and leptin revisited: adiposity signals with overlapping physiological and intracellular signaling capabilities. Front Neuroendocrinol 2003; 24(1):1–10.

154. Marks JL, Porte D, Jr, Stahl WL, Baskin DG. Localization of insulin receptor mRNA in rat brain by in situ hybridization. Endocrinology 1990; 127(6):3234–3236.

155. Woods SC, Lotter EC, McKay LD, Porte D, Jr. Chronic intracerebroventricular infusion of insulin reduces food intake and body weight of baboons. Nature 1979; 282(5738):503–505.

156. Bruning JC, Gautam D, Burks DJ, Gillette J, Schubert M, Orban PC et al. Role of brain insulin receptor in control of body weight and reproduction. Science 2000; 289(5487):2122–2125.

157. Cohen P, Zhao C, Cai X, Montez JM, Rohani SC, Feinstein P et al. Selective deletion of leptin receptor in neurons leads to obesity. J Clin Invest 2001; 108(8):1113–1121.

158. Kaiyala KJ, Prigeon RL, Kahn SE, Woods SC, Schwartz MW. Obesity induced by a high-fat diet is associated with reduced brain insulin transport in dogs. Diabetes 2000; 49(9):1525–1533.

159. Benoit SC, Air EL, Coolen LM, Strauss R, Jackman A, Clegg DJ et al. The catabolic action of insulin in the brain is mediated by melanocortins. J Neurosci 2002; 22(20):9048–9052.

160. Schwartz MW, Sipols AJ, Marks JL, Sanacora G, White JD, Scheurink A et al. Inhibition of hypothalamic neuropeptide Y gene expression by insulin. Endocrinology 1992; 130(6):3608–3616.
161. White JD, Olchovsky D, Kershaw M, Berelowitz M. Increased hypothalamic content of preproneuropeptide-Y messenger ribonucleic acid in streptozotocin-diabetic rats. Endocrinology 1990; 126(2):765–772.
162. Bagdade JD, Bierman EL, Porte D, Jr. The significance of basal insulin levels in the evaluation of the insulin response to glucose in diabetic and nondiabetic subjects. J Clin Invest 1967; 46(10):1549–1557.
163. Larsson LI, Sundler F, Hakanson R. Immunohistochemical localization of human pancreatic polypeptide (HPP) to a population of islet cells. Cell Tissue Res 1975; 156(2):167–171.
164. Asakawa A, Inui A, Yuzuriha H, Ueno N, Katsuura G, Fujimiya M et al. Characterization of the effects of pancreatic polypeptide in the regulation of energy balance. Gastroenterology 2003; 124(5):1325–1336.
165. Whitcomb DC, Taylor IL, Vigna SR. Characterization of saturable binding sites for circulating pancreatic polypeptide in rat brain. Am J Physiol 1990; 259(4 Pt 1):G687–G691.
166. Hwang JJ, Chan JL, Ntali G, Malkova D, Mantzoros CS. Leptin does not directly regulate the pancreatic hormones, amylin and pancreatic polypeptide: interventional studies in humans. Diabetes Care 2008; 31:945–951.
167. Ueno N, Inui A, Iwamoto M, Kaga T, Asakawa A, Okita M et al. Decreased food intake and body weight in pancreatic polypeptide-overexpressing mice. Gastroenterology 1999; 117(6):1427–1432.
168. Malaisse-Lagae F, Carpentier JL, Patel YC, Malaisse WJ, Orci L. Pancreatic polypeptide: a possible role in the regulation of food intake in the mouse. Hypothesis. Experientia 1977; 33(7):915–917.
169. McLaughlin CL, Baile CA. Obese mice and the satiety effects of cholecystokinin, bombesin and pancreatic polypeptide. Physiol Behav 1981; 26(3):433–437.
170. Batterham RL, Le Roux CW, Cohen MA, Park AJ, Ellis SM, Patterson M et al. Pancreatic polypeptide reduces appetite and food intake in humans. J Clin Endocrinol Metab 2003; 88(8):3989–3992.
171. Berntson GG, Zipf WB, O'Dorisio TM, Hoffman JA, Chance RE. Pancreatic polypeptide infusions reduce food intake in Prader–Willi syndrome. Peptides 1993; 14(3):497–503.
172. Clark JT, Kalra PS, Crowley WR, Kalra SP. Neuropeptide Y and human pancreatic polypeptide stimulate feeding behavior in rats. Endocrinology 1984; 115(1):427–429.
173. Fujimoto S, Inui A, Kiyota N, Seki W, Koide K, Takamiya S et al. Increased cholecystokinin and pancreatic polypeptide responses to a fat-rich meal in patients with restrictive but not bulimic anorexia nervosa. Biol Psychiatry 1997; 41(10):1068–1070.
174. Uhe AM, Szmukler GI, Collier GR, Hansky J, O'Dea K, Young GP. Potential regulators of feeding behavior in anorexia nervosa. Am J Clin Nutr 1992; 55(1):28–32.
175. Glaser B, Zoghlin G, Pienta K, Vinik AI. Pancreatic polypeptide response to secretin in obesity: effects of glucose intolerance. Horm Metab Res 1988; 20(5):288–292.
176. Lassmann V, Vague P, Vialettes B, Simon MC. Low plasma levels of pancreatic polypeptide in obesity. Diabetes 1980; 29(6):428–430.
177. Zipf WB, O'Dorisio TM, Cataland S, Dixon K. Pancreatic polypeptide responses to protein meal challenges in obese but otherwise normal children and obese children with Prader–Willi syndrome. J Clin Endocrinol Metab 1983; 57(5):1074–1080.
178. Zipf WB, O'Dorisio TM, Cataland S, Sotos J. Blunted pancreatic polypeptide responses in children with obesity of Prader–Willi syndrome. J Clin Endocrinol Metab 1981; 52(6):1264–1266.
179. Meryn S, Stein D, Straus EW. Fasting- and meal-stimulated peptide hormone concentrations before and after gastric surgery for morbid obesity. Metabolism 1986; 35(9):798–802.
180. Wisen O, Bjorvell H, Cantor P, Johansson C, Theodorsson E. Plasma concentrations of regulatory peptides in obesity following modified sham feeding (MSF) and a liquid test meal. Regul Pept 1992; 39(1):43–54.
181. Marco J, Zulueta MA, Correas I, Villanueva ML. Reduced pancreatic polypeptide secretion in obese subjects. J Clin Endocrinol Metab 1980; 50(4):744–747.
182. Koska J, DelParigi A, de Court, Weyer C, Tataranni PA. Pancreatic polypeptide is involved in the regulation of body weight in Pima Indian male subjects. Diabetes 2004; 53(12):3091–3096.
183. Lutz TA. Amylinergic control of food intake. Physiol Behav 2006.
184. Lutz TA, Mollet A, Rushing PA, Riediger T, Scharrer E. The anorectic effect of a chronic peripheral infusion of amylin is abolished in area postrema/nucleus of the solitary tract (AP/NTS) lesioned rats. Int J Obes Relat Metab Disord 2001; 25(7):1005–1011.

185. Rushing PA, Hagan MM, Seeley RJ, Lutz TA, D'Alessio DA, Air EL et al. Inhibition of central amylin signaling increases food intake and body adiposity in rats. Endocrinology 2001; 142(11):5035.
186. Woods SC, Lutz TA, Geary N, Langhans W. Pancreatic signals controlling food intake; insulin, glucagon and amylin. Philos Trans R Soc Lond B Biol Sci 2006; 361(1471):1219–1235.
187. Rushing PA. Central amylin signaling and the regulation of energy homeostasis. Curr Pharm Des 2003; 9(10):819–825.
188. Reidelberger RD, Kelsey L, Heimann D. Effects of amylin-related peptides on food intake, meal patterns, and gastric emptying in rats. Am J Physiol Regul Integr Comp Physiol 2002; 282(5):R1395–R1404.
189. Osto M, Wielinga PY, Alder B, Walser N, Lutz TA. Modulation of the satiating effect of amylin by central ghrelin, leptin and insulin. Physiol Behav 2007; 91(5):566–572.
190. Roth JD, Hughes H, Kendall E, Baron AD, Anderson CM. Antiobesity effects of the beta-cell hormone amylin in diet-induced obese rats: effects on food intake, body weight, composition, energy expenditure, and gene expression. Endocrinology 2006; 147(12):5855–5864.
191. Schmitz O, Brock B, Rungby J. Amylin agonists: a novel approach in the treatment of diabetes. Diabetes 2004; 53(Suppl 3):S233–S238.
192. Hollander P, Maggs DG, Ruggles JA, Fineman M, Shen L, Kolterman OG et al. Effect of pramlintide on weight in overweight and obese insulin-treated type 2 diabetes patients. Obes Res 2004; 12(4):661–668.
193. Hollander P, Maggs DG, Ruggles JA, Fineman M, Shen L, Kolterman OG et al. Effect of pramlintide on weight in overweight and obese insulin-treated type 2 diabetes patients. Obes Res 2004; 12(4):661–668.
194. Aronne L, Fujioka K, Aroda V, Chen K, Halseth A, Kesty NC et al. Progressive reduction in body weight after treatment with the amylin analog pramlintide in obese subjects: a phase 2, randomized, placebo-controlled, dose-escalation study. J Clin Endocrinol Metab 2007; 92(8):2977–2983.
195. Kojima M, Hosoda H, Date Y, Nakazato M, Matsuo H, Kangawa K. Ghrelin is a growth-hormone-releasing acylated peptide from stomach. Nature 1999; 402(6762):656–660.
196. Toshinai K, Date Y, Murakami N, Shimada M, Mondal MS, Shimbara T et al. Ghrelin-induced food intake is mediated via the orexin pathway. Endocrinology 2003; 144(4):1506–1512.
197. Cummings DE, Purnell JQ, Frayo RS, Schmidova K, Wisse BE, Weigle DS. A preprandial rise in plasma ghrelin levels suggests a role in meal initiation in humans. Diabetes 2001; 50(8):1714–1719.
198. Cummings DE, Weigle DS, Frayo RS, Breen PA, Ma MK, Dellinger EP et al. Plasma ghrelin levels after diet-induced weight loss or gastric bypass surgery. N Engl J Med 2002; 346(21):1623–1630.
199. Cummings DE, Frayo RS, Marmonier C, Aubert R, Chapelot D. Plasma ghrelin levels and hunger scores in humans initiating meals voluntarily without time- and food-related cues. Am J Physiol Endocrinol Metab 2004; 287(2):E297–E304.
200. Tschop M, Weyer C, Tataranni PA, Devanarayan V, Ravussin E, Heiman ML. Circulating ghrelin levels are decreased in human obesity. Diabetes 2001; 50(4):707–709.
201. English PJ, Ghatei MA, Malik IA, Bloom SR, Wilding JP. Food fails to suppress ghrelin levels in obese humans. J Clin Endocrinol Metab 2002; 87(6):2984.
202. Chan JL, Bullen J, Lee JH, Yiannakouris N, Mantzoros CS. Ghrelin levels are not regulated by recombinant leptin administration and/or three days of fasting in healthy subjects. J Clin Endocrinol Metab 2004; 89(1):335–343.
203. Nakazato M, Murakami N, Date Y, Kojima M, Matsuo H, Kangawa K et al. A role for ghrelin in the central regulation of feeding. Nature 2001; 409(6817):194–198.
204. Wren AM, Small CJ, Abbott CR, Dhillo WS, Seal LJ, Cohen MA et al. Ghrelin causes hyperphagia and obesity in rats. Diabetes 2001; 50(11):2540–2547.
205. Wren AM, Seal LJ, Cohen MA, Brynes AE, Frost GS, Murphy KG et al. Ghrelin enhances appetite and increases food intake in humans. J Clin Endocrinol Metab 2001; 86(12):5992.
206. Zigman JM, Nakano Y, Coppari R, Balthasar N, Marcus JN, Lee CE et al. Mice lacking ghrelin receptors resist the development of diet-induced obesity. J Clin Invest 2005; 115(12):3564–3572.
207. Wortley KE, del Rincon JP, Murray JD, Garcia K, Iida K, Thorner MO et al. Absence of ghrelin protects against early-onset obesity. J Clin Invest 2005; 115(12):3573–3578.
208. Wortley KE, Anderson KD, Garcia K, Murray JD, Malinova L, Liu R et al. Genetic deletion of ghrelin does not decrease food intake but influences metabolic fuel preference. Proc Natl Acad Sci USA 2004; 101(21):8227–8232.

209. Sun Y, Ahmed S, Smith RG. Deletion of ghrelin impairs neither growth nor appetite. Mol Cell Biol 2003; 23(22):7973–7981.

210. Sun Y, Wang P, Zheng H, Smith RG. Ghrelin stimulation of growth hormone release and appetite is mediated through the growth hormone secretagogue receptor. Proc Natl Acad Sci USA 2004; 101(13):4679–4684.

211. Dong J, Peeters TL, De Smet B, Moechars D, Delporte C, Vanden Berghe P et al. Role of endogenous ghrelin in the hyperphagia of mice with streptozotocin-induced diabetes. Endocrinology 2006; 147(6):2634–2642.

212. Sun Y, Asnicar M, Saha PK, Chan L, Smith RG. Ablation of ghrelin improves the diabetic but not obese phenotype of ob/ob mice. Cell Metab 2006; 3(5):379–386.

213. Neary NM, Small CJ, Wren AM, Lee JL, Druce MR, Palmieri C et al. Ghrelin increases energy intake in cancer patients with impaired appetite: acute, randomized, placebo-controlled trial. J Clin Endocrinol Metab 2004; 89(6):2832–2836.

214. Wynne K, Giannitsopoulou K, Small CJ, Patterson M, Frost G, Ghatei MA et al. Subcutaneous ghrelin enhances acute food intake in malnourished patients who receive maintenance peritoneal dialysis: a randomized, placebo-controlled trial. J Am Soc Nephrol 2005; 16(7):2111–2118.

215. Tatemoto K, Mutt V. Isolation of two novel candidate hormones using a chemical method for finding naturally occurring polypeptides. Nature 1980; 285(5764):417–418.

216. Adrian TE, Ferri GL, Bacarese-Hamilton AJ, Fuessl HS, Polak JM, Bloom SR. Human distribution and release of a putative new gut hormone, peptide YY. Gastroenterology 1985; 89(5):1070–1077.

217. Tatemoto K, Carlquist M, Mutt V. Neuropeptide Y – a novel brain peptide with structural similarities to peptide YY and pancreatic polypeptide. Nature 1982; 296(5858):659–660.

218. Anini Y, Fu-Cheng X, Cuber JC, Kervran A, Chariot J, Roz C. Comparison of the postprandial release of peptide YY and proglucagon-derived peptides in the rat. Pflugers Arch 1999; 438(3):299–306.

219. Korner J, Leibel RL. To eat or not to eat – how the gut talks to the brain. N Engl J Med 2003; 349(10):926–928.

220. Challis BG, Coll AP, Yeo GS, Pinnock SB, Dickson SL, Thresher RR et al. Mice lacking pro-opiomelanocortin are sensitive to high-fat feeding but respond normally to the acute anorectic effects of peptide-YY(3-36). Proc Natl Acad Sci USA 2004; 101(13):4695–4700.

221. Pittner RA, Moore CX, Bhavsar SP, Gedulin BR, Smith PA, Jodka CM et al. Effects of PYY[3–36] in rodent models of diabetes and obesity. Int J Obes Relat Metab Disord 2004; 28(8):963–971.

222. Degen L, Oesch S, Casanova M, Graf S, Ketterer S, Drewe J et al. Effect of peptide YY3-36 on food intake in humans. Gastroenterology 2005; 129(5):1430–1436.

223. Chelikani PK, Haver AC, Reidelberger RD. Intravenous infusion of peptide YY (3–36) potently inhibits food intake in rats. Endocrinology 2005; 146(2):879–888.

224. Batterham RL, Cowley MA, Small CJ, Herzog H, Cohen MA, Dakin CL et al. Gut hormone PYY(3–36) physiologically inhibits food intake. Nature 2002; 418(6898):650–654.

225. Sileno AP, Brandt GC, Spann BM, Quay SC. Lower mean weight after 14 days intravenous administration peptide YY3–36 (PYY3–36) in rabbits. Int J Obes (Lond) 2006; 30(1):68–72.

226. Corp ES, McQuade J, Krasnicki S, Conze DB. Feeding after fourth ventricular administration of neuropeptide Y receptor agonists in rats. Peptides 2001; 22(3):493–499.

227. Hagan MM, Castaneda E, Sumaya IC, Fleming SM, Galloway J, Moss DE. The effect of hypothalamic peptide YY on hippocampal acetylcholine release in vivo: implications for limbic function in binge-eating behavior. Brain Res 1998; 805(1/2):20–28.

228. Batterham RL, Cohen MA, Ellis SM, Le Roux CW, Withers DJ, Frost GS et al. Inhibition of food intake in obese subjects by peptide YY3-36. N Engl J Med 2003; 349(10):941–948.

229. Chan JL, Stoyneva V, Kelesidis T, Raciti P, Mantzoros CS. Peptide YY levels are decreased by fasting and elevated following caloric intake but are not regulated by leptin. Diabetologia 2006; 49(1):169–173.

230. Chan JL, Mun EC, Stoyneva V, Mantzoros CS, Goldfine AB. Peptide YY levels are elevated after gastric bypass surgery. Obesity (Silver Spring) 2006; 14(2):194–198.

231. Halford JC. Obesity drugs in clinical development. Curr Opin Invest Drugs 2006; 7(4):312–318.

232. Drucker DJ, Philippe J, Mojsov S, Chick WL, Habener JF. Glucagon-like peptide I stimulates insulin gene expression and increases cyclic AMP levels in a rat islet cell line. Proc Natl Acad Sci USA 1987; 84(10):3434–3438.

233. Tang-Christensen M, Vrang N, Larsen PJ. Glucagon-like peptide containing pathways in the regulation of feeding behaviour. Int J Obes Relat Metab Disord 2001; 25(Suppl 5):S42–S47.

234. Turton MD, O'Shea D, Gunn I, Beak SA, Edwards CM, Meeran K et al. A role for glucagon-like peptide-1 in the central regulation of feeding. Nature 1996; 379(6560):69–72.

235. Meeran K, O'Shea D, Edwards CM, Turton MD, Heath MM, Gunn I et al. Repeated intracerebroventricular administration of glucagon-like peptide-1-(7-36) amide or exendin-(9-39) alters body weight in the rat. Endocrinology 1999; 140(1):244–250.

236. Greig NH, Holloway HW, De Ore KA, Jani D, Wang Y, Zhou J et al. Once daily injection of exendin-4 to diabetic mice achieves long-term beneficial effects on blood glucose concentrations. Diabetologia 1999; 42(1):45–50.

237. Szayna M, Doyle ME, Betkey JA, Holloway HW, Spencer RG, Greig NH et al. Exendin-4 decelerates food intake, weight gain, and fat deposition in Zucker rats. Endocrinology 2000; 141(6):1936–1941.

238. Scrocchi LA, Hill ME, Saleh J, Perkins B, Drucker DJ. Elimination of glucagon-like peptide 1R signaling does not modify weight gain and islet adaptation in mice with combined disruption of leptin and GLP-1 action. Diabetes 2000; 49(9):1552–1560.

239. Scrocchi LA, Brown TJ, MaClusky N, Brubaker PL, Auerbach AB, Joyner AL et al. Glucose intolerance but normal satiety in mice with a null mutation in the glucagon-like peptide 1 receptor gene. Nat Med 1996; 2(11):1254–1258.

240. Meier JJ, Gallwitz B, Schmidt WE, Nauck MA. Glucagon-like peptide 1 as a regulator of food intake and body weight: therapeutic perspectives. Eur J Pharmacol 2002; 440(2/3):269–279.

241. Verdich C, Flint A, Gutzwiller JP, Naslund E, Beglinger C, Hellstrom PM et al. A meta-analysis of the effect of glucagon-like peptide-1 (7–36) amide on ad libitum energy intake in humans. J Clin Endocrinol Metab 2001; 86(9):4382–4389.

242. Naslund E, King N, Mansten S, Adner N, Holst JJ, Gutniak M et al. Prandial subcutaneous injections of glucagon-like peptide-1 cause weight loss in obese human subjects. Br J Nutr 2004; 91(3):439–446.

243. Bullock BP, Heller RS, Habener JF. Tissue distribution of messenger ribonucleic acid encoding the rat glucagon-like peptide-1 receptor. Endocrinology 1996; 137(7):2968–2978.

244. Badman MK, Flier JS. The gut and energy balance: visceral allies in the obesity wars. Science 2005; 307(5717):1909–1914.

245. Schmidt PT, Naslund E, Gryback P, Jacobsson H, Hartmann B, Holst JJ et al. Peripheral administration of GLP-2 to humans has no effect on gastric emptying or satiety. Regul Pept 2003; 116(1–3):21–25.

246. Miyawaki K, Yamada Y, Ban N, Ihara Y, Tsukiyama K, Zhou H et al. Inhibition of gastric inhibitory polypeptide signaling prevents obesity. Nat Med 2002; 8(7):738–742.

247. Buse JB, Henry RR, Han J, Kim DD, Fineman MS, Baron AD. Effects of exenatide (exendin-4) on glycemic control over 30 weeks in sulfonylurea-treated patients with type 2 diabetes. Diabetes Care 2004; 27(11):2628–2635.

248. DeFronzo RA, Ratner RE, Han J, Kim DD, Fineman MS, Baron AD. Effects of exenatide (exendin-4) on glycemic control and weight over 30 weeks in metformin-treated patients with type 2 diabetes. Diabetes Care 2005; 28(5):1092–1100.

249. Kendall DM, Riddle MC, Rosenstock J, Zhuang D, Kim DD, Fineman MS et al. Effects of exenatide (exendin-4) on glycemic control over 30 weeks in patients with type 2 diabetes treated with metformin and a sulfonylurea. Diabetes Care 2005; 28(5):1083–1091.

250. Kuehn BM. New diabetes drugs target gut hormones. JAMA 2006; 296(4):380–381.

251. Drucker DJ, Nauck MA. The incretin system: glucagon-like peptide-1 receptor agonists and dipeptidyl peptidase-4 inhibitors in type 2 diabetes. Lancet 2006; 368(9548):1696–1705.

252. Ristic S, Byiers S, Foley J, Holmes D. Improved glycaemic control with dipeptidyl peptidase-4 inhibition in patients with type 2 diabetes: vildagliptin (LAF237) dose response. Diabetes Obes Metab 2005; 7(6):692–698.

253. Charbonnel B, Karasik A, Liu J, Wu M, Meininger G. Efficacy and safety of the dipeptidyl peptidase-4 inhibitor sitagliptin added to ongoing metformin therapy in patients with type 2 diabetes inadequately controlled with metformin alone. Diabetes Care 2006; 29(12):2638–2643.

254. Aschner P, Kipnes MS, Lunceford JK, Sanchez M, Mickel C, Williams-Herman DE. Effect of the dipeptidyl peptidase-4 inhibitor sitagliptin as monotherapy on glycemic control in patients with type 2 diabetes. Diabetes Care 2006; 29(12):2632–2637.

255. Raz I, Hanefeld M, Xu L, Caria C, Williams-Herman D, Khatami H. Efficacy and safety of the dipeptidyl peptidase-4 inhibitor sitagliptin as monotherapy in patients with type 2 diabetes mellitus. Diabetologia 2006; 49(11):2564–2571.

256. Rosenstock J, Brazg R, Andryuk PJ, Lu K, Stein P. Efficacy and safety of the dipeptidyl peptidase-4 inhibitor sitagliptin added to ongoing pioglitazone therapy in patients with type 2 diabetes: a 24-week, multicenter, randomized, double-blind, placebo-controlled, parallel-group study. Clin Ther 2006; 28(10):1556–1568.

257. Balas B, Baig MR, Watson C, Dunning BE, Ligueros-Saylan M, Wang Y et al. The dipeptidyl peptidase IV inhibitor vildagliptin suppresses endogenous glucose production and enhances islet function after single dose administration in type 2 diabetic patients. J Clin Endocrinol Metab 2007; 92(4):1249–1255.

258. Pi-Sunyer FX, Schweizer A, Mills D, Dejager S. Efficacy and tolerability of vildagliptin monotherapy in drug-naive patients with type 2 diabetes. Diabetes Res Clin Pract 2007; 76(1):132–138.

259. Pratley RE, Jauffret-Kamel S, Galbreath E, Holmes D. Twelve-week monotherapy with the DPP-4 inhibitor vildagliptin improves glycemic control in subjects with type 2 diabetes. Horm Metab Res 2006; 38(6):423–428.

260. Le Quellec A, Kervran A, Blache P, Ciurana AJ, Bataille D. Oxyntomodulin-like immunoreactivity: diurnal profile of a new potential enterogastrone. J Clin Endocrinol Metab 1992; 74(6):1405–1409.

261. Dakin CL, Gunn I, Small CJ, Edwards CM, Hay DL, Smith DM et al. Oxyntomodulin inhibits food intake in the rat. Endocrinology 2001; 142(10):4244–4250.

262. Dakin CL, Small CJ, Batterham RL, Neary NM, Cohen MA, Patterson M et al. Peripheral oxyntomodulin reduces food intake and body weight gain in rats. Endocrinology 2004; 145(6):2687–2695.

263. Cohen MA, Ellis SM, Le Roux CW, Batterham RL, Park A, Patterson M et al. Oxyntomodulin suppresses appetite and reduces food intake in humans. J Clin Endocrinol Metab 2003; 88(10):4696–4701.

264. Wynne K, Park AJ, Small CJ, Patterson M, Ellis SM, Murphy KG et al. Subcutaneous oxyntomodulin reduces body weight in overweight and obese subjects: a double-blind, randomized, controlled trial. Diabetes 2005; 54(8):2390–2395.

265. Wynne K, Park AJ, Small CJ, Meeran K, Ghatei MA, Frost GS et al. Oxyntomodulin increases energy expenditure in addition to decreasing energy intake in overweight and obese humans: a randomised controlled trial. Int J Obes (Lond) 2006; 30(12):1729–1736.

266. Go VLW. The physiology of cholecystokinin. Gut hormones. Edinburgh: Chruchill Livingstone, 1978: 203.

267. Kissileff HR, Carretta JC, Geliebter A, Pi-Sunyer FX. Cholecystokinin and stomach distension combine to reduce food intake in humans. Am J Physiol Regul Integr Comp Physiol 2003; 285(5):R992–R998.

268. Moran TH, McHugh PR. Cholecystokinin suppresses food intake by inhibiting gastric emptying. Am J Physiol 1982; 242(5):R491–R497.

269. Corp ES, Curcio M, Gibbs J, Smith GP. The effect of centrally administered CCK-receptor antagonists on food intake in rats. Physiol Behav 1997; 61(6):823–827.

270. Beglinger C, Degen L, Matzinger D, D'Amato M, Drewe J. Loxiglumide, a CCK-A receptor antagonist, stimulates calorie intake and hunger feelings in humans. Am J Physiol Regul Integr Comp Physiol 2001; 280(4):R1149–R1154.

271. West DB, Fey D, Woods SC. Cholecystokinin persistently suppresses meal size but not food intake in free-feeding rats. Am J Physiol 1984; 246(5 Pt 2):R776–R787.

272. McLaughlin CL, Baile CA, Buonomo FC. Effect of CCK antibodies on food intake and weight gain in Zucker rats. Physiol Behav 1985; 34(2):277–282.

273. Meereis-Schwanke K, Klonowski-Stumpe H, Herberg L, Niederau C. Long-term effects of CCK-agonist and -antagonist on food intake and body weight in Zucker lean and obese rats. Peptides 1998; 19(2):291–299.

274. Matson CA, Reid DF, Cannon TA, Ritter RC. Cholecystokinin and leptin act synergistically to reduce body weight. Am J Physiol Regul Integr Comp Physiol 2000; 278(4):R882–R890.

275. Merali Z, McIntosh J, Anisman H. Role of bombesin-related peptides in the control of food intake. Neuropeptides 1999; 33(5):376–386.

276. Flynn FW. Fourth ventricular injection of selective bombesin receptor antagonists facilitates feeding in rats. Am J Physiol 1993; 264(1 Pt 2):R218–R221.

277. Gutzwiller JP, Drewe J, Hildebrand P, Rossi L, Lauper JZ, Beglinger C. Effect of intravenous human gastrin-releasing peptide on food intake in humans. Gastroenterology 1994; 106(5):1168–1173.

278. Battey JF, Way JM, Corjay MH, Shapira H, Kusano K, Harkins R et al. Molecular cloning of the bombesin/gastrin-releasing peptide receptor from Swiss 3T3 cells. Proc Natl Acad Sci USA 1991; 88(2):395–399.

279. Gibbs J, Kulkosky PJ, Smith GP. Effects of peripheral and central bombesin on feeding behavior of rats. Peptides 1981; 2(Suppl 2):179–183.

280. Gibbs J, Fauser DJ, Rowe EA, Rolls BJ, Rolls ET, Maddison SP. Bombesin suppresses feeding in rats. Nature 1979; 282(5735):208–210.

281. Smith GP, Jerome C, Gibbs J. Abdominal vagotomy does not block the satiety effect of bombesin in the rat. Peptides 1981; 2(4):409–411.

282. Lieverse RJ, Jansen JB, van de ZA, Samson L, Masclee AA, Rovati LC et al. Bombesin reduces food intake in lean man by a cholecystokinin-independent mechanism. J Clin Endocrinol Metab 1993; 76(6):1495–1498.

283. Ohki-Hamazaki H, Watase K, Yamamoto K, Ogura H, Yamano M, Yamada K et al. Mice lacking bombesin receptor subtype-3 develop metabolic defects and obesity. Nature 1997; 390(6656):165–169.

284. Green PH, Glickman RM, Riley JW, Quinet E. Human apolipoprotein A-IV. Intestinal origin and distribution in plasma. J Clin Invest 1980; 65(4):911–919.

285. Liu M, Doi T, Shen L, Woods SC, Seeley RJ, Zheng S et al. Intestinal satiety protein apolipoprotein AIV is synthesized and regulated in rat hypothalamus. Am J Physiol Regul Integr Comp Physiol 2001; 280(5):R1382–R1387.

286. Tso P, Liu M, Kalogeris TJ, Thomson AB. The role of apolipoprotein A-IV in the regulation of food intake. Annu Rev Nutr 2001; 21:231–254.

287. Tso P, Liu M. Apolipoprotein A-IV, food intake, and obesity. Physiol Behav 2004; 83(4):631–643.

288. Tso P, Liu M. Ingested fat and satiety. Physiol Behav 2004; 81(2):275–287.

289. Fujimoto K, Machidori H, Iwakiri R, Yamamoto K, Fujisaki J, Sakata T et al. Effect of intravenous administration of apolipoprotein A-IV on patterns of feeding, drinking and ambulatory activity of rats. Brain Res 1993; 608(2):233–237.

290. Fujimoto K, Fukagawa K, Sakata T, Tso P. Suppression of food intake by apolipoprotein A-IV is mediated through the central nervous system in rats. J Clin Invest 1993; 91(4):1830–1833.

291. Erlanson-Albertsson C, York D. Enterostatin – a peptide regulating fat intake. Obes Res 1997; 5(4):360–372.

292. York DA, Lin L, Thomas SR, Braymer HD, Park M. Procolipase gene expression in the rat brain: source of endogenous enterostatin production in the brain. Brain Res 2006; 1087(1):52–59.

293. Okada S, York DA, Bray GA, Erlanson-Albertsson C. Enterostatin (Val-Pro-Asp-Pro-Arg), the activation peptide of procolipase, selectively reduces fat intake. Physiol Behav 1991; 49(6):1185–1189.

294. Ookuma K, Barton C, York DA, Bray GA. Effect of enterostatin and kappa-opioids on macronutrient selection and consumption. Peptides 1997; 18(6):785–791.

295. Lin L, Umahara M, York DA, Bray GA. Beta-casomorphins stimulate and enterostatin inhibits the intake of dietary fat in rats. Peptides 1998; 19(2):325–331.

296. Nogueiras R, Tschop M. Biomedicine. Separation of conjoined hormones yields appetite rivals. Science 2005; 310(5750):985–986.

297. Zhang JV, Ren PG, Avsian-Kretchmer O, Luo CW, Rauch R, Klein C et al. Obestatin, a peptide encoded by the ghrelin gene, opposes ghrelin's effects on food intake. Science 2005; 310(5750):996–999.

298. Nogueiras R, Pfluger P, Tovar S, Arnold M, Mitchell S, Morris A et al. Effects of obestatin on energy balance and growth hormone secretion in rodents. Endocrinology 2007; 148(1):21–26.

299. Holst B, Egerod KL, Schild E, Vickers SP, Cheetham S, Gerlach LO et al. GPR39 signaling is stimulated by zinc ions but not by obestatin. Endocrinology 2007; 148(1):13–20.

300. Gale SM, Castracane VD, Mantzoros CS. Energy homeostasis, obesity and eating disorders: recent advances in endocrinology. J Nutr 2004; 134(2):295–298.

301. Collins S, Kuhn CM, Petro AE, Swick AG, Chrunyk BA, Surwit RS. Role of leptin in fat regulation. Nature 1996; 380(6576):677.

302. Haynes WG, Morgan DA, Walsh SA, Mark AL, Sivitz WI. Receptor-mediated regional sympathetic nerve activation by leptin. J Clin Invest 1997; 100(2):270–278.

303. Hucking K, Hamilton-Wessler M, Ellmerer M, Bergman RN. Burst-like control of lipolysis by the sympathetic nervous system in vivo. J Clin Invest 2003; 111(2):257–264.

304. Halaas JL, Boozer C, Blair-West J, Fidahusein N, Denton DA, Friedman JM. Physiological response to long-term peripheral and central leptin infusion in lean and obese mice. Proc Natl Acad Sci USA 1997; 94(16):8878–8883.

305. Chan JL, Mietus JE, Raciti PM, Goldberger AL, Mantzoros CS. Short-term fasting-induced autonomic activation and changes in catecholamine levels are not mediated by changes in leptin levels in healthy humans. Clin Endocrinol (Oxf) 2007; 66(1):49–57.

306. Kamohara S, Burcelin R, Halaas JL, Friedman JM, Charron MJ. Acute stimulation of glucose metabolism in mice by leptin treatment. Nature 1997; 389(6649):374–377.

307. Haque MS, Minokoshi Y, Hamai M, Iwai M, Horiuchi M, Shimazu T. Role of the sympathetic nervous system and insulin in enhancing glucose uptake in peripheral tissues after intrahypothalamic injection of leptin in rats. Diabetes 1999; 48(9):1706–1712.

308. Minokoshi Y, Haque MS, Shimazu T. Microinjection of leptin into the ventromedial hypothalamus increases glucose uptake in peripheral tissues in rats. Diabetes 1999; 48(2):287–291.

309. Bates SH, Dundon TA, Seifert M, Carlson M, Maratos-Flier E, Myers MG, Jr. LRb-STAT3 signaling is required for the neuroendocrine regulation of energy expenditure by leptin. Diabetes 2004; 53(12):3067–3073.

310. Lee JH, Chan JL, Sourlas E, Raptopoulos V, Mantzoros CS. r-metHuLeptin therapy in replacement doses improves insulin resistance and metabolic profile in patients with lipoatrophy and metabolic syndrome induced by the highly active antiretroviral therapy (HAART). J Clin Endocrinol Metab 2006; 91(7):2605–2611.

311. Oral EA, Simha V, Ruiz E, Andewelt A, Premkumar A, Snell P et al. Leptin-replacement therapy for lipodystrophy. N Engl J Med 2002; 346(8):570–578.

312. Papathanassoglou E, El Haschimi K, Li XC, Matarese G, Strom T, Mantzoros C. Leptin receptor expression and signaling in lymphocytes: kinetics during lymphocyte activation, role in lymphocyte survival, and response to high fat diet in mice. J Immunol 2006; 176(12):7745–7752.

313. Chan JL, Moschos SJ, Bullen J, Heist K, Li X, Kim YB et al. Recombinant methionyl human leptin administration activates signal transducer and activator of transcription 3 signaling in peripheral blood mononuclear cells in vivo and regulates soluble tumor necrosis factor-{alpha} receptor levels in humans with relative leptin deficiency. J Clin Endocrinol Metab 2005; 90(3):1625–1631.

314. Matarese G, Moschos S, Mantzoros CS. Leptin in immunology. J Immunol 2005; 174(6):3137–3142.

315. Strobel A, Issad T, Camoin L, Ozata M, Strosberg AD. A leptin missense mutation associated with hypogonadism and morbid obesity. Nat Genet 1998; 18(3):213–215.

316. Farooqi IS, Jebb SA, Langmack G, Lawrence E, Cheetham CH, Prentice AM et al. Effects of recombinant leptin therapy in a child with congenital leptin deficiency. N Engl J Med 1999; 341(12):879–884.

317. Ozata M, Ozdemir IC, Licinio J. Human leptin deficiency caused by a missense mutation: multiple endocrine defects, decreased sympathetic tone, and immune system dysfunction indicate new targets for leptin action, greater central than peripheral resistance to the effects of leptin, and spontaneous correction of leptin-mediated defects. J Clin Endocrinol Metab 1999; 84(10):3686–3695.

318. Mantzoros CS. The role of leptin in human obesity and disease: a review of current evidence. Ann Intern Med 1999; 130(8):671–680.

319. Munzberg H, Myers MG, Jr. Molecular and anatomical determinants of central leptin resistance. Nat Neurosci 2005; 8(5):566–570.

320. Bjorbaek C, Elmquist JK, Frantz JD, Shoelson SE, Flier JS. Identification of SOCS-3 as a potential mediator of central leptin resistance. Mol Cell 1998; 1(4):619–625.

321. El Haschimi K, Lehnert H. Leptin resistance – or why leptin fails to work in obesity. Exp Clin Endocrinol Diabetes 2003; 111(1):2–7.

322. Farooqi IS, Keogh JM, Kamath S, Jones S, Gibson WT, Trussell R et al. Partial leptin deficiency and human adiposity. Nature 2001; 414(6859):34–35.
323. Chan JL, Bluher S, Yiannakouris N, Suchard MA, Kratzsch J, Mantzoros CS. Regulation of circulating soluble leptin receptor levels by gender, adiposity, sex steroids, and leptin: observational and interventional studies in humans. Diabetes 2002; 51(7):2105–2112.
324. Boden G, Chen X, Mozzoli M, Ryan I. Effect of fasting on serum leptin in normal human subjects. J Clin Endocrinol Metab 1996; 81(9):3419–3423.
325. Jimerson DC, Mantzoros C, Wolfe BE, Metzger ED. Decreased serum leptin in bulimia nervosa. J Clin Endocrinol Metab 2000; 85(12):4511–4514.
326. Audi L, Mantzoros CS, Vidal-Puig A, Vargas D, Gussinye M, Carrascosa A. Leptin in relation to resumption of menses in women with anorexia nervosa. Mol Psychiatry 1998; 3(6):544–547.

4   Central Integration of Environmental and Endogenous Signals Important in the Regulation of Food Intake and Energy Expenditure

Iosif Kelesidis, Theodore Kelesidis, and Christos S. Mantzoros

KEY POINTS

- The worsening global epidemic of obesity has necessitated intensification of research into the mechanisms of appetite regulation.
- Obesity can be viewed as the result of a classic gene–environment interaction where the human genotype is susceptible to environmental influences that affect energy intake and energy expenditure. The obesity epidemic can also be viewed as a problem of energy balance.
- Food intake and energy expenditure are processes dependent on information relayed to a central network of sensing and processing neurons through hard-wired neural, metabolic, and hormonal signals from the periphery.
- Complex pathways that modulate energy balance involve mainly hormonal signals released by the gut and other organs in the periphery that convey information on energy status, as well as appetite centers in the hypothalamus and brain stem.
- Our understanding of the neuronal pathways that initiate changes in ingestive behavior or energy expenditure as well as our knowledge of the detailed signaling modalities underlying central body weight regulation still remain largely unknown.
- Careful clarification of how behavioral and environmental factors interact to produce energy balance (and in states of energy excess how the system fails to achieve energy balance, with the end result being weight gain) is required in order to understand the etiology of obesity.
- Modification of a combination of these factors may be able to reverse the epidemic of obesity and help the population achieve energy balance and a healthy body weight.
- The purpose of this chapter is to summarize our current understanding of the central pathways regulating energy homeostasis. These neuronal pathways in the central nervous system receive and integrate signals from the periphery that convey information about the status of energy fluxes and stores. Understanding these mechanisms will provide insights for the development of new treatment options for obesity.

From: *Nutrition and Health: Nutrition and Metabolism*
Edited by: C.S. Mantzoros, DOI: 10.1007/978-1-60327-453-1_4,
© Humana Press, a part of Springer Science+Business Media, LLC 2009

Key Words: Obesity, Energy homeostasis, Energy expenditure, Signals

1. CENTRAL REGULATION OF ENERGY HOMEOSTASIS

Discovery of the fat hormone leptin as part of an "adipostatic" endocrine system of body weight regulation has elucidated our understanding of body weight homeostasis *(1)* and has increased our knowledge of how peripheral endocrine organs and the central nervous system (CNS) interact in the control of energy homeostasis. Peripherally generated signals are integrated in the brain in a complex manner, resulting in activation of both anorexigenic and orexigenic pathways to regulate energy balance. The molecular elucidation of this complex system has improved our understanding of energy homeostasis.

Peripheral signals such as nutrients (mainly lipids and carbohydrates) participate in the regulation of energy homeostasis by activation of intracellular second messenger pathways through surface enzymes *(2)* and ion channels *(3,4)* expressed in hypothalamic neurons. In addition, the short-term regulation of feeding is accomplished by conduction of information from chemoreceptors (mainly CCK) or stretch receptors to brainstem through neural afferent signals from the periphery, conveyed mainly via the vagus nerve, which innervates densely the gastrointestinal tract (Fig. 1). All these peripheral signals are integrated in the CNS through complex neural structures, which are described below.

1.1. Structures in the CNS Mediating Energy Homeostasis

The hypothalamus plays a central role in the integration of peripheral signals in the current energy homeostasis model *(2)*. Within the hypothalamus, the arcuate nucleus (ARC) is a major site of peripheral signal integration, as it is considered to be the key sensor of peripheral energy input (reviewed in *(3)*).

Peripheral signals act mainly on two distinct neuronal populations. One population co-expresses the orexigenic neuropeptides agouti-related peptide (AgRP) and neuropeptide Y (NPY); the other population releases cocaine- and amphetamine-regulated transcript and pro-opiomelanocortin, both of which inhibit feeding (Fig. 1). Both of these populations project to the paraventricular nucleus (PVN) and other nuclei involved in energy regulation *(4,5)*.

In states of positive energy balance, neurochemical signaling inhibits orexigenic centers and activates anorexigenic centers, while during negative energy states the opposite occurs. Energy-modulating neuropeptides as well as receptors for peripheral hormones, including leptin and insulin, as well as several sensors of nutrient intake and expenditure have been identified in brain stem neurons *(3)*. Therefore, the brain stem appears to also play an important role in the integration of signals of energy availability *(6)*. Obviously, the energy homeostasis circuit is controlled at several levels and not only in the CNS.

1.2. Hypothalamic Structure and Neuronal Pathways Regulating Appetite

Most individuals maintain stable body weight over long periods of time despite wide daily variations of food intake and energy expenditure (EE). For this to happen, food intake and EE must be constantly adjusted and precisely balanced over time. Currently, the emphasis in the regulation of body weight and endocrine function is placed on neuronal circuits, composed of specific neuropeptides, rather than specific hypothalamic nuclei that have been thought to play a major role in the past (see Fig. 1).

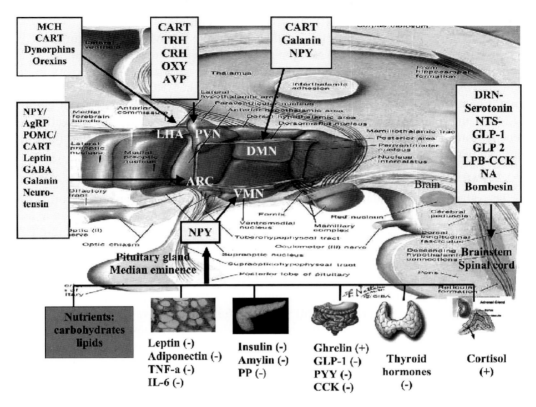

Fig. 1. Integration of peripheral signals in the hypothalamus and the central nervous system. The interaction between the various components of this complex system is noted, as are the neuropeptides that are expressed in each part of this complex circuit. *ARC* arcuate nucleus, *AVP* vasopressin, *AgRP* agouti related protein, *CART* cocaine- and amphetamine-regulated transcript, *CCK* cholecystokinin, *CRH* corticotropin releasing hormone, *DMN* dorsomedial nucleus, *DRN* dorsal reticular nucleus, *GABA* γ-aminobutyric acid, *GLP-1/2* glucagon-like peptide 1/2, *IL-6* interleukin-6, *LHA* lateral hypothalamus, *LPB* lateral parabrachial nucleus, *NA* noradrenalin, *NTS* nucleus of the solitary tract, *OXY* oxytocin, *PVN* paraventricular nucleus, *PP* pancreatic polypeptide, *POMC* pro-opiomelanocortin, *TNF-α* tumor necrosis factor alpha, *TRH* thyrotropin-releasing hormone, *VMN* ventromedial nucleus. + indicates orexigenic effect; −, anorexigenic effect; ?, unknown effect.

1.2.1. THE ARCUATE NUCLEUS

The arcuate nucleus (ARC), one of the hypothalamic nuclei, is thought to play a pivotal role in the integration of signals regulating appetite. This is because the immediate surroundings of the ARC are not being shielded by the blood–brain barrier and this allows unrestricted access to afferent inputs *(8)*.

Neuropeptide Y and pro-opiomelanocortin neurons in the hypothalamic ARC are prototypic metabolic sensors. Both use glucose as a signaling molecule, and both have receptors for peripheral hormones, including insulin and leptin *(8)*. The pro-opiomelanocortin neurons produce α-melanocyte-stimulating hormone whose release and binding to melanocortin-3 and -4 receptors in the PVN and lateral hypothalamus reduces food intake and increases EE mainly through projections from these nuclei to autonomic and neuroendocrine effector systems *(9)*. Firing of NPY neurons releases both NPY and AgRP; NPY *(10)* is an anabolic peptide that strongly stimulates ingestive behaviors and minimizes EE, whereas AgRP acts as a functional antagonist of catabolic melanocortin receptors. Under homeostatic conditions, leptin and insulin levels reflect the amount of adiposity in the body*(7,11)*. In addition to input from insulin and leptin, the ARC also senses changes in energy balance conveyed by the gastric/gastrointestinal-system-secreted hormone ghrelin *(12)* and the intestinal hormone peptide YY 3–36 (PYY 3–36) *(13)*. By activating its receptor on NPY/AgRP neurons, ghrelin stimulates food intake; currently ghrelin is the only known circulating hormone to exert an orexigenic effect *(14)*.

1.2.2. PARAVENTRICULAR NUCLEUS

The other main hypothalamic areas identified as effectors of peripheral information are the paraventricular nucleus (PVN), the lateral hypothalamus perifornical area, and the ventromedial and dorsomedial nuclei *(15,16)*. These structures are divided into two categories. The lateral area constitutes the orexigenic limb, whereas the ventromedial, dorsomedial, and paraventricular nuclei constitute the anorexigenic part of the hypothalamus. The PVN, located adjacent to the third ventricle, acts to integrate neuropeptide signals from numerous CNS regions, including the ARC and brain stem *(17)*. The PVN plays a major role in integration of all signaling functions that regulate energy homeostasis *(18,19)*. This brain area seems to house neurons that mainly promote negative energy balance and play an important role in energy homeostasis, at least in part, by conveying input from the ARC to other key brain areas *(20)*. Certainly more research is needed to fully elucidate the role PVN plays in energy homeostasis.

1.2.3. DORSOMEDIAL NUCLEUS/HYPOTHALAMUS

The dorsomedial nucleus (DMN) plays a significant role in the modulation of energy intake. Destruction of the DMN results in hyperphagia and obesity, although less dramatic than in response to VMN lesioning. Injection of orexigenic peptides, NPY, galanin, and GABA, into the DMN increases food intake *(21)*, Similar to all other nuclei important in energy regulation, the DMN has extensive connections with other hypothalamic nuclei. It receives projections from AgRP/NPY neurons from the ARC but also contains NPY-expressing cell bodies. Administration of melanocortin agonists in the DMN has been shown to reduce both local NPY expression and suckling-induced hyperphagia in rats most likely because of proximal localization of α-MSH immunoreactive fibers to these NPY-expressing cells *(22)*.

1.2.4. LATERAL HYPOTHALAMIC AREA AND PERIFORNICAL AREA

The lateral hypothalamic area and perifornical area (LHA/PFA) are other hypothalamic areas involved in energy homeostasis. The PFA seems to be one of the most sensitive areas for NPY-induced feeding, apparently more so than the PVN *(15)*. The LHA/PFA contains melanin-concentrating hormone (MCH) expressing neurons *(16)*, and among the key LHA neurons involved in body weight regulation are those that express either orexin *(23)* or MCH *(24)*. Data from animal studies support an important role for MCH because targeted deletion of MCH *(25)* or its receptor *(26)* causes a weight-reduced, lean, hypermetabolic phenotype whereas central administration *(24)* and/or transgenic overexpression of this peptide increases food intake *(22,24)*. The LHA/PFA also contains neurons expressing prepro-orexin and releasing the peptide products orexin

A and B (also called hypocretins 1 and 2) *(3,23)*. Orexin neurons project widely through the CNS to several areas, including the PVN, ARC, nucleus tractus solitarius (NTS), and dorsal motor nucleus of the vagus *(27)*, i.e., to areas associated with arousal and attention as well as feeding. The mechanisms by which the MCH and orexin neurons in the LHA integrate CNS and peripheral signals to influence energy homeostasis remain to be fully clarified *(3)*. However, major targets are currently considered the endocrine and autonomic nervous system, the cranial nerve motor nuclei, and cortical structures. Finally, neurons in the LHA (mainly orexin-containing) may play an important role in narcolepsy *(28)* and arguably an important role, by extension, in sleep regulation.

1.2.5. Ventromedial Hypothalamus

The ventromedial hypothalamus (VMH) has been known for many years to play a role in energy homeostasis. The VMH receives NPY, AgRP, and α-MSH immunoreactive projections from neurons in the ARC, and in turn, VMH neurons project onto both hypothalamic nuclei (e.g., dorsomedial hypothalamus) and brain stem regions (e.g., NTS). Brain-derived neurotrophic factor (BDNF), a neurotrophic factor that has recently been linked to weight loss *(29)*, is highly expressed in the VMH, and its expression is regulated both by food deprivation and melanocortin agonists *(29)*. Mice with reduced BDNF receptor expression or reduced BDNF signaling have increased food intake and body weight *(29)*. Therefore, BDNF neurons in the VMH may act as an additional downstream pathway through which nutritional status and the melanocortin system modulate energy homeostasis. Finally, data from recent studies *(30)* strongly support the view that BDNF plays a role as an anorexigenic factor in the dorsal vagal complex.

1.2.6. Brainstem/Nucleus Tractus Solitarius

The brain stem seems to play an important role in signal integration of energy availability *(3)*. Caudal brainstem includes several sensors of nutrient intake and expenditure, as well as receptors of peripheral hormones, including leptin and insulin *(3)*. Extensive reciprocal connections exist between the hypothalamus and brain stem, particularly the NTS. The NTS is in close anatomical proximity to the area postrema, a circumventricular organ with an incomplete blood–brain barrier *(3)*. Like the ARC, the NTS is therefore in an ideal position to respond to peripheral circulating signals, but in addition, it also receives vagal afferents from the gastrointestinal tract and afferents from the glossopharyngeal nerves *(31)*. In addition to glucagon-like peptide 1 (GLP-1) (see below), NPY neurons from the brain stem project forward to the PVN, and extracellular NPY levels within the NTS are modulated by feeding *(32)*. Other important structures found in the NTS include NPY-binding sites (Y1 and Y5 receptors), melanocortin system *(33)*, and MC4R *(3)*.

1.3. Synaptic Plasticity in Energy Balance Regulation

Recently, the scientific community realized that the system involving hypothalamic neuropeptide systems is far from being static. There is a rapid synaptic remodeling *(34)*, and according to recent studies *(34)*, changing metabolic states can cause alterations in neuronal interactions by changes of the wiring of synapses and hypothalamic metabolic circuits. In these studies, fasting resulted in a balance of stimulatory and inhibitory synapses on orexin and NPY neurons that favored increasing activity of these neurons. On the other hand, inhibitory interneurons of the same regions (neurons that would inhibit either orexin or NPY neuronal activity) exhibited a synaptic balance during fasting that would support neuronal inactivation, thereby further enhancing the activity level of orexin and NPY perikarya. These observations raise the notion that metabolic signals, leptin in particular, may have an acute effect on synaptic plasticity within the appetite centers. Recent data suggest that leptin-mediated plasticity in the ob/ob hypothalamus may underlie some of the hormone's behavioral effects (34). Similarly, the effects of an orexigenic hormone, ghrelin, and anorexigenic hormone, estradiol, have also been studied. It appears that synaptic plasticity is not leptin-specific since rearrangement of synapses has also been observed in response to ghrelin and estradiol in a leptin-independent manner (34). These observations raised the intriguing possibility that altered synaptic plasticity could be an important way through which peripheral metabolic hormones may influence brain functions in the long term.

1.4. Central Neuropeptides Regulating Energy Balance

The CNS structures responsible for regulating energy homeostasis mediate their effects through the release of specific neuropeptides which, although grouped into orexigenic and anorexigenic subcategories, act in a coordinated manner, either synergistically or antagonistically (summarized in Table 1). Several orexigenic neuropeptides have been identified, which are expressed centrally and integrate peripheral signals to reduce EE and/or increase energy intake, the most important being NPY, agouti-related protein (AgRP), MCH, orexin, and galanin (GAL). On the other hand, signals of a positive energy balance are integrated centrally via anorexigenc neuropeptides, including α-melanocyte-stimulating hormone (α-MSH), cocaine- and amphetamine-regulated transcript, galanin-like peptide, the corticotrophin-releasing hormone family of peptides, serotonin, and dopamine. The above peptides are presented briefly in Table 1.

1.5. Other Systems

1.5.1. GLUCAGON-LIKE PEPTIDE 1

The NTS contains NPY, melanocortin, and GLP-1 neuronal circuits. GLP-1 forms the major brain stem circuit known to regulate energy homeostasis. In the CNS, GLP-1 is synthesized exclusively in the caudal NTS, and these preproglucagon neurons also express leptin receptors. GLP1 immunoreactive fibers then project widely, but particularly to the PVN and DMN, with fewer projections to the ARC. GLP-1 receptor expression is also widespread, both within the hypothalamus (PVN, dorsomedial hypothalamus, and supraoptic nucleus) and in the brain stem. Central administration of GLP-1, either into the third or fourth ventricle, potently reduces fasting and NPY-induced food intake (35). These data have suggested a role of not only circulating but also endogenous hypothalamic GLP-1 in energy homeostasis.

1.5.2. OPIOIDS

The opioid system appears to play a significant role in energy homeostasis. Release of opioids, such as endorphins, during food intake could enhance the pleasure of eating. Opioids released in response to ingestion of sweet and other palatable foods can increase central opioidergic activity and exogenously administered opioids generally increase food intake (36). Microinjection of opioid agonists into the nucleus accumbens, an important part of the reward circuit, stimulates the preferential consumption of highly

Table 1

Centrally expressed neuropeptides important in energy homeostasis

Peptide	Receptors	Expression Area	Factors that upregulate expression	Factors that downregulate expression	Function
Orexigenic neuropeptides					
Neuropeptide Y (NPY) (138) (139, 140)	Six known NPY receptors (main are NPY1 and NPY5 receptors) (141)	Expressed throughout the CNS, but especially in hypothalamic nuclei and the locus ceruleus of the brainstem Co-localized with agouti related protein (AgRP) in the arcuate nucleus	A state of negative energy balance (142) Ghrelin, increases the expression of NPY and AgRP in the arcuate nucleus (14) Corticosterone (CORT) (143–146) Hypoglycemia (147–149)	Positive energy balance, associated with increased leptin and insulin levels (152) PYY inhibits NPY expression in the arcuate nucleus via the Y2-receptor (13)	NPY is the most potent orexigen known, and repeated third ventricle or PVN injection of NPY causes marked hyperphagia and obesity Central administration of NPY increases food intake, decreases energy expenditure, decreases sympathetic outflow to brown adipose tissue, and increases lipogenesis (139, 153) NPY stimulates basal plasma insulin and morning plasma cortisol (54), effects which are independent of increased food intake
Agouti-related protein (AgRP)	Mediates its effects mainly by blocking α-MSH from binding to MC4R and MC3R in the brain (139)	Co-expressed with NPY in the arcuate nucleus (139,154,155)	Increased Ghrelin and CORT levels (10, 156, 157) Declining carbohydrate stores and hypoglycaemia AgRP and NPY potentiate each other's effect on feeding behavior (158)	Rising leptin and insulin levels (10, 156, 157)	Central administration of AgRP in rodents increases feeding and body weight (159,160) AgRP also affects energy expenditure and thermogenesis via the TRH system, such that exogenous AgRP in rats results in a decreased TSH and total T4 simulating the hypothyroid state present during fasting (161) Activation of ARC NPY/AgRP neurons potently stimulates feeding via a number of pathways: the orexigenic effect of NPY released in the PVN, AgRP

(continued)

Table 1
(continued)

Peptide	Receptors	Expression Area	Factors that upregulate expression	Factors that downregulate expression	Function
					antagonism of MC3R/MC4R in the PVN, and local release of NPY and GABA within the ARC to inhibit the arcuate POMC neurons via Y1 and GABA receptors, respectively
Melanin-concentrating hormone (MCH)	Melanin Concentrating Hormone Receptor 1 (MCH1-R) and 2 (MCH2-R) (139,162)	Lateral hypothalamus (LHA) and the zona incerta	Fasting Insulin(163) Declining fatty acid levels(164,165) Ghrelin and glucose do not influence its expression to a significant extent (166)	Rising leptin levels	Central administration of MCH causes hyperphagia (24) MCH knockout mice have reduced weight and are lean due to hypophagia (139), and possibly increased energy expenditure (162) Mice with targeted disruption of MCH1-R display excessive feeding, hyperactivity, increased metabolic rate, and resistance to diet induced obesity (25). This resistance to weight gain in the setting of hyperphagia suggests that MCH may promote a positive energy balance mainly by decreasing activity and energy expenditure, rather than by increasing nutrient intake
Orexins (also known as hypocretins) Orexin A Orexin B	Orexin A has high affinity for the orexin-1 receptor, which is highly	Lateral hypothalamus and perifornical area orexin neurons project widely through the CNS	Similar to NPY and AgRP, they are stimulated by a negative energy balance and by rising levels of		Central orexin neurons express both neuropeptide (mainly NPY) receptors and leptin receptors and hence may be able to integrate actions of both CNS and peripheral signals Major targets of these

	expressed in the VMH. Orexins A and B have equal affinities for the orexin-2 receptor, which is expressed primarily within the PVN	to areas including the PVN, ARC, NTS, and dorsal motor nucleus of the vagus and to areas associated with arousal and attention as well as feeding	glucocorticoids and Ghrelin (23,158, 167–171)
			Hypoglycaemia and insulin also exert a stimulatory effect on the expression of orexin mRNA (172,173)
			Leptin does not significantly regulate orexin levels, with obesity and hyperphagia (hyperleptinemic states) actually being associated with increased levels of these neuropeptides (167, 174–177)
			neuropeptides are currently considered the endocrine and autonomic nervous system, the cranial nerve motor nuclei, and cortical structures
			The considerable rise in orexin mRNA observed in response to declining blood sugar and the subsequent stimulating effects of orexins on locomotor activity and searching behavior suggests a role in hypothalamic arousal (167, 172, 178–180)
Galanin (GAL)	GALR1, GALR2 (181–184)	Hypothalamus, primarily in the PVN and ARC nuclei, as well as the LHA and periformical area (181)	High-fat diets (185–187)
			Declining glucose levels fail to elicit changes in GAL mRNA expression (188)
			Exogenous administration of GAL stimulates feeding behavior, decreases energy expenditure and decreases sympathetic nervous system activity (189)
			GAL has a role in regulating carbohydrate metabolism in the setting of a high-fat diet (190)

(continued)

Table 1
(continued)

Peptide	Receptors	Expression Area	Factors that upregulate expression	Factors that downregulate expression	Function
Anorexigenic peptides Melanocortins are cleaved from propiomelanocortin (POMC): α-melanocyte stimulating hormone (α-MSH) γ-MSH (191)	G-protein-coupled receptors (MCR) are expressed throughout the body	MC3R, expressed in many areas of the CNS and in several peripheral sites, and MC4R, expressed mostly in the CNS (192), are the receptors most relevant to energy regulation. Five melanocortin receptors have been identified, MC1R-MC5R, however, MC3R and MC4R are most likely to play a role in energy homeostasis.	Peripheral signals of energy abundance, such as insulin and leptin (11, 193) In contrast to the orexigenic peptides, dietary nutrients exert no regulatory control over POMC expression (194–196)		Decrease of energy intake and increase of energy expenditure (197) MC4R knockout mice are obese MC4R antagonists administered centrally decrease food intake dramatically (191) MC3R knockout mice have reduced lean body mass and increased fat mass, despite hypophagia and normal metabolic rates (198) Central administration of MC4R agonists suppresses food intake, while administration of antagonists results in hyperphagia Furthermore, several MC4R mutations have been identified in obese humans (199, 200), accounting for approximately 5% of morbid obesity in children (46, 201), (201) Melanocortin agonists reduce both food intake and body weight in several mouse models of obesity (197, 202), and their role in humans is being evaluated in ongoing trials

Cocaine and amphetamine regulated transcript (CART)	No specific receptor has been identified to date	Arcuate nucleus, lateral hypothalamus and paraventricular nuclei (203)	Elevated levels of leptin, insulin and glucocorticoids (204) High-fat diets also exert a stimulatory effect on CART mRNA expression	Food deprivation	Direct intracerebroventricular CART administration decreases nocturnal, as well as fasting induced food intake in rodents (139) Neurons synthesizing CART are indirectly responsible for the effects of leptin through sympathetic nervous system activation (205) CART may also act as a modulator of the rebound thermogenic effect taking place in states of hypothermia (206, 207)
Galanin-like peptide (GALP)	GALR2 (208)	Arcuate nucleus	GALP mRNA levels increase in response to leptin and food restriction (209) Glucose administration has been shown to increase GALP entry into the brain (210)		Central injection of this hormone results in decreased feeding and body weight (211) Additionally, a thermogenic response has been observed following acute administration of GALP (212)
Corticotropin Releasing Hormone (CRH) family of peptides: Corticotropin Releasing Factor (CRF) Endogenous CRF receptor ligands, the urocortins (213)	CRF receptor	PVN (CRF)	CRF mRNA expression is tightly controlled by CORT levels (214, 215)		The CRH family of peptides: they promote negative energy balance, they continue to maintain tight glycemic control through the effects of adrenal steroids. (216–221) CRF regulates ACTH release from the anterior pituitary and subsequent release of CORT from the adrenal glands (220, 222)

(continued)

Table 1
(continued)

Peptide	Receptors	Expression Area	Factors that upregulate expression	Factors that downregulate expression	Function
					Interventional studies have demonstrated that central administration of CRF results in hypophagia, increased energy expenditure, increased blood glucose, and decreased insulin secretion
Serotonin (5-HT)					Important anorexigenic role by mediating leptin's weight reducing effect (223) and by stimulating POMC neurons to release α-MSH (224) 5-HT2C receptor knockout mice have decreased oxygen consumption, increased food intake and increased body weight (223). Several anti-obesity drugs act by increasing 5-HT receptor signaling Increasing the availability of 5-HT by affecting its release and reuptake in the synaptic cleft, or the direct activation of the 5-HT receptors, reduces food consumption, whereas decreasing 5-HT receptor activation produces the opposite effect Arena Pharmaceuticals is currently developing APD356, a new selective 5-HT2C receptor agonist for obesity. Also in development is Wyeth's 5-HT2C agonist WAY–16390915

Catecholamines	Central α_1 or β_2 adrenergic (β–ARs) receptors	Activation of 1 and, 2-adrenergic receptors inhibits food intake
		Beta-adrenergic receptors are considered the most important receptors in the adrenergic family for regulation of energy expenditure in response to dietary excess. Ablation of all three β-Rs in mice results in obesity, which is largely due to lower energy expenditure, and this effect is enhanced when mice are challenged with caloric excess (48). Thus, these mice are mildly obese on a regular diet but become massively obese on a high fat diet. These data are further supported by the fact that mutations of β-Rs are clearly associated with human obesity
Dopamine (DA)	Dopamine receptor isoforms (D_1–D_5)	Tyrosine hydroxylase gene replacement, and hence dopamine replacement, into the caudate putamen restores feeding, while gene therapy into either the caudate putamen or nucleus accumbens (NAc) restores preference for a palatable diet	Plays a central role in energy intake, as seen in the abnormal feeding associated with pharmacological depletion and / or genetic disruption of dopamine synthesis (223)
			Striatal extracellular DA increases with food intake in normal weight subjects (225), but in obese subjects there is reduced brain DA activity, which may predispose them to excessive food intake (225). Further studies are needed to define the specific dopamine receptor isoforms (D_1–D_5) that will have the most significant weight reducing effects, while avoiding behavioral side effects or addiction

palatable sucrose and fat *(37)*. Conversely, opioid antagonists administered into the nucleus accumbens reduce preferentially sucrose ingestion in comparison to other less palatable substances *(37)*. Several studies indicate that there are interactions of opioids with other appetite-regulating processes *(38)*.

1.5.3. THE CANNABINOID SYSTEM

Among the several novel antiobesity strategies currently under development, it was hoped that pharmacological antagonism of the anabolic cannabinoid-1 receptor could potentially be the first to come into clinical use. The cloning of the G-protein-coupled cannabinoid-1 receptor (CB1R) provided valuable information about the mechanisms of action of the principal active constituent of cannabis, δ9-tetrahydrocannabinol *(39)*. The lipids anandamide and 2-arachidonoyl glycerol, which are known as endocannabinoids, are natural ligands for CB1R. CB1R mediates the anabolic effects of exogenous and endogenous cannabinoids *(40)*. Anabolic and prodiabetic actions of endocannabinoids include the following: (1) in the hypothalamus, increase of orexigenic and decrease of anorexigenic neuropeptides; (2) in mesolimbic reward centers, enhancement of food palatability and reward reinforcement; (3) in the hindbrain, blunting of nausea and GI satiation signals transmitted from the vagus nerve; (4) in the GI tract, inhibition of satiation signals and potentiation of hunger signals transmitted to vagal sensory nerve terminals, as well as facilitation of nutrient absorption; (5) in adipose tissue and liver, stimulation of lipogenesis; and (6) in muscle, impairment of glucose uptake *(40)*.

Given the major anabolic actions of CB1R, it is not surprising that pharmacological antagonism of this receptor promotes weight loss. A specific CB1R antagonist, rimonabant, was created only a few years after the receptor was discovered and was followed by the discovery of other antagonists such as taranabant. Through its actions in the hypothalamus, hindbrain, mesolimbic reward centers, and vagus nerve, rimonabant enhances anorexia, potentiates satiation signals, and lessens the motivation to consume palatable, rewarding foods. Together, these effects reduce food intake and body weight. Beneficial effects of rimonabant on body weight, adiposity, and other features of the metabolic syndrome have been confirmed in phase III human trials lasting up to 2 years *(41–43)* which led many European nations to approve this agent as a new drug for obesity. The approval in the USA has been delayed, however, owing to concerns about a potential for psychiatric side effects. It remains to be seen whether rimonabant or taranabant or both will eventually be approved for obesity and the metabolic syndrome.

2. ENERGY EXPENDITURE IN ENERGY HOMEOSTASIS

According to the first law of thermodynamics, the total energy of a system plus the surroundings remains constant. Obesity can result, therefore, from a relative increase in energy intake (food) compared to EE. The regulation of EE and its role in body weight homeostasis has not been very well studied to date. Potent physiologic mechanisms maintain body weight within a narrow "set point" and regulate energy balance with accuracy in most humans *(44)*, as demonstrated by under- and overfeeding studies *(45)*. Certain thermogenic mechanisms, such as leptin-induced increases in EE *(46,47)* and diet-induced thermogenesis, a critically important antiobesity mechanism as per studies in rodents *(48,49)*, have evolved in mammals to allow burning up of excess energy *(50,51)*. Human studies suggest that increased sympathetic nervous system (SNS) activity, decreased parasympathetic nervous system activity, and an inferred form of physical activity known as non-exercise activity thermogenesis (NEAT) lead to an increase in EE in overfeeding states and obesity *(52–55)*. However, many more studies are needed to determine the importance of thermogenic, antiobesity mechanisms in humans *(48)*.

2.1. Components of Energy Expenditure

EE can be categorized into obligatory (basal) and adaptive (facultative) thermogenesis. Obligatory EE includes all processes that are involved in the maintenance of basic metabolic and physiologic processes, including the maintenance of ion gradients, muscle tone, digestion, and blood flow (standard metabolic rate). Adaptive thermogenesis includes cold and diet-induced thermogenesis. For example, although thyroid hormone (TH) is required for up to 30% of standard metabolic rate, adaptive increases in TH are required for normal cold-induced thermogenesis *(56)*. Physical activity can also have long-lasting effects on resting metabolic rate *(57)*. Approximate contributions of the various EE components are resting metabolic rate (70%), physical activity (20%), facultative (10%), with physical activity representing the most variable component *(58)*.

2.2. The Role of Regulation of Energy Expenditure in the Development of Obesity

Mammals have potent homeostatic mechanisms, which maintain body weight by changing food intake and EE *(59)*. Only relative differences in EE might explain predisposition to obesity since obese patients have increased EE when compared to lean subjects *(56)*. Although there are data demonstrating that increased food intake causes obesity, there has been less evidence that decreased EE may specifically lead to obesity. Differences in EE have been proposed to be associated with the development of obesity over a period of years *(60)* while genetic factors may play a major role in controlling EE *(52,61)*. However, other reports do not support the hypothesis that abnormal regulation of EE leads to obesity *(58,62,63)*. For example, several studies have failed to find obesity-promoting mechanisms to explain differences between lean and obese subjects, including SNS nerve activity *(64)*, catecholamine turnover *(65)*, lipolysis *(66)*, the thermic effect of food, *(58)* and THs *(67)*. In summary, the hypothesis that relatively low EE contributes to the development of obesity has been supported by a few but not all studies. It remains unclear whether stimulation of EE in humans will eventually prove to be a useful approach for antiobesity therapy.

2.3. Regulation of Energy Expenditure

Regulation of EE depends on many factors, including physical activity, changes in energy intake/diet, THs, SNS, adrenergic receptors, futile cycles, and intermediary metabolism genes.

2.3.1. Physical Activity

Increasing physical activity represents an effective method to resist obesity in the setting of increased food intake; it has effects on EE both acutely, with large increases in maximal oxygen consumption, and chronically via increased mitochondrial proliferation

(68). In humans, a combination of decreased food intake and physical activity is most successful for sustained weight loss *(69)*. Overfeeding studies in lean humans showed that the majority of increased EE in response to caloric excess occurs via increased non-exercise activity thermogenesis (NEAT), a separate category of physical activity that is related to adiposity which includes all tasks of daily living *(70)*, and not via increases in thermic effect of food, or coordinated physical activity *(55)*. Further research into the regulation of physical activity as a specific mechanism to control body fat stores is still needed.

Although there are limited data available based on measurements of everyday, real life physical activity at the population level, it appears that energy intake has increased and physical activity has decreased more than enough to explain the increasing prevalence of obesity in the population *(71)*. A related controversial issue in the area is how much physical activity should be recommended for prevention of weight gain, for weight loss, and/or for prevention of weight regain after weight loss. In this respect, several studies have shown that very large increases in physical activity are necessary to avoid weight regain after weight loss *(72)* while very small increases may prevent weight gain *(59)*.

2.3.2. CHANGES IN ENERGY INTAKE/DIET

Diet composition

The role of diet composition on body weight is an area of controversy in the field of obesity research. Diet composition can affect body weight in individuals who are in energy balance. In a recent review, Astrup et al. *(73)* found that body weight is reduced slightly as dietary fat content of the diet is lowered in individuals who were in energy balance. Reducing dietary fat without food restriction may affect both energy intake and EE in small ways, since voluntary intake may be lower with low- vs. high-fat diets *(74,75)*. Increasing dietary carbohydrate and reducing dietary fat could also be expected to produce a slight increase in the thermic effect of food *(75)*, since carbohydrate produces more thermic effect than fat does, but this remains to be conclusively shown. The impact of high- vs. low-glycemic diets as well as of protein diets on energy balance is still the focus of intensive research efforts *(76,77)*.

Diet composition during negative energy balance

Diet composition may have different effects depending on whether subjects are in energy balance or whether they are in positive or negative energy balance. During equivalent negative energy balance, there might be little difference in altering the fat/carbohydrate ratio of the diet and there seems to be similar body weight and body fat loss with high- and low-fat diets when total energy intake is fixed at a level below energy requirements *(78)*. However, there are several reports of differences in weight loss with high- and low-fat diets when energy intake is not fixed *(79,80)*, suggesting that diet composition may affect satiety or hunger during dieting. A recent meta-analysis *(81)* concluded that nonenergy-restricted, low-carbohydrate diets were at least as effective as low-fat diets over a period of 1 year. Lowering dietary fat has little impact during negative energy balance. Therefore, in general, low-fat diets have not been found to lead to greater weight loss than diets higher in fat content.

Diet composition during positive energy balance

During positive energy balance, diet composition can have a relatively larger effect on energy balance. Studies have shown that excess energy is efficiently stored in the body regardless of its source, but it has been proposed that excess energy from dietary fat is stored more efficiently than excess energy from carbohydrates *(82)*. This area is of significant interest and the focus of intensive research efforts.

2.3.3. THYROID HORMONES

Thyroid hormones (TH; including T_4 and T_3) play a significant role in regulating EE. Thyroid hormones mediate ~30% of basal thermogenesis and stimulate numerous anabolic and catabolic pathways (reviewed in *(83)*). Low TH levels in response to dietary restriction are associated with reduced EE during weight loss and act to resist body weight change in obesity *(84)*. These changes in TH levels are also associated with changes in EE and SNS. All these alterations are to a certain degree due to falling leptin levels in response to weight loss *(84)*, but the extent to which falling leptin mediates the alterations in TH in response to food deprivation and whether leptin administration in replacement doses would improve weight loss maintenance remain to be seen.

2.3.4. SYMPATHETIC NERVOUS SYSTEM AND ADRENERGIC RECEPTORS

The SNS is another significant regulator of EE (reviewed in *(85)*). β-Adrenergic receptors (AR) are apparently the most important receptors in the adrenergic family for regulation of EE in response to dietary excess but other receptors are also important in EE regulation *(86)*. Several studies support the model of altered EE in response to caloric excess, and resistance to obesity. In most rodent models of obesity there is low SNS activity, which can be associated with propensity for future weight gain *(85,87)*, and activation of this pathway by β-AR agonists is effective in reducing obesity in mice *(88,89)*. Numerous attempts to alter SNS function (by surgical, chemical, immunological, and genetic means) failed to affect body weight, however, and thus the importance of SNS-mediated diet-induced thermogenesis lacks support *(90–92)*. On the other hand, ablation of all 3 β-ARs in mice (β-less mice) results in obesity that is entirely due to lower EE, and this deficit is enhanced when mice are challenged with caloric excess *(48)*. These results are supported by genetic studies in humans reporting mutations in β-ARs that are associated with human obesity *(86,93)*. In contrast, the development of β-AR agonists for the treatment of obesity has failed to result in any usable compounds in studies in humans.

2.3.5. FUTILE CYCLES

EE in mammals can be regulated by thermogenic futile cycles that can involve various metabolic pathways, including the glycolysis pathway *(94)*, as well as calcium *(95–97)*, sodium, and proton cycling in cells. Although lipogenic/lipolytic futile cycles are stimulated in white adipose tissue (WAT) in response to peroxisome proliferator-activated receptor (PPAR) agonists *(98)*, futile cycles have not yet been shown to play a significant role in mammalian body weight regulation, however.

2.3.6. INTERMEDIARY METABOLISM GENES THAT REGULATE EE AND BODY WEIGHT

There is increasing evidence that EE in mammals is controlled at numerous, rate-limiting, and, in some cases, leptin-mediated steps in glucose and fatty acid metabolism. In many rodent models loss of function of key synthetic enzymatic steps in fatty acid synthesis results in increased EE, reduced body weight, and obesity resistance *(99–102)*. In humans, polymorphisms in the rate-limiting enzyme for triglyceride synthesis are associated with lean kindreds *(103)*. AMP kinase, which is regulated by leptin, is an emerging, central mediator of these critical steps in fatty acid metabolism and affects appetite and EE *(104,105)*.

2.4. Thermogenic Tissues

Many tissues have the metabolic potential to mediate thermogenesis as a specific response to increased body weight and adipose stores.

2.4.1. BROWN ADIPOSE TISSUE

Brown adipose tissue (BAT) plays a critical role in thermogenesis and body weight regulation in rodents *(106)*, but may not represent an attractive target for antiobesity treatment because of its apparent absence in adult humans. BAT is a highly thermogenic form of adipose tissue *(107)*. Stimulation of β-ARs by catecholamines or synthetic β-AR agonists markedly stimulates EE, primarily in BAT *(50)*. β-AR agonists have not been proven to be effective as potential treatment options for human obesity, because of low abundance of the $β_3$-AR in human tissues, or lack of specificity for the human $β_3$-AR, or intolerable side effects because of the high doses needed. These considerations have made the use of β-AR agonists for human obesity uncertain *(108)*. High fat feeding also results in marked BAT hypertrophy and increased EE, suggesting that BAT plays a role in resisting obesity *(49,50)*. Subsequent isolation and cloning of a 32-kDa protein, then-called thermogenin, initiated a search for the function of such proteins (uncoupling proteins, or UCPs) that uncouple oxidative phosphorylation and thus have the capacity to produce heat *(109)*. Some studies *(110,111)* have supported a role for UCPs in more specialized forms of thermogenesis, but other studies have revealed controversial results. Others have emphasized the existence of a paradox: BAT is necessary for normal body weight regulation, but the major thermogenic protein, UCP-1, is not apparently absolutely required *(112)*. This paradox may be solved by either finding another thermogenic mediator in BAT or investigating other tissues as potential mediators of diet-induced thermogenesis.

2.4.2. WHITE ADIPOSE TISSUE

White adipose tissue (WAT) clearly participates actively in many metabolic processes *(113)* via regulation of glucose uptake, lipolysis, response to adrenergic stimulation, and release of numerous cytokines (leptin, ASP, adiponectin, resistin) *(114)*. Furthermore, although the metabolic rate of WAT is often cited as low, strong evidence indicates that significant overall EE derives from WAT *(115)*. Secreted WAT-specific cytokines, including leptin, adiponectin, resistin, and other substances, are reviewed in previously published papers *(113)*. Our current understanding is that WAT can be viewed not only as a storage depot, but as an important endocrine organ that profoundly affects EE and body weight. WAT represents an important potential antiobesity target via increased EE.

2.5. Approaches to Treat Obesity via Manipulation of EE

Appropriate strategies for weight loss would be to either prevent positive energy balance and stop the gradual weight gain of the population or treat obesity in those already affected. This involves producing negative energy balance to produce weight loss, followed by achieving energy balance permanently at a lowered body weight. In the following paragraphs, we discuss the above approaches. The major antiobesity pathways that have been targeted for manipulation of EE include mitochondrial uncoupling, the activation of the SNS, and TH use. With the possible exception of the medicines discussed below, none of these has been successful in treating human obesity because of either intolerable side effects or lack of efficacy, as judged by prevention of further weight gain, 5–10% loss of weight, metabolic improvement, and/or long-term maintenance *(116)*.

2.5.1. UNCOUPLING OXIDATIVE PHOSPHORYLATION

Compounds that short circuit the mitochondrial membrane potential, called uncouplers, had preceded the isolation and characterization of endogenous UCPs. These compounds (2,4-dinotrophenol, for example), which are effective treatments for obesity through their ability to increase oxygen consumption, have been abandoned because of a narrow therapeutic window and intolerable side effects *(117)*.

2.5.2. HORMONES

Leptin

Leptin is an adipocyte-derived cytokine that stimulates numerous pathways in the CNS, including weight loss. Exogenously administered leptin results in decreased food intake in leptin-deficient humans and, presumably via the SNS, in modest (if any) increase in EE and fat mobilization. The majority of obese human patients have elevated leptin levels in serum, however, indicating that there is resistance to leptin. The effect of exogenous leptin on body weight loss in humans is highly variable across a wide patient population, most likely because of already high leptin levels in obese patients reflecting a variable degree of tolerance or resistance to its effects *(118)*. Although leptin-deficient patients respond markedly to leptin treatment, these patients are extremely rare *(119)*. In addition, it is possible that certain patients with partial leptin deficiency may also respond to exogenous leptin treatment *(120,121)*, but this remains to be studied in the future.

Thyroid hormone

Activation of TH receptor β increases metabolic rate and causes weight loss in mice, and thus may become a drug target for obesity *(122)*. Subtype-specific compounds that are selective for a single thyroid receptor isoform are potential approaches to making antiobesity compounds *(123)*, but this is currently only an emerging area of research.

2.5.3. SYMPATHOMIMETICS

Ephedrine is a sympathomimetic agent that increases numerous SNS activity responses, including heart rate, blood pressure, and basal metabolic rate, probably through direct activation of adrenergic receptors. Its usefulness is limited by cardiovascular side effects and relatively low efficacy in the treatment of obesity, although in combination with caffeine it may show greater efficacy *(124)*.

Sibutramine is a nonselective NE/serotonin reuptake inhibitor that acts both as an appetite suppressant *(125)* and activator of SNS activity via the β_3-AR *(126)*. Sibutramine is currently indicated for obesity treatment in the absence of known cardiovascular disease (see relevant chapter below) *(127)*. Dose-limiting toxicity and potential side effects include increased heart rate and blood pressure. Patients should be screened for evidence of underlying atherosclerotic heart disease and need to be followed periodically while on sibutramine.

Nicotine stimulates norepinephrine release from sympathetic nerve terminals, resulting in modest (5%) thermogenesis *(128)*. Smoking cessation may have contributed to the increase in the prevalence of obesity because of withdrawal of nicotine, which acts as both an appetite suppressant and stimulator of thermogenesis *(129)*.

Caffeine stimulates thermogenesis by inhibition of adenosine receptors on tissues, resulting in increased intracellular cAMP levels and lipolysis *(130)*. Caffeine may be useful, to a small extent, as a treatment for obesity, especially in combination with other compounds such as ephedrine or nicotine *(128)*, and long-term studies have shown beneficial effects of endogenous insulin sensitizers, including adiponectin, on the metabolic syndrome and diabetes. Caffeine intake is not currently included among the recommended treatments for obesity, however.

The ability of β-AR agonists to reverse obesity in rodent models led to great hopes that these could become effective treatments in humans *(89)*. $β_3$-Agonists, in particular, would seem to be ideal targets for drug development, because their expression is restricted to adipose tissue and they effectively reduce body weight in rodents *(107)*. The potential mechanisms of action of β-agonists are multiple, including increased mitochondrial function and abundance, differentiation of BAT in WAT depots, lipolysis, and increased fatty acid oxidation. However, the future of β-agonists as effective antiobesity treatments remains unclear as outlined above *(131,132)*.

2.5.4. PRODUCING NEGATIVE ENERGY BALANCE AND WEIGHT LOSS

Food restriction is practically the primary driver of weight loss in humans; any diet that results in ingesting fewer calories will produce weight loss. Although it is also possible to lose weight with physical activity alone *(133,134)*, it is difficult for most people to exercise enough to achieve a degree of negative energy balance that would result in significant weight loss. This is also why adding physical activity to food restriction produces only a minimal additional amount of weight loss *(133,134)*. Unfortunately, weight tends to be regained in most people regardless of the composition of the diet used for weight loss *(79,80)*. It has been estimated that long-term success in obesity treatment is about 20% or less if success was defined as maintaining a 10% reduction in body weight for at least 1 year *(135)*. The mechanisms underlying the ability of the organism to defend a given body weight are under intensive investigation.

2.5.5. WEIGHT LOSS MAINTENANCE

Although there are several studies about factors that contribute to weight loss, we have very little evidence to understand the factors that contribute to weight loss maintenance. In a descriptive study by Klem et al. *(72)*, although most (>90%) participants reported that they used both food restriction and physical activity to lose weight, there was little similarity in the types of diets used for weight loss *(72)*. Conversely, in this study many similarities were seen in the behaviors and strategies used to maintain weight loss. The four that stand out are as follows:

- Eating a moderately low-fat, high-carbohydrate diet. This is consistent with previous work suggesting that low-fat diets should be better than high-fat diets in preventing positive energy balance *(75)*.
- Consistent self-monitoring of body weight, food intake, and physical activity. This is consistent with other reports that self-monitoring facilitates long-term success in weight management *(136)*.
- Eating breakfast every day. This is consistent with a growing body of data showing that eating breakfast facilitates maintenance of a healthy body weight *(137)*.
- Very high levels of physical activity.

2.6. Therapeutic Implications/Future Directions

The exploding obesity pandemic certainly suggests that efficient and safe behavioral and pharmacological approaches to treat obesity are needed. Efforts to clarify the mechanisms underlying energy homeostasis have provided a pathway for identifying and studying targets for drug development in the treatment of obesity and related metabolic disorders. As an example, identifying the mechanisms underlying neuronal resistance to adiposity signals has clear therapeutic implications; drugs that prevent or reverse this resistance can be predicted to favor the defence of a reduced level of body fat. A more detailed understanding of the pathogenesis of human obesity hopefully will ultimately guide the development of efficacious treatment options that could benefit the affected individuals.

REFERENCES

1. Zhang Y, Proenca R, Maffei M, Barone M, Leopold L, Friedman JM. Positional cloning of the mouse obese gene and its human homologue. Nature 1994; 372(6505):425–432.
2. Barsh GS, Schwartz MW. Genetic approaches to studying energy balance: perception and integration. Nat Rev Genet 2002; 3(8):589–600.
3. Horvath TL, Diano S, Tschop M. Brain circuits regulating energy homeostasis. Neuroscientist 2004; 10(3):235–246.
4. Kalra SP, Dube MG, Pu S, Xu B, Horvath TL, Kalra PS. Interacting appetite-regulating pathways in the hypothalamic regulation of body weight. Endocr Rev 1999; 20(1):68–100.
5. Saper CB, Chou TC, Elmquist JK. The need to feed: homeostatic and hedonic control of eating. Neuron 2002; 36(2):199–211.
6. Berthoud HR. Multiple neural systems controlling food intake and body weight. Neurosci Biobehav Rev 2002; 26(4):393–428.
7. Schwartz MW, Seeley RJ, Woods SC, Weigle DS, Campfield LA, Burn P et al. Leptin increases hypothalamic pro-opiomelanocortin mRNA expression in the rostral arcuate nucleus. Diabetes 1997; 46(12):2119–2123.
8. Benoit SC, Air EL, Coolen LM, Strauss R, Jackman A, Clegg DJ et al. The catabolic action of insulin in the brain is mediated by melanocortins. J Neurosci 2002; 22(20):9048–9052.
9. Fan W, Boston BA, Kesterson RA, Hruby VJ, Cone RD. Role of melanocortinergic neurons in feeding and the agouti obesity syndrome. Nature 1997; 385(6612):165–168.
10. Hahn TM, Breininger JF, Baskin DG, Schwartz MW. Coexpression of AgRP and NPY in fasting-activated hypothalamic neurons. Nat Neurosci 1998; 1(4):271–272.
11. Cowley MA, Smart JL, Rubinstein M, Cerdan MG, Diano S, Horvath TL et al. Leptin activates anorexigenic POMC neurons through a neural network in the arcuate nucleus. Nature 2001; 411(6836):480–484.
12. Kojima M, Hosoda H, Date Y, Nakazato M, Matsuo H, Kangawa K. Ghrelin is a growth-hormone-releasing acylated peptide from stomach. Nature 1999; 402(6762):656–660.
13. Batterham RL, Cowley MA, Small CJ, Herzog H, Cohen MA, Dakin CL et al. Gut hormone PYY(3–36) physiologically inhibits food intake. Nature 2002; 4186898.:650–654.
14. Nakazato M, Murakami N, Date Y, Kojima M, Matsuo H, Kangawa K et al. A role for ghrelin in the central regulation of feeding. Nature 2001; 409(6817):194–198.
15. Stanley BG, Magdalin W, Seirafi A, Thomas WJ, Leibowitz SF. The perifornical area: the major focus of (a) patchily distributed hypothalamic neuropeptide Y-sensitive feeding system(s). Brain Res 1993; 604(1/2):304–317.
16. Marsh DJ, Weingarth DT, Novi DE, Chen HY, Trumbauer ME, Chen AS et al. Melanin-concentrating hormone 1 receptor-deficient mice are lean, hyperactive, and hyperphagic and have altered metabolism. Proc Natl Acad Sci USA 2002; 99(5):3240–3245.
17. Giraudo SQ, Billington CJ, Levine AS. Feeding effects of hypothalamic injection of melanocortin 4 receptor ligands. Brain Res 1998; 809(2):302–306.

18. Fekete C, Legradi G, Mihaly E, Huang QH, Tatro JB, Rand WM et al. α-Melanocyte-stimulating hormone is contained in nerve terminals innervating thyrotropin-releasing hormone-synthesizing neurons in the hypothalamic paraventricular nucleus and prevents fasting-induced suppression of prothyrotropin-releasing hormone gene expression. J Neurosci 2000; 20(4):1550–1558.

19. Sarkar S, Lechan RM. Central administration of neuropeptide Y reduces alpha-melanocyte-stimulating hormone-induced cyclic adenosine 5′-monophosphate response element binding protein (CREB) phosphorylation in pro-thyrotropin-releasing hormone neurons and increases CREB phosphorylation in corticotropin-releasing hormone neurons in the hypothalamic paraventricular nucleus. Endocrinology 2003; 144(1):281–291.

20. Tokunaga K, Fukushima M, Kemnitz JW, Bray GA. Comparison of ventromedial and paraventricular lesions in rats that become obese. Am J Physiol 1986; 251(6 Pt 2):R1221–R1227.

21. Stanley BG, Daniel DR, Chin AS, Leibowitz SF. Paraventricular nucleus injections of peptide YY and neuropeptide Y preferentially enhance carbohydrate ingestion. Peptides 1985; 6(6):1205–1211.

22. Chen P, Williams SM, Grove KL, Smith MS. Melanocortin 4 receptor-mediated hyperphagia and activation of neuropeptide Y expression in the dorsomedial hypothalamus during lactation. J Neurosci 2004; 24(22):5091–5100.

23. Sakurai T, Amemiya A, Ishii M, Matsuzaki I, Chemelli RM, Tanaka H et al. Orexins and orexin receptors: a family of hypothalamic neuropeptides and G protein-coupled receptors that regulate feeding behavior. Cell 1998; 92(5):1.

24. Qu D, Ludwig DS, Gammeltoft S, Piper M, Pelleymounter MA, Cullen MJ et al. A role for melanin-concentrating hormone in the central regulation of feeding behaviour. Nature 1996; 380(6571):243–247.

25. Shimada M, Tritos NA, Lowell BB, Flier JS, Maratos-Flier E. Mice lacking melanin-concentrating hormone are hypophagic and lean. Nature 1998; 396(6712):670–674.

26. Chen Y, Hu C, Hsu CK, Zhang Q, Bi C, Asnicar M et al. Targeted disruption of the melanin-concentrating hormone receptor-1 results in hyperphagia and resistance to diet-induced obesity. Endocrinology 2002; 143(7):2469–2477.

27. de Lecea L, Kilduff TS, Peyron C, Gao X, Foye PE, Danielson PE et al. The hypocretins: hypothalamus-specific peptides with neuroexcitatory activity. Proc Natl Acad Sci USA 1998; 95(1):322–327.

28. Williams CJ, Hu FB, Patel SR, Mantzoros CS. Sleep duration and snoring in relation to biomarkers of cardiovascular disease risk among women with type 2 diabetes. Diabetes Care 2007; 30(5):1233–1240.

29. Xu B, Goulding EH, Zang K, Cepoi D, Cone RD, Jones KR et al. Brain-derived neurotrophic factor regulates energy balance downstream of melanocortin-4 receptor. Nat Neurosci 2003; 6(7):736–742.

30. Bariohay B, Lebrun B, Moyse E, Jean A. Brain-derived neurotrophic factor plays a role as an anorexigenic factor in the dorsal vagal complex. Endocrinology 2005; 146(12):5612–5620.

31. Kalia M, Sullivan JM. Brainstem projections of sensory and motor components of the vagus nerve in the rat. J Comp Neurol 1982; 211(3):248–265.

32. Dumont Y, Fournier A, Quirion R. Expression and characterization of the neuropeptide Y Y5 receptor subtype in the rat brain. J Neurosci 1998; 18(15):5565–5574.

33. Grauerholz BL, Jacobson JD, Handler MS, Millington WR. Detection of pro-opiomelanocortin mRNA in human and rat caudal medulla by RT-PCR. Peptides 1998; 19(5):939–948.

34. Horvath TL. Synaptic plasticity in energy balance regulation. Obesity (Silver Spring) 2006; 14Suppl 5):228S–233S.

35. Yoshihara T, Honma S, Honma K. Effects of restricted daily feeding on neuropeptide Y release in the rat paraventricular nucleus. Am J Physiol 1996; 2704 Pt 1):E589–E595.

36. Si EC, Bryant HU, Yim GK. Opioid and non-opioid components of insulin-induced feeding. Pharmacol Biochem Behav 1986; 244):899–903.

37. Zhang M, Balmadrid C, Kelley AE. Nucleus accumbens opioid, GABAergic, and dopaminergic modulation of palatable food motivation: contrasting effects revealed by a progressive ratio study in the rat. Behav Neurosci 2003; 117(2):202–211.

38. Mercer ME, Holder MD. Food cravings, endogenous opioid peptides, and food intake: a review. Appetite 1997; 29(3):325–352.

39. Matsuda LA, Lolait SJ, Brownstein MJ, Young AC, Bonner TI. Structure of a cannabinoid receptor and functional expression of the cloned cDNA. Nature 1990; 346(6284):561–564.

40. Pagotto U, Marsicano G, Cota D, Lutz B, Pasquali R. The emerging role of the endocannabinoid system in endocrine regulation and energy balance. Endocr Rev 2006; 27(1):73–100.

41. Van Gaal LF, Rissanen AM, Scheen AJ, Ziegler O, Rossner S. Effects of the cannabinoid-1 receptor blocker rimonabant on weight reduction and cardiovascular risk factors in overweight patients: 1-year experience from the RIO-Europe study. Lancet 2005; 365(9468):1389–1397.

42. Pi-Sunyer FX, Aronne LJ, Heshmati HM, Devin J, Rosenstock J. Effect of rimonabant, a cannabinoid-1 receptor blocker, on weight and cardiometabolic risk factors in overweight or obese patients: RIO-North America: a randomized controlled trial. JAMA 2006; 295(7):761–775.

43. Despres JP, Golay A, Sjostrom L. Effects of rimonabant on metabolic risk factors in overweight patients with dyslipidemia. N Engl J Med 2005; 353(20):2121–2134.

44. Friedman JM. A war on obesity, not the obese. Science 2003; 299(5608):856–858.

45. Rosenbaum M, Leibel RL, Hirsch J. Obesity. N Engl J Med 1997; 337(6):396–407.

46. O'Rahilly S, Farooqi IS, Yeo GS, Challis BG. Minireview: human obesity-lessons from monogenic disorders. Endocrinology 2003; 144(9):3757–3764.

47. Halaas JL, Boozer C, Blair-West J, Fidahusein N, Denton DA, Friedman JM. Physiological response to long-term peripheral and central leptin infusion in lean and obese mice. Proc Natl Acad Sci USA 1997; 94(16):8878–8883.

48. Bachman ES, Dhillon H, Zhang CY, Cinti S, Bianco AC, Kobilka BK et al. betaAR signaling required for diet-induced thermogenesis and obesity resistance. Science 2002; 297(5582):843–845.

49. Glick Z, Teague RJ, Bray GA. Brown adipose tissue: thermic response increased by a single low protein, high carbohydrate meal. Science 1981; 213(4512):1125–1127.

50. Rothwell NJ, Stock MJ. A role for brown adipose tissue in diet-induced thermogenesis. Nature 1979; 281(5726):31–35.

51. Stock MJ. Gluttony and thermogenesis revisited. Int J Obes Relat Metab Disord 1999; 23(11): 1105–1117.

52. Bouchard C, Tremblay A, Despres JP, Nadeau A, Lupien PJ, Theriault G et al. The response to long-term overfeeding in identical twins. N Engl J Med 1990; 322(21):1477–1482.

53. Stunkard AJ, Harris JR, Pedersen NL, McClearn GE. The body-mass index of twins who have been reared apart. N Engl J Med 1990; 322(21):1483–1487.

54. Saad MF, Alger SA, Zurlo F, Young JB, Bogardus C, Ravussin E. Ethnic differences in sympathetic nervous system-mediated energy expenditure. Am J Physiol 1991; 261(6 Pt 1):E789–E794.

55. Levine JA, Eberhardt NL, Jensen MD. Role of nonexercise activity thermogenesis in resistance to fat gain in humans. Science 1999; 283(5399):212–214.

56. de Jesus LA, Carvalho SD, Ribeiro MO, Schneider M, Kim SW, Harney JW et al. The type 2 iodothyronine deiodinase is essential for adaptive thermogenesis in brown adipose tissue. J Clin Invest 2001; 108(9):1379–1385.

57. Speakman JR, Selman C. Physical activity and resting metabolic rate. Proc Nutr Soc 2003; 62(3):621–634.

58. Ravussin E, Swinburn BA. Pathophysiology of obesity. Lancet 1992; 340(8816):404–408.

59. Hill JO, Wyatt HR, Reed GW, Peters JC. Obesity and the environment: where do we go from here. Science 2003; 299(5608):853–855.

60. Ravussin E, Lillioja S, Knowler WC, Christin L, Freymond D, Abbott WG et al. Reduced rate of energy expenditure as a risk factor for body-weight gain. N Engl J Med 1988; 318(8):467–472.

61. Bogardus C, Lillioja S, Ravussin E, Abbott W, Zawadzki JK, Young A et al. Familial dependence of the resting metabolic rate. N Engl J Med 1986; 315(2):96–100.

62. Weyer C, Pratley RE, Salbe AD, Bogardus C, Ravussin E, Tataranni PA. Energy expenditure, fat oxidation, and body weight regulation: a study of metabolic adaptation to long-term weight change. J Clin Endocrinol Metab 2000; 85(3):1087–1094.

64. Scherrer U, Randin D, Tappy L, Vollenweider P, Jequier E, Nicod P. Body fat and sympathetic nerve activity in healthy subjects. Circulation 1994; 89(6):2634–2640.

65. Rumantir MS, Vaz M, Jennings GL, Collier G, Kaye DM, Seals DR et al. Neural mechanisms in human obesity-related hypertension. J Hypertens 1999; 17(8):1125–1133.

66. Jansson PA, Larsson A, Smith U, Lonnroth P. Glycerol production in subcutaneous adipose tissue in lean and obese humans. J Clin Invest 1992; 89(5):1610–1617.

67. Kokkoris P, Pi-Sunyer FX. Obesity and endocrine disease. Endocrinol Metab Clin North Am 2003; 32(4):895–914.
68. Irrcher I, Adhihetty PJ, Joseph AM, Ljubicic V, Hood DA. Regulation of mitochondrial biogenesis in muscle by endurance exercise. Sports Med 2003; 33(11):783–793.
69. Jakicic JM. Exercise in the treatment of obesity. Endocrinol Metab Clin North Am 2003; 32(4):967–980.
70. Levine J, Baukol P, Pavlidis I. The energy expended in chewing gum. N Engl J Med 1999; 341(27):2100.
71. Brown WJ, Williams L, Ford JH, Ball K, Dobson AJ. Identifying the energy gap: magnitude and determinants of 5-year weight gain in midage women. Obes Res 2005; 13(8):1431–1441.
72. Klem ML, Wing RR, McGuire MT, Seagle HM, Hill JO. A descriptive study of individuals successful at long-term maintenance of substantial weight loss. Am J Clin Nutr 1997; 66(2):239–246.
73. Astrup A, Ryan L, Grunwald GK, Storgaard M, Saris W, Melanson E et al. The role of dietary fat in body fatness: evidence from a preliminary meta-analysis of ad libitum low-fat dietary intervention studies. Br J Nutr 2000; 83(Suppl 1):S25–S32.
74. Thomas CD, Peters JC, Reed GW, Abumrad NN, Sun M, Hill JO. Nutrient balance and energy expenditure during ad libitum feeding of high-fat and high-carbohydrate diets in humans. Am J Clin Nutr 1992; 55(5):934–942.
75. Hill JO, Drougas H, Peters JC. Obesity treatment: can diet composition play a role. Ann Intern Med 1993; 119(7 Pt 2):694–697.
76. Due A, Toubro S, Skov AR, Astrup A. Effect of normal-fat diets, either medium or high in protein, on body weight in overweight subjects: a randomised 1-year trial. Int J Obes Relat Metab Disord 2004; 28(10):1283–1290.
77. Ludwig DS. Dietary glycemic index and obesity. J Nutr 2000; 130(2S Suppl):280S–283S.
78. Golay A, Allaz AF, Morel Y, de Tonnac N, Tankova S, Reaven G. Similar weight loss with low- or high-carbohydrate diets. Am J Clin Nutr 1996; 63(2):174–178.
79. Stern L, Iqbal N, Seshadri P, Chicano KL, Daily DA, McGrory J et al. The effects of low-carbohydrate versus conventional weight loss diets in severely obese adults: one-year follow-up of a randomized trial. Ann Intern Med 2004; 140(10):778–785.
80. Samaha FF, Iqbal N, Seshadri P, Chicano KL, Daily DA, McGrory J et al. A low-carbohydrate as compared with a low-fat diet in severe obesity. N Engl J Med 2003; 348(21):2074–2081.
81. Nordmann AJ, Nordmann A, Briel M, Keller U, Yancy WS, Jr, Brehm BJ et al. Effects of low-carbohydrate vs low-fat diets on weight loss and cardiovascular risk factors: a meta-analysis of randomized controlled trials. Arch Intern Med 2006; 166(3):285–293.
82. Horton TJ, Drougas H, Brachey A, Reed GW, Peters JC, Hill JO. Fat and carbohydrate overfeeding in humans: different effects on energy storage. Am J Clin Nutr 1995; 62(1):19–29.
83. Silva JE. The thermogenic effect of thyroid hormone and its clinical implications. Ann Intern Med 2003; 139(3):205–213.
84. Rosenbaum M, Hirsch J, Murphy E, Leibel RL. Effects of changes in body weight on carbohydrate metabolism, catecholamine excretion, and thyroid function. Am J Clin Nutr 2000; 71(6):1421–1432.
85. Snitker S, Macdonald I, Ravussin E, Astrup A. The sympathetic nervous system and obesity: role in aetiology and treatment. Obes Rev 2000; 1(1):5–15.
86. Lowell BB, Bachman ES. Beta-adrenergic receptors, diet-induced thermogenesis, and obesity. J Biol Chem 2003; 278(32):29385–29388.
87. Tataranni PA, Young JB, Bogardus C, Ravussin E. A low sympathoadrenal activity is associated with body weight gain and development of central adiposity in Pima Indian men. Obes Res 1997; 5(4): 341–347.
88. Arch JR, Ainsworth AT, Cawthorne MA, Piercy V, Sennitt MV, Thody VE et al. Atypical beta-adrenoceptor on brown adipocytes as target for anti-obesity drugs. Nature 1984; 309(5964):163–165.
89. Himms-Hagen J, Cui J, Danforth E, Jr, Taatjes DJ, Lang SS, Waters BL et al. Effect of CL-316,243, a thermogenic beta 3-agonist, on energy balance and brown and white adipose tissues in rats. Am J Physiol 1994; 266(4 Pt 2):R1371–R1382.
90. Levin BE, Triscari J, Marquet E, Sullivan AC. Dietary obesity and neonatal sympathectomy. I. Effects on body composition and brown adipose. Am J Physiol 1984; 247(6 Pt 2):R979–R987.

91. Rohrer DK, Chruscinski A, Schauble EH, Bernstein D, Kobilka BK. Cardiovascular and metabolic alterations in mice lacking both beta1- and beta2-adrenergic receptors. J Biol Chem 1999; 274(24):16701–16708.

92. Susulic VS, Frederich RC, Lawitts J, Tozzo E, Kahn BB, Harper ME et al. Targeted disruption of the beta 3-adrenergic receptor gene. J Biol Chem 1995; 270(49):29483–29492.

93. Bachman ES, Hampton TG, Dhillon H, Amende I, Wang J, Morgan JP et al. The metabolic and cardiovascular effects of hyperthyroidism are largely independent of beta-adrenergic stimulation. Endocrinology 2004; 145(6):2767–2774.

94. Leite A, Neto JA, Leyton JF, Crivellaro O, el Dorry HA. Phosphofructokinase from bumblebee flight muscle. Molecular and catalytic properties and role of the enzyme in regulation of the fructose 6-phosphate/fructose 1,6-bisphosphate cycle. J Biol Chem 1988; 263(33):17527–17533.

95. Block BA, O'Brien J, Meissner G. Characterization of the sarcoplasmic reticulum proteins in the thermogenic muscles of fish. J Cell Biol 1994; 127(5):1275–1287.

96. Denborough M. Malignant hyperthermia. Lancet 1998; 352(9134):1131–1136.

97. Ducreux S, Zorzato F, Muller C, Sewry C, Muntoni F, Quinlivan R et al. Effect of ryanodine receptor mutations on interleukin-6 release and intracellular calcium homeostasis in human myotubes from malignant hyperthermia-susceptible individuals and patients affected by central core disease. J Biol Chem 2004; 279(42):43838–43846.

98. Guan HP, Li Y, Jensen MV, Newgard CB, Steppan CM, Lazar MA. A futile metabolic cycle activated in adipocytes by antidiabetic agents. Nat Med 2002; 8(10):1122–1128.

99. Ntambi JM, Miyazaki M, Stoehr JP, Lan H, Kendziorski CM, Yandell BS et al. Loss of stearoyl-CoA desaturase-1 function protects mice against adiposity. Proc Natl Acad Sci USA 2002; 99(17):11482–11486.

100. Smith SJ, Cases S, Jensen DR, Chen HC, Sande E, Tow B et al. Obesity resistance and multiple mechanisms of triglyceride synthesis in mice lacking Dgat. Nat Genet 2000; 25(1):87–90.

101. Stone SJ, Myers HM, Watkins SM, Brown BE, Feingold KR, Elias PM et al. Lipopenia and skin barrier abnormalities in DGAT2-deficient mice. J Biol Chem 2004; 279(12):11767–11776.

102. Abu-Elheiga L, Matzuk MM, Abo-Hashema KA, Wakil SJ. Continuous fatty acid oxidation and reduced fat storage in mice lacking acetyl-CoA carboxylase 2. Science 2001; 291(5513):2613–2616.

103. Ludwig EH, Mahley RW, Palaoglu E, Ozbayrakci S, Balestra ME, Borecki IB et al. DGAT1 promoter polymorphism associated with alterations in body mass index, high density lipoprotein levels and blood pressure in Turkish women. Clin Genet 2002; 62(1):68–73.

104. Minokoshi Y, Kim YB, Peroni OD, Fryer LG, Muller C, Carling D et al. Leptin stimulates fatty-acid oxidation by activating AMP-activated protein kinase. Nature 2002; 415(6869):339–343.

105. Minokoshi Y, Alquier T, Furukawa N, Kim YB, Lee A, Xue B et al. AMP-kinase regulates food intake by responding to hormonal and nutrient signals in the hypothalamus. Nature 2004; 428(6982):569–574.

106. Lowell BB, Susulic V, Hamann A, Lawitts JA, Himms-Hagen J, Boyer BB et al. Development of obesity in transgenic mice after genetic ablation of brown adipose tissue. Nature 1993; 366(6457):740–742.

107. Robidoux J, Martin TL, Collins S. Beta-adrenergic receptors and regulation of energy expenditure: a family affair. Annu Rev Pharmacol Toxicol 2004; 44:297–323.

108. Weyer C, Gautier JF, Danforth E, Jr. Development of beta 3-adrenoceptor agonists for the treatment of obesity and diabetes – an update. Diabetes Metab 1999; 251):11–21.

109. Nicholls DG. A history of UCP1. Biochem Soc Trans 2001; 29Pt 6):751–755.

110. Zhang CY, Baffy G, Perret P, Krauss S, Peroni O, Grujic D et al. Uncoupling protein-2 negatively regulates insulin secretion and is a major link between obesity, beta cell dysfunction, and type 2 diabetes. Cell 2001; 1056):745–755.

111. Arsenijevic D, Onuma H, Pecqueur C, Raimbault S, Manning BS, Miroux B et al. Disruption of the uncoupling protein-2 gene in mice reveals a role in immunity and reactive oxygen species production. Nat Genet 2000; 26(4):435–439.

112. Clapham JC, Arch JR, Chapman H, Haynes A, Lister C, Moore GB et al. Mice overexpressing human uncoupling protein-3 in skeletal muscle are hyperphagic and lean. Nature 2000; 406(6794):415–418.

113. Havel PJ. Update on adipocyte hormones: regulation of energy balance and carbohydrate/lipid metabolism. Diabetes 2004; 53(Suppl 1):S143–S151.

114. Klaus S. Adipose tissue as a regulator of energy balance. Curr Drug Targets 2004; 5(3):241–250.

115. Goran MI, Kaskoun M, Johnson R. Determinants of resting energy expenditure in young children. J Pediatr 1994; 125(3):362–367.

116. Campfield LA, Smith FJ, Burn P. Strategies and potential molecular targets for obesity treatment. Science 1998; 280(5368):1383–1387.

117. Harper JA, Dickinson K, Brand MD. Mitochondrial uncoupling as a target for drug development for the treatment of obesity. Obes Rev 2001; 2(4):255–265.

118. Gura T. Obesity drug pipeline not so fat. Science 2003; 299(5608):849–852.

119. O'Rahilly S. Leptin: defining its role in humans by the clinical study of genetic disorders. Nutr Rev 2002; 60(10 Pt 2):S30–S34.

120. Farooqi IS, Keogh JM, Kamath S, Jones S, Gibson WT, Trussell R et al. Partial leptin deficiency and human adiposity. Nature 2001; 414(6859):34–35.

121. Heymsfield SB, Greenberg AS, Fujioka K, Dixon RM, Kushner R, Hunt T et al. Recombinant leptin for weight loss in obese and lean adults: a randomized, controlled, dose-escalation trial. JAMA 1999; 282(16):1568–1575.

122. Grover GJ, Mellstrom K, Ye L, Malm J, Li YL, Bladh LG et al. Selective thyroid hormone receptor-beta activation: a strategy for reduction of weight, cholesterol, and lipoprotein (a) with reduced cardiovascular liability. Proc Natl Acad Sci USA 2003; 100(17):10067–10072.

123. Wagner RL, Huber BR, Shiau AK, Kelly A, Cunha Lima ST, Scanlan TS et al. Hormone selectivity in thyroid hormone receptors. Mol Endocrinol 2001; 15(3):398–410.

124. Daly PA, Krieger DR, Dulloo AG, Young JB, Landsberg L. Ephedrine, caffeine and aspirin: safety and efficacy for treatment of human obesity. Int J Obes Relat Metab Disord 1993; 17(Suppl 1):S73–S78.

125. Yanovski SZ, Yanovski JA. Obesity. N Engl J Med 2002; 346(8):591–602.

126. Connoley IP, Liu YL, Frost I, Reckless IP, Heal DJ, Stock MJ. Thermogenic effects of sibutramine and its metabolites. Br J Pharmacol 1999; 126(6):1487–1495.

127. Thearle M, Aronne LJ. Obesity and pharmacologic therapy. Endocrinol Metab Clin North Am 2003; 32(4):1005–1024.

128. Jessen AB, Toubro S, Astrup A. Effect of chewing gum containing nicotine and caffeine on energy expenditure and substrate utilization in men. Am J Clin Nutr 2003; 77(6):1442–1447.

129. Hofstetter A, Schutz Y, Jequier E, Wahren J. Increased 24-hour energy expenditure in cigarette smokers. N Engl J Med 1986; 314(2):79–82.

130. Astrup A, Toubro S, Christensen NJ, Quaade F. Pharmacology of thermogenic drugs. Am J Clin Nutr 1992; 55(1 Suppl):246S–248S.

131. Arch JR. Beta(3)-adrenoceptor agonists: potential, pitfalls and progress. Eur J Pharmacol 2002; 440(2/3):99–107.

132. Hu B, Jennings LL. Orally bioavailable beta 3-adrenergic receptor agonists as potential therapeutic agents for obesity and type-II diabetes. Prog Med Chem 2003; 41:167–194.

133. Wing RR. Physical activity in the treatment of the adulthood overweight and obesity: current evidence and research issues. Med Sci Sports Exerc 1999; 31(11 Suppl):S547–S552.

134. Ross R, Dagnone D, Jones PJ, Smith H, Paddags A, Hudson R et al. Reduction in obesity and related comorbid conditions after diet-induced weight loss or exercise-induced weight loss in men. A randomized, controlled trial. Ann Intern Med 2000; 133(2):92–103.

135. McGuire MT, Wing RR, Hill JO. The prevalence of weight loss maintenance among American adults. Int J Obes Relat Metab Disord 1999; 23(12):1314–1319.

136. Boutelle KN, Kirschenbaum DS. Further support for consistent self-monitoring as a vital component of successful weight control. Obes Res 1998; 6(3):219–224.

137. Rampersaud GC, Pereira MA, Girard BL, Adams J, Metzl JD. Breakfast habits, nutritional status, body weight, and academic performance in children and adolescents. J Am Diet Assoc 2005; 105(5):743–760.

138. Allen YS, Adrian TE, Allen JM, Tatemoto K, Crow TJ, Bloom SR et al. Neuropeptide Y distribution in the rat brain. Science 1983; 221(4613):877–879.

139. Hillebrand JJ, de Wied D, Adan RA. Neuropeptides, food intake and body weight regulation: a hypothalamic focus. Peptides 2002; 23(12):2283–2306.

140. Sawchenko PE, Pfeiffer SW. Ultrastructural localization of neuropeptide Y and galanin immuno-reactivity in the paraventricular nucleus of the hypothalamus in the rat. Brain Res 1988; 474(2):231–245.

141. Hu Y, Bloomquist BT, Cornfield LJ, DeCarr LB, Flores-Riveros JR, Friedman L et al. Identification of a novel hypothalamic neuropeptide Y receptor associated with feeding behavior. J Biol Chem 1996; 271(42):26315–26319.

142. Shiraishi T, Oomura Y, Sasaki K, Wayner MJ. Effects of leptin and orexin-A on food intake and feeding related hypothalamic neurons. Physiol Behav 2000; 71(3/4):251–261.

143. Akabayashi A, Watanabe Y, Wahlestedt C, McEwen BS, Paez X, Leibowitz SF. Hypothalamic neuropeptide Y, its gene expression and receptor activity: relation to circulating corticosterone in adrenalectomized rats. Brain Res 1994; 665(2):201–212.

144. McKibbin PE, Cotton SJ, McCarthy HD, Williams G. The effect of dexamethasone on neuropeptide Y concentrations in specific hypothalamic regions. Life Sci 1992; 51(16):1301–1307.

145. Stanley BG, Lanthier D, Chin AS, Leibowitz SF. Suppression of neuropeptide Y-elicited eating by adrenalectomy or hypophysectomy: reversal with corticosterone. Brain Res 1989; 501(1):32–36.

146. Tempel DL, Leibowitz SF. Adrenal steroid receptors: interactions with brain neuropeptide systems in relation to nutrient intake and metabolism. J Neuroendocrinol 1994; 6(5):479–501.

147. Giraudo SQ, Kotz CM, Grace MK, Levine AS, Billington CJ. Rat hypothalamic NPY mRNA and brown fat uncoupling protein mRNA after high-carbohydrate or high-fat diets. Am J Physiol 1994; 266(5 Pt 2):R1578–R1583.

148. Wang J, Akabayashi A, Dourmashkin J, Yu HJ, Alexander JT, Chae HJ et al. Neuropeptide Y in relation to carbohydrate intake, corticosterone and dietary obesity. Brain Res 1998; 802(1/2):75–88.

149. Welch CC, Kim EM, Grace MK, Billington CJ, Levine AS. Palatability-induced hyperphagia increases hypothalamic dynorphin peptide and mRNA levels. Brain Res 1996; 721(1/2):126–131.

150. Campfield LA, Smith FJ. Blood glucose dynamics and control of meal initiation: a pattern detection and recognition theory. Physiol Rev 2003; 83(1):25–58.

151. Campfield LA, Smith FJ, Rosenbaum M, Hirsch J. Human eating: evidence for a physiological basis using a modified paradigm. Neurosci Biobehav Rev 1996; 20(1):133–137.

152. Krysiak R, Obuchowicz E, Herman ZS. Interactions between the neuropeptide Y system and the hypothalamic-pituitary-adrenal axis. Eur J Endocrinol 1999; 140(2):130–136.

153. Billington CJ, Briggs JE, Grace M, Levine AS. Effects of intracerebroventricular injection of neuropeptide Y on energy metabolism. Am J Physiol 1991; 260(2 Pt 2):R321–R327.

154. Baskin DG, Hahn TM, Schwartz MW. Leptin sensitive neurons in the hypothalamus. Horm Metab Res 1999; 31(5):345–350.

155. Broberger C, Johansen J, Johansson C, Schalling M, Hokfelt T. The neuropeptide Y/agouti gene-related protein (AGRP) brain circuitry in normal, anorectic, and monosodium glutamate-treated mice. Proc Natl Acad Sci USA 1998; 95(25):15043–15048.

156. Chen P, Li C, Haskell-Luevano C, Cone RD, Smith MS. Altered expression of agouti-related protein and its colocalization with neuropeptide Y in the arcuate nucleus of the hypothalamus during lactation. Endocrinology 1999; 140(6):2645–2650.

157. Mizuno TM, Mobbs CV. Hypothalamic agouti-related protein messenger ribonucleic acid is inhibited by leptin and stimulated by fasting. Endocrinology 1999; 140(2):814–817.

158. Wirth MM, Giraudo SQ. Agouti-related protein in the hypothalamic paraventricular nucleus: effect on feeding. Peptides 2000; 21(9):1369–1375.

159. Small CJ, Kim MS, Stanley SA, Mitchell JR, Murphy K, Morgan DG et al. Effects of chronic central nervous system administration of agouti-related protein in pair-fed animals. Diabetes 2001; 50(2):248–254.

160. Ghilardi N, Ziegler S, Wiestner A, Stoffel R, Heim MH, Skoda RC. Defective STAT signaling by the leptin receptor in diabetic mice. Proc Natl Acad Sci USA 1996; 93(13):6231–6235.

161. Kim MS, Small CJ, Stanley SA, Morgan DG, Seal LJ, Kong WM et al. The central melanocortin system affects the hypothalamo-pituitary thyroid axis and may mediate the effect of leptin. J Clin Invest 2000; 105(7):1005–1011.

162. Tritos NA, Maratos-Flier E. Two important systems in energy homeostasis: melanocortins and melanin-concentrating hormone. Neuropeptides 1999; 33(5):339–349.

163. Bahjaoui-Bouhaddi M, Fellmann D, Griffond B, Bugnon C. Insulin treatment stimulates the rat melanin-concentrating hormone-producing neurons. Neuropeptides 1994; 27(4):251–258.

164. Sergeev VG, Akmaev IG. Effects of blockers of carbohydrate and lipid metabolism on expression of mRNA of some hypothalamic neuropeptides. Bull Exp Biol Med 2000; 130(8):766–768.

165. Sergeyev V, Broberger C, Gorbatyuk O, Hokfelt T. Effect of 2-mercaptoacetate and 2-deoxy-d-glucose administration on the expression of NPY, AGRP, POMC, MCH and hypocretin/orexin in the rat hypothalamus. NeuroReport 2000; 11(1):117–121.

166. Toshinai K, Mondal MS, Nakazato M, Date Y, Murakami N, Kojima M et al. Upregulation of ghrelin expression in the stomach upon fasting, insulin-induced hypoglycemia, and leptin administration. Biochem Biophys Res Commun 2001; 281(5):1220–1225.

167. Cai XJ, Widdowson PS, Harrold J, Wilson S, Buckingham RE, Arch JR et al. Hypothalamic orexin expression: modulation by blood glucose and feeding. Diabetes 1999; 48(11):2132–2137.

168. Mondal MS, Nakazato M, Date Y, Murakami N, Yanagisawa M, Matsukura S. Widespread distribution of orexin in rat brain and its regulation upon fasting. Biochem Biophys Res Commun 1999; 256(3):495–499.

169. Stricker-Krongrad A, Beck B. Modulation of hypothalamic hypocretin/orexin mRNA expression by glucocorticoids. Biochem Biophys Res Commun 2002; 296(1):129–133.

170. Lawrence CB, Snape AC, Baudoin FM, Luckman SM. Acute central ghrelin and GH secretagogues induce feeding and activate brain appetite centers. Endocrinology 2002; 143(1):155–162.

171. Olszewski PK, Li D, Grace MK, Billington CJ, Kotz CM, Levine AS. Neural basis of orexigenic effects of ghrelin acting within lateral hypothalamus. Peptides 2003; 24(4):597–602.

172. Griffond B, Risold PY, Jacquemard C, Colard C, Fellmann D. Insulin-induced hypoglycemia increases preprohypocretin (orexin) mRNA in the rat lateral hypothalamic area. Neurosci Lett 1999; 262(2):77–80.

173. Moriguchi T, Sakurai T, Nambu T, Yanagisawa M, Goto K. Neurons containing orexin in the lateral hypothalamic area of the adult rat brain are activated by insulin-induced acute hypoglycemia. Neurosci Lett 1999; 264(1/3):101–104.

174. Beck B, Richy S. Hypothalamic hypocretin/orexin and neuropeptide Y: divergent interaction with energy depletion and leptin. Biochem Biophys Res Commun 1999; 258(1):119–122.

175. Taheri S, Mahmoodi M, Opacka-Juffry J, Ghatei MA, Bloom SR. Distribution and quantification of immunoreactive orexin A in rat tissues. FEBS Lett 1999; 457(1):157–161.

176. Wortley KE, Chang GQ, Davydova Z, Leibowitz SF. Peptides that regulate food intake: orexin gene expression is increased during states of hypertriglyceridemia. Am J Physiol Regul Integr Comp Physiol 2003; 284(6):R1454–R1465.

177. Yamamoto Y, Ueta Y, Date Y, Nakazato M, Hara Y, Serino R et al. Down regulation of the prepro-orexin gene expression in genetically obese mice. Brain Res Mol Brain Res 1999; 65(1):14–22.

178. Briski KP, Sylvester PW. Hypothalamic orexin-A-immunpositive neurons express Fos in response to central glucopenia. NeuroReport 2001; 12(3):531–534.

179. Cai XJ, Evans ML, Lister CA, Leslie RA, Arch JR, Wilson S et al. Hypoglycemia activates orexin neurons and selectively increases hypothalamic orexin-B levels: responses inhibited by feeding and possibly mediated by the nucleus of the solitary tract. Diabetes 2001; 50(1):105–112.

180. Yamanaka A, Beuckmann CT, Willie JT, Hara J, Tsujino N, Mieda M et al. Hypothalamic orexin neurons regulate arousal according to energy balance in mice. Neuron 2003; 38(5):701–713.

181. Gundlach AL, Burazin TC, Larm JA. Distribution, regulation and role of hypothalamic galanin systems: renewed interest in a pleiotropic peptide family. Clin Exp Pharmacol Physiol 2001; 28(1/2):100–105.

182. Leibowitz SF. Brain peptides and obesity: pharmacologic treatment. Obes Res 1995; 3(Suppl 4):573S–589S.

183. Tempel DL, Leibowitz SF. Diurnal variations in the feeding responses to norepinephrine, neuropeptide Y and galanin in the PVN. Brain Res Bull 1990; 25(6):821–825.

184. Wynick D, Bacon A. Targeted disruption of galanin: new insights from knock-out studies. Neuropeptides 2002; 36(2/3):132–144.

185. Akabayashi A, Koenig JI, Watanabe Y, Alexander JT, Leibowitz SF. Galanin-containing neurons in the paraventricular nucleus: a neurochemical marker for fat ingestion and body weight gain. Proc Natl Acad Sci USA 1994; 91(22):10375–10379.

186. Leibowitz SF, Akabayashi A, Wang J. Obesity on a high-fat diet: role of hypothalamic galanin in neurons of the anterior paraventricular nucleus projecting to the median eminence. J Neurosci 1998; 18(7):2709–2719.

187. Odorizzi M, Max JP, Tankosic P, Burlet C, Burlet A. Dietary preferences of Brattleboro rats correlated with an overexpression of galanin in the hypothalamus. Eur J Neurosci 1999; 11(9):3005–3014.

188. Wang J, Akabayashi A, Yu HJ, Dourmashkin J, Alexander JT, Silva I et al. Hypothalamic galanin: control by signals of fat metabolism. Brain Res 1998; 804(1):7–20.

189. Kyrkouli SE, Stanley BG, Leibowitz SF. Galanin: stimulation of feeding induced by medial hypothalamic injection of this novel peptide. Eur J Pharmacol 1986; 122(1):159–160.

190. Nemeth PM, Rosser BW, Choksi RM, Norris BJ, Baker KM. Metabolic response to a high-fat diet in neonatal and adult rat muscle. Am J Physiol 1992; 262(2 Pt 1):C282–C286.

191. MacNeil DJ, Howard AD, Guan X, Fong TM, Nargund RP, Bednarek MA et al. The role of melanocortins in body weight regulation: opportunities for the treatment of obesity. Eur J Pharmacol 2002; 450(1):93–109.

192. Gantz I, Fong TM. The melanocortin system. Am J Physiol Endocrinol Metab 2003; 284(3): E468–E474.

193. Kieffer TJ, Habener JF. The adipoinsular axis: effects of leptin on pancreatic beta-cells. Am J Physiol Endocrinol Metab 2000; 278(1):E1–E14.

194. Clegg DJ, Benoit SC, Air EL, Jackman A, Tso P, D'Alessio D et al. Increased dietary fat attenuates the anorexic effects of intracerebroventricular injections of MTII. Endocrinology 2003; 144(7) :2941–2946.

195. Harrold JA, Williams G, Widdowson PS. Changes in hypothalamic agouti-related protein (AGRP), but not alpha-MSH or pro-opiomelanocortin concentrations in dietary-obese and food-restricted rats. Biochem Biophys Res Commun 1999; 258(3):574–577.

196. Torri C, Pedrazzi P, Leo G, Muller EE, Cocchi D, Agnati LF et al. Diet-induced changes in hypothalamic pro-opio-melanocortin mRNA in the rat hypothalamus. Peptides 2002; 23(6):1063–1068.

197. Pierroz DD, Ziotopoulou M, Ungsunan L, Moschos S, Flier JS, Mantzoros CS. Effects of acute and chronic administration of the melanocortin agonist MTII in mice with diet-induced obesity. Diabetes 2002; 51(5):1337–1345.

198. Chen AS, Marsh DJ, Trumbauer ME, Frazier EG, Guan XM, Yu H et al. Inactivation of the mouse melanocortin-3 receptor results in increased fat mass and reduced lean body mass. Nat Genet 2000; 26(1):97–102.

199. Yeo GS, Farooqi IS, Aminian S, Halsall DJ, Stanhope RG, O'Rahilly S. A frameshift mutation in MC4R associated with dominantly inherited human obesity. Nat Genet 1998; 20(2):111–112.

200. Vaisse C, Clement K, Guy-Grand B, Froguel P. A frameshift mutation in human MC4R is associated with a dominant form of obesity. Nat Genet 1998; 20(2):113–114.

201. Farooqi IS, Keogh JM, Yeo GS, Lank EJ, Cheetham T, O'Rahilly S. Clinical spectrum of obesity and mutations in the melanocortin 4 receptor gene. N Engl J Med 2003; 348(12):1085–1095.

202. Bluher S, Ziotopoulou M, Bullen JW, Jr, Moschos SJ, Ungsunan L, Kokkotou E et al. Responsiveness to peripherally administered melanocortins in lean and obese mice. Diabetes 2004; 53(1):82–90.

203. Hurd YL, Fagergren P. Human cocaine- and amphetamine-regulated transcript (CART) mRNA is highly expressed in limbic- and sensory-related brain regions. J Comp Neurol 2000; 425(4): 583–598.

204. Kristensen P, Judge ME, Thim L, Ribel U, Christjansen KN, Wulff BS et al. Hypothalamic CART is a new anorectic peptide regulated by leptin. Nature 1998; 393(6680):72–76.

205. Elias CF, Lee C, Kelly J, Aschkenasi C, Ahima RS, Couceyro PR et al. Leptin activates hypothalamic CART neurons projecting to the spinal cord. Neuron 1998; 21(6):1375–1385.

206. Savontaus E, Conwell IM, Wardlaw SL. Effects of adrenalectomy on AGRP, POMC, NPY and CART gene expression in the basal hypothalamus of fed and fasted rats. Brain Res 2002; 958(1):130–138.

207. Vrang N, Larsen PJ, Tang-Christensen M, Larsen LK, Kristensen P. Hypothalamic cocaine-amphetamine regulated transcript (CART) is regulated by glucocorticoids. Brain Res 2003; 965(1/2):45–50.

208. Larm JA, Gundlach AL. Galanin-like peptide (GALP) mRNA expression is restricted to arcuate nucleus of hypothalamus in adult male rat brain. Neuroendocrinology 2000; 72(2):67–71.

209. Jureus A, Cunningham MJ, McClain ME, Clifton DK, Steiner RA. Galanin-like peptide (GALP) is a target for regulation by leptin in the hypothalamus of the rat. Endocrinology 2000; 141(7):2703–2706.

210. Kastin AJ, Akerstrom V, Hackler L. Food deprivation decreases blood galanin-like peptide and its rapid entry into the brain. Neuroendocrinology 2001; 74(6):423–432.

211. Krasnow SM, Fraley GS, Schuh SM, Baumgartner JW, Clifton DK, Steiner RA. A role for galanin-like peptide in the integration of feeding, body weight regulation, and reproduction in the mouse. Endocrinology 2003; 144(3):813–822.

212. Lawrence CB, Baudoin FM, Luckman SM. Centrally administered galanin-like peptide modifies food intake in the rat: a comparison with galanin. J Neuroendocrinol 2002; 14(11):853–860.

213. Richard D, Lin Q, Timofeeva E. The corticotropin-releasing factor family of peptides and CRF receptors: their roles in the regulation of energy balance. Eur J Pharmacol 2002; 440(2/3):189–197.

214. Cai A, Wise PM. Age-related changes in the diurnal rhythm of CRH gene expression in the paraventricular nuclei. Am J Physiol 1996; 270(2 Pt 1):E238–E243.

215. Moldow RL, Fischman AJ. Circadian rhythm of corticotropin releasing factor-like immunoreactivity in rat hypothalamus. Peptides 1984; 5(6):1213–1215.

216. Arase K, York DA, Shimizu H, Shargill N, Bray GA. Effects of corticotropin-releasing factor on food intake and brown adipose tissue thermogenesis in rats. Am J Physiol 1988; 255(3 Pt 1):E255–E259.

217. Egawa M, Yoshimatsu H, Bray GA. Effect of corticotropin releasing hormone and neuropeptide Y on electrophysiological activity of sympathetic nerves to interscapular brown adipose tissue. Neuroscience 1990; 34(3):771–775.

218. Glowa JR, Barrett JE, Russell J, Gold PW. Effects of corticotropin releasing hormone on appetitive behaviors. Peptides 1992; 13(3):609–621.

219. Inui A. Transgenic approach to the study of body weight regulation. Pharmacol Rev 2000; 52(1):35–61.

220. Richard D, Huang Q, Timofeeva E. The corticotropin-releasing hormone system in the regulation of energy balance in obesity. Int J Obes Relat Metab Disord 2000; 24 Suppl 2:S36–S39.

221. Rothwell NJ. Central effects of CRF on metabolism and energy balance. Neurosci Biobehav Rev 1990; 14(3):263–271.

222. Whitnall MH. Regulation of the hypothalamic corticotropin-releasing hormone neurosecretory system. Prog Neurobiol 1993; 40(5):573–629.

223. Schwartz MW, Woods SC, Porte D, Jr, Seeley RJ, Baskin DG. Central nervous system control of food intake. Nature 2000; 404(6778):661–671.

224. Heisler LK, Cowley MA, Kishi T, Tecott LH, Fan W, Low MJ et al. Central serotonin and melanocortin pathways regulating energy homeostasis. Ann NY Acad Sci 2003; 994:169–174.

225. Wang GJ, Volkow ND, Fowler JS. The role of dopamine in motivation for food in humans: implications for obesity. Expert Opin Ther Targets 2002; 6(5):601–609.

5

Insulin Resistance in States of Energy Excess: Underlying Pathophysiological Concepts

Susann Blüher and Christos S. Mantzoros

KEY POINTS

- The epidemic of obesity and associated metabolic and cardiovascular disorders are of increasing prevalence and, thus, importance.
- Despite significant progress made during this past decade, the pathophysiological mechanisms underlying the development of these diseases are still poorly understood.
- A dysfunctional adipose tissue is currently considered the "conditio sine qua non" for the development of the metabolic syndrome; this may result from either an a priori limited or an exhausted storage capacity of adipocytes in states of lipoatrophy or chronic energy excess, respectively.
- The latter is associated with hypertrophy of adipocytes and when coupled with excessive fat deposition in muscle and liver leads to a derangement in the release of fatty acids, hormones, adipokines, proinflammatory cytokines, and other molecules, which, in turn, result in insulin resistance and a low grade inflammation.
- According to our current understanding, chronic inflammation may contribute further toward the development of both insulin resistance and artherosclerosis.
- Impairment of insulin action in the periphery and activation of certain immunological responses lead over time to the special features and comorbidites of the metabolic syndrome.
- This chapter provides information on factors and molecules involved in the pathogenesis of insulin resistance and other aspects of the metabolic syndrome and discusses our present understanding of the role adipokines, free fatty acids, and inflammatory markers play in the development of this syndrome.

Key Words: Obesity, Metabolic syndrome, Insulin resistance, Pathophysiology, Adipokines, Body fat distribution

1. INTRODUCTION

An epidemic of obesity is evolving not only in most industrial countries, but also in many developing countries around the world. Obesity substantially increases the risk for metabolic, cardiovascular, and orthopedic comorbidites. The degree of body fat

From: *Nutrition and Health: Nutrition and Metabolism*
Edited by: C.S. Mantzoros, DOI: 10.1007/978-1-60327-453-1_5,
© Humana Press, a part of Springer Science+Business Media, LLC 2009

mass accumulation depends on several factors including ethnic background and genetic makeup, gender, and age, but also neuroendocrine, environmental and societal parameters. Gonadal steroids may play a major role in the distribution of body fat. At the onset of puberty, men become more muscular and have less fat, whereas women start to have a higher percentage of body fat in relation to their muscle mass. These differences persist throughout life and are reflected in the typical male and female fat distribution pattern. With advancing age, both gonadal steroid and growth hormone secretion decline, resulting in increased accumulation of visceral fat, particularly in men. In women, higher serum testosterone concentrations are usually associated with increased visceral fat. Thus, the decline in growth hormone and the loss of estrogen at the time of menopause may explain the relatively rapid increase in visceral fat in postmenopausal women. Differences in adipose tissue cellularity have also been suggested as a possible link between obesity and diabetes. Obese people with large subcutaneous abdominal adipocyte size are on average more hyperinsulinemic and glucose intolerant than those with a similar degree of adiposity but with relatively smaller subcutaneous abdominal adipocyte size *(1)*.

According to the department of Health and Human Services, 30% of the US population was obese in 2001 with prevalence rates in other developed nations either being similar or following very closely. The prevalence of overweight or obesity in western populations is currently approximately 60% but among type 2 diabetic patients it is as high as 80% *(2,3)*. It is anticipated that, if the same trend continues, more than 80% of American adults will be either overweight or obese by 2020.

In general terms, obesity is the result of excessive energy stored in fat. An increased fat mass is associated with an increase in fat cell size (hypertrophy) and/or fat cell amount (hyperplasia). Obesity leads to the development of a cluster of metabolic and other disturbances, collectively called the metabolic/insulin resistance syndrome, which include (or predispose to) lipid abnormalities, arterial hypertension, impaired glucose tolerance or diabetes, a proinflammatory state, and coagulation abnormalities, all of which lead in turn to metabolic and cardiovascular diseases as well as certain malignancies *(4–6)*.

Several explanations for the development of the metabolic syndrome have been proposed, including ectopic fat accumulation, which apparently accompanies the obese state, as well as dysregulation and dysfunction of adipose tissue, which, in turn, secretes abnormal amounts of cytokines and hormones collectively called adipokines *(7–9)*. A major determinant in the development of the metabolic syndrome seems to be not only the total amount of energy stored as fat but also the body fat distribution, since visceral obesity is much more closely associated with the metabolic/insulin resistance syndrome than overall obesity *(5,6)*.

This chapter focuses on pathways linking obesity to the features of the metabolic syndrome and discusses underlying pathophysiological mechanisms.

2. THE METABOLIC SYNDROME

2.1. Insulin Resistance

Insulin resistance, a state in which normal circulating levels of insulin fail to produce its expected physiological effects, usually refers to the reduced ability of insulin to regulate carbohydrate homeostasis by regulating glucose uptake and/or glucose production. The resistance in carbohydrate metabolism results in increased insulin production, which in turn may produce excessive effects of insulin in other pathways *(5,10)*. Thus, the consequences of insulin resistance are different in different tissues affected: in muscle, insulin resistance leads to impaired inward transmembrane glucose transport *(11)*, whereas in the liver, insulin resistance is mainly associated with increased neoglucogenesis and suppressed glycogenolysis as well as impaired liver glucose uptake *(12)*. In adipose tissue (both visceral and subcutaneous), insulin resistance is manifested as a reduced insulin-mediated glucose uptake *(13)*. Insulin resistance in metabolically active tissues leads to compensatory hyperinsulinemia. Other tissues affected by peripheral insulin resistance include the ovaries, where insulin resistance may result in the polycystic ovary syndrome, and vascular cells in which the development of artherosclerosis is the major complication. In addition, it is well established that insulin resistance may promote carcinogenesis in several tissues *(14)*.

2.2. Overweight and Obesity vs Weight Reduction

Up to 60% of the population and up to 80% of type 2 diabetics are currently either overweight or obese *(3)*. Follow up for several years of either middle-aged women in the Nurses Health Study or men in the Health Professionals Follow-up Study has clearly shown that the risk of developing type 2 diabetes is rising in parallel with an increasing degree of overweight and obesity. In accordance, weight reduction is associated with decreased incidence of type 2 diabetes *(4)*. In the Nurses Health Study, a weight loss of 5 kg or more reduced the risk of developing type 2 diabetes by approximately 50% *(4)*. This observation was later also documented in interventional studies including the Diabetes Prevention Program (DPP), where an approximate 7% of weight reduction, maintained for an average duration of 2.8 years, was associated with a 58% reduction in the risk of developing type 2 diabetes in the prediabetic individuals with impaired glucose tolerance (IGT) *(15)*.

2.3. Body Fat Distribution/Fat Storage and Secretory Capacity of Different Fat Depots

The distribution of adipose tissue is a major determinant of the metabolic risk profile. In addition, it has been proposed that the fact that functional capacity of the adipose tissue varies among subjects might offer an explanation for the incomplete overlap between the metabolic syndrome and obesity.

Although the subcutaneous adipose tissue is the site of main energy storage, when the storage capacity in subcutaneous fat is exhausted, the visceral fat takes over and lipids are also deposited in several other organs including muscle and liver. Individual and gender differences define the storage capacity of subcutaneous fat depots and thus the moment in which energy starts to be stored in visceral fat. In general, men have a lower subcutaneous fat storage capacity and start to accumulate fat in the visceral depot earlier than women *(5,6)*. In concordance with these differences of functional capacity of adipose tissue, individuals with upper body fat accumulation or higher visceral fat mass are more insulin resistant than those with a predominantly lower body fat accumulation and more subcutaneous fat. This has been attributable not only to the increased sensitivity of visceral fat to lipolytic stimuli, but also to altered secretion of adipokines by visceral fat *(16–19)*. Visceral fat is more active in terms of accepting and releasing free fatty acids (FFAs) and is characterized by a different pattern of adipocytokine secretion *(20)*.

Thus, central or visceral obesity is associated more closely than overall obesity with higher risk to develop insulin resistance and related metabolic disorders and leads to an altered plasma lipid composition (5–7).

Subcutaneous fat is the main energy storage site in addition to producing certain levels of adipokines. Visceral fat cells produce excessive amounts of proinflammatory adipokines including tumor necrosis factor α (TNFα), interleukin 6 (IL-6), plasminogen activator inhibitor 1 (PAI-1), and/or decreased amounts of insulin sensitizing, antiinflammatory adipokines such as adiponectin (21–23). These differences in the gene expression profile between visceral and subcutaneous fat may account for the diverging metabolic risk between the two fat depots. Out of the 1,660 genes expressed in adipose tissue, 297 (17.9%) genes have shown a twofold or higher difference in their expression between the visceral and subcutaneous fat depots. Many of these genes are involved in glucose homeostasis and insulin action, such as the peroxisome proliferator activator receptor γ (PPAR γ), or in lipid metabolism, such as the HMG CoA synthase and hormone-sensitive lipase (23).

2.4. Dietary Patterns and Physical Activity

Healthy dietary patterns, including the low glycemic index diets and Mediterannean type diets have received much recognition over the past few years for their association with substantial health benefits. A cross-sectional study evaluating plasma markers and dietary data from 987 diabetic women from the Nurses' Health Study (NHS) revealed that women following a Mediterranean-type dietary pattern albeit older tended to have lower body mass indexes and waist circumferences, and had higher total energy intakes, physical activities, and plasma adiponectin concentrations. Of the several components of the Mediterranean dietary pattern score, alcohol, nuts, and whole grains showed the strongest association with adiponectin concentrations (24). The significance of high circulating adiponectin levels in the context of features of the metabolic syndrome is discussed later on, but women in the NHS adhering closely to a Mediterranean dietary pattern had, in addition to higher adiponectin levels, lower levels of proinflammatory adipokines, lower degrees of insulin resistance, and lower risk for diabetes and cardiovascular disease. In contrast, high glycemic index diet and higher consumption of sugar-sweetened beverages, observed mainly in relation to a Western dietary pattern, are clearly associated with a greater magnitude of weight gain and an increased risk for developing type 2 diabetes (25–27). Recent studies suggest that long-term coffee consumption is associated with a reduction in long-term weight gain and a statistically significantly lower risk for type 2 diabetes (28–30). A higher nut consumption has also been described to offer potential benefits in lowering risk of type 2 diabetes in women (31). Finally, in addition to dietary patterns, physical activity significantly improves insulin resistance, insulin sensitivity, and the metabolic syndrome, in part by altering circulating adiponectin and expression of adiponectin as well as adiponectin receptor mRNA in muscle, as discussed later on (32).

3. DYSFUNCTION AND DYSREGULATION OF ADIPOSE TISSUE

The prevalence of the metabolic/insulin resistance syndrome continues to increase with the exploding prevalence of overweight and obesity. This is the case in several racial and ethnic groups including Americans among whom the prevalence of the metabolic syndrome is estimated to be as high as 40% *(2–6)*. Several studies have demonstrated that weight reduction through increased physical activity, pharmacotherapy, or bariatric surgery is associated with a highly significant reduced risk to develop any component of the metabolic syndrome, including impaired glucose tolerance and type 2 diabetes *(15,33–35)*.

Emerging data strongly support the view that adipose tissue dysregulation and dysfunction might play a role of major significance in the pathogenesis of the insulin resistance syndrome. A dysfunctional adipose tissue associated with hypertrophy of adipocytes and coupled with excessive fat deposition in muscle and liver is currently considered a "conditio sine qua non" for the development of the metabolic syndrome *(5,6)*. These alterations lead to a derangement in the release of fatty acids, hormones, adipokines, cytokines, and other molecules as discussed in more detail below.

4. INSULIN RESISTANCE AS A CHRONIC INFLAMMATORY PROCESS

Mechanisms inducing a low-grade systemic inflammation have been recently suggested to be one of the putative links between obesity, adipose tissue dysfunction, and the development of insulin resistance *(7,36)*. Although the exact signals and the mechanisms that trigger the inflammatory response remain incompletely understood, chronic inflammation is apparently not only associated with, but is also most probably causally related to the development of insulin resistance. It has been shown that accumulation of macrophages in adipocytes leads to an activation of inflammatory pathways *(10,37,38)*. Markers of chronic inflammation such as C-reactive protein (CRP), fibrinogen, TNFα and IL-6, and/or circulating triglyceride levels are elevated in serum of obese subjects and can predict the future development of impaired glucose tolerance and type 2 diabetes *(39,40)*.

Although the question of how the hypertrophic adipocytes are linked to the recruitment of macrophages into the adipose tissue and the establishment of a proinflammatory state remains to be fully elucidated, and the consequences of these changes are far better understood. The two most important harmful cytokines involved in this process are currently thought to be TNFα and IL-6, whereas adiponectin appears to be the most protective adipocytokine. Both harmful adipokines impair insulin signaling (at the level of the insulin receptor or at postreceptor levels including the Insulin Receptor Substrates level) as well as actions of insulin *(7,41)*. The fact that the number of macrophages in human adipose tissue correlates positively with the degree of obesity strengthens the hypothesis that macrophage infiltration into adipose tissue may contribute to the development of dysregulated adipose tissue function and initiate the process of chronic inflammation *(7)*.

A major focus of research has been the question whether dysfunctional and inflamed adipose tissue can be converted into "healthy" adipose tissue again and whether the progression of metabolic dysfunction can be stopped or reversed by modulation of the inflammatory profile in adipose tissue. In this context, several studies have shown that administration of thiazolidinediones (TZD), which act by binding to and activating peroxisome proliferator-activated receptors (PPARγ), is capable of reversing inflammatory properties and lipid abnormalities besides the direct and indirect effects of TZDs to improve insulin resistance, including increase of circulating levels of adiponectin, an endogenous insulin sensitizer *(42)*. Importantly, TZDs improve glycemic control and enhance insulin sensitivity despite the paradoxical weight gain seen with TZD treatment.

The latter seems to be attributable to the fact that TZDs may redistribute fat within the body by reducing visceral and hepatic fat mass and increasing subcutaneous fat depots. Since TZDs may also lead to fluid retention, osteoporosis, and other complications, it has been proposed that development of non-thiazolidinedione, selective PPARγ modulators (SPARMs) could hopefully lead to availability of effective medications that could result in increasing adiponectin levels and insulin sensitization without any side effects *(43)*. INT-131, a compound in development by Intekrin is the one in the most advanced stages of development in this area.

5. IMPACT OF FREE FATTY ACIDS AND LIPID METABOLISM ON INSULIN RESISTANCE: EFFECTS OF LIPOTOXICITY

Insulin inhibits lipolysis in adipose tissue and promotes the transfer of FFAs from circulating lipoproteins to the adipose tissue. Thus, in states of insulin resistance, FFA levels increase in the circulation due to unrestrained lipolysis and decreased clearance of FFAs in the periphery; this phenomenon leads also to an increase of triglycerides (TG) *(10)*. Circulating levels of FFAs are increased in obese subjects and have been proposed to be a major contributor to peripheral insulin resistance *(44,45)* initiating thus a vicious cycle. Chronically elevated serum FFA levels stimulate gluconeogenesis, induce insulin resistance at the level of liver and muscle, and impair insulin secretion in genetically predisposed individuals *(43)*. Increased FFA levels also tend to increase triglyceride accumulation in both liver and skeletal muscle, and this correlates with the degree of insulin resistance in these tissues *(46,47)*. Serum triglycerides, which are in a state of constant turnover, and their metabolites such as acyl coenzymes A, ceramides, and diacylglycerol also contribute toward both impaired hepatic and peripheral insulin action. In addition, nonesterified fatty acids are raised in obese subjects (both, diabetic and nondiabetic) following enhanced adipocyte lipolysis. Increased fatty acid concentrations lead to enhanced insulin secretion in the short term and significant (even total) inhibition of insulin secretion as early as 24 h thereafter *(48,49)*. This sequence of events is frequently called lipotoxicity *(50)*. Accumulating evidence suggests that such lipotoxicity may also be an important contributor to the pancreatic β cell dysfunction seen in type 2 diabetic patients *(48,51)*. Since the magnitude of the effects of lipotoxicity has been questioned by some investigators, this area remains an active area of research.

As previously described, when the classical fat depots are filled to capacity, other storage depots may be used for the storage of excess fat, namely liver and muscle. The failure of adipose tissue to take up more fat absorbed by the digestive tract leads to an excessive postprandial lipid flux toward muscle and liver and to a decreased clearance of triglyceride rich lipoprotein particles. The interplay of these particles with HDL and LDL cholesterol leads to the typical dyslipidemic profile, whereas the increased availability of (FFAs) has direct effects on the liver *(9,52)*.

6. LIPODYSTROPHY AND INSULIN RESISTANCE

Similar to states of energy excess leading to obesity, congenital forms of lipodystrophy in humans, i.e., states characterized by selective loss of subcutaneous and visceral fat, are also associated with metabolic abnormalities (hyperglycemia, insulin resistance, dyslipidemia) in humans *(53)*. Insufficient adipose tissue storage capacity may in turn lead to excessive energy storage in fat, skeletal muscle, and liver. This is in turn linked to the development of severe insulin resistance in these organs. Patients with generalized lipodystrophy represent thus another model of human ectopic fat deposition. In accordance with the concept of ectopic fat accumulation as a contributing factor for obesity-associated insulin resistance and related metabolic disorders, these subjects also have abnormal secretion of proinflammatory cytokines and abnormally low circulating levels of two adipokines, i.e., leptin and adiponectin *(53)*. The impact of an abnormal secretion pattern of those adipokines on lipid metabolism and the pathogenesis of the metabolic syndrome is discussed later on.

Recent studies support the concept that insulin resistance in one of the contributing factors to the development of dyslipidemia seen in the metabolic syndrome *(10)*, but it has also been proposed that elevated FFAs and triglyceride levels also contribute to exaggeration of insulin resistance through a lipotoxicity mechanism. Moreover, the classic diabetic dyslipidemia could be considered as the main clinical manifestation of adipose tissue failure, i.e., lack of adipose tissue storage capacity either directly (lipoatrophy) or indirectly i.e., because existing adipose tissue stores are filled to capacity *(9,54)*.

7. THE ROLE OF ADIPOKINES IN INSULIN RESISTANCE

The discovery of the adipocyte secreted hormone leptin in December 1994 has resulted in a dramatically altered view of the role the adipose tissue plays in human physiology. In addition to its classical physiological functions (heat insulation, mechanical cushioning, storage site for triglycerides), the adipose tissue is now recognized as an active endocrine organ that produces a variety of bioactive peptides (adipokines) as well as inflammatory and antiinflammatory molecules including leptin, adiponectin, TNFα, IL-6, IL-18, CRP, PAI-1, and many others *(7,9,55)*. Some of these molecules are almost exclusively expressed in adipose tissue (e.g., leptin, adiponectin), while others are produced by both adipose tissue and adipose tissue-resident macrophages as well as other organs or systems (e.g., TNFα, IL-6, PAI-1). With the exception of adiponectin, which is decreased, all other adipokines and inflammatory markers are increased in overweight and obese individuals.

7.1. Adiponectin

Adiponectin is an adipocyte secreted endogenous insulin sensitizer almost exclusively expressed in adipocytes. Adiponectin expression is higher in subcutaneous than in visceral fat, which might offer an explanation for the negative correlation between circulating adiponectin levels and insulin resistance *(56)*. This negative correlation is independent of body mass index *(57)*. Circulating adiponectin levels are reduced in obesity, insulin resistance, and type 2 diabetes *(58)*. In contrast to most other adipokines, adiponectin exerts profound beneficial actions including insulin sensitizing, antidiabetogenic, anti-inflammatory/-proliferative, and anti-atherogenic effects. Up to now, two adiponectin receptors (AdipoR1 and AdipoR2) have been described and are mainly expressed in liver and muscle *(59–66)*. Adiponectin increases fatty acid oxidation in skeletal muscle, promotes glucose utilization, and reduces hepatic glucose production, resulting thus in an increase of insulin sensitivity *(9,67)*. Animal studies have shown that adiponectin deficiency plays an important role in the pathogenesis of insulin resistance, as adiponectin knockout mice develop insulin resistance that is reversed by adiponectin administration *(61)*. In addition, circulating adiponectin levels correlate positively with insulin sensitivity in rodents and humans and predict the development of insulin resistance, diabetes, and cardiovascular disease as well as certain malignancies associated with obesity and the metabolic syndrome *(62,63, 68–71)*.

In addition to its insulin-sensitizing effects, adiponectin has antiinflammatory properties and may also protect against development or progression of atherosclerosis *(72,73)*. Thus, observational studies have shown that not only adiponectin, but also AdipoR1 and AdipoR2 are all associated with body composition, insulin sensitivity, and metabolic parameters. A healthy diet, i.e. α low glycemic index diet *(74,75)* and a mediterannean type diet *(76)* also increase circulating adiponectin levels. Intensive, but probably not moderate physical training increases circulating adiponectin and mRNA expression of its receptors in muscle, and this may in turn mediate the improvement of insulin resistance and the metabolic syndrome in response to exercise *(32)*. A 7% reduction in body weight by lifestyle modification for 6 months results in a significant increase in plasma adiponectin levels in obese type 2 diabetic patients with insulin resistance *(77)*. These effects of weight loss and lifestyle modification on adiponectin levels are in agreement with the observation that these interventions decrease the risk for diabetes and that subjects with high adiponectin concentrations are less likely to develop type 2 diabetes than those with lower concentrations *(78)*.

The role of the two adiponectin receptors, AdipoR1 and AdipoR2, in the regulation of energy homeostasis and glucose metabolism is now being extensively studied in rodents and humans. The development of obesity by hypercaloric feeding in mice is associated with an altered expression/secretion profile of adiponectin and its receptors in muscle and liver *(79)*. In addition, adiponectin and both adiponectin receptors seem to be involved in the improvement of insulin sensitivity associated with ciliary neurotrophic factor (CNTF)-induced weight loss *(80)*. The mechanisms by which adiponectin improves insulin sensitivity have not yet been fully elucidated. One proposed mechanism is the activation of adenosine monophosphate-activated protein kinase (AMPK) in skeletal muscle and liver, in addition to enhancing insulin-stimulated glucose uptake into fat and muscle and suppressing hepatic glucose production as well as stimulating fatty acid oxidation. Through the stimulation of fatty acid oxidation, circulating FFAs are further decreased and the actions of insulin are improved *(72)*.

7.2. Leptin

Leptin is the prototype adipokine, which is almost exclusively expressed in adipose tissue and more so in subcutaneous fat *(81)*. According to our current understanding, leptin's main function is to inform several organs of the organism that there is "enough energy to sustain life." This hormone exerts direct effects in metabolically active tissues and/or indirect effects by activating hypothalamic centers via leptin receptors. Circulating leptin levels are increased in obese subjects and decreased in leaner subjects and/or in response to food deprivation *(82)*. Its key functions include the regulation of food intake/energy expenditure, the regulation of neuroendocrine and immune function, and the modulation of glucose and fat metabolism by improving insulin sensitivity and reducing intracellular lipids *(55,66)*.

Animal studies have shown that leptin administration has an insulin sensitizing effect in muscle cells and adipocytes *(83–85)*. In humans, mutations of the leptin gene have been associated with severe obesity, glucose intolerance, and insulin resistance, which are reversed by leptin administration *(86–88)*. The long-term effects of leptin replacement have been intensely studied in uncontrolled studies in patients with rare syndromes of complete, mostly congenital, lipoatrophy and severe insulin resistance or partial lipoatrophy and milder insulin resistance/metabolic syndrome induced by administration of highly active antiretrovirals (HAART) in HIV positive patients. Leptin administration in replacement doses significantly improved glycemia, dyslipidemia, and hepatic steatosis in these hypoleptinemic patients with severe insulin resistance *(89,90)* and improved lipidemia and insulin resistance in HIV positive patients *(91,92)*.

Whether elevated leptin levels contribute toward the development of the inflammation associated with obesity, type 2 diabetes, and atherosclerosis needs to be fully elucidated. Suggested pathways include direct actions on macrophages to augment their phagocytic activity and to increase production of other inflammatory cytokines *(93,94)*. However, initial studies in humans do not support a role for increased leptin levels in this respect. The exact role of leptin in influencing and regulating neuroendocrine and immune function as well as energy homeostasis remains a subject of intense research efforts *(55,66,95)*.

7.3. Resistin

Resistin is an adipokine that has been proposed to correlate closely with hepatic insulin resistance, and circulating resistin levels and resistin expression in adipose tissue was proposed to be increased in type 2 diabetes and obesity *(96–98)*. However, recent data on a potential association between resistin and insulin resistance have been controversial. Additional studies are needed to fully understand the molecular and cellular mechanisms of action of this adipokine *(99,100)*.

7.4. Visfatin

Visfatin is a recently discovered adipokine. It was first described in 2005 and seems to be associated to the pathogenesis of obesity and impaired glucose homeostasis. In the initial visfatin study, it was proposed that the protein is mainly produced in visceral adipose tissue and that its expression is increased in states of insulin resistance. The authors also reported that visfatin directly binds to the insulin receptor and that it excerts insulin-like effects in vivo and in vitro *(101)*. Meanwhile other groups have reported that visfatin is also produced by a variety of other cells and that it acts as a multifunctional protein and enzyme *(9)*. To date, the role of visfatin in adipogenesis and glucose homeostasis remains controversial. The distinct role of visfatin in the pathogenesis of insulin resistance and its impact in states of energy excess needs to be fully elucidated by carefully designed studies in the future.

7.5. Retinol-Binding-Protein 4 (RBP4)

Another promising adipocytokine, the role of which also remains to be fully elucidated, is retinol-binding-protein 4 (RBP4). RBP4, the only transporter protein for vitamin A, retinol, has been proposed to be elevated in obesity and type 2 diabetes and is decreased with inflammation or infection *(102)*. RBP4 was discovered as a molecule that may regulate the expression of glucose transporter 4 (GLUT4), the most important insulin-stimulated glucose transporter, which is increased in states of insulin resistance and leads to an impaired glucose uptake into adipocytes and progressing glucose intolerance. Several but not all groups have also reported that there is an association between RBP4 and insulin resistance, obesity, and other features of the metabolic syndrome (lipid profile, HOMA index, arterial hypertension, proinflammatory markers like CRP or IL-6) *(9)*. The exact mechanism underlying these associations needs to be studied in more detail. Since data on the role of RBP4 in humans are controversial, more studies of this molecule are clearly needed to fully understand its physiological role in energy homeostasis and insulin resistance.

7.6. Tumor Necrosis Factor a (TNFα)

TNFα is a potent proinflammatory cytokine implicated in the development of insulin resistance and type 2 diabetes as well as atherosclerosis *(103)*. Circulating TNFα levels and/or levels of the soluble TNFα receptor, a long-term marker of TNFα systemic activation, are increased in both obese nondiabetic individuals *(104)* and in type 2 diabetes *(105)*. TNFα is structurally similar but functionally opposite to adiponectin, and these molecules are reciprocally regulated. Studies in genetically obese animals suggest that increased release of TNFα from adipocytes may play a major and direct role in the impairment of insulin action *(106,107)*. TNFα influences insulin signaling through impairing serine phosphorylation of insulin receptor and insulin receptor substrate-1, inhibiting thus insulin action at the organ level through autocrine and paracrine mechanisms *(108)*. TNFα may also alter glucose transporter physiology and thus impair insulin sensitivity and glucose metabolism.

7.7. Interleukin 6 (IL-6)

IL-6 is another important proinflammatory cytokine, which may also influence insulin resistance. Similar to TNFα, IL-6 regulates hepatic production of CRP and other acute phase proteins. In animal studies, IL-6 has been implicated in the development of insulin resistance in muscle and may also be involved in β cell apoptosis *(109)*. IL-6 levels are elevated in type 2 diabetic subjects and correlate with severity of inflammation as well as glucose intolerance *(110,111)*. The interrelationship between the two proinflammatory cytokines, TNFα and IL-6, is complex, since not only TNFα stimulates IL-6 production and consequently CRP production, but IL-6 also exerts a feed back inhibitory effect on TNFα production *(112)*. Intervention programs that mainly increase IL-6, such as physical activity, may have an antiinflammatory effect through suppression of TNFα, which is one of the major inducers of inflammation *(113)*.

7.8. Plasminogen Activator Inhibitor-1 (PAI-1)

Plasminogen activator inhibitor-1 (PAI-1) is another cytokine that may link obesity to type 2 diabetes and cardiovascular disease. This serine protease inhibits the fibrinolytic cascade. Elevated PAI-1 levels cause an imbalance accelerating the atherosclerotic process *(114)*. Adipose tissue is one of the major sources of PAI-1, and circulating levels are elevated in obese and diabetic subjects. It has also been noted that hyperinsulinemia, which usually accompanies insulin resistant states, is a potent stimulus for PAI-1 production by adipose tissue *(115,116)*.

8. SUMMARY AND CONCLUSIONS

Obesity-related insulin resistance and the metabolic syndrome is a complex state the pathophysiology of which remains poorly understood. The prevalence of the metabolic syndrome has been increasing during the past few years, and this has generated a tremendous research activity in this area. However, even more intense research is needed to further elucidate the molecular and cellular mechanisms underlying this important public health problem and to potentially provide better therapeutic options for the patients suffering from this syndrome.

REFERENCES

1. Weyer C, Foley JE, Bogardus PA, Tataranni REP. Enlarged subcutaneous abdominal adipocyte size, but not obesity itself, predicts type 2 diabetes independent of insulin resistance. Diabetologia 2000; 43: 1498–1506.
2. Tunstall-Pedoe H. Preventing Chronic Diseases. A Vital Investment: WHO Global Report. Geneva: World Health Organization, 2005, pp 200. CHF 30.00. ISBN 92 4 1563001. Also published on http://www.who.int/chp/chronic_disease_report/en/Int J Epidemiol 2006.
3. Mokad AH, Ford ES, Bowman BA, et al. Prevalence of obesity, diabetes and obesity-related health risk factors 2001. JAMA 2003; 289: 76–79.
4. Field AE, Coakley EH, Must A, et al. Impact of overweight on the risk of developing common chronic diseases during a 10-year period. Arch Int Med 2001; 161: 1581–1586.
5. Fulop T, Tessier D, Carpentier A. The metabolic syndrome. Path Biol 2006; 54: 375–386.
6. Laclaustra M, Corella D, Ordovas JM. Metabolic syndrome pathophysiology: The role of adipose tissue. Nutr Metab Cardiovasc Dis 2007; 17: 125–139.
7. Murdolo G, Smith U. The dysregulated adipose tissue: A connecting link between insulin resistance, type 2 diabetes mellitus and atherosclerosis. Nutr Metab Card Dis 2006; 16: S35–S38.
8. Yang X, Jansson PA, Nagaev I, et al. Evidence of impaired adipogenesis in insulin resistance. Biochem Biophys Res Commun 2004; 317: 1045–1051.
9. Kiess W, Petzold S, Töpfer M, Garten A, Blüher S, Kapellen Th, Körner A, Kratzsch J. Adipocytes and adipose tissue. Best Pract Res Clin Endocrinol Metab 2008; 22: 135–153.
10. Sweeney L, Brennan AM, Mantzoros CS. Metabolic syndrome. In Regensteiner J, Reusc J, Stewart J and Veves A. (editors): Diabetes and Exercise. Humana Press 2009 (in press).
11. Bonadonna RC, Del Prato S, Saccomani MB et al. Transmembrane glucose transport in skeletal muscle of patients with non-insulin dependent diabetes. J Clin Invest 1993; 92: 486–494.
12. Gastaldelli A, Baldi S, Pettiti M et al. Influence of obesity and type 2 diabetes on gluconeogenesis and output in humans: a quantitative study. Diabetes 2000; 49: 1367–1373.
13. Virtanen KA, Iozzo P, Hallsten K. Increased fat mass compensates for insulin resistance in abdominal obesity and type 2 diabetes: a positron-emitting tomography study. Diabetes 2005; 54: 2720–2726.
14. Barb D, Pazaitou-Panayiotou K, Mantzoros CS. Adiponectin: a link between obesity and cancer. Expert Opin Investig Drugs 2006; 15: 917–931.
15. Knowler WC, Barrett-Conner E, Fowler E, et al. Reduction in the incidence of type 2 diabetes with lifestyle intervention or metformin. NEJM 2002; 346: 393–403
16. Albu JB, Kovera AJ, Johnson JA. Fat distribution and health in obesity. Ann NY Acad Sci 2000; 904: 491–501.
17. Zeirath JR, Livingston JN, Thorne J, et al. Regional difference in insulin inhibition of non-esterified fatty acid release from human adipocytes: relation to insulin receptor hosphorylation and intracellular signaling through the insulin receptor substrate-1-pathway. Diabetologia 1998; 41: 1343–1354.
18. Arner P. Regional differences in protein production by human adipose tissue. Biochem Soc Trans 2001; 29: 72–75.
19. Motoshima H, Wu X, Sinha MK, et al. Differential regulation of adiponectin secretion from cultured human omental and subcutaneous adipocytes: effects of insulin and rosiglitazone. J Clin Endocrinol Metab 2002; 87: 5662–5667.

20. Desprès JP. Is visceral obesity the cause of the metabolic syndrome. Ann Med 2006; 38: 52–63.

21. Sewter CP, Blows F, Vidal Puig A, O'Rahilly S. Regional differences in the response of human pre-adipocytes to PPARγ and RXRα agonists. Diabetes 2002; 51: 7218–7223.

22. Bouchard C, Depress JP, Mauriege P. Genetics and nongenetic determinants of regional fat distribution. Endocr Rev 1993; 14: 72–93.

23. Perusse L, Rice T, Chagnon YC, et al. A genome-wide scan for abdominal fat assessed by computed tomography in the Quebec Family Study. Diabetes 2001; 50: 614–621.

24. Mantzoros CS, Li T, Manson JE, Meigs JB, Hu FB. Circulating adiponectin levels are associated with better glycemic control, more favorable lipid profile, and reduced inflammation in women with type 2 diabetes. J Clin Endocrinol Metab 2005; 90: 4542–4548.

25. Schulze MB, Liu S, Rimm EB, Manson JE, Willett WC, Hu FB. Glycemic index, glycemic load, and dietary fiber intake and incidence of type 2 diabetes in younger and middle-aged women. Am J Clin Nutr 2004; 80: 348–356.

26. Schulze MB, Manson JE, Ludwig DS, Colditz GA, Stampfer MJ, Willett WC, Hu FB. Sugar-sweetened beverages, weight gain, and incidence of type 2 diabetes in young and middle-aged women. JAMA 2004; 292: 927–934.

27. Schulze MB, Fung TT, Manson JE, Willett WC, Hu FB. Dietary patterns and changes in body weight in women. Obesity (Silver Spring) 2006; 14: 1444–1453.

28. Van Dam RM and Hu FB. Coffee consumption and risk of type 2 diabetes: a systematic review. JAMA 2005; 294: 97–104.

29. Lopez-Garcia E, van Dam RM, Rajpathak S, Willett WC, Manson JE, Hu FB. Changes in caffeine intake and long-term weight change in men and women. Am J Clin Nutr 2006; 83: 674–680.

30. Williams CJ, Fargnoli JL, Hwang JJ, van Dam RM, Blackburn GL, Hu FB, Mantzoros CS. Coffee consumption is associated with higher plasma adiponectin concentrations in women with or without type 2 diabetes: a prospective cohort study. Diabetes Care 2008; 31: 504–507.

31. Jiang R, Manson JE, Stampfer MJ, Liu S, Willett WC, Hu FB. Nut and peanut butter consumption and risk of type 2 diabetes in women. JAMA 2002; 288: 2554–2560.

32. Blüher M, Bullen JW, Lee JH, et al. Circulating adiponectin and expression of adiponectin receptors in human skeletal muscle: Associations with metabolic parameters and insulin resistance and regulation by physical training. J Clin Endocrinol Metab 2006; 91: 2310–2316.

33. Helmrich SP, Ragland DR, Leung RW et al. Physical activity and reduced occurrence of non-insulin dependent diabetes mellitus. N Engl J Med 1991; 325: 147–152.

34. Sjostrom CD, Lissner L, Wedel H, et al. Reduction in incidence of diabetes, hypertension and lipid disturbances after intentional weight loss induced by bariatric surgery: the SOS Intervention Study. Obes Res 1999; 7: 477–484.

35. Dixon JB, O'Brien PE. Health outcomes of severely obese type 2 diabetic subjects 1 year after laparoscopic adjustable gastric banding. Diabetes Care 2002; 25(2): 358–63.

36. Hoekstra T, Geleijnse JM, Schouten EG, Kok FJ, Kluft C. Relationship of C-reactive protein with components of the metabolic syndrome in normal-weight and overweight elderly. Nutr Metab Cardiovasc Dis 2005; 15: 270–278.

37. Weisberg SP, McCann D, Desai M, et al. Obesity is associated with macrophage accumulation in adipose tissue. J Clin Invest 2003; 112: 1798–1808.

38. Xu H, Barnes GT, Yang Q, et al. Chronic inflammation in fat plays a crucial role in the development of obesity-related insulin resistance. J Clin Invest 2003; 112: 1821–1830.

39. Pickup JC, Mattock MB, Chusney GD, et al. NIDDM as a disease of the innate immune system: associations of the acute phase reactants and interleukin-6 with metabolic syndrome X. Diabetologia 1997; 40: 1286–1292.

40. Shai I, Schulze MB, Manson JE, Rexrode KM, Stampfer MJ, Mantzoros C, Hu FB. A prospective study of soluble tumor necrosis factor-alpha receptor II (sTNF-RII) and risk of coronary heart disease among women with type 2 diabetes. Diabetes Care 2005; 28: 1376–1382.

41. Rotter V, Nagaev I, Smith U. Interleukin-6 (IL-6) induces insulin resistance in 3T3-L1 adipocytes and is, like IL-8 and tumor necrosis factor-α, overexpressed in human fat cells from insulin-resistant subjects. J Biol Chem 2003; 278: 45777–45784.

42. Dandona P, Aljada A. A rational approach to pathogenesis and treatment of type 2 diabetes mellitus, insulin resistance, inflammation, and artherosclerosis. Am J Cardiol 2002; 90: 27G–33G.

43. Bays H, Mandarino L, DeFronzo RA. Role of the adipocyte, free fatty acids, and ectopic fat in the pathogenesis of type 2 diabetes mellitus: Peroxismal proliferatiors-activated receptor agonists provide a rational therapeutic approach. J Clin Endocrinol Metab 2004; 89: 463–478.

44. Boden G, Chen X. Effects of fat on glucose uptake and utilization in patients with non-insulin dependent diabetes. J Clin Invest 1995; 96: 1261–1268.

45. Paolisso G, Tataranni PA, Foley JE, et al. A high concentration of fasting plasma non-esterified fatty acids is a risk factor for the development of NIDDM. Diabetologia 1995; 38: 1213–1217.

46. Greco AV, Mingrone G, Giancaterini A, et al. Insulin resistance in morbid obesity. Reversal with intramyocellular fat depletion. Diabetes 2002; 51: 144–151.

47. Seppala-Lindroos A, Vehkavaara S, Hakkinen A-M, et al. Fat accumulation in the liver is associated with defects in insulin suppression of glucose production and serum free fatty acids independent of obesity in normal men. J Clin Endocrinol Metab 2002; 87: 3023–3028.

48. Robertson RP, Harmon J, Tran OP, Poitout V. Beta-cell glucose toxicity, lipotoxicity, and chronic oxidative stress in type 2 diabetes. Diabetes 2004; 53: S119–S124.

49. Stumvoll M, Goldstein BJ, van Haeften TW. Type 2 diabetes: principles of pathogenesis and therapy. Lancet 2005; 365: 1333–1346.

50. Unger RH. Lipotoxicity in the pathogenesis of obesity-dependent NIDDM: genetic and clinical implications. Diabetes 1996; 45: 273–283.

51. Shimabukuro M, Zhou YT, Leve M, Unger RH. Fatty acid induced β cell apoptosis. Proc Natl Acad Sci USA 1998; 95: 2498–2502.

52. Avramoglu RK, Basciano H, Aedli K. Lipid andlipoprotein dysregulation in insulin resistant states. Clin Chim Acta 2006; 368: 1–19.

53. Mantzoros CS. Syndromes of severe insulin resistance. In De Groot L (editor): Endocrinology, 5th Edition. Philadelphia: Saunders, 2005, pp. 1133–1149.

54. Ginsberg HN. New perspective on atherogenesis: Role of abnormal triglyceride-rich lipoprotein metabolism. Circulation 2002; 106: 2137–2142.

55. Fruhbeck G, Gomez-Ambrosi J, Muruzabal FJ, Burrell MA. The adipocyte: A model for integration of endocrine and metabolic signaling in energy metabolism regulation. Am J Physiol 2001; 280: E827–47.

56. Hotta K, Funahashi T, Bodkin NL, et al. Circulating concentrations of the adipocyte protein adiponectin are decreased in parallel with reduced insulin sensitivity during the progression to type 2 diabetes in rhesus monkeys. Diabetes 2001; 50: 1126–1133.

57. Yang WS, Lee WJ, Funahashi T, Tanaka S, Matsuzawa Y, Chao CL, Chen CL, Tai TY, Chaung LM. Weight reduction increases plasma levels of an adipose-derived anti-inflammatory protein, adiponectin. J Clin Endocrinol Metab 2001; 86: 3815–3819.

58. Brennan AM, Mantzoros CS. Leptin and adiponectin: Their role in diabetes. Curr Diab Rep 2007; 7: 1–2.

59. Yamauchi T, Kamon J, Waki H, et al. The fat derived hormone adiponectin reverses insulin resistance associated with both lipoatrophy and obesity. Nat Med 2001; 7: 941–946.

60. Nadler ST, Stoehr JP, Schueler KL, et al. The expression of adipogenic genes is decreased in obesity and diabetes mellitus. Proc Natl Acad Sci 2000; 97: 11371–11376.

61. Maeda N, Shimomura I, Kishida K, et al. Diet-induced insulin resistance in mice lacking adiponectin/ACRP30. Nat Med 2002; 8: 731–737.

62. Weyer C, Funahashi T, Tanaka S, Hotta K, Matsuzawa Y, Pratley RE, Tataranni AP. Hypoadiponectinemia in obesity and type 2 diabetes: close association with insulin resistance and hyperinsulinemia. J Clin Endocrinol Metab 2001; 86: 1930–1935.

63. Abbasi F, Chu JW, Mclaughlin T, Lamendola C, Reaven G, Hayden JM, Reaven P. Obesity versus insulin resistance in modulation of plasma adiponectin concentration. Diabetes 2002; 52(suppl 1): A81.

64. Arita Y, Kihara S, Ouchi N, et al. Paradoxical decrease of an adipose – specific protein, adiponectin, in obesity. Biochem Biopys Res Commun 1999; 257: 79–83.

65. Hotta K, Funahashi T, Arita Y, et al. Plasma concentration of a novel adipose-specific protein, adiponectin, in type 2 diabetic patients. Arterioscler Thromb Vasc Biol 2000; 20: 1595–1599.

66. Ronti T, Lupattelli G, Mannarino E. The endocrine function of adipose tissue: an update. Clin Endocrinol (Oxf) 2006; 64: 355–365.

67. Spyridopoulos TN, Petridou E, Skalkidou A, Dessypris N, Chrousos GP, Mantzoros CS. and the Obesity and Cancer Oncology Group. Low adiponectin levels are associated with renal cell carcinoma: A case-control study. Int J Cancer 2007; 120: 1573–1578.

68. Michalakis K, Williams KJ, Mitsiades N, Blakeman J, Balafouta-Tselenis S, Giannopoulos A, Mantzoros CS. Serum adiponectin concentrations and tissue expression of adiponectin receptors are reduced in patients with prostate cancer: A case-control study. Cancer Epidemiol Biomarkers Prev 2007; 16: 308–313.

69. Korner A, Pazaitou- Panayiotou K, Kelesidis T, et al. Total and high molecular weight adiponectin in breast cancer: in vitro and in vivo studies. J Clin Endocrinol Metab 2007; 92: 1041–1048.

70. Tworoger SS, Eliassen AH, Kelesidis T, Colditz GA, Willett WC, Mantzoros CS Hankinson SE, . Plasma adiponectin concentrations and risk of incident breast cancer J Clin Endocrin Metab 2007; 92: 1510–1516.

71. Kelesidis I, Kelesidis T, Mantzoros CS. Adiponectin and cancer: a systematic review. Br J Cancer 2006; 94: 1221–1225.

72. Yamauchi T, Kamon J, Minokoshi Y, et al. Adiponectin stimulates glucose utilization and fatty-acid oxidation by activating AMP-activated protein kinase. Nat Med 2002; 8: 1288–1295.

73. Yokota T, Oritani K, Takahashi I, Ishikawa J, Matsuyama A, Ouchi N. Adiponectin, a new member of the family of soluble defense collagens, negatively regulated the growth of myelmonocytic progenitors and the functions of macrophages. Blood 2000; 96: 1723–1732.

74. Qi L, van Darn RM, Liu S, Franz M, Mantzoros C, Hu FB. Whole-grain, bran, and cereal fiber intakes and markers of systemic inflammation in diabetic women. Diabetes Care 2006; 29: 207–211.

75. Qi L, Meigs JB, Liu S, Manson JE, Mantzoros C, Hu FB. Dietary fibers and glycemic load, obesity, and plasma adiponectin levels in women with type 2 diabetes. Diabetes Care 2006; 29: 1501–1515.

76. Manztoros CS, Williams CJ, Manson JE, Meigs JB, Hu FB. Adherence to the Mediterranean dietary pattern is positively associated with plasma adiponectin concentrations in diabetic women. Am J Clin Nutr 2006; 84: 328–335.

77. Monzillo LU, Hamdy O, Horton ES, et al. Effect of lifestyle modification on adipokine levels in obese subjects with insulin resistance. Obes Res 2003; 11: 1048–1054.

78. Lindsay RS, Funahashi T, Hanson RL, Matsuwaza Y, Tanaka S, Tataranni PA, Knowler WC, Krakoff J. Adiponectin and development of type 2 diabetes in the Pima Indian population. Lancet 2002; 360: 57–58.

79. Bullen J, Bluher S, Kelesidis T, Mantzoros CS. Regulation of adiponectin and its receptors in response to development of diet induced obesity in mice. Am J Physiol Endocrinol Metab 2007; 292: E1079–E1086.

80. Blüher S, Bullen J, Mantzoros C. Altered levels of adiponectin and adiponectin receptors may underlie the effect of ciliary neurotrophic factor (CNTF) to enhance insulin sensitivity in diet induced obese mice. Horm Metab Res 2008; 40: 225–227.

81. Brennan AM, Mantzoros CS. The role of leptin in human physiology and pathophysiology: emerging clinical applications in leptin deficient states. Nature (Clinical Practice Endocrinology and Metabolism) 2006; 2: 1–5.

82. Lonnqvist F, Arner P, Nordfors L, Schalling M. Overexpression of the obese (ob) gene in adipose tissue of human obese subjects. Nat Med 1995; 1: 950–993.

83. Ceddia Rb, William Jr WN, Curi R. Comparing effects of leptin and insulin on glucose metabolism in skeletal muscle: Evidence for an effect of leptin on glucose uptake and decarboxylation. Int J Obesity Related Metab Disord 1999; 23: 75–82.

84. Kamohara S, Burcelin R, Halaas JL, Freidman JM. Acute stimulation of glucose metabolism in mice by leptin treatment. Nature 1997; 389: 374–77.

85. Muoio DM, Dohm GL. Peripheral metabolic actions of leptin. Best Practice Res Clin Endocrinol Metab 2002; 16: 653–66.

86. Clement K, Vaisse C, Lahlou N, et al. A mutation in the human leptin receptor gene causes obesity and pituitary dysfunction. Nature 1998; 392: 398–401.

87. Farooqui IS, Jebb SA, Langmack G, et al. Effects of recombinant leptin therapy in a child with congenital leptin deficiency. N Engl J Med 1999; 341: 879–884.

88. Mantzoros CS, Flier JS. Editorial: Leptin as a therapeutic agent-trials and tribulations. J Clin Endocrinol Metab 2000; 85: 4000–4002.

89. Oral EA, Simha V, Ruiz E, et al. Leptin replacement therapy for lipodystrophy. N Engl J Med 2002; 346: 57–78.

90. Javor ED, Cochran EK, Musso C, et al. Long-term efficacy of leptin replacement in patients with generaliszed lipodystrophy. Diabetes 2005; 54: 1994–2002.

91. Lee JH, Chan JL, Sourlas E, Raptopoulos V, Mantzoros CS. Recombinant methionyl human leptin therapy in replacement doses improves insulin resistance and metabolic profile in patients with lipoatrophy and metabolic syndrome induced by the highly active antiretroviral therapy. J Clin Endocrinol Metab 2006; 91: 2605–2611.

92. Tsiodras S, Mantzoros C. The role of leptin and adiponectin in the HAART induced metabolic syndrome. Am J Infect Dis 2006; 2: 141–152.

93. Santos-Alvarez J, Goberna R, Sanchez-Margalet V. Human leptin stimulates proliferation and activation of human circulating monocytes. Cell Immunol 1999; 194: 6–11.

94. Giansford T, Willson TA, Metcalf D, et al. Leptin can induce proliferation, differentiation, and functional activation of hemopoietic cells. Proc Natl Acad Sci USA 1996; 93: 14564–14568.

95. Chan JL, Mantzoros CS. Role of leptin in energy-deprivation states: normal human physiology and clinical implications for hypothalamic amenorrhoea and anorexia nervosa. Lancet 2005; 366: 74–85.

96. Smith SR, Bai F, Charbonneau C, et al. A promoter genotype and oxidative stress potentially link resistin to human insulin resistance. Diabetes 2003; 52: 1611–1618.

97. Wang H, Chu WS, Hemphill C, Elbein SC. Human resistin gene: molecular scanning and evaluation of association with insulin sensitivity and type 2 diabetes in Caucasians. J Clin Endocrinol Metab 2002; 87: 2520–2524.

98. Vidal-Puig A, O'Rahilly S, Resistin: a new link between obesity and insulin resistance. Clin Endocrionol (Oxf) 2001; 55: 437–438.

99. Lee JH, Bullen Jr JW, Stoyneva VL, Mantzoros CS. Circulating resistin in lean, obese, and insulin-resistant mouse models: lack of association with insulinemia and glycemia. Am J Physiol Endocrinol Metab 2005; 288: E625–E632.

100. Lee JH, Chan JL, Yiannakouris N, et al. Circulating resistin levels are not associated with obesity or insulin resistance in humans and are not regulated by fasting or leptin administration: cross-sectional and interventional studies in normal, insulin-resistant, and diabetic subjects. J Clin Endocrinol Metab 2003; 88: 4848–4856.

101. Fukuhara A, Matsuda M, Nishizawa M, et al. Visfatin: a protein secreted by visceral fat that mimics the effects of insulin. Science 2005; 307: 426–430.

102. Yang Q, Graham TE, Mody N, et al. Serum retinol binding protein 4 contributes to insulin resistance in obesity and type 2 diabetes. Nature 2005; 21; 436: 356–362.

103. Uzui H, Harpf A, Liu M, et al. Increased expression of membrane type 3-matrix metalloproteinase in human atherosclerotic plaque: role of activated macrophages and inflammatory cytokines. Circulation 2002; 106: 3024–3030.

104. Hotamisligil GS, Arner P, Caro JF, et al. Increased adipose tissue expression of tumor necrosis factor-alpha in human obesity and insulin resistance. J Clin Invest 1995; 95: 2409–1245.

105. Miyazaki Y, Pipek R, Mandarino LJ, DeFronzo RA. Tumor necrosis factor α and insulin resistance in obese type 2 diabetic patients. Int J Obesity 2003; 27: 88–94.

106. Hotamisligil GS, Peraldi P, Budavari A, et al. IRS-1 mediated inhibition of insulin receptor tyrosine kinase activity in TNF-α and obesity induced insulin resistance. Science 1996; 271: 665–668.

107. Uysal KT, Wiesbrock SM, Marino MW, Hotamisligil GS. Protection from obesity-induced insulin resistance in mice lacking TNF-alpha function. Nature 1997; 389: 610–614.

108. Hofmann C, Lorenz K, Braithwaite SS, et al. Altered gene expression for tumor necrosis factor-alpha and its receptors during drug and dietary modulation of insulin resistance. Endocrinology 1994; 134: 264–270.

109. Sandler S, Bendtzen K, Eizirik DL, Welsh M. Interleukin-6 affects insulin secretion and glucose metabolism of rat pancreatic islets in vitro. Endocrinology 1990; 126: 1288–1294.

110. Pradhan AD, Manson JE, Rifai N, et al. C-Reative protein, interleukin 6 and the risk of developing type 2 diabetes. JAMA 2001; 286: 327–334.

111. Pickup JC, Chusney GD, Thomas SM, Burt D. Plasma interleukin 6, tumor necrosis factor and blood cytokine production in type 2 diabetes. Life Sci 2000; 67: 291–300.

112. Suzuki K, Nakaji S, Yamada M, et al. Systemic inflammatory response to exhaustive exercise. Cytokine kinetics. Exerc Immunol Rev 2002; 8: 6–48.

113. Starkie R, Ostrowski SR, Jauffred S, et al. Exercise and IL-6 infusion inhibit endotoxin-nduced

TNF-alpha production in humans. FASEB J 2003; 17: 884–886.
114. Yudkin JS. Abnormalities of coagulation and fibrinolysis in insulin resistance. Evidence for a common antecedent? Diabetes Care 1999; 22: C25–C30.
115. Alessi MC, Bastelica D, Morange P, et al. Plasminogen activator inhibitor 1, transforming growth factor-β1 amd ABMI are closely associated in human adipose tissue during morbid obesity. Diabetes 2000; 49: 1374–1380.
116. Alessi MC, Peiretti F, Morange P, et al. Production of plasminogen activator inhibitor1 by human adipose tissue: possible link between visceral fat accumulation and vascular disease. Diabetes 1997; 46: 860–867.

III

PUBLIC HEALTH PERSPECTIVE

6 Targeting Childhood Obesity Through Lifestyle Modification

Eirini Bathrellou and Mary Yannakoulia

KEY POINTS

- Evidence regarding the efficacy of intervention programs targeting childhood obesity suggests that treatment should focus on dietary and physical activity changes, along with behavior modification and parental support.
- Different types of dietary interventions, aiming at negative energy balance and improvement of dietary habits, have been applied, such as calorie limit combined with an exchange food system, low energy balanced diets, or even ad libitum low-glycemic diets.
- The physical activity component includes an increase in structured or nonstructured activities and a decrease in sedentary activities. To support the child to implement and maintain the desired lifestyle changes, behavior modification techniques have been incorporated in the treatment programs, most common of which are self-monitoring, goal setting, stimulus control, and problem solving.
- Parental involvement is recommended to provide support to the child's effort, although several types of parental roles have been evaluated with variable success.
- Currently no consensus has been reached on the most effective intervention, and most studies report short-term results with limited generalizability.
- There is an urgent need for well-designed randomized trials to evaluate the long-term effectiveness of lifestyle interventions for the management of children's overweight.

Key Words: Childhood Obesity, Dietary intake, Physical activity, Behavior modification, Parental involvement, Low-glycemic diets

1. INTRODUCTION

Childhood obesity has been recognized as a public health priority for many countries. Prevalence of overweight has increased in Europe, the United States, and many other parts of the world *(1–3)*. During the last decades, all industrialized and many low-income countries have doubled or even tripled their numbers, while countries which traditionally confronted undernutrition problems now encounter obesity problems as well *(4)*. In addition, comparisons of the distribution of body mass index (BMI) between earlier and later

From: *Nutrition and Health: Nutrition and Metabolism*
Edited by: C.S. Mantzoros, DOI: 10.1007/978-1-60327-453-1_6,
© Humana Press, a part of Springer Science+Business Media, LLC 2009

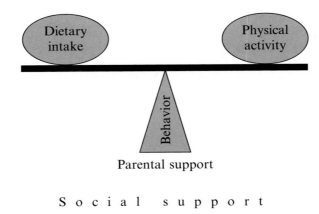

Fig. 1. Interaction of the parameters targeted for the management of children's overweight.

studies show a greater shift in the upper part of the distribution, implying that heavier children have now become even heavier *(5)*.

This global epidemic would not have justified the alarming interest of scientists, health care professionals, and the general public on the prevention and treatment of childhood obesity, if it were not for its multilevel consequences. Obesity has both short and long-term health consequences, affecting the child both in its present and future adult life *(6)*. One of the most well documented short-term effects refers to the cardiovascular risk factors, namely hypertension, dyslipidemia, endothelial dysfunction, hyperinsulinemia, and insulin resistance *(7–9)*. Metabolic syndrome, a clustering of cardiovascular risk factors frequently seen in adults, has also been identified in children and it correlates with obesity status *(10–12)*. Childhood obesity also has harmful psychosocial and economic consequences *(13,14)*, and it tracks well into adulthood *(15,16)*.

Even though genetic predisposition and environmental influences interact to cause excess weight, the accelerated increase in the prevalence of childhood obesity during the last decades cannot be explained by a genetic shift *(17)*. It rather reflects profound changes in environmental factors, resulting in positive energy balance. Thus, treatment should focus on the modifiable factors of the energy equilibrium, i.e., dietary intake and physical activity. Several approaches have been proposed for inducing dietary and physical activity changes, along with behavior modification and the participation of parents (Fig. 1). Purpose of this chapter is to discuss these approaches in the context of lifestyle interventions in managing overweight in children.

2. DIETARY CHANGES

Although hypocaloric diets have been widely used in achieving weight loss, the optimal type of diet remains unknown. Research in adults indicates that short-term success can be achieved with diets varying widely in composition, from very low-fat to very low-carbohydrate content; however, most individuals experience weight regain over the long term *(18–21)*. In children, combinations of calorie limits and food exchange systems have been applied. The traffic light diet is a food exchange system, first developed by Epstein and colleagues *(22)*; foods are divided into three categories according to their energy and fat content: greens can be consumed freely, oranges should be consumed with caution, and reds should be avoided. A daily or weekly number of servings for each of these food groups is, then, recommended. The traffic light diet has evolved in terms of number of calories or red foods *(23)*, allowing for a higher calorie limit (up to 1,500 kcal) and more red foods *(24)*, while modified versions have been developed using either a specific diet *(25,26)* or no calorie limit *(27)*.

A low energy diet, ranging in calorie content from 1,200 to 2,000 kcal, applied either as a tailored or an exchange-based regime, has been also used *(25,28–32)*. Most of the recommended diets so far were characterized as "prudent" or "balanced," with a caloric deficit of around 30% less of the reported intake or 15% less than the estimated required intake, providing approximately 30% of calories from fat. However, available evidence from randomized trials do not support current recommendations for low-fat energy restricted diets *(33)*.

Less restrictive dietary interventions have been successfully undertaken. Recent guidelines suggest that dietary treatment should focus on eating behaviors, such as breakfast skipping and meal frequency, eating out and portion size *(34)*, rather than calorie restriction per se. The need for putting less restraint in the dietary manipulation is also supported by evidence indicating that flexible, not rigid, dietary restraint is associated with lower BMI values and a more successful long-term weight control, both in adults and children *(35,36)*, as well as by concerns that obese children are at high risk for developing eating disorders or show resistance to treatment *(37)*. Under this perspective, nonprescription approaches, promoting the concept of "eating differently, not necessarily less" and a healthy eating *(38,39)*, or focusing on ad libitum low-glycemic diets have been investigated. With regard to the latter, Ebbeling et al. examined the long-term effects of a reduced glycemic load, nonenergy restricted diet with those of a reduced-fat, externally imposed hypocaloric diet, in a small-scale randomized controlled trial of 16 obese adolescents *(40)*. Over 12 months, BMI and fat mass significantly decreased in the reduced-glycemic load diet group, whereas neither measure changed significantly in the conventional diet group. Furthermore, insulin resistance, as assessed by the homeostasis model assessment, increased less with the low-glycemic load diet, even after statistical adjustment for BMI. These findings indicate that reducing the glycemic load or index of a diet, without externally imposing energy restriction, may yield several health benefits in young people. Adolescents, in particular, may more easily adhere to such a dietary pattern, as they may feel less hungry and also more flexible in their dietary choices, thus reaching more easily a negative energy balance allowing for a weight loss.

3. PHYSICAL ACTIVITY INTERVENTIONS

Including a physical activity-related component in weight management programs for overweight children is of major importance, because of its obvious effect on energy balance and its beneficial impact on cardiovascular risk factors, even independently of weight reduction *(41,42)*. Recommendations regarding physical activity in children target a generally active lifestyle, and suggest at least 60 min of moderate intensity physical activity, if possible everyday, and not exceeding 2 h of daily screen time *(34)*. Within school setting, individual or team noncompetitive sports, and recreational activities are suggested *(43)*, as well as an active participation in physical education classes *(44)*.

Results of a 10-year follow up suggest that physical activity as a lifestyle change is a promising, feasible, and convenient way for managing overweight in children *(45)*. On the one hand, both structured and nonstructured activities have been beneficial in reducing BMI in children *(46)*. On the other hand, targeting sedentary activities has been proven at least as *(47)* or even more *(48)* effective in reducing percent overweight in children compared with targeting an increase in physical activity per se. It has, further, been proposed that changes in physical activity habits in children reach a plateau: a set-point of physical activity competence may exist within each child, irrespective of the environmental opportunities *(49)*, acting as a mediator of his/her physical activity levels.

4. BEHAVIOR MODIFICATION

Both dietary intake and physical activity constitute the result of numerous corresponding behaviors; therefore, studying behavior in the context of combating obesity has attracted great scientific interest. The beneficial effect of adding behavioral modification techniques in a conventional program for the treatment of childhood obesity has been originally described in the early 1990s *(50,51)*, and has been confirmed many times ever since *(52)*. Behavioral and cognitive-behavioral components have been considered as important components of the lifestyle treatment programs *(53)*. There is also some preliminary evidence proposing that the use of a motivational interviewing style by pediatricians and dietitians may be another promising office-based strategy for preventing overweight children to become obese *(54)*, even though its efficacy as a treatment modality has not been proven yet *(55)*.

Several techniques have been used in the childhood obesity treatment programs under the aim of modifying eating patterns and increasing physical activity levels. These include contracting, self-monitoring, stimulus control, goal setting, reinforcement, parental training, homework exercises, problem solving, and overcoming stressful situations. Although it is difficult to isolate a specific technique and assess its effectiveness, some of them have been evaluated and proven to have a beneficial effect in pediatric populations, like self-monitoring *(56)*, stimulus control *(57)*, and problem-solving *(58)*.

5. THE ROLE OF PARENTS

Parents affect children's eating and physical activity patterns by several means, namely formulating children's environment, being role models, and controlling their dietary intake *(59)*. Parental participation is considered as an essential component in a program aiming at modifying child's lifestyle habits and combating obesity. A great body of research investigates the most effective parental role. Epstein and colleagues highly supported the role of parents as targets for managing their own weight along with their child's effort to manage body weight *(45)*: a significantly higher reduction in percent overweight of children was revealed after 10 years of follow-up when parents and children were both targeted for weight loss compared to when only children were targeted. Israel et al. found that when parents were helpers, rather than cotargets, the therapeutic outcome was slightly enhanced *(60)*. Moreover, training children in self-regulatory techniques compared with assigning parents most responsibility for change was proven essential in maintaining percent overweight loss after treatment *(29)*. In the studies of Golan and colleagues, parents were the exclusive agents of change, without any direct child involvement *(61)*. It was found that this approach was more efficient in managing children's weight compared with the approach of children being the exclusive agents.

As studies are not conclusive with regard to the most effective parental role or the exact degree of parental involvement, recommendations so far suggest a rather supportive role of parents, with less involvement as the child gets older *(17)*, and this is the most widely adopted approach *(25,32,39,62,63)*.

6. IMPLEMENTATION OF PROGRAMS

The structure of the programs targeting childhood obesity varies greatly. In most cases, therapeutic programs are conducted in groups *(25,60,62–65)*, and seldom in individual sessions *(28,39)* or in conjunction *(38,57)*. Although data comparing individualized and group treatment are scarce, there seems to be a slight advantage in favor of the group format. Goldfield et al. *(66)* compared the effectiveness of the same family-based behavioral treatment conducted only in groups or in a mixed format, combining group and individualized sessions. As weight outcomes did not differ between the two approaches, group only format was proven more cost-effective. Moreover, Braet and Van Winckel *(39)* found a favorable long-term tendency for the group approach, when it was compared with an individualized, and to a summer camp approach. Diverging from the conventional setup, and in the context of applying a more cost-effective approach with greater generalization and dissemination, innovative delivery approaches using media technologies have also been evaluated. Frequent telephone and mail contact were proven feasible and effective in promoting use of behavioral skills for weight control in a group of adolescents, when compared with a single-advice typical care session *(67)*. An interactive Website-based behavioral treatment was effective in improving some weight-related parameters in the short term, but Web hits decreased dramatically in the long-term *(68)*.

The length of the intervention ranges from 6 weeks to 18 months, with the majority of studies lasting between 3 and 6 months *(23)*. Sessions are usually conducted on a weekly basis. Combinations of weekly and biweekly *(29)* or even monthly *(45)* sessions has also been applied, lengthening intervention time. As long-term effectiveness is the ultimate outcome of obesity interventions, addressing weight loss maintenance postinterventionally emerges as a necessity, in accordance to adult studies which, in this regard, propose the extension of treatment contact or content *(69)*. Wilfley et al. *(70)* successfully tested the efficacy of adding an active maintenance phase following a standard family-based behavioral treatment, in a randomized controlled trial. Interestingly, both maintenance methods studied, i.e., behavioral skills or social facilitation, produced many benefits, either in weight or psychosocial outcomes, compared with no maintenance approach. Still, a decline in treatment effectiveness was observed, regardless of the treatment duration or content, suggesting the need for the development of continuous care models for children.

7. CONCLUDING REMARKS

As the degree of obesity of children who participate in weight control programs has increased over the last two decades, in accordance to the increase in childhood obesity rates observed in the general population, it is not surprising that more children in the earlier studies were below the criteria for being at risk for overweight or overweight after treatment *(71)*. As young people nowadays live in a more obesogenic environment, promoting greater food intake and more sedentary activities, contemporary programs need to be more powerful to produce treatment effects similar to those observed in the studies during 1970s and 1980s.

A lot of work needs to be done in refining existing programs. An earlier review concluded that the reduction of sedentary behavior appeared to be the most effective intervention for achieving and maintaining weight loss in children and that the degree of parental involvement in childhood obesity interventions remains uncertain *(72)*. A more recent pointed out that, although the combination of diet, exercise, behavioral techniques, and parental involvement remains the cornerstone for improving the effectiveness of a weight-loss program, there is still a limited number of studies including a control group *(73)*. Furthermore, most studies are small and noncomparable, they report short-term results with limited generalizability, rarely reporting health outcomes, such as cardiovascular risk factors *(74)*. With regard to diet, interventions including dietetic treatment can be effective, but there are not many quality studies undertaken to date, with adequate long-term follow-up data *(23)*. Therefore, there is an urgent need for well-designed randomized trials to evaluate the lasting effectiveness of dietary interventions *(33)* and lifestyle programs.

In conclusion, for the time being, the combination of the four parameters discussed, i.e., dietary and physical activity changes, behavioral modification and parental support, constitute the best available therapeutic strategy for childhood obesity. The most recent recommendations on the treatment of childhood obesity are based on this scheme *(34)*, proposed though to be implemented at different settings, from a primary care provider to a multidisciplinary team, and supplemented when needed with more invasive strategies.

REFERENCES

1. Ebbeling, C.B., D.B. Pawlak, and D.S. Ludwig. Childhood obesity: public-health crisis, common sense cure. Lancet, 2002, 360(9331): p. 473–82.
2. Jackson-Leach, R. and T. Lobstein. Estimated burden of paediatric obesity and co-morbidities in Europe. Part 1. The increase in the prevalence of child obesity in Europe is itself increasing. Int J Pediatr Obes, 2006, 1(1): p. 26–32.
3. Ogden, C.L., et al. Prevalence of overweight and obesity in the United States, 1999–2004. JAMA, 2006, 295(13): p. 1549–55.
4. Wang, Y. and T. Lobstein. Worldwide trends in childhood overweight and obesity. Int J Pediatr Obes, 2006, 1(1): p. 11–25.
5. Flegal, K.M. and R.P. Troiano. Changes in the distribution of body mass index of adults and children in the US population. Int J Obes Relat Metab Disord, 2000, 24(7): p. 807–18.
6. Reilly, J.J., et al. Health consequences of obesity. Arch Dis Child, 2003, 88(9): p. 748–52.
7. Freedman, D.S., et al. The relation of overweight to cardiovascular risk factors among children and adolescents: the Bogalusa Heart Study. Pediatrics, 1999, 103(6 Pt 1): p. 1175–82.
8. Giannini, C., et al. Obese related effects of inflammatory markers and insulin resistance on increased carotid intima media thickness in pre-pubertal children. Atherosclerosis, 2008, 197(1): p. 448–56.
9. Valle Jimenez, M., et al. Endothelial dysfunction is related to insulin resistance and inflammatory biomarker levels in obese prepubertal children. Eur J Endocrinol, 2007, 156(4): p. 497–502.
10. Weiss, R., et al. Obesity and the metabolic syndrome in children and adolescents. N Engl J Med, 2004, 350(23): p. 2362–74.
11. Invitti, C., et al. Metabolic syndrome in obese Caucasian children: prevalence using WHO-derived criteria and association with nontraditional cardiovascular risk factors. Int J Obes (Lond), 2006, 30(4): p. 627–33.
12. Pervanidou, P., C. Kanaka-Gantenbein, and G.P. Chrousos. Assessment of metabolic profile in a clinical setting. Curr Opin Clin Nutr Metab Care, 2006, 9(5): p. 589–95.

13. Strauss, R.S. and H.A. Pollack. Social marginalization of overweight children. Arch Pediatr Adolesc Med, 2003, 157(8): p. 746–52.
14. Wang, G. and W.H. Dietz. Economic burden of obesity in youths aged 6 to 17 years: 1979–1999. Pediatrics, 2002, 109(5): p. E81–1.
15. Whitaker, R.C., et al. Predicting obesity in young adulthood from childhood and parental obesity. N Engl J Med, 1997, 337(13): p. 869–73.
16. Deshmukh-Taskar, P., et al. Tracking of overweight status from childhood to young adulthood: the Bogalusa Heart Study. Eur J Clin Nutr, 2006, 60(1): p. 48–57.
17. Barlow, S.E. Expert committee recommendations regarding the prevention, assessment, and treatment of child and adolescent overweight and obesity: summary report. Pediatrics, 2007, 120(Suppl 4): p. S164–92.
18. Baron, J.A., et al. A randomized controlled trial of low carbohydrate and low fat/high fiber diets for weight loss. Am J Public Health, 1986, 76(11): p. 1293–6.
19. McManus, K., L. Antinoro, and F. Sacks. A randomized controlled trial of a moderate-fat, low-energy diet compared with a low fat, low-energy diet for weight loss in overweight adults. Int J Obes Relat Metab Disord, 2001, 25(10): p. 1503–11.
20. Foster, G.D., et al. A randomized trial of a low-carbohydrate diet for obesity. N Engl J Med, 2003, 348(21): p. 2082–90.
21. Stern, L., et al. The effects of low-carbohydrate versus conventional weight loss diets in severely obese adults: one-year follow-up of a randomized trial. Ann Intern Med, 2004, 140(10): p. 778–85.
22. Epstein, L.H., et al. Child and parent weight loss in family-based behavior modification programs. J Consult Clin Psychol, 1981, 49(5): p. 674–85.
23. Collins, C.E., et al. Measuring effectiveness of dietetic interventions in child obesity: a systematic review of randomized trials. Arch Pediatr Adolesc Med, 2006, 160(9): p. 906–22.
24. Epstein, L.H., et al. The effect of reinforcement or stimulus control to reduce sedentary behavior in the treatment of pediatric obesity. Health Psychol, 2004, 23(4): p. 371–80.
25. Reinehr, T., et al. Long-term follow-up of overweight children: after training, after a single consultation session, and without treatment. J Pediatr Gastroenterol Nutr, 2003, 37(1): p. 72–4.
26. Jiang, J.X., et al. A two year family based behaviour treatment for obese children. Arch Dis Child, 2005, 90(12): p. 1235–8.
27. Duffy, G. and S.H. Spence. The effectiveness of cognitive self-management as an adjunct to a behavioural intervention for childhood obesity: a research note. J Child Psychol Psychiatry, 1993, 34(6): p. 1043–50.
28. Flodmark, C.E., et al. Prevention of progression to severe obesity in a group of obese schoolchildren treated with family therapy. Pediatrics, 1993, 91(5): p. 880–4.
29. Israel, A.C., et al. An evaluation of enhanced self-regulation training in the treatment of childhood obesity. J Pediatr Psychol, 1994, 19(6): p. 737–49.
30. Golan, M., et al. Parents as the exclusive agents of change in the treatment of childhood obesity. Am J Clin Nutr, 1998, 67(6): p. 1130–5.
31. Eliakim, A., et al. The effect of a combined intervention on body mass index and fitness in obese children and adolescents – a clinical experience. Eur J Pediatr, 2002, 161(8): p. 449–54.
32. Nemet, D., et al. Short- and long-term beneficial effects of a combined dietary-behavioral-physical activity intervention for the treatment of childhood obesity. Pediatrics, 2005, 115(4): p. e443–9.
33. Gibson, L.J., et al. Lack of evidence on diets for obesity for children: a systematic review. Int J Epidemiol, 2006, 35(6): p. 1544–52.
34. Spear, B.A., et al. Recommendations for treatment of child and adolescent overweight and obesity. Pediatrics, 2007, 120(Suppl 4): p. S254–88.
35. Westenhoefer, J. Establishing dietary habits during childhood for long-term weight control. Ann Nutr Metab, 2002, 46(Suppl 1): p. 18–23.
36. Westenhoefer, J., A.J. Stunkard, and V. Pudel. Validation of the flexible and rigid control dimensions of dietary restraint. Int J Eat Disord, 1999, 26(1): p. 53–64.
37. Decaluwe, V. and C. Braet. The cognitive behavioural model for eating disorders: a direct evaluation in children and adolescents with obesity. Eat Behav, 2005, 6(3): p. 211–20.
38. Braet, C. Treatment of obese children: a new rationale. Clin Child Psychol Psychiatry, 1999, 4: p. 579–591.

39. Braet, C. and M. Van Winckel. Long-term follow-up of a cognitive behavioral treatment program for obese children. Behav Ther, 2000, 31: p. 55–74.

40. Ebbeling, C.B., et al. A reduced-glycemic load diet in the treatment of adolescent obesity. Arch Pediatr Adolesc Med, 2003, 157(8): p. 773–9.

41. Nassis, G.P., et al. Aerobic exercise training improves insulin sensitivity without changes in body weight, body fat, adiponectin, and inflammatory markers in overweight and obese girls. Metabolism, 2005, 54(11): p. 1472–9.

42. Meyer, A.A., et al. Improvement of early vascular changes and cardiovascular risk factors in obese children after a six-month exercise program. J Am Coll Cardiol, 2006, 48(9): p. 1865–70.

43. American Academy of Pediatrics. Physical fitness and activity in schools. Pediatrics, 2000, 105(5): p. 1156–7.

44. Carrel, A.L., et al. Improvement of fitness, body composition, and insulin sensitivity in overweight children in a school-based exercise program: a randomized, controlled study. Arch Pediatr Adolesc Med, 2005, 159(10): p. 963–8.

45. Epstein, L.H., et al. Ten-year follow-up of behavioral, family-based treatment for obese children. JAMA, 1990, 264(19): p. 2519–23.

46. Berkey, C.S., et al. One-year changes in activity and in inactivity among 10- to 15-year-old boys and girls: relationship to change in body mass index. Pediatrics, 2003, 111(4 Pt 1): p. 836–43.

47. Epstein, L.H., et al. Decreasing sedentary behaviors in treating pediatric obesity. Arch Pediatr Adolesc Med, 2000, 154(3): p. 220–6.

48. Epstein, L.H., et al. Effects of decreasing sedentary behavior and increasing activity on weight change in obese children. Health Psychol, 1995, 14(2): p. 109–15.

49. Wilkin, T.J., et al. Variation in physical activity lies with the child, not his environment: evidence for an 'activitystat' in young children (EarlyBird 16). Int J Obes (Lond), 2006, 30(7): p. 1050–5.

50. Epstein, L.H., et al. Comparison of family-based behavior modification and nutrition education for childhood obesity. J Pediatr Psychol, 1980, 5(1): p. 25–36.

51. Epstein, L.H., et al. Effects of family-based behavioral treatment on obese 5-to-8-year-old children. Behavior Therapy, 1985, 16: p. 205–212.

52. Jelalian, E. and B.E. Saelens. Empirically supported treatments in pediatric psychology: pediatric obesity. J Pediatr Psychol, 1999, 24(3): p. 223–48.

53. Powers, S.W., J.S. Jones, and B.A. Jones. Behavioral and cognitive-behavioral interventions with pediatric populations. Clin Child Psychol Psychiatry, 2005, 10(1): p. 65–77.

54. Schwartz, R.P., et al. Office-based motivational interviewing to prevent childhood obesity: a feasibility study. Arch Pediatr Adolesc Med, 2007, 161(5): p. 495–501.

55. Resnicow, K., R. Davis, and S. Rollnick. Motivational interviewing for pediatric obesity: Conceptual issues and evidence review. J Am Diet Assoc, 2006, 106(12): p. 2024–33.

56. Kirschenbaum, D.S., J.N. Germann, and B.H. Rich. Treatment of morbid obesity in low-income adolescents: effects of parental self-monitoring. Obes Res, 2005, 13(9): p. 1527–9.

57. Golan, M., M. Fainaru, and A. Weizman. Role of behaviour modification in the treatment of childhood obesity with the parents as the exclusive agents of change. Int J Obes Relat Metab Disord, 1998, 22(12): p. 1217–24.

58. Graves, T., A.W. Meyers, and L. Clark. An evaluation of parental problem-solving training in the behavioral treatment of childhood obesity. J Consult Clin Psychol, 1988, 56(2): p. 246–50.

59. Johnson-Taylor, W.L. and J.E. Everhart. Modifiable environmental and behavioral determinants of overweight among children and adolescents: report of a workshop. Obesity (Silver Spring), 2006, 14(6): p. 929–66.

60. Israel, A.C., L.C. Solotar, and E. Zimand. An investigation of two parental involvement roles in the treatment of obese children. Int J Eat Disord, 1990, 9: p. 557–564.

61. Golan, M. and S. Crow. Targeting parents exclusively in the treatment of childhood obesity: long-term results. Obes Res, 2004, 12(2): p. 357–61.

62. Levine, M.D., et al. Is family-based behavioral weight control appropriate for severe pediatric obesity? Int J Eat Disord, 2001, 30(3): p. 318–28.

63. Korsten-Reck, U., et al. Freiburg Intervention Trial for Obese Children (FITOC): results of a clinical observation study. Int J Obes (Lond), 2005, 29(4): p. 356–61.

64. Brownell, K.D., J.H. Kelman, and A.J. Stunkard. Treatment of obese children with and without their mothers: changes in weight and blood pressure. Pediatrics, 1983, 71(4): p. 515–23.

65. Epstein, L.H., J.N. Roemmich, and H.A. Raynor. Behavioral therapy in the treatment of pediatric obesity. Pediatr Clin North Am, 2001, 48(4): p. 981–93.

66. Goldfield, G.S., et al. Cost-effectiveness of group and mixed family-based treatment for childhood obesity. Int J Obes Relat Metab Disord, 2001, 25(12): p. 1843–9.

67. Saelens, B.E., et al. Behavioral weight control for overweight adolescents initiated in primary care. Obes Res, 2002, 10(1): p. 22–32.

68. Williamson, D.A., et al. Two-year internet-based randomized controlled trial for weight loss in African-American girls. Obesity (Silver Spring), 2006, 14(7): p. 1231–43.

69. Jeffery, R.W., et al. Long-term maintenance of weight loss: current status. Health Psychol, 2000, 19(1 Suppl): p. 5–16.

70. Wilfley, D.E., et al. Efficacy of maintenance treatment approaches for childhood overweight: a randomized controlled trial. JAMA, 2007, 298(14): p. 1661–73.

71. Epstein, L.H., et al. Family-based obesity treatment, then and now: twenty-five years of pediatric obesity treatment. Health Psychol, 2007, 26(4): p. 381–91.

72. Glenny, A.M., et al. The treatment and prevention of obesity: a systematic review of the literature. Int J Obes Relat Metab Disord, 1997, 21(9): p. 715–37.

73. Snethen, J.A., M.E. Broome, and S.E. Cashin. Effective weight loss for overweight children: a meta-analysis of intervention studies. J Pediatr Nurs, 2006, 21(1): p. 45–56.

74. Whitlock, E.P., et al. Screening and interventions for childhood overweight: a summary of evidence for the US Preventive Services Task Force. Pediatrics, 2005, 116(1): p. e125–44.

7 Diet and Physical Activity in the Prevention of Obesity

Frank B. Hu

KEY POINTS

- Numerous epidemiologic and clinical studies have examined the role of dietary factors in the development of obesity.
- Cumulative evidence indicates that there is no "magic bullet" for weight control. Rather, many individual dietary factors each exert a modest effect on body weight, and over time cumulative effects of small changes in daily energy balance lead to weight gain and obesity.
- On the one hand, there is some evidence that higher consumption of whole grains, fruits, and vegetables is beneficial for weight control. On the other hand, higher intake of sugar-sweetened beverages is associated with both weight gain and type 2 diabetes risk.
- Emerging evidence suggests potential weight control benefits by lowering refined carbohydrates and glycemic loads, but prospective data are limited.
- Epidemiologic studies have provided strong evidence that sedentary such as prolonged TV watching is an important risk factor for obesity and type 2 diabetes, whereas increasing physical activity including brisk walking is associated with weight maintenance and a lower risk of obesity and type 2 diabetes.
- Given the obesogenic environment in which we live, characterized by the abundance of energy dense, processed and highly convenient foods, and sedentary lifestyle, it is critical to change our nutrition and physical activity environment and social norms. Otherwise, the effects of any kind of weight loss or maintenance diets are difficult to sustain.

Key Words: Obesity, Weight loss, Diet, Exercise, Fat, Carbohydrate, Protein, Whole grains, Fruits andvegetables, Glycemic load

Obesity has reached epidemic proportions in the US. On the basis of the NHANES 2003–2004 data, the prevalence of the conditions in US adults is estimated at 66.3 and 32.2%, respectively *(1)*. The prevalence of morbid obesity (BMI > 40 kg/m^2) is approximately 4.8%. There has been a marked upward trend in obesity over the past several decades in both men and women.

From: *Nutrition and Health: Nutrition and Metabolism*
Edited by: C.S. Mantzoros, DOI: 10.1007/978-1-60327-453-1_7,
© Humana Press, a part of Springer Science+Business Media, LLC 2009

Overweight and obesity are central to the metabolic syndrome and the single most important risk factor for type 2 diabetes. Obesity is associated with increased incidence of cardiovascular disease, cancer, and mortality from all-causes. The US Surgeon General in 2001 issued a Call to Action, pointing out that "Overweight and obesity may soon cause as much preventable disease and death as cigarette smoking" in the United States. Approximately 300,000 US deaths a year currently are associated with obesity and overweight (compared with more than 400,000 deaths a year associated with cigarette smoking) *(2)*.

Obesity is a complex problem resulting from a combination of genetic, behavioral, environmental, cultural, and socioeconomic influences. Although behavioral and environmental factors are considered primary determinants of obesity, specific dietary lifestyle factors have not been clearly defined. In this chapter, we review epidemiologic and clinical evidence regarding dietary factors and several popular diets and their effects on obesity and weight loss. Also we review epidemiologic evidence regarding the role of physical activity in preventing weight gain.

1. DIETARY FAT

Hypothetically, as dietary fat is the most energy-dense macronutrient in the diet, over-consumption of energy could result if food intake is not regulated *(3)*. In addition, the enhanced palatability of high-fat foods could impact regulation of the volume of food intake, leading to increased energy intake and weight gain. Findings from short-term feeding studies have also suggested that as carbohydrate produces a greater thermogenic effect than fat, dietary fat might be used more efficiently and accumulate as body fat *(4)*. However, when studies are extended to 4 days, no differences in stored energy is observed, which would not be the case if fat truly is being used more efficiently relative to carbohydrate. Over 20 years ago, Flatt *(5)* proposed that carbohydrate intake is regulated, unlike fat, therefore individuals on high-fat diets in theory consume more energy than those on low-fat diets to obtain required amounts of carbohydrate. To date, few data exist that support these claims, and the hypothesis itself is flawed since excess carbohydrate intake can be converted to fat, which is then stored *(3)*.

Although several cross-sectional studies suggested a positive association between dietary fat intake and obesity, few prospective cohort studies have examined long-term relationships between dietary fat and body fatness or weight gain, and among those that have, the results have been highly inconsistent *(6,7)*. These studies have varied considerably in size, duration of follow-up, age groups, covariates adjusted in the statistical analyses, and dietary assessment methods.

In a 6-year study of 361 Swedish women, Heitmann and colleagues *(8)* found a significant association between high dietary fat intake and BMI in predisposed women ($P = 0.003$) but not obese women with lean parents or lean women with or without obese parents. There was a relationship between dietary fat and BMI in genetically predisposed women after adjustment for total energy intake, smoking habits, physical activity, and menopausal status, but subgroup analysis was limited by the very small sample size ($n = 56$).

A much larger study by Field and colleagues *(9)* examined the association between dietary fat and 8-year weight gain among 41,518 women in the Nurses' Health Study

(NHS). Data showed a positive relationship between weight change and increased intake of animal fat, saturated fat, and trans fat, especially in overweight women. There was a weak positive association between total fat consumption and weight gain, no association with increases in percentages of energy from mono or polyunsaturated fats, and no evidence that parental weight status modified the relationship between dietary fat and weight gain. The effects of fat on body weight vary according to type of fat. These differences may reflect biological actions of these fats on insulin resistance and fat accumulation. In that the amount of energy provided by different types of fat is the same, the varied effects may also reflect confounding of the association between diet and body weight by other dietary and lifestyle factors.

Only one prospective study (of 16, 587 US men aged 40–75 in the Health Professionals' Follow-up Study) has examined the association between dietary fat intake and 9-year change in waist circumference. Multivariate analyses by Koh-Banerjee and colleagues *(10)* found that total fat intake was not associated with gain in waist circumference. However, a significant association was found between increasing consumption of trans fat and gain in waist circumference, even after further adjustment for concurrent changes in BMI. Although confounding by other dietary factors related to high intake of trans fat (e.g., fast-food and breakfast habits) cannot be ruled out, these data suggest potentially detrimental effects of trans fat on fat accumulation.

1.1. Low-Fat Diets and Weight Loss

To date, a large spectrum of randomized trials have been published that offer a less confounded evaluation of low-fat diets in relation to body weight than the many ecologic and cross-sectional studies that have examined this association (see review by Malik and Hu *(11)*). A metaanalysis *(12)* of 28 short-term trials suggests that a 10% decrease in total energy from fat can reduce bodyweight by 16 g/day, which is extrapolated to a weight reduction of 8.8 kg by 18 months and 23.4 kg by 4 years *(3)*. Longer-term trials, however, do not substantiate these predictions. In a qualitative review by Willett *(3)*, several clinical and intervention trials of the effect of low-fat diets (ranging from 18 to 40% of energy) on weight, including nine long-term trials ranging from 12 to 24 months, were evaluated. This review suggests that diets lower in fat can result in modest reductions in body weight in the short-term but studies lasting for 1 year or more show that 18–40% of energy intake from fat has a negligible effect on body weight *(3)*.

Similar findings were observed in the Women's Health Initiative Dietary Modification Trial (WHI) *(13)*, a randomized intervention trial comparing an ad libitum low-fat dietary pattern with usual diet in 48,835 postmenopausal women in the US with a mean follow-up of 7.5 years. The intervention group was instructed to reduce total fat intake to 20% of total energy intake by increasing fruit, vegetable, and whole grain consumption, and received intensive behavioral modification sessions led by nutritionists. The control group received a copy of *Dietary Guidelines for Americans (14)* and followed their usual diet. Neither group was given instructions to lose weight. Overall results suggested that although the intervention group lost weight in the first year compared with the control group (2.2 kg; *P* < 0.01), the difference in weight loss between the two groups was negligible at the end of follow-up (year 9) over an average of 7.5 years (0.4 kg at 7.5 years; Fig. 1) *(13)*.The authors suggest the trial provides evidence that fat restriction does not lead to weight gain, refuting claims that low-fat, high-carbohydrate

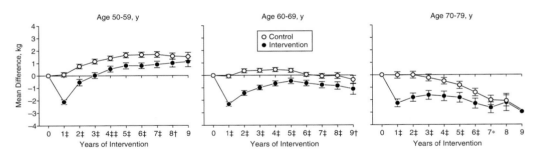

Fig. 1. Differences from baseline in body weight by low-fat diet vs. usual diet, and age at screening. The error bars indicate 95% CIs. *Numbers* at baseline for intervention and control in the 50- to 59-year group were 7,206 and 10,797, respectively; 60–69 years, 9,086 and 13,626; 70–79 years, 3,249 and 4,871. Adapted from *(13)*.

diets are driving the obesity trend *(13)*.However, few older women are supposed to gain weight. A major limitation of the study was that the authors did not differentiate between types of fats and carbohydrates.

2. DIETARY CARBOHYDRATES

Low-fat, high-carbohydrate diets generally produce higher postprandial glucose and insulin responses. However, similar to total fat, the total percentage of energy derived from carbohydrates in the diet has generally not been found to predict diabetes risk. Metabolic consequences of carbohydrate intake depend not only on their quantity but also on their quality. The glycemic response of a given carbohydrate load depends on the food sources, which has led to the development of the glycemic index (GI), ranking foods by their ability to raise postprandial blood glucose levels *(15)*. The GI quantifies the glycemic response by a standard amount of carbohydrates from a food relative to the response by the same amount of carbohydrates from white bread or glucose. The overall GI of a diet has been found to be associated with an increased diabetes risk in some prospective observational studies *(16)*. However, the relevance of the concept of GI is indirectly supported by the reduction in diabetes incidence observed with acarbose, an alpha-glucosidase inhibitor that slows down the digestion of carbohydrates *(17)*.

Effects of carbohydrate-rich foods on insulin resistance and diabetes risk may also depend on fiber content and type. Several epidemiologic studies found that diets rich in whole grains or cereal fiber may protect against type 2 diabetes *(16)*. Controlled feeding studies have found benefits of whole grains, when compared with refined grains, on insulin sensitivity and glucose metabolism. This effect may be partially mediated by positive effects on body weight – studies generally support an inverse association between intake of whole grains and body weight *(18)*. In addition, fiber tends to slow down gastrointestinal absorption, resulting in a lower GI of whole-grain products compared with their refined-grain counterparts, but other mechanisms by which whole grains influence glucose metabolism are likely to play a role as well, e.g., short-chain fatty acid production and micronutrient content.

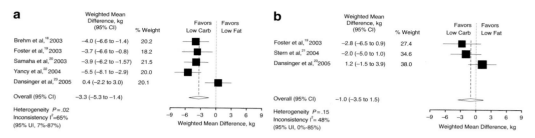

Fig. 2. Weighted mean differences in weight loss after (**a**) 6 months and (**b**) 12 months of follow-up from a metaanalysis *(30)* comparing the effects of ad libitum low-carbohydrate diets versus low-fat energy-restricted diets on weight loss. Adapted from *(19)*.

2.1. Low-Carbohydrate Diets

Given the vast popularity of low-carbohydrate diets, a large number of studies, mostly randomized controlled trials, have been conducted to evaluate the efficacy of carbohydrate-restricted diets compared with fat-restricted diets on weight loss. A metaanalysis *(19)* compared the effects of ad libitum low-carbohydrate diets (allowing a maximum intake of 60 g of carbohydrates per day or 10% energy) with those of low-fat (30% energy), energy-restricted diets on weight loss *(19)*. In total, five randomized controlled trials (*n* = 447) were analyzed, with 6–12 months follow-up. The authors found that after 6 months, participants randomized to a low-carbohydrate diet had lost more weight than those randomized to a low-fat diet (weighted mean difference 3.3 kg, 95% CI −5.3 to −1.4 kg) *(19)*. Notably, after 12 months this difference dissipated (weighted mean difference −1.0 kg, 95% CI −3.5 to 1.5 kg; Fig. 2) *(19)*. This metaanalysis also compared the effect of the two dietary patterns on cardiovascular disease risk factors and found that after 6 months triglyceride and HDL cholesterol level changes were more favorable in the low-carbohydrate diet group, but total cholesterol and LDL cholesterol level changes were more favorable in the low-fat group. Overall, existing trials of low-carbohydrate diets/high-fat diets have shown greater short-term weight loss (within 6 months) than low-fat diets; however, most studies have been small and inconclusive. Similar findings have been shown for low-carbohydrate/high-protein diets (generally 25% energy) *(20)*.

3. MEDITERRANEAN-TYPE DIETS

The Mediterranean dietary pattern emphasizes moderate consumption of fat (~40% energy) primarily from foods high in monounsaturated fatty acids, such as olive oil and encourages consumption of fruits, vegetables, tree nuts, legumes, whole grains, and fish as well as moderate consumption of alcohol *(21)*. A review of trials assessing the effect of the Mediterranean diet on disease prevention identified three studies that evaluated change in body weight *(22)*. Of these, only the trial by McManus et al. *(23)* was able to provide sound evidence for a beneficial role of the Mediterranean diet on weight loss. In their trial, individuals were randomized to either a moderate-fat energy-restricted diet (35% energy from fat) or a low-fat energy-restricted diet (20% energy from fat). After 18 months, the moderate-fat group had decreases in body weight (4.1 kg), BMI (1.6 kg/m^2), and waist circumference (6.9 cm) while the low-fat group had increases of 2.9 kg, 1.4 kg/m^2, and 2.6 cm, respectively (*P* < 0.001). After extending the study for an additional year, mean weight loss in the moderate fat group was significantly greater than that in the low fat group, illustrating the sustainability of a Mediterranean dietary pattern compared with traditional low-fat recommendations. Though compelling as they are, these results need to be further substantiated, and it should be noted that the dropout rate among participants was relatively high. Similarly a study by Esposito et al. *(24)*, which randomized individuals with the metabolic syndrome to either a prudent diet (total fat < 30% energy) or Mediterranean diet, found that after 2 years, mean (SD) body weight loss was higher in patients in the Mediterranean diet group (4.0 [1.1] kg) than in the low-fat diet group (1.2 [0.6] kg; $P < .001$). However, it is difficult to differentiate whether these findings are a consequence of the more intensive weight loss counseling received by the Mediterranean diet group relative to the low-fat diet group. Of particular interest was the finding that levels of inflammatory markers were significantly reduced in individuals on the Mediterranean diet compared with individuals on the low-fat diet. Such findings have recently been corroborated by Estruch et al. *(25)* who evaluated the short-term effects of two ad libitum Mediterranean diets (supplemented with either 1 L/week of free virgin olive oil or 30 g/day of free tree nuts (walnuts, almonds, and hazelnuts)) versus those of an ad libitum low-fat diet on intermediate markers of cardiovascular disease. Compared with participants in the low-fat diet group, after 3 months those in the two Mediterranean diet groups had decreased systolic and diastolic blood pressure, blood glucose levels, and inflammatory markers and increased HDL levels. Despite much higher amounts of dietary fat in the Mediterranean diet groups, supplemented with olive oil or nuts, there was no difference in body weight between the intervention and low-fat groups.

One of the most desirable features of the Mediterranean diet relative to traditional low-fat diets is its ability to improve cardiovascular disease risk factors. However, given the large number of carbohydrate-rich foods consumed in the Mediterranean diet, such a dietary pattern should include mostly low-GI carbohydrates. Though not explicitly studied, it has been suggested that traditional Mediterranean diets may enhance weight loss by providing a sustainable dietary pattern that offers a variety of healthy, portion-controlled, palatable foods.

4. INDIVIDUAL FOODS AND BEVERAGES

4.1. Nuts

Substantial evidence from epidemiologic studies and clinical trials indicates that high nut consumption has beneficial effects on blood lipids and cardiovascular risk *(16)*. A major concern is that because of their high fat content and high energy density, higher consumption of nuts may cause weight gain and obesity. However, several cross-sectional analyses of large cohort studies, including the Adventist Health Study *(26)* and the NHS *(27)*, have shown that people who consume nuts regularly tend to weigh less than those who rarely consume them.

A 28-month prospective study conducted in Spain found an association between higher nut consumption and lower risk of weight gain. Compared with those who never or almost never ate nuts, participants who ate nuts two or more times per week had a 31% (relative risk, 0.69; 95% CI, 0.53–0.90) lower risk of gaining at least 5 kg during the follow-up. Overall, participants who frequently consumed nuts gained an average of

0.42 kg less than those who rarely consumed nuts *(28)*. In the NHS, nut consumption was inversely associated with risk of type 2 diabetes after adjustment for age, BMI, family history of diabetes, physical activity, smoking and alcohol, and total energy intake *(29)*. The multivariate relative risk of women who consumed nuts at least five times per week (1 oz. serving size) compared with those who never/almost never ate nuts was 0.73 (95% CI, 0.60–0.89, *P* for trend <0.001). Sixteen-year average weight gain was also slightly lower among those who consumed nuts at least five times per week compared with those who rarely ate them (6.2 kg vs. 6.5 kg, respectively).

Several trials of nut consumption without constraints on body weight have shown no significant weight changes in groups assigned higher consumption of nuts *(30)*. Three months of follow-up in the PREDIMED Study, which was conducted in Spain, found that Mediterranean diets supplemented with tree nuts improved cardiovascular risk factors but did not lead to weight gain when compared with a low-fat diet *(25)*. Wien and colleagues *(31)* also demonstrated that substitution of almonds (84 g/day) for carbohydrates in a formula-based low-calorie diet resulted in greater weight loss during a 24-week intervention among 65 overweight and obese adults.

These epidemiologic and clinical trial data indicate that in free-living subjects, higher nut consumption does not cause greater weight gain; rather, incorporating nuts into hypocaloric diets may be beneficial for weight control. The mechanisms for these observations are unclear but could be related to higher amounts of protein and fiber in nuts, which may enhance satiety and suppress hunger *(32)*. In dietary practice, the majority of energy contained in nuts appears to be balanced by reductions in other sources of energy, especially carbohydrates. This may explain the lack of predicted weight gain in nut-supplemented diets *(33)*. Increased fecal loss of fat due to incomplete mastication of nuts leads to loss of available energy; this has also been suggested as an explanation for the lack of expected weight gain among those who eat nuts *(30)*.

4.2. Whole Grains

Grains are staple foods in most societies. In traditional diets, grain were typically consumed either in whole intact form or as coarse flours produced from stone grinding. Grinding or milling using modern technology produces fine flours with very small particle size. Milling also removes most of the bran and much of the germ. The resulting refined grain products contain more starch but lose substantial amount of dietary fiber, vitamins, minerals, essential fatty acids, and phytochemicals. Because of loss of the outer bran layer and pulverization of the endosperm, refined grains are digested and absorbed more rapidly than whole grain products and tend to cause more rapid and larger increases in levels of blood glucose and insulin. Thus, whole grain products such as whole wheat breads, brown rice, oats, and barley usually have lower glycemic index (GI) values than refined grains *(12)*. Whole grains are also rich in fiber, antioxidant vitamins, magnesium, and phytochemicals.

During 12 years of follow-up in the NHS, Liu and colleagues *(34)* examined the relationship between changes in intakes of dietary fiber and whole or refined-grain products and weight gain. Increased consumption of whole grains was associated with a lower mean 4-year weight gain (1.58 kg in the lowest quintile and 1.07 kg in the highest quintile; *P* for trend < 0.0001). In contrast, increased intake of refined grains was related to greater weight gain (from 0.99 to 1.65 kg; *P* for trend <0.0001). These findings are consistent with those in a related study on associations between whole-grain, bran, and cereal-fiber consumption and weight in a cohort of men from the HPFS *(35)*. During 8 years of follow-up, increased whole-grain intake was inversely associated with long-term weight gain (*P* for trend <0.0001). There was also a dose–response relationship; each 40 g/day increment in whole-grain intake from all foods reduced weight gain by 0.49 kg. Bran from fortified-grain foods further reduced the risk of weight gain (*P* for trend = 0.01) by 0.36 kg for every 20 g/day increase in consumption. Correction for measurement errors in assessing dietary changes strengthened these associations (each 40 g/day increment in whole-grain intake from all foods reduced weight gain by 1.1 kg).

4.3. Sugar Sweetened Beverages

Sugar-sweetened beverages have received growing attention as potential contributors to the obesity and diabetes epidemic because of dramatically increased consumption in the past several decades. Energy contained in beverages seems less well detected by the body, and subsequent food intake is poorly adjusted to account for the energy intake from beverages. Sugar-sweetened beverages have been associated with weight gain in clinical studies and observational studies among children and adults *(36)*. The high sugar loads from sugar-sweetened beverages may also have detrimental effects on glucose metabolism leading to diabetes, beyond their potential contribution to obesity. In the Nurses' Health Study II, a higher consumption of sugar-sweetened beverages was associated with a greater magnitude of weight gain and an increased risk for development of type 2 diabetes in women *(37)* (Fig. 3). After adjustment for potential confounders, women consuming one or more sugar-sweetened soft drinks per day had an RR of type

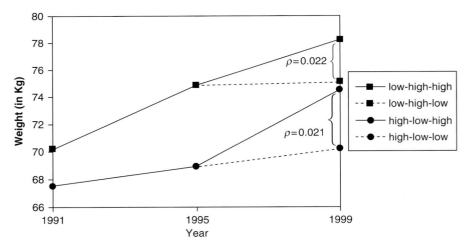

Fig. 3. Mean weight in 1991, 1995, and 1999 according to trends in sugar-sweetened soft drink consumption in 1,969 women who changed consumption between 1991 and 1995 and either changed or maintained level of consumption until 1999. Low and high intakes were defined as ≤1 per week and ≥1 per day. The number of subjects were: low–high–high = 323, low–high–low = 461, high–low–high = 110, and high–low–low = 746. Groups with similar intake in 1991 and 1995 were combined for estimates for these time points. Means were adjusted for age, alcohol intake, physical activity, smoking, postmenopausal hormone use, oral contraceptive use, cereal fiber intake, and total fat intake at each time point. Adapted from *(37)*.

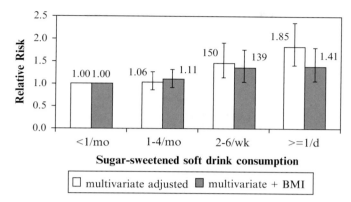

Fig. 4. Multivariate relative risks (RRs) of type 2 diabetes according to sugar-sweetened soft drink consumption in the Nurses' Health Study II 1991–1999. Multivariate RRs were adjusted for age, alcohol (0, 0.1–4.9, 5.0–9.9, 10+ g/day), physical activity (quintiles), family history of diabetes, smoking (never, past, current), postmenopausal hormone use (never, ever), oral contraceptive use (never, past, current), intake (quintiles) of cereal fiber, magnesium, trans fat, polyunsaturated:saturated fat, and consumption of sugar-sweetened soft drinks, diet soft drinks, fruit juice, and fruit punch (other than the main exposure, depending on model). Adapted from *(37)*.

2 diabetes of 1.83 (95% CI: 1.42–2.36; *P* < .001 for trend) compared with those who consumed less than one of these beverages per month. The RR for extreme categories further controlling for BMI was 1.39 (95% CI: 1.07–1.76; *P* for trend = 0.012) (Fig. 4). This finding suggests that BMI accounted for about half of the excess risk.

5. PHYSICAL ACTIVITY

Midlife weight gain is a widespread phenomenon in most populations. Hill and colleagues *(38)* estimated that US adults have been gaining an average of 0.45–0.90 kg/year in the decades since the epidemic of obesity started. Likewise, Brown and colleagues *(39)* estimated that middle-aged Australian women add an average of 0.5 kg/year. For most people, midlife weight gain reflects gain in body fat, sometimes accompanied by loss of lean body mass with aging. Because weight loss and maintenance are very difficult for obese individuals, finding ways to prevent age-related weight gain is of critical importance.

Over the 4-year follow-up period in the Health Professionals' Follow-up Study *(40)* men who increased vigorous exercise (including jogging, running, lap swimming, bicycling and rowing, calisthenics and racquet sports) to 1.5 h/week, decreased TV viewing, and stopped eating between meals, lost an average of 1.4 kg, compared with a weight gain of 1.4 kg among the overall population. Those who maintained a relatively high level of vigorous physical activity over time (at least 1.5 h/week) had the lowest prevalence of obesity as well as the smallest increase in body weight (Fig. 5). These data suggest that increasing and maintaining vigorous activity and decreasing TV use are important to prevent weight gain over 4 years.

Schmitz and colleagues *(41)* examined the longitudinal relationship between changes in physical activity and weight gain during 10 years of follow-up among 5,115 black

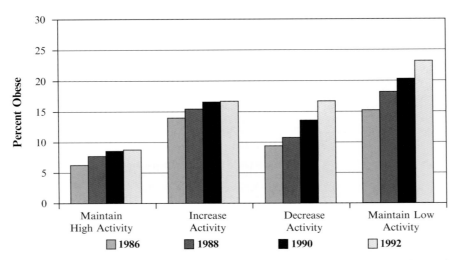

Fig. 5. Prevalence of obesity (BMI 27.8) over time for different patterns of recreational vigorous physical activity. This figure is based on 3,666 nonsmoking, non-hypertensive, and nonhypercholesterolemic men aged 45–54 years (in 1986). Adapted from *(40)*.

and white men and women aged 18–30 years at baseline in the Coronary Artery Risk Development in Young Adults (CARDIA) Study. After adjustment for secular trend, age, clinic site, education, smoking, alcohol intake, parity, percentage of energy intake from fat, and changes in these variables over time, increasing physical activity was significantly associated with decreasing weight gain in all four race and sex subgroups. Specifically, increasing high-intensity activity (requiring 6 MET hours) by 2 h/week offset observed weight gain for all groups but black men. The benefits of exercise in preventing weight gain were much greater for obese subjects than for those of normal weight at baseline. In addition, an increase in physical activity in the 2–3 years of follow-up was associated with a slowing of weight gain during the subsequent 5-year follow-up; the average attenuation of 5-year weight gain was approximately 1 kg among those who increased their activity in the first 2–3 years of follow-up (by 1 h/week of high intensity activity) relative to those who decreased their activity. These results suggest that increasing physical activity slows long-term weight gain.

In a subsequent analysis of data from the Nurses' Health Study *(42)*, we examined the relationship between walking, sedentary behavior (especially prolonged TV watching), and risk of obesity and type 2 diabetes among 50,277 healthy nonobese women at baseline in 1992. During 6 years of follow-up, 3,757 (7.5%), the women who had a BMI of less than 30 kg/m^2 in 1992 became obese (BMI 30 kg/m^2). In the multivariate analyses adjusting for age, smoking, exercise level, dietary factors, and other covariates, each brisk walk for 1 h/day was associated with a 24% (95% CI, 19–29%) reduction in obesity, and standing or walking around at home (2 h/day) with a 9% (95% CI, 6–12%) reduction in obesity. In contrast, each 2 h/day increment in TV watching was associated with a 23% (95% CI, 17–30%) increase in obesity; and each 2 h/day increment in sitting at work was associated with a 5% (95% CI, 0–10%) increase in obesity. There was a significant association between brisk walking and reduced risk of type 2 diabetes. Conversely, time spent watching TV was associated with increased diabetes risk. It was estimated that in this cohort, 30% (95% CI, 24–36%)

of new cases of obesity and 43% (95% CI, 32–52%) of new cases of diabetes could be prevented by adopting a relatively active lifestyle (<10 h/week of TV watching and 30 min/day of brisk walking).

6. SUMMARY

Although diet is widely believed to play a major role in obesity, the impact of specific dietary factors remains elusive. Cumulative epidemiologic and clinical-trial evidence indicates that there is no "magic bullet" for weight control. Rather, many individual dietary factors each exert a modest effect on body weight, and over time, cumulative effects of small changes in daily energy balance lead to weight gain and obesity (43). Although dietary fat has long been considered the main culprit behind obesity, large prospective cohort studies and long-term randomized clinical trials have not demonstrated a major role of dietary fat in obesity. In contrast, emerging evidence suggests potential weight control benefits by lowering refined carbohydrates and glycemic loads, but prospective data are limited. Increasing consumption of protein is also thought to be of potential benefit; however, long-term data on protein and body weight are lacking.

Currently, there is no conclusive evidence that one popular diet is superior to another in long-term weight control. Clearly, one diet does not fit all. Thus, when prescribing such diets to patients, it is important to consider cultural habits and food preference to maximize long-term adherence (11). For most patients, rapid weight loss should not be the goal for dietary therapy. Instead, dietary recommendations should target gradual and sustained weight loss and long-term benefits on cardiovascular health. Toward this end, one should choose healthy sources of fats and whole grain products, which are known to be cardio-protective and may also enhance weight loss. Substitution of healthy sources of protein for refined carbohydrates and added sugar can be also beneficial for body weight and cardiovascular risk factors. Such macronutrient choices underpin the role of Mediterranean-style diets in improving cardiovascular disease risk and reducing major chronic diseases.

Compelling evidence supports that sedentary lifestyle indicated by prolonged TV watching is an important risk factor for obesity and type 2 diabetes, whereas increasing physical activity is associated with weight maintenance and a lower risk of obesity and type 2 diabetes. There are at least two explanations for the observed positive association between TV watching and diabetes risk. First, TV watching is directly related to obesity and weight gain, probably due to lower energy expenditure (i.e. less physical activity) and higher caloric intake. Second, participants who spent more time watching TV tended to eat more red meat, processed meat, snacks, refined grains, and sweets and less vegetables, fruits, and whole grains. Such an eating pattern, which is linked to commercial advertisements and food cues appearing on TV, may adversely affect diabetes risk.

Most of adults in the US do not engage in regular exercise and substantial proportion of the population is completely sedentary. Also, past several decades have seen an increasing trend of sedentary behaviors, especially prolong TV watching. The combination of lack of exercise and increasing sedentary behavior at least partially contributes to the increasing epidemic of obesity and type 2 diabetes in the US and worldwide. Public health campaign is urgently needed not only to promote increasing physical activity but also to reduce sedentary behaviors especially prolonged TV watching in both adults and children.

Given the obesogenic environment in which we live, characterized by the abundance of energy dense, processed, and highly convenient foods and sedentary lifestyle, we should realize that without changing our nutrition and physical activity environment, for most people, the effects of any kind of weight loss or maintenance diets are difficult to sustain *(11)*.

REFERENCES

1. Ogden C.L., Carroll M.D., Curtin L.R., et al. Prevalence of overweight and obesity in the United States, 1999–2004. JAMA 2006;295:1549–55.
2. Allison D.B., Fontaine K.R., Manson J.E., et al. Annual deaths attributable to obesity in the United States. JAMA 1999;282:1530–8.
3. Willett W.C. Dietary fat plays a major role in obesity: no. Obes Rev 2002;3:59–68.
4. Astrup A. Dietary composition, substrate balances and body fat in subjects with a predisposition to obesity. Int J Obes Relat Metab Disord 1993;17 Suppl 3:S32–6; discussion S41–2.
5. Flatt J.P., Ravussin E., Acheson K.J., et al. Effects of dietary fat on postprandial substrate oxidation and on carbohydrate and fat balances. J Clin Invest 1985;76:1019–24.
6. Lissner L., Heitmann B.L. Dietary fat and obesity: evidence from epidemiology. Eur J Clin Nutr 1995;49:79–90.
7. Seidell J.C. Dietary fat and obesity: an epidemiologic perspective. Am J Clin Nutr 1998;67(3 Suppl):546S–50S.
8. Heitmann B.L., Lissner L., Sorensen T.I., et al. Dietary fat intake and weight gain in women genetically predisposed for obesity. Am J Clin Nutr 1995;61:1213–7.
9. Field A.E., Willett W.C., Lissner L., et al. Dietary fat and weight gain among women in the Nurses' Health Study. Obesity (Silver Spring) 2007;15(4):967–76.
10. Koh-Banerjee P., Chu N.F., Spiegelman D., et al. Prospective study of the association of changes in dietary intake, physical activity, alcohol consumption, and smoking with 9-y gain in waist circumference among 16 587 US men. Am J Clin Nutr 2003;78:719–27.
11. Malik V.S., Hu F.B. Popular weight-loss diets: from evidence to practice. Nat Clin Pract Cardiovasc Med 2007;4:34–41.
12. Bray G.A., Popkin B.M. Dietary fat intake does affect obesity! Am J Clin Nutr 1998;68:1157–73.
13. Howard B.V., Manson J.E., Stefanick M.L., et al. Low-fat dietary pattern and weight change over 7 years: the Women's Health Initiative Dietary Modification Trial. JAMA 2006;295:39–49.
14. Agriculture UDo. Dietary Guidelines for Americans. 3rd ed. Washington, DC: US Departments of Agriculture and Health and Human Services; 1990. Home and Garden Bulletin No. 232.
15. Jenkins D.J., Wolever T.M., Taylor R.H., et al. Glycemic index of foods: a physiological basis for carbohydrate exchange. Am J Clin Nutr 1981;34:362–6.
16. Hu F.B., Willett W.C. Optimal diets for prevention of coronary heart disease. JAMA 2002;288:2569–78.
17. Chiasson J.L., Josse R.G., Gomis R., et al. Acarbose for prevention of type 2 diabetes mellitus: the STOP-NIDDM randomised trial. Lancet 2002;359:2072–7.
18. Koh-Banerjee P., Rimm E.B. Whole grain consumption and weight gain: a review of the epidemiological evidence, potential mechanisms and opportunities for future research. Proc Nutr Soc 2003;62:25–9.
19. Nordmann A.J., Nordmann A., Briel M., et al. Effects of low-carbohydrate vs low-fat diets on weight loss and cardiovascular risk factors: a meta-analysis of randomized controlled trials. Arch Intern Med 2006;166:285–93.
20. Hu F.B. Protein, body weight, and cardiovascular health. Am J Clin Nutr 2005;82:242S–7S.
21. Willett W.C., Sacks F., Trichopoulou A., et al. Mediterranean diet pyramid: a cultural model for healthy eating. Am J Clin Nutr 1995;61:1402S–6S.
22. Serra-Majem L., Roman B., Estruch R. Scientific evidence of interventions using the Mediterranean diet: a systematic review. Nutr Rev 2006;64:S27–47.

23. McManus K., Antinoro L., Sacks F. A randomized controlled trial of a moderate-fat, low-energy diet compared with a low fat, low-energy diet for weight loss in overweight adults. Int J Obes Relat Metab Disord 2001;25:1503–11.

24. Esposito K., Marfella R., Ciotola M., et al. Effect of a mediterranean-style diet on endothelial dysfunction and markers of vascular inflammation in the metabolic syndrome: a randomized trial. JAMA 2004;292:1440–6.

25. Estruch R., Martinez-Gonzalez MA, Corella D, et al. Effects of a Mediterranean-style diet on cardiovascular risk factors: a randomized trial. Ann Intern Med 2006;145:1–11.

26. Fraser G.E., Sabate J., Beeson W.L., et al. A possible protective effect of nut consumption on risk of coronary heart disease. The Adventist Health Study. Arch Intern Med 1992;152:1416–24.

27. Hu F.B., Stampfer M.J., Manson J.E., et al. Frequent nut consumption and risk of coronary heart disease in women: prospective cohort study. BMJ 1998;317:1341–5.

28. Bes Rastrollo M., Sabate J., Gomez-Garcia E., et al. Nut consumption and weight gain in a Mediterranean cohort: The SUN Study. Obesity (Silver Spring) 2007;15(1):107–16.

29. Jiang R., Manson J.E., Stampfer M.J., et al. Nut and peanut butter consumption and risk of type 2 diabetes in women. JAMA 2002;288:2554–60.

30. Sabate J. Nut consumption and body weight. Am J Clin Nutr 2003;78(3 Suppl):647S–50S.

31. Wien M.A., Sabate J.M., Ikle D.N., et al. Almonds vs complex carbohydrates in a weight reduction program. Int J Obes Relat Metab Disord 2003;27:1365–72.

32. Alper C.M., Mattes R.D. Effects of chronic peanut consumption on energy balance and hedonics. Int J Obes Relat Metab Disord 2002;26:1129–37.

33. Fraser G.E., Bennett H.W., Jaceldo K.B., et al. Effect on body weight of a free 76 Kilojoule (320 calorie) daily supplement of almonds for six months. J Am Coll Nutr 2002;21:275–83.

34. Liu S., Willett W.C., Manson J.E., et al. Relation between changes in intakes of dietary fiber and grain products and changes in weight and development of obesity among middle-aged women. Am J Clin Nutr 2003;78:920–7.

35. Koh-Banerjee P., Franz M., Sampson L., et al. Changes in whole-grain, bran, and cereal fiber consumption in relation to 8-y weight gain among men. Am J Clin Nutr 2004;80:1237–45.

36. Malik V.S., Schulze M.B., Hu F.B. Intake of sugar-sweetened beverages and weight gain: a systematic review. Am J Clin Nutr 2006;84:274–88.

37. Schulze M.B., Manson J.E., Ludwig D.S., et al. Sugar-sweetened beverages, weight gain, and incidence of type 2 diabetes in young and middle-aged women. JAMA 2004;292:927–34.

38. Hill J.O., Wyatt H.R., Reed G.W., et al. Obesity and the environment: where do we go from here. Science 2003;299:853–5.

39. Brown W.J., Williams L., Ford J.H., et al. Identifying the energy gap: magnitude and determinants of 5-year weight gain in midage women. Obes Res 2005;13:1431–41.

40. Coakley E.H., Rimm E.B., Colditz G., et al. Predictors of weight change in men: results from the Health Professionals Follow-up Study. Int J Obes Relat Metab Disord 1998;22:89–96.

41. Schmitz K.H., Jacobs D.R., Jr., Leon A.S., et al. Physical activity and body weight: associations over ten years in the CARDIA study. Coronary Artery Risk Development in Young Adults. Int J Obes Relat Metab Disord 2000;24:1475–87.

42. Hu F.B., Li T.Y., Colditz G.A., et al. Television watching and other sedentary behaviors in relation to risk of obesity and type 2 diabetes mellitus in women. JAMA 2003;289:1785–91.

43. Hu F.B. Chapter 14. Diet, Nutrition, and Obesity. In Obesity Epidemiology, edited by Hu FB. Oxford University Press. New York 2008;275–300.

8 Diet and Exercise in the Prevention and Management of the Metabolic Syndrome

Mary Yannakoulia, Evaggelia Fappa, Janice Jin Hwang, and Christos S. Mantzoros

KEY POINTS

- The metabolic syndrome (MetSyn) encompasses a constellation of metabolic abnormalities that are thought to place patients at higher risk for cardiovascular morbidity.
- Many definitions have been proposed, and although the exact mechanisms underlying the syndrome remain unclear, increased abdominal fat correlated with dyslipidemia, insulin resistance, and hyperinsulinemia are believed to be the core of its pathophysiology.
- Its increasing prevalence urged the need for preventing and managing strategies. Prevention of the syndrome includes keeping body weight within the normal range, exercise training, and consumption of a moderate carbohydrate diet, with moderate consumption of mono or polyunsaturated fatty acids (omega-3 polyunsaturated fatty acids).
- Current guidelines for the clinical management propose lifestyle changes (diet and physical activity) as a first-line intervention. However, research in this area is limited.
- Weight loss has been recognized as an important issue in the management of MetSyn, in addition to exercise training and diet quality.
- Short-term success of lifestyle intervention programs has been observed, though they failed to sustain long-term effectiveness.
- Multiple follow-up booster sessions proved more effective in maintaining lifestyle changes than one counseling session at the end of follow-up.
- In conclusion, diet and physical activity have a pivotal role in the prevention and management of the MetSyn. Hence, it is of major importance to explore strategies to improve adherence and ensure that patients achieve and maintain lifestyle changes.

Key Words: Metabolic syndrome, Weight loss, Lifestyle intervention, Diet, Physical activity, Adherence, Behavior modification

From: *Nutrition and Health: Nutrition and Metabolism*
Edited by: C.S. Mantzoros, DOI: 10.1007/978-1-60327-453-1_8,
© Humana Press, a part of Springer Science+Business Media, LLC 2009

1. INTRODUCTION

The metabolic syndrome (MetSyn), also known as syndrome X or insulin resistance syndrome, constitutes a constellation of symptoms, including obesity, insulin resistance/ glucose intolerance, dyslipidemia, and hypertension, and it is associated with a two to fourfold increase in cardiovascular morbidity and stroke (1). The increasing prevalence of MetSyn is concurrent with the alarming increase in the prevalence of obesity and type 2 diabetes. On the basis of the US population data from 1988 to 1994, the prevalence increased from 6.7% among participants aged 20 through 29 years to 43.5 and 42.0% for participants aged 60 through 69 years and aged at least 70 years respectively, reaching an overall percentage of 24.5% (2). Although there has been a controversy surrounding the exact definition of the syndrome, there is incontrovertible evidence that the risk factors associated with the MetSyn should and need to be addressed in concert. In this chapter, the risk factors will be summarized and the literature examining prevention and clinical management of the syndrome will be discussed.

2. DEFINITION AND PATHOPHYSIOLOGY OF THE METABOLIC SYNDROME

Although several criteria exist, most criteria include metabolic risk factors, such as abdominal/central obesity, hypertriglyceridemia, low levels of high density lipoprotein (HDL) cholesterol, hypertension, and elevated fasting glucose levels. Gerald Reaven first described "syndrome X" in 1988 proposing insulin resistance to be the critical factor of the syndrome, predisposing patients to hypertension, hyperlipidemia, and type 2 diabetes mellitus (3). Ten years later the World Health Organization published the first criteria for the syndrome (4). Since then, a number of definitions have been proposed (5–7). They could be categorized in two groups depending on the leading cause of the syndrome, being either visceral obesity or insulin resistance. The different definitions may lead to research and clinical problems, such as difficulties in comparability between studies or misclassification of patients.

The pathophysiology of the MetSyn is complex and remains, in most part, unknown. A full review of the current literature is beyond the scope of this chapter (8) Briefly, increased abdominal fat correlates with dyslipidemia (9–13), insulin resistance, and hyperinsulinemia (14) via mechanisms involving increased free fatty acids (15,16) and/or changes in levels of adipokines, such as adiponectin (17–21), resistin (22–24), and leptin (25–28). These factors, along with the proinflammatory state associated with obesity (29,30), may create an unfavorable proatherogenic milieu (31).

Park and colleagues identified risk factors associated with the MetSyn, including older age, postmenopausal status, Mexican American ethnicity, higher body mass index, current smoking, low household income, high carbohydrate intake, no alcohol consumption, and physical inactivity (32). Few randomized control trials specifically examining incidence or resolution of MetSyn have been conducted so far (33–44); however, there is overwhelming evidence showing that management of the individual components of the syndrome can delay or prevent the onset of diabetes, hypertension, and cardiovascular disease.

3. PREVENTION OF RISK FACTORS FOR METABOLIC SYNDROME: THE ROLE OF PHYSICAL FITNESS/ACTIVITY AND OF DIETARY FACTORS

A cornerstone of prevention lies in avoiding excess body weight *(45)*. Excess body weight increases the risk for diabetes *(46–49)*, hypertension *(50,51)*, and cardiovascular disease *(49,52)*. An in-depth examination of the current treatment options for obesity can be found in Chaps. 15 and 16. In addition to decreasing the risk of adverse metabolic sequel, weight loss is also associated with decreased levels of inflammatory markers *(53–57)*.

3.1. Physical Fitness and Physical Activity

Several observational studies revealed associations between physical fitness and likelihood of death from cardiovascular disease. Blair et al. examined 10,224 men and 3,120 women for an average of 8 years follow-up and found that the rate of mortality was 64/10,000 person-years in the least fit men, compared with 18.6/10,000 person-years in the most fit men *(58)*. Corresponding values for women were 39.5/10,000 person-years to 8.5/10,000 person-years. These trends remained significant after adjustment for age, smoking habits, cholesterol levels, systolic blood pressure, fasting blood glucose levels, parental history of coronary heart disease, and follow-up interval. The same scientific group has subsequently published several similar prospective studies showing that low fitness was an independent predictor of mortality in all body mass index groups after adjustment for other mortality predictors *(59)*.

Another prospective cohort study followed 936 women who required coronary angiography for a median of 3.9 years *(60)*. Self reported higher physical fitness scores were found to be associated with fewer coronary artery disease (CAD) risk factors, less angiographic CAD, and lower risk for adverse cardiovascular events. Furthermore, asymptomatic men with low cardiorespiratory fitness levels have been shown to be more likely to develop MetSyn *(61)*.

Most studies to date suggest that exercise confers additional health benefits beyond those achieved from weight loss or changes in body fat ratios. Chronic exercise is associated with improvements in triglycerides *(62,63)*, and even a single bout of exercise has been shown to induce favorable changes in lipid metabolism of healthy men *(64)*. Physical training reduces skeletal muscle lipid levels and insulin resistance regardless of body mass index *(65,66)*. In addition, exercise may also exert favorable effects on adipokines, such as adiponectin and other inflammatory markers, without significant changes in body weight *(67,68)*.

3.2. Dietary Factors

Several dietary parameters have been related to MetSyn risk factors. Regarding lipid metabolism, *trans*-fatty acids are associated with increased low density lipoprotein (LDL) and decreased HDL cholesterol levels *(69)*, whereas omega-3 fatty acids, in the form of fish oils, were effective in lowering triglyceride levels (and blood pressure) in people with mild hypertension *(70)*. Even though there has been a controversy among studies regarding the effect of polyunsaturated fatty acids consumption on glycemic control *(71,72)*, substituting saturated for unsaturated fatty acids increases insulin sensitivity in healthy men and women *(73)*. Additionally, it has been shown that *trans*-fatty acids increased risk of diabetes *(74)*. However, restricting saturated fatty acids and replacing with carbohydrates leads to lower HDL levels as well, so as to keep fat consumption relatively high and at the same time avoiding adverse effects on health, substituting saturated with mono or polyunsaturated fat seems to provide the optimal result *(75)*.

On the topic of carbohydrates, it seems that glycemic and insulinemic responses to ingestion of carbohydrates depend on the glycemic index or load *(76)*. More precisely, subjects in the highest quintile of glycemic load diet compared with lowest quintile subjects had higher triglyceride and lower HDL cholesterol levels *(77,78)*. High glycemic index foods increase the demand for insulin, creating additional stress on beta-cell function and impairing glucose tolerance *(79)*. Alternatively, low/moderate carbohydrate diets (from 60 g of carbohydrates/day to 40% of energy from carbohydrates) were associated with improvements in HDL cholesterol and triglycerides compared with high carbohydrate or low fat diets; however, changes in LDL cholesterol were not in favor of low as opposed to moderate carbohydrate diets *(80,81)*. A decrease in glycemic load with the use of acarbose, an alpha-glucosidase inhibitor that slows the digestion and absorption of starch, led to a significant decrease in blood pressure and an increased reversion of impaired to normal glucose tolerance *(82,83)*.

Regarding alcohol consumption, 30 g/day of alcohol intake reduced fasting insulin concentration and triglyceride concentration, and increased insulin sensitivity compared with no consumption *(84)*. A prospective cohort from the Quebec Cardiovascular Study followed 1,966 cardiovascular heart disease free men for 13 years and found that men who consumed ≥ 15.2 g of alcohol/day had elevated plasma HDL cholesterol concentrations ($P < 0.001$), and lower plasma concentrations of insulin ($P = 0.01$), C-reactive protein ($P = 0.01$), and fibrinogen ($P < 0.001$) than men who consumed <1.3 g of alcohol/day *(85)*. On the contrary, high (greater than 3 drinks/day) alcohol consumption is associated with hypertension, but this association has not been consistently shown with moderate amounts of intake *(86)*.

Beyond individual nutrients or foods, holistic approaches targeting overall lifestyle changes provide interesting results. The Diabetes Prevention Program randomized trial compared the effects of placebo, metformin, and intensive lifestyle intervention (including moderate intensity physical activity such as brisk walking for at least 150 min/week) on prevention of the MetSyn in 3,234 subjects with impaired glucose tolerance. After 3 years, the cumulative incidence of MetSyn was 51, 45, and 34% in the placebo, metformin, and lifestyle groups, respectively *(87)*. Incidence of the MetSyn was reduced by 41% in the lifestyle group and by 17% in the metformin group, compared with placebo. Interestingly, the effects of lifestyle intervention on MetSyn prevention appeared to be more strongly related to decreased waist circumference and improvements in blood pressure as opposed to dyslipidemia. The Finnish Diabetes Prevention Study, similarly, found that intensive lifestyle intervention resulted in improved glucose levels, lipid markers, and body mass index after 3 years compared with controls *(88)*.

4. CLINICAL MANAGEMENT OF METABOLIC SYNDROME

The high prevalence of the MetSyn and its ability to detect people at risk for cardiovascular disease or type II diabetes mellitus led the National Cholesterol Education Program to publish, in 2001, clinical management guidelines. Recommendations include weight reduction and increase in physical activity as first-line intervention beyond this, specific treatments are proposed against the lipid and the nonlipid components of the MetSyn *(6)*. Long-term lifestyle changes constitute, therefore, the cornerstone for the management of MetSyn.

4.1. Weight Loss and Energy Deficit

A few studies have evaluated the efficacy of lifestyle modification in resolving the syndrome. In the majority of them, weight reduction was the main goal and, most likely, the underlying mechanism leading to improvement in MetSyn parameters. Weight loss was found to favorably affect all the individual components *(51,89,90)*: it is associated with a significant improvement in glucose control and lipid and nonlipid abnormalities *(33,34)*. Ten percent weight loss, compared with lower rates, has been documented to result in greater reductions in the MetSyn components, with patients going beyond the 10% reduction experiencing greater short and long-term (16 months) benefits *(35)*. Interestingly, benefits from weight loss may be present even at high posttreatment body mass index levels (≥ 30 kg/m^2) *(36,91)*.

Caloric restriction along with a low-fat or a high omega-3/low saturated fatty acids diet were found to have a beneficial effect on the MetSyn *(37–39)*. A hypocaloric, prudent dietary pattern, rich in fruits and vegetables, consumed for a period of 24 weeks, has also been successfully applied for the management of MetSyn *(40)*. Furthermore, great energy deficits, achieved by very low calorie diets, with or without exercise, resulted in favorable changes to the components of the MetSyn *(36,41)*, as did the supplementary use of orlistat, a pancreatic lipase inhibitor, for achieving energy restriction *(42)*.

4.2. Diet Quality

Research is limited with regard to the effect of dietary manipulation of macronutrient content in patients with MetSyn. Although some evidence support the view that the modest weight loss, rather than the macronutrient composition per se, induces changes in MetSyn parameters *(44)*, there are studies that have found improvements in blood lipid profile and pressure by modifying macronutrient composition of the diet but not energy balance and keeping stable body weight *(92,93)*.

Although people on a low-fat, high-carbohydrate diet have greater odds of having MetSyn, compared with those on a low-carbohydrate, high-fat diet *(94)*, this is in disagreement with data from patients having the MetSyn. When a high-carbohydrate, low-fat diet was compared with a high-fat and protein, low carbohydrate diet, all the components of MetSyn decreased significantly with both diets (except of HDL cholesterol, which remained unchanged) *(95)*. On the basis of the fact that low-carbohydrate diet was associated with a greater decrease in the prevalence of hypertension and hypertriacylglycerolemia, it has been proposed that tailoring dietary interventions to the specific presentation of the MetSyn may be the best way of reducing the risk factors for cardiovascular disease *(95)*.

Apart from the effect of individual macronutrients, dietary patterns have also been examined in relation to MetSyn parameters. In one study, consumption of a Mediterranean-style diet was shown to improve endothelial function and significantly reduce markers of systemic vascular inflammation in MetSyn patients, even with modest weight loss *(43)*. Participants in the Mediterranean diet intervention showed a reduction in the components of the syndrome to that extent that the overall prevalence of MetSyn was reduced by approximately one half. The authors commented that, as the analysis was adjusted for changes in body weight, the overall reduction in the prevalence of the metabolic syndrome probably represents a conservative measure. Adoption of a Mediterranean-style diet rich in whole grains, fruits, vegetables, legumes, walnuts, and olive oil is a safe and effective strategy in reducing both the prevalence of MetSyn and its associated cardiovascular risk. Furthermore, another dietary pattern, the DASH diet (Dietary Approach to Stop Hypertension), has been shown to favorably influence MetSyn parameters, and particularly blood pressure. Adoption of a DASH diet, in the context of an intensive behavioral intervention including the established lifestyle modifications for lowering blood pressure, may be a key feature to achieve a decline in blood pressure in MetSyn patients *(96)*.

4.3. Physical Activity

The beneficial effects of physical activity on MetSyn are well established: increases in physical activity improve individual metabolic parameters or combinations of them *(33,37,97)*, either directly or by promoting weight reduction. MetSyn resolved in 30% of patients after 20 weeks of supervised aerobic exercise training *(98)*. In addition, 8 weeks of low-intensity endurance exercise induced a moderate decrease in insulin resistance *(99)*. As weight loss constitutes an important therapeutic goal for the treatment of MetSyn, increase and maintenance of physical activity levels further contributes to this goal by supporting weight loss maintenance *(100)*.

The type of physical activity varies greatly among studies, from nonprescribed ad libitum physical activity *(35,36,43)* to supervised exercise, specified in terms of duration and type *(33,34,37–40)*. Resistance and aerobic exercise have been proven to be equally effective in improving metabolic parameters *(101)*. Concerning, the intensity and amount of aerobic exercise, a modest amount of moderate-intensity exercise, in the absence of dietary changes, significantly improved MetSyn and, thus, supported the recommendation that adults should get 30 min of moderate-intensity exercise every day *(102)*. Furthermore, there was an indication that moderate-intensity may be better than vigorous-intensity exercise for improving MetSyn.

Changes in physical activity were among the principal goals of most lifestyle interventions for MetSyn, in addition to dietary modifications *(33–40,43)*. In one study, adding an exercise component to a dietary intervention led to a significant reduction only in systolic blood pressure compared with the nonexercise, diet-only group *(33)*. Alternatively, adding a dietary modification component to an exercise intervention had beneficial effects on several parameters, namely weight reduction, fasting glucose levels, and diastolic blood pressure *(37)*. Furthermore, combining diet and exercise had additive effects on the resolution of MetSyn compared with either treatment alone *(103)*. It should be pointed out, however, that, in those interventions that include both exercise changes and dietary modifications, improvements in MetSyn components were not specifically attributed to the exercise or the dietary component *(33–40,43)*, and we cannot draw conclusions on the relative significance of these two lifestyle parameters.

The effect of physical activity has also been examined in relation to the maintenance of changes. To further improve MetSyn parameters or maintain achieved changes, the addition of exercise at the end of a weight-reduction program has been found to be as effective as dietary therapy alone; in other words, physical activity did not confer further benefit to the parameters studied *(91)*. The authors postulated that either the exercise dose was too small or the adherence to the exercise sessions was not at the prescribed levels. Nevertheless, there is accumulating evidence in support to that long-term maintenance of weight loss is facilitated by regular physical activity *(104–106)*. This is of great value considering that body weight is an important factor affecting MetSyn parameters.

4.4. Adherence to the Therapeutic Intervention

Adoption of a healthy balanced diet requires behavioral changes in relation to meal planning, food selection, food preparation, portion control, and appropriate responses to eating challenges. Long-term adherence is required and its importance has been extensively discussed in the context of obesity or diabetes *(107–109)*. However, evidence regarding MetSyn is limited. Greater adherence has been correlated with greater decreases in MetSyn parameters *(40)*. Anderssen et al. *(39)* reported significant improvements in MetSyn components in the group of "good responders," i.e. those belonging to the highest tertile of change for body weight and oxygen uptake. This finding could be translated as "best adherence, best results."

With regard to maintenance, although significant changes in MetSyn parameters have been observed in the short-term *(34,37,40,109)*, in the absence of posttreatment booster sessions, subjects tend to maintain only part of the changes achieved or, for some components, they even return to their initial status *(38)*. On the contrary, when active follow-up was included in the treatment (as three to four follow-up visits per year for 20 months), a further improvement in MetSyn components was achieved *(35)*.

As noted earlier, low adherence to prescribed exercise sessions was suggested to mediate the modest changes observed in the components of the MetSyn *(91)*. In a study by Singh et al. *(40)*, control and intervention groups were given written advice to increase physical activity, whereas the intervention group also participated in a supervised exercise program. Improvement in the MetSyn components was achieved only in the intervention group, consistent with the finding that this group experienced a greater increase in physical activity, i.e., greater compliance to the program. Therefore, most investigators preferably use supervised exercise treatment *(33,34,37–39)*, instead of an ad libitum exercise component *(35,36,43)*.

5. CONCLUSION

There is a growing body of literature supporting the important role of diet and physical activity in the prevention and management of the MetSyn. To date, most of the lifestyle interventions had a favorable effect on the MetSyn; dietary changes constitute the core of the treatment, weight reduction plays a key role, and exercise confers an additional favorable effect. Nonetheless, it is of major importance to explore strategies to improve adherence and ensure that patients achieve and maintain lifestyle changes.

REFERENCES

1. Levantesi G, Macchia A, Marfisi R, et al. Metabolic syndrome and risk of cardiovascular events after myocardial infarction. J Am Coll Cardiol 2005;46:277–83.
2. Ford ES, Giles WH, Dietz WH. Prevalence of the metabolic syndrome among US adults: findings from the third National Health and Nutrition Examination Survey. JAMA 2002;287:356–9.

3. Reaven GM. Banting lecture 1988. Role of insulin resistance in human disease. Diabetes 1988;37: 1595–607.

4. Alberti KG, Zimmet PZ. Definition, diagnosis and classification of diabetes mellitus and its complications. Part 1: diagnosis and classification of diabetes mellitus provisional report of a WHO consultation. Diabet Med 1998;15:539–53.

5. Balkau B, Charles MA. Comment on the provisional report from the WHO consultation. European Group for the Study of Insulin Resistance (EGIR). Diabet Med 1999;16:442–3.

6. Executive Summary of the Third Report of the National Cholesterol Education Program (NCEP) Expert Panel on Detection, Evaluation, and Treatment of High Blood Cholesterol in Adults (Adult Treatment Panel III). Expert Panel on Detection, Evaluation, and Treatment of High Blood Cholesterol in Adults. JAMA 2001;285:2486–97.

7. Bloomgarden ZT. American Association of Clinical Endocrinologists (AACE) consensus conference on the insulin resistance syndrome: 25–26 August 2002, Washington, DC. Diabetes Care 2003;26:1297–303.

8. Moller DE, Kaufman KD. Metabolic syndrome: a clinical and molecular perspective. Annu Rev Med 2005;56:45–62.

9. Avramoglu RK, Basciano H, Adeli K. Lipid and lipoprotein dysregulation in insulin resistant states. Clin Chim Acta 2006;368:1–19.

10. Balasubramanyam A, Sekhar RV, Jahoor F, Jones PH, Pownall HJ. Pathophysiology of dyslipidemia and increased cardiovascular risk in HIV lipodystrophy: a model of 'systemic steatosis'. Curr Opin Lipidol 2004;15:59–67.

11. Grundy SM. Atherogenic dyslipidemia associated with metabolic syndrome and insulin resistance. Clin Cornerstone 2006;8 Suppl 1:S21–7.

12. Lewis GF, Carpentier A, Adeli K, Giacca A. Disordered fat storage and mobilization in the pathogenesis of insulin resistance and type 2 diabetes. Endocr Rev 2002;23:201–29.

13. Schondorf T, Maiworm A, Emmison N, Forst T, Pfutzner A. Biological background and role of adiponectin as marker for insulin resistance and cardiovascular risk. Clin Lab 2005;51:489–94.

14. Third Report of the National Cholesterol Education Program (NCEP) Expert Panel on Detection, Evaluation, and Treatment of High Blood Cholesterol in Adults (Adult Treatment Panel III) final report. National Cholesterol Education Program (NCEP) Expert Panel on Detection, Evaluation, and Treatment of High Blood Cholesterol in Adults (Adult Treatment Panel III). Circulation 2002;106:3143–421.

15. Boden G. Role of fatty acids in the pathogenesis of insulin resistance and NIDDM. Diabetes 1997;46:3–10.

16. Boden G, Shulman GI. Free fatty acids in obesity and type 2 diabetes: defining their role in the development of insulin resistance and beta-cell dysfunction. Eur J Clin Invest 2002;32 Suppl 3:14–23.

17. Berg AH, Combs TP, Du X, Brownlee M, Scherer PE. The adipocyte-secreted protein Acrp30 enhances hepatic insulin action. Nat Med 2001;7:947–53.

18. Berg AH, Combs TP, Scherer PE. ACRP30/adiponectin: an adipokine regulating glucose and lipid metabolism. Trends Endocrinol Metab 2002;13:84–9.

19. Combs TP, Berg AH, Obici S, Scherer PE, Rossetti L. Endogenous glucose production is inhibited by the adipose-derived protein Acrp30. J Clin Invest 2001;108:1875–81.

20. Yamauchi T, Hara K, Kubota N, et al. Dual roles of adiponectin/Acrp30 in vivo as an anti-diabetic and anti-atherogenic adipokine. Curr Drug Targets Immune Endocr Metabol Disord 2003;3:243–54.

21. Yamauchi T, Kamon J, Ito Y, et al. Cloning of adiponectin receptors that mediate antidiabetic metabolic effects. Nature 2003;423:762–9.

22. Banerjee RR, Rangwala SM, Shapiro JS, et al. Regulation of fasted blood glucose by resistin. Science 2004;303:1195–8.

23. Rajala MW, Qi Y, Patel HR, et al. Regulation of resistin expression and circulating levels in obesity, diabetes, and fasting. Diabetes 2004;53:1671–9.

24. Steppan CM, Bailey ST, Bhat S, et al. The hormone resistin links obesity to diabetes. Nature 2001;409:307–12.

25. Chu NF, Chang JB, Shieh SM. Plasma leptin, fatty acids, and tumor necrosis factor-receptor and insulin resistance in children. Obes Res 2003;11:532–40.

26. Lee JH, Chan JL, Sourlas E, Raptopoulos V, Mantzoros CS. Recombinant methionyl human leptin therapy in replacement doses improves insulin resistance and metabolic profile in patients with lipoatrophy

and metabolic syndrome induced by the highly active antiretroviral therapy. J Clin Endocrinol Metab 2006;91:2605–11.

27. Lichnovska R, Gwozdziewiczova S, Chlup R, Hrebicek J. Serum leptin in the development of insulin resistance and other disorders in the metabolic syndrome. Biomed Pap Med Fac Univ Palacky Olomouc Czech Repub 2005;149:119–26.

28. Zimmet P, Boyko EJ, Collier GR, de Courten M. Etiology of the metabolic syndrome: potential role of insulin resistance, leptin resistance, and other players. Ann N Y Acad Sci 1999;892:25–44.

29. Hotamisligil GS, Shargill NS, Spiegelman BM. Adipose expression of tumor necrosis factor-alpha: direct role in obesity-linked insulin resistance. Science 1993;259:87–91.

30. Spiegelman BM, Hotamisligil GS. Through thick and thin: wasting, obesity, and TNF alpha. Cell 1993;73:625–7.

31. Moller DE, Chang PY, Yaspelkis BB, III, Flier JS, Wallberg-Henriksson H, Ivy JL. Transgenic mice with muscle-specific insulin resistance develop increased adiposity, impaired glucose tolerance, and dyslipidemia. Endocrinology 1996;137:2397–405.

32. Park YW, Zhu S, Palaniappan L, Heshka S, Carnethon MR, Heymsfield SB. The metabolic syndrome: prevalence and associated risk factor findings in the US population from the Third National Health and Nutrition Examination Survey, 1988–1994. Arch Intern Med 2003;163:427–36.

33. Christ M, Iannello C, Iannello PG, Grimm W. Effects of a weight reduction program with and without aerobic exercise in the metabolic syndrome. Int J Cardiol 2004;97:115–22.

34. Villareal DT, Miller BV, III, Banks M, Fontana L, Sinacore DR, Klein S. Effect of lifestyle intervention on metabolic coronary heart disease risk factors in obese older adults. Am J Clin Nutr 2006;84:1317–23.

35. Muzio F, Mondazzi L, Sommariva D, Branchi A. Long-term effects of low-calorie diet on the metabolic syndrome in obese nondiabetic patients. Diabetes Care 2005;28:1485–6.

36. Case CC, Jones PH, Nelson K, O'Brian Smith E, Ballantyne CM. Impact of weight loss on the metabolic syndrome. Diabetes Obes Metab 2002;4:407–14.

37. Watkins LL, Sherwood A, Feinglos M, et al. Effects of exercise and weight loss on cardiac risk factors associated with syndrome X. Arch Intern Med 2003;163:1889–95.

38. Lindahl B, Nilsson TK, Asplund K, Hallmans G. Intense nonpharmacological intervention in subjects with multiple cardiovascular risk factors: decreased fasting insulin levels but only a minor effect on plasma plasminogen activator inhibitor activity. Metabolism 1998;47:384–90.

39. Anderssen SA, Hjermann I, Urdal P, Torjesen PA, Holme I. Improved carbohydrate metabolism after physical training and dietary intervention in individuals with the "atherothrombogenic syndrome". Oslo Diet and Exercise Study (ODES). A randomized trial. J Intern Med 1996;240:203–9.

40. Singh RB, Singh NK, Rastogi SS, Mani UV, Niaz MA. Effects of diet and lifestyle changes on atherosclerotic risk factors after 24 weeks on the Indian Diet Heart Study. Am J Cardiol 1993;71:1283–8.

41. Niskanen L, Laaksonen DE, Punnonen K, Mustajoki P, Kaukua J, Rissanen A. Changes in sex hormone-binding globulin and testosterone during weight loss and weight maintenance in abdominally obese men with the metabolic syndrome. Diabetes Obes Metab 2004;6:208–15.

42. Brook RD, Bard RL, Glazewski L, et al. Effect of short-term weight loss on the metabolic syndrome and conduit vascular endothelial function in overweight adults. Am J Cardiol 2004;93:1012–6.

43. Esposito K, Marfella R, Ciotola M, et al. Effect of a mediterranean-style diet on endothelial dysfunction and markers of vascular inflammation in the metabolic syndrome: a randomized trial. JAMA 2004;292:1440–6.

44. Poppitt SD, Keogh GF, Prentice AM, et al. Long-term effects of ad libitum low-fat, high-carbohydrate diets on body weight and serum lipids in overweight subjects with metabolic syndrome. Am J Clin Nutr 2002;75:11–20.

45. Higgins M, Kannel W, Garrison R, Pinsky J, Stokes J, III. Hazards of obesity – the Framingham experience. Acta Med Scand Suppl 1988;723:23–36.

46. Knowler WC, Barrett-Connor E, Fowler SE, et al. Reduction in the incidence of type 2 diabetes with lifestyle intervention or metformin. N Engl J Med 2002;346:393–403.

47. Hu FB. Sedentary lifestyle and risk of obesity and type 2 diabetes. Lipids 2003;38:103–8.

48. Hu FB, Manson JE, Stampfer MJ, et al. Diet, lifestyle, and the risk of type 2 diabetes mellitus in women. N Engl J Med 2001;345:790–7.

49. Stampfer MJ, Hu FB, Manson JE, Rimm EB, Willett WC. Primary prevention of coronary heart disease in women through diet and lifestyle. N Engl J Med 2000;343:16–22.

50. Huang Z, Willett WC, Manson JE, et al. Body weight, weight change, and risk for hypertension in women. Ann Intern Med 1998;128:81–8.

51. Neter JE, Stam BE, Kok FJ, Grobbee DE, Geleijnse JM. Influence of weight reduction on blood pressure: a meta-analysis of randomized controlled trials. Hypertension 2003;42:878–84.

52. Manson JE, Colditz GA, Stampfer MJ, et al. A prospective study of maturity-onset diabetes mellitus and risk of coronary heart disease and stroke in women. Arch Intern Med 1991;151:1141–7.

53. Visser M, Bouter LM, McQuillan GM, Wener MH, Harris TB. Elevated C-reactive protein levels in overweight and obese adults. JAMA 1999;282:2131–5.

54. Albert MA, Ridker PM. The role of C-reactive protein in cardiovascular disease risk. Curr Cardiol Rep 1999;1:99–104.

55. Morrow DA, Ridker PM. C-Reactive protein, inflammation, and coronary risk. Med Clin North Am 2000;84:149–61, ix.

56. Ridker PM, Hennekens CH, Buring JE, Rifai N. C-Reactive protein and other markers of inflammation in the prediction of cardiovascular disease in women. N Engl J Med 2000;342:836–43.

57. Bougoulia M, Triantos A, Koliakos G. Effect of weight loss with or without orlistat treatment on adipocytokines, inflammation, and oxidative markers in obese women. Hormones (Athens) 2006;5:259–69.

58. Blair SN, Kohl HW, III, Paffenbarger RS, Jr., Clark DG, Cooper KH, Gibbons LW. Physical fitness and all-cause mortality. A prospective study of healthy men and women. JAMA 1989;262:2395–401.

59. Wei M, Kampert JB, Barlow CE, et al. Relationship between low cardiorespiratory fitness and mortality in normal-weight, overweight, and obese men. JAMA 1999;282:1547–53.

60. Wessel TR, Arant CB, Olson MB, et al. Relationship of physical fitness vs body mass index with coronary artery disease and cardiovascular events in women. JAMA 2004;292:1179–87.

61. Orakzai RH, Orakzai SH, Nasir K, et al. Association of increased cardiorespiratory fitness with low risk for clustering of metabolic syndrome components in asymptomatic men. Arch Med Res 2006;37:522–8.

62. Simonelli C, Eaton RP. Reduced triglyceride secretion: a metabolic consequence of chronic exercise. Am J Physiol 1978;234:E221–7.

63. Simonelli C, Eaton RP. Cardiovascular and metabolic effects of exercise: the strong case for conditioning. Postgrad Med 1978;63:71–7.

64. Tsekouras YE, Yanni AE, Bougatsas D, Kavouras SA, Sidossis LS. A single bout of brisk walking increases basal very low-density lipoprotein triacylglycerol clearance in young men. Metabolism 2007;56:1037–43.

65. Duncan GE, Perri MG, Theriaque DW, Hutson AD, Eckel RH, Stacpoole PW. Exercise training, without weight loss, increases insulin sensitivity and postheparin plasma lipase activity in previously sedentary adults. Diabetes Care 2003;26:557–62.

66. Goodpaster BH, He J, Watkins S, Kelley DE. Skeletal muscle lipid content and insulin resistance: evidence for a paradox in endurance-trained athletes. J Clin Endocrinol Metab 2001;86:5755–61.

67. Ring-Dimitriou S, Paulweber B, von Duvillard SP, et al. The effect of physical activity and physical fitness on plasma adiponectin in adults with predisposition to metabolic syndrome. Eur J Appl Physiol 2006;98:472–81.

68. Nassis GP, Papantakou K, Skenderi K, et al. Aerobic exercise training improves insulin sensitivity without changes in body weight, body fat, adiponectin, and inflammatory markers in overweight and obese girls. Metabolism 2005;54:1472–9.

69. Ascherio A, Katan MB, Zock PL, Stampfer MJ, Willett WC. Trans fatty acids and coronary heart disease. N Engl J Med 1999;340:1994–8.

70. Toft I, Bonaa KH, Ingebretsen OC, Nordoy A, Jenssen T, Effects of n-3 polyunsaturated fatty acids on glucose homeostasis and blood pressure in essential hypertension. A randomized, controlled trial. Ann Intern Med 1995;123:911–8.

71. Glauber H, Wallace P, Griver K, Brechtel G. Adverse metabolic effect of omega-3 fatty acids in non-insulin-dependent diabetes mellitus. Ann Intern Med 1988;108:663–8.

72. Popp-Snijders C, Schouten JA, Heine RJ, van der Meer J, van der Veen EA. Dietary supplementation of omega-3 polyunsaturated fatty acids improves insulin sensitivity in non-insulin-dependent diabetes. Diabetes Res 1987;4:141–7.

73. Vessby B, Unsitupa M, Hermansen K, et al. Substituting dietary saturated for monounsaturated fat impairs insulin sensitivity in healthy men and women: The KANWU Study. Diabetologia 2001;44:312–9.

74. Salmeron J, Hu FB, Manson JE, et al. Dietary fat intake and risk of type 2 diabetes in women. Am J Clin Nutr 2001;73:1019–26.

75. Montoya MT, Porres A, Serrano S, et al. Fatty acid saturation of the diet and plasma lipid concentrations, lipoprotein particle concentrations, and cholesterol efflux capacity. Am J Clin Nutr 2002;75:484–91.

76. Willett W, Manson J, Liu S. Glycemic index, glycemic load, and risk of type 2 diabetes. Am J Clin Nutr 2002;76:274S–80S.

77. Liu S, Manson JE, Buring JE, Stampfer MJ, Willett WC, Ridker PM. Relation between a diet with a high glycemic load and plasma concentrations of high-sensitivity C-reactive protein in middle-aged women. Am J Clin Nutr 2002;75:492–8.

78. Liu S, Manson JE, Stampfer MJ, et al. Dietary glycemic load assessed by food-frequency questionnaire in relation to plasma high-density-lipoprotein cholesterol and fasting plasma triacylglycerols in postmenopausal women. Am J Clin Nutr 2001;73:560–6.

79. Ludwig DS. The glycemic index: physiological mechanisms relating to obesity, diabetes, and cardiovascular disease. JAMA 2002;287:2414–23.

80. Nordmann AJ, Nordmann A, Briel M, et al. Effects of low-carbohydrate vs low-fat diets on weight loss and cardiovascular risk factors: a meta-analysis of randomized controlled trials. Arch Intern Med 2006;166:285–93.

81. Abbasi F, McLaughlin T, Lamendola C, et al. High carbohydrate diets, triglyceride-rich lipoproteins, and coronary heart disease risk. Am J Cardiol 2000;85:45–8.

82. Chiasson JL, Josse RG, Gomis R, Hanefeld M, Karasik A, Laakso M. Acarbose for prevention of type 2 diabetes mellitus: the STOP-NIDDM randomised trial. Lancet 2002;359:2072–7.

83. Chiasson JL, Josse RG, Gomis R, Hanefeld M, Karasik A, Laakso M. Acarbose treatment and the risk of cardiovascular disease and hypertension in patients with impaired glucose tolerance: the STOP-NIDDM trial. JAMA 2003;290:486–94.

84. Davies MJ, Baer DJ, Judd JT, Brown ED, Campbell WS, Taylor PR. Effects of moderate alcohol intake on fasting insulin and glucose concentrations and insulin sensitivity in postmenopausal women: a randomized controlled trial. JAMA 2002;287:2559–62.

85. Gigleux I, Gagnon J, St-Pierre A, et al. Moderate alcohol consumption is more cardioprotective in men with the metabolic syndrome. J Nutr 2006;136:3027–32.

86. Klatsky AL. Alcohol and cardiovascular disease – more than one paradox to consider. Alcohol and hypertension: does it matter? Yes. J Cardiovasc Risk 2003;10:21–4.

87. Orchard TJ, Temprosa M, Goldberg R, et al. The effect of metformin and intensive lifestyle intervention on the metabolic syndrome: the Diabetes Prevention Program randomized trial. Ann Intern Med 2005;142:611–9.

88. Lindstrom J, Louheranta A, Mannelin M, et al. The Finnish Diabetes Prevention Study (DPS): lifestyle intervention and 3-year results on diet and physical activity. Diabetes Care 2003;26:3230–6.

89. Dattilo AM, Kris-Etherton PM. Effects of weight reduction on blood lipids and lipoproteins: a meta-analysis. Am J Clin Nutr 1992;56:320–8.

90. Hubbard RS, Beck EC. Changes in the glucose tolerance of obese subjects after weight reduction. J Clin Invest 1939;18:783–9.

91. Kukkonen-Harjula KT, Borg PT, Nenonen AM, Fogelholm MG. Effects of a weight maintenance program with or without exercise on the metabolic syndrome: a randomized trial in obese men. Prev Med 2005;41:784–90.

92. Appel LJ, Sacks FM, Carey VJ, et al. Effects of protein, monounsaturated fat, and carbohydrate intake on blood pressure and serum lipids: results of the OmniHeart randomized trial. JAMA 2005;294:2455–64.

93. Kris-Etherton PM, Pearson TA, Wan Y, et al. High-monounsaturated fatty acid diets lower both plasma cholesterol and triacylglycerol concentrations. Am J Clin Nutr 1999;70:1009–15.

94. Wannamethee SG, Shaper AG, Whincup PH. Modifiable lifestyle factors and the metabolic syndrome in older men: Effects of lifestyle changes. J Am Geriatr Soc 2006;54:1909–14.

95. Muzio F, Mondazzi L, Harris WS, Sommariva D, Branchi A. Effects of moderate variations in the macronutrient content of the diet on cardiovascular disease risk factors in obese patients with the metabolic syndrome. Am J Clin Nutr 2007;86:946–51.

96. Lien LF, Brown AJ, Ard JD, et al. Effects of PREMIER lifestyle modifications on participants with and without the metabolic syndrome. Hypertension 2007;50:609–16.

97. Corcoran MP, Lamon-Fava S, Fielding RA. Skeletal muscle lipid deposition and insulin resistance: effect of dietary fatty acids and exercise. Am J Clin Nutr 2007;85:662–77.

98. Katzmarzyk PT, Leon AS, Wilmore JH, et al. Targeting the metabolic syndrome with exercise: evidence from the HERITAGE Family Study. Med Sci Sports Exerc 2003;35:1703–9.

99. Dumortier M, Brandou F, Perez-Martin A, Fedou C, Mercier J, Brun JF. Low intensity endurance exercise targeted for lipid oxidation improves body composition and insulin sensitivity in patients with the metabolic syndrome. Diabetes Metab 2003;29:509–18.

100. Votruba SB, Horvitz MA, Schoeller DA. The role of exercise in the treatment of obesity. Nutrition 2000;16:179–88.

101. Fenkci S, Sarsan A, Rota S, Ardic F. Effects of resistance or aerobic exercises on metabolic parameters in obese women who are not on a diet. Adv Ther 2006;23:404–13.

102. Johnson JL, Slentz CA, Houmard JA, et al. Exercise training amount and intensity effects on metabolic syndrome (from Studies of a Targeted Risk Reduction Intervention through Defined Exercise). Am J Cardiol 2007;100:1759–66.

103. Anderssen SA, Carroll S, Urdal P, Holme I. Combined diet and exercise intervention reverses the metabolic syndrome in middle-aged males: results from the Oslo Diet and Exercise Study. Scand J Med Sci Sports 2007;17:687–95.

104. Jakicic JM, Otto AD. Physical activity considerations for the treatment and prevention of obesity. Am J Clin Nutr 2005;82:226S–9S.

105. Johannsen DL, Redman LM, Ravussin E. The role of physical activity in maintaining a reduced weight. Curr Atheroscler Rep 2007;9:463–71.

106. Schoeller DA, Shay K, Kushner RF. How much physical activity is needed to minimize weight gain in previously obese women? Am J Clin Nutr 1997;66:551–6.

107. McManus K, Antinoro L, Sacks F. A randomized controlled trial of a moderate-fat, low-energy diet compared with a low fat, low-energy diet for weight loss in overweight adults. Int J Obes Relat Metab Disord 2001;25:1503–11.

108. Yannakoulia M. Eating behavior among type 2 diabetic patients: a poorly recognized aspect in a poorly controlled disease. Rev Diabet Stud 2006;3:11–6.

109. Oh EG, Hyun SS, Kim SH, et al. A randomized controlled trial of therapeutic lifestyle modification in rural women with metabolic syndrome: a pilot study. Metabolism 2008;57:255–61.

9 Diet and Physical Activity in Cancer Prevention

Alicja Wolk

KEY POINTS

- Cancer confers a major disease burden worldwide, especially in affluent societies.
- Cancer incidence and mortality between low risk and high risk countries differs several-fold.
- These differences are ascribed such environmental factors as lifelong dietary behaviors, physical inactivity, weight gain, alcohol consumption, and the use of tobacco.
- Through a healthy diet, optimal levels of physical activity and by maintaining normal body weight, a large proportion of cancers may be prevented.

Key Words: Cancer, Diet, Food consumption, Incidence, Mortality, Physical activity, Obesity, Prevention, Recommendations, Trends

1. INTRODUCTION

Cancer confers a major disease burden worldwide, but there are marked geographical variations in cancer incidence overall and in cancers of specific organ sites. Worldwide, approximately 10 million people are diagnosed with cancer annually, and more than 6 million die of the disease every year; currently over 22 million people in the world are cancer patients. The total cancer burden is highest in affluent societies, mainly due to a high incidence of tumors associated with Western lifestyle and smoking, i.e., tumors of the prostate, breast, colorectum, and lung *(1)*. Cancer incidence and mortality between low risk and high risk countries differs by several fold.

2. TEMPORAL CHANGES IN CANCER INCIDENCE AND MORTALITY

Trends for cancer mortality during 1950–2000 and cancer incidence in 2002 for the United States, Europe, and Japan are presented in Figs. 1 and 2. Cancer incidence and mortality have been steadily rising throughout the century in most areas of the world. However, over the last few years in North America and in Western Europe, some decline

From: *Nutrition and Health: Nutrition and Metabolism*
Edited by: C.S. Mantzoros, DOI: 10.1007/978-1-60327-453-1_9,
© Humana Press, a part of Springer Science+Business Media, LLC 2009

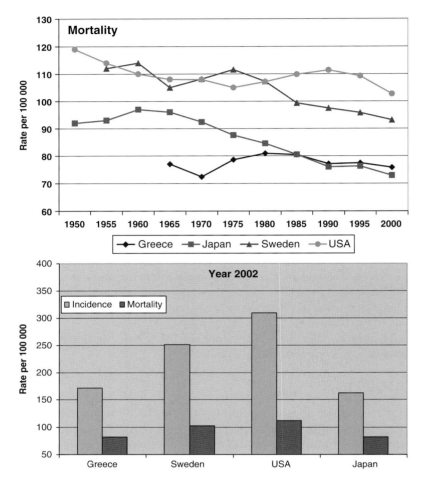

Fig. 1. Time trends in mortality from all cancer and incidence rates of all cancer in 2002 among women.

in cancer mortality has been observed. Thus, age-standardized cancer mortality rates for all neoplasms in the USA declined by 3.1% in both sexes combined between 1990 and 1995 *(1)*. Approximately half of the decline was attributed to the leveling of lung and other tobacco-related cancer epidemics, and the rest to several factors, including reduced exposure to occupational carcinogens, prevention and early diagnosis, and improved treatment. In Europe as well as in North America and Japan, between 80 and 90% of lung cancers in men, and between 55 and 80% of lung cancers in women, are attributable to cigarette smoking. Taking into account all tobacco-related cancers, between 25 and 30% of all cancers in Europe and the USA are due to tobacco smoking. Because of the length of the latency period, tobacco-related cancers observed today are mainly related to cigarette smoking patterns several decades ago *(1)*. Another major factor, identified almost three decades ago as a factor contributing to cancer risk, is diet *(2)*.

Comparing the incidence and mortality rates between the different countries we have to keep in mind that Greek data may be less reliable than Swedish, and the data from the United States and from Japan are reasonably reliable. The Greek data may overestimate

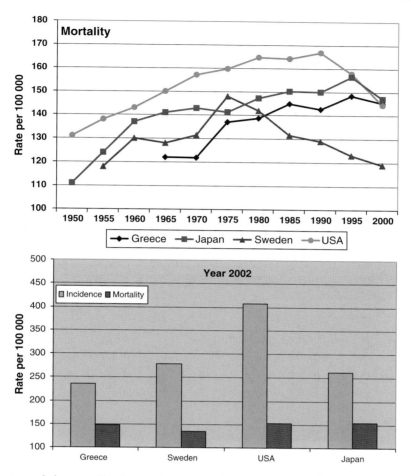

Fig. 2. Time trends in mortality from all cancer and incidence rates of all cancer in 2002 among men.

actual rates, because regional registries exist in the more developed regions that are usually characterized by higher cancer rates *(3)*.

Later we present time trends for prostate, breast, and colorectal cancer mortality between 1950 and 2000 as well as incidence of these cancer sites in 2002 for the four chosen countries representing different geographical regions (Figs. 3–5). The differences between Japan and Sweden as well as the USA are striking for prostate and breast cancer incidence and mortality, with Sweden having the highest and still increasing prostate cancer mortality *(4)*.

While breast cancer mortality is decreasing in the USA and Sweden, and there is a suggestion that the increasing trend in Greece has changed, the opposite trend is seen in Japan. The difference in mortality rates between the USA and Japan has changed from almost five-fold in the 1950s to about 2.5-fold in 2000.

Mortality rates for colon cancer in the USA, although systematically decreasing since the mid 1980s, are still higher than in Japan and Greece where rates continue to increase.

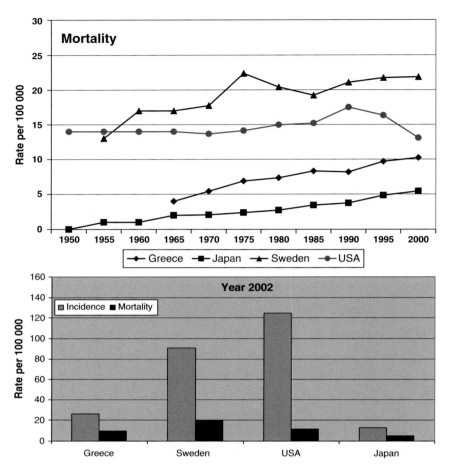

Fig. 3. Time trends in mortality rates from prostate cancer and incidence rates of prostate cancer in 2002.

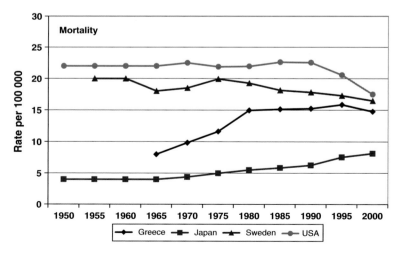

Fig. 4. Time trends in mortality rates from breast cancer and incidence rates of breast cancer in 2002.

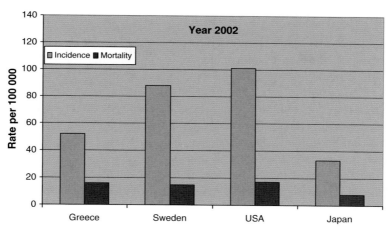

Fig. 4. (continued)

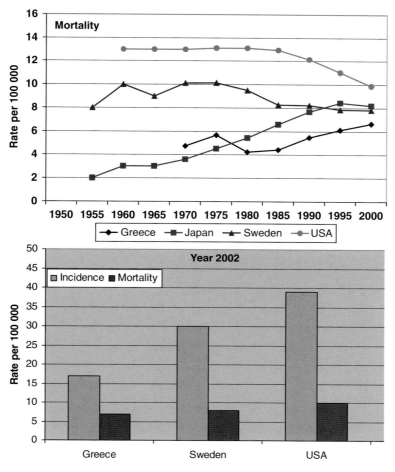

Fig. 5. Time trends in mortality rates from colon cancer and incidence rates of colorectal cancer in women and men in 2002.

3. MODIFIABLE CAUSES OF CANCER

Already in 1964, an expert committee of the World Health Organization concluded that many common fatal cases of cancer could be potentially prevented by changes in lifestyle and other environmental factors, including dietary deficiencies, hormonal factors, and some environmental carcinogens (5). On the basis of the epidemiological observation that migrants tend to acquire the cancer rates of their new country, Doll and Peto concluded that differences in cancer rates can be attributed in part to environmental factors such as smoking, diet, and others.

On the basis of comparisons of high and low incidence countries, they concluded that 75–80% of cancers diagnosed in the United States in 1970 theoretically could have been avoided (2). Their highest estimates were for poor dietary habits (approximately 35%) and smoking (30%), as shown in Fig. 6.

The question was what made the United States population different from low risk populations, at that time. The question why the US has higher cancer incidence rates than Greece, Japan, or Sweden is still not fully answered. The environmental factors that differ between these countries are many and include mainly lifelong dietary behaviors, physical inactivity, lifelong weight gain, alcohol consumption, and the use of tobacco.

Although the conclusion by Doll and Peto was provocative at that time, because of limited data from analytical and rigorously performed epidemiological studies, it is still true today, more than 25 years later.

Accumulated evidence from thousands of observational epidemiological studies have confirmed the contribution of specific lifestyle factors to the etiology of cancer and have expanded the list of cancer risk factors to include also obesity and physical inactivity. The previously estimated 75–80% reduction in cancer burden was a theoretical maximum, and Doll and Peto acknowledged that it was rather unlikely that any society could change lifestyle enough – even over many years – to decrease cancer incidence by this amount. However, the new estimates indicate that more than 50% of all cancer

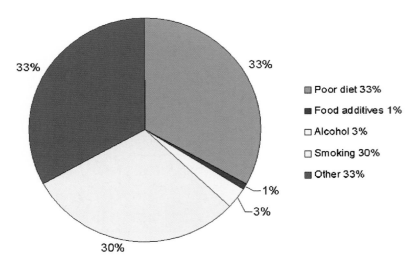

Fig. 6. Proportions of cancer attributed to nongenetic factors. Estimated proportions that could have been avoided in each category of factors as estimated by Doll and Peto (2).

cases could be prevented by achievable changes *(6)*. Evidence indicates that in the United States (Fig. 7), obesity accounts for some 15% of all cancer cases, physical inactivity for 5% of cases, poor diet for 10–25% of cases, alcohol consumption for 4% of cancer cases, and tobacco use for 30% *(7)*.

For the great majority of people who do not use tobacco, weight control, dietary choices, and the levels of physical activity are the most important modifiable determinants of cancer risk *(8–10)*. Although genetic factors influence the risk of cancer, most of the variations in cancer risk across populations and among individuals are due to factors that are not inherited *(11,12)*. Such modifiable lifestyle-related factors as no smoking, maintaining a healthy weight, staying physically active throughout life, and consuming a healthy diet can substantially reduce one's lifetime risk for developing cancer *(10,13)*. It is important to point out that the same healthy behaviors are also associated with reduced risk of developing cardiovascular disease.

As is shown in Figs. 3–5, cancer rates especially for prostate and breast cancer, differ several fold between Western and Asian countries, similar to differences in food consumption (Fig. 8a–d). Differences in food patterns between the four countries described in this chapter are large. In Greece there is much higher per capita availability of vegetables, roots and tubers, fruits, pulses, and nuts than in the three other countries (Fig. 8a, b). In Sweden there is the highest per capita availability of milk and coffee (Fig. 8c, d); Japan is leading regarding the per capita availability of fish and tea (Fig. 8c, d), and USA is leading in red meat availability (Fig. 8c).

Differences in prevalence of obesity between the four countries are several fold, with Japan having the lowest and USA the highest prevalence (Fig. 9). Overweight and obesity have reached epidemic proportions globally along with an adoption of a life-style characterized by a combination of excessive food intake and inadequate physical activity. The dramatic rise in prevalence of obesity and increasing inactivity has been accompanied by increases in the incidence and prevalence of type 2 diabetes. There is accumulating evidence that diabetes is associated with an increased risk for cancer at several sites *(14)*.

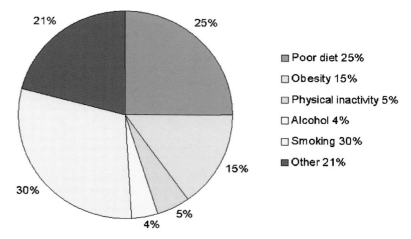

Fig. 7. Proportion of cancer attributable to modifiable lifestyle factors in the United States according to recent estimates.

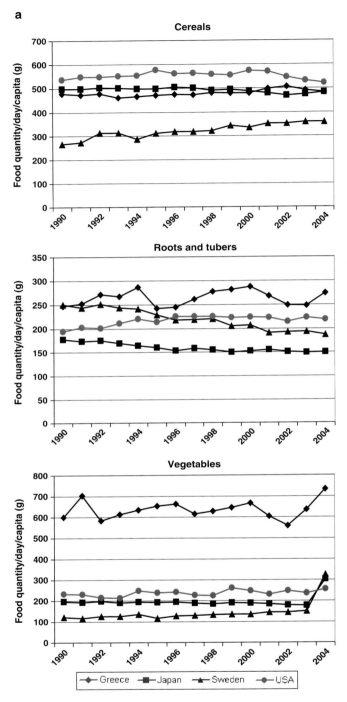

Fig. 8. (**a**) Time trends in mean per capita availability (in g/day) of selected food groups – cereals, roots and tubers, and vegetables – in Greece, Sweden, USA and Japan. (**b**) Time trends in mean per capita availability (in g/day) of selected food groups – fruits and berries, pulses, and nuts – in Greece, Sweden, USA, and Japan. (**c**) Time trends in mean per capita availability (in g/day) of selected food groups – fish, red meat, and milk – in Greece, Sweden, USA, and Japan. (**d**) Time trends in mean per capita availability (in g/day) of selected food groups – coffee, tea and matè, and sugar crops – in Greece, Sweden, USA, and Japan.

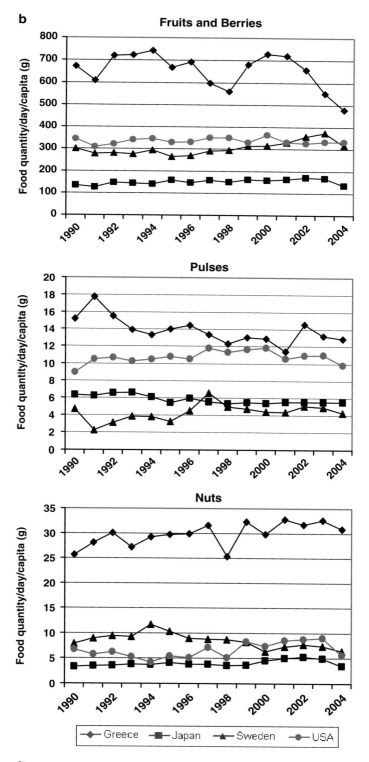

Fig. 8. (continued)

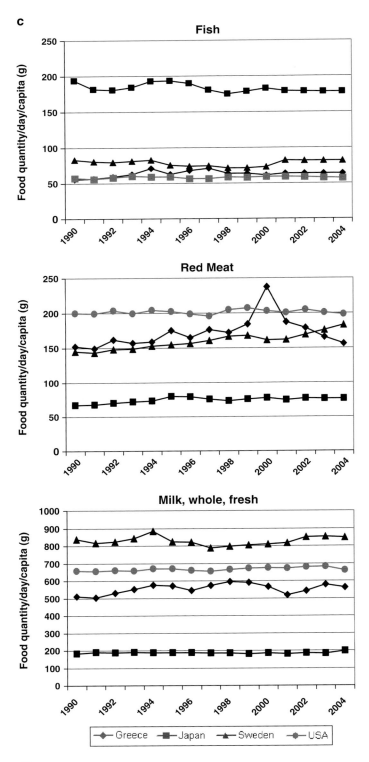

Fig. 8. (continued)

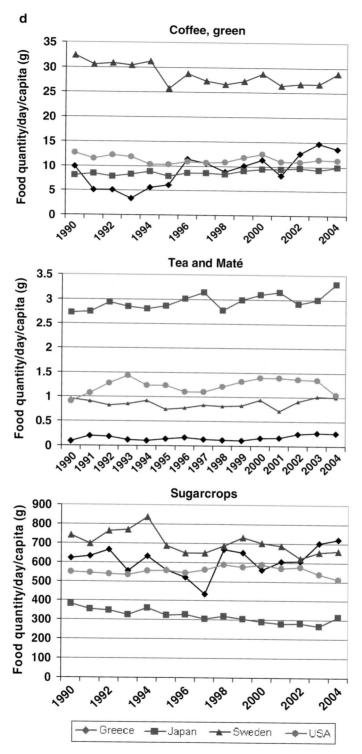

d

Fig. 8. (continued)

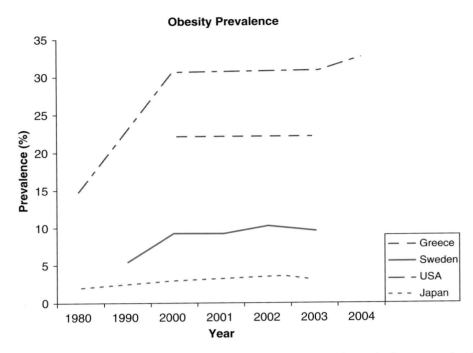

Fig. 9. Time trends in obesity prevalence among adult women and men in four countries from different geographic regions.

Differences in physical activity and inactivity between the countries described in this chapter are presented in Fig. 10. As shown in Fig. 11a, b, temporal changes in decreasing physical activity between the 1930s and the 1990s among Swedish women and men are very striking in all age groups *(16,17)*. Especially pronounced is the decreasing demand for occupational physical activity and decreasing energy expenditure related to walking.

Furthermore, there are differences between the four countries in alcohol consumption and tobacco use (Fig. 12). Temporal changes in these modifiable lifestyle factors that have been shown to be associated with cancer risk – namely food consumption patterns, obesity, physical inactivity, smoking and alcohol – are paralleled by changes in cancer incidence. Prevalence of smoking in Sweden and USA has been decreasing in both women and men (Fig. 12). Policy and community interventions have been especially successful in Swedish men.

4. DIET AND CANCER

This review on diet and cancer is limited to the three cancer sites with the highest incidence in developed countries.

4.1. Prostate Cancer

Prostate cancer (PC) is the most frequent cancer among men in North America as well as in Northern and Western Europe. Causes of the disease are essentially unknown, although it is estimated in studies of twins that hereditability of PC is approximately

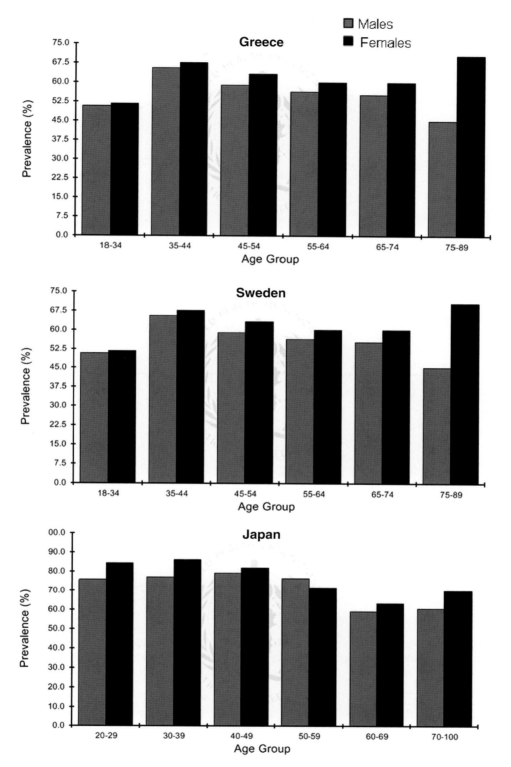

Fig. 10. Prevalence of physical inactivity (unspecified) by age groups in Greece, Sweden, and Japan *(15)*.

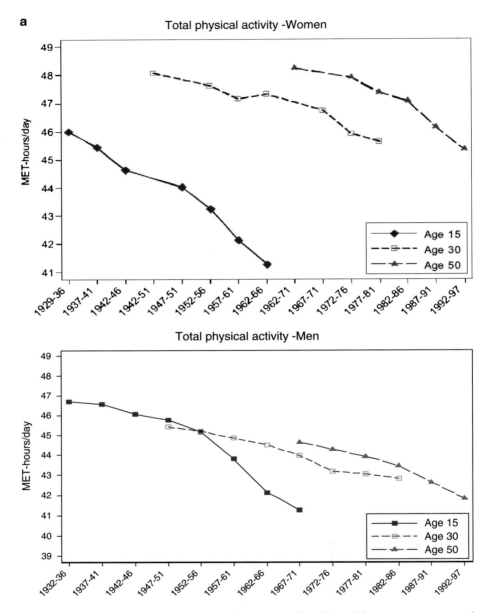

Fig. 11. (a) Temporal trends in physical activity among Swedish adolescents, women and men. **(b)** Temporal trends in specific types of physical activity among Swedish adolescent girls and boys, women and men.

42%, the highest of all studied cancers *(11)*. There is approximately a 40-fold difference in the reported incidence and a 12-fold difference in mortality of PC between various geographic areas and populations *(21)*. Diet is suspected to play a major role in the initiation, promotion, and progression of PC. Among the dietary factors that have

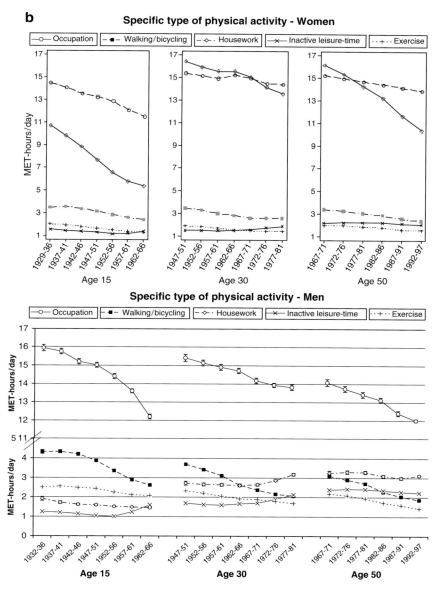

Fig. 11. (continued)

most consistently been associated with increased risk of PC development are meat and milk products.

High consumption of meat, particularly red or processed meat, generally is associated with moderate to severe increases in risk of PC by 30 or more percent in most studies *(22)*, although conflicting evidence exists *(23)*. Those few studies that have separately analyzed the association, not only with total prostate cancer but also with advanced and metastatic tumors, have reported even higher risk estimates for the advanced stages

Temporal changes in prevalence of smoking

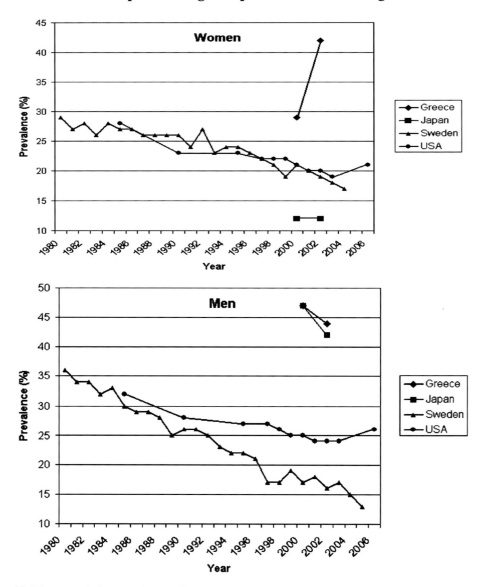

Fig. 12. Time trends in prevalence of smoking among women and men in four countries *(18–20).*

of the disease *(24)*. A two-fold increase was found for advanced cancer and a 2.2-fold increase in metastatic cancer compared with 40–50% increase for total PC. These results suggest a possible role of meat in the progression of PC. The mechanisms by which meat consumption might affect the risk of prostate cancer remain unknown. It has been speculated that the observed positive association may reflect the high intake of fat, especially that of total fat; in Asian countries with a low incidence of the disease, total intake of fat is much lower than in countries with high incidence, although findings of total dietary fat and specific fat types are mixed *(24)*. Another speculation is that meat that is grilled or pan-fried at high temperatures contains heterocyclic amines that have been found to contain carcinogens in animal studies on rat prostates *(25)*. A recent prospective study has indeed shown that an average consumption of more than 10 g/day of very well done meat, compared with no consumption at all, is associated with a statistically significant 70% increased risk of incident prostate cancer *(26)*. Red meat is a major source of zinc, which is known to be essential for testosterone synthesis *(27)*. The use of zinc supplements of more than 100 mg/day and for more than 10 years was associated with more than two-fold increase in risk of PC compared with nonusers *(28)*. High consumption of red meat and a high zinc and protein intake was also associated with a higher circulating concentration of insulin-like growth factor 1 (IGF-1) *(29)*. Interestingly, high IGF-1 levels have consistently been associated with high incidence of PC *(30)*.

Milk products also appear to consistently be associated with increased risk of PC. Those few studies that have analyzed advanced and metastasized PC separately suggested that the association might be stronger for the more advanced cancers than for all PC *(22)*. This might indicate a possible role of dairy products in the progression of this neoplasm. The mechanisms behind these observed associations are not known. Many studies indicate that calcium, the main dietary component of dairy products, may play an important role in PC development. In the Health Professionals follow-up study, men who consumed more than 2,000 mg/day of calcium had an approximately five-fold increased risk of developing metastatic and fatal PC compared with those consuming less than 500 mg/day *(31,32)*. High consumption of low-fat milk has been associated with a higher concentration of circulating IGF-1 *(33)*. Another possibility is that branched fatty acids present mainly in milk fat, and also in beef, may up-regulate the α-methylacyl Co A racemase (*AMACR*) gene, previously shown to be over-expressed in PC tumors, and not in healthy prostates *(34)*.

There are also other dietary factors that are thought to be protective. Although there is a general health recommendation to eat five or more servings of fruits and vegetables per day, the accumulated evidence does not support any reduced risk of prostate cancer *(35)*. However, several epidemiological studies have reported that some vegetables, specifically tomatoes, and lycopene (the predominant carotenoid found in serum), from tomatoes mainly, are associated with lower risk of PC. Indeed, a review of four studies of serum lycopene and incidence of PC report a significant reduction in risk (25–80%) *(36)*. In a meta-analysis of 21 studies, high consumption of tomatoes resulted in a 10–20% risk reduction *(37)*. There is also a suggestion that other carotenoids lower the risk *(24)*. Several epidemiological studies have reported an inverse relationship with cruciferous vegetables (specifically cabbage, broccoli, cauliflower, and brussel-sprouts) and the risk of developing PC *(24)*, whereas the European Prospective Investigation into Cancer (EPIC) did not *(38)*. In the Health Professionals follow-up study, an inverse association was only observed for early stage cancer in younger men, suggesting that cruciferous vegetables may be important early on in the carcinogenesis process *(39)*. Anticarcinogenic phytochemicals that are present in cruciferous vegetables (indole-3-carbinol and isothiocyanates) can induce antioxidative enzymes and counteract oxidative damage. They have also been shown to have proapoptotic, antiproliferative, and antimetastatic properties in animal models of PC *(40)*.

Furthermore, other phytochemicals found in fruits and vegetables, tea, and red wine, namely polyphenols and isoflavones, have been shown in experimental studies to have antioxidant, antiproliferative, antiangiogenesic, or proapoptotic effects (24,41). Given the promising results from in vitro and animal studies on these phytochemicals, epidemiological studies are needed.

The most promising micronutrients regarding nutritional protective factors are vitamin E and selenium. Vitamin E, an antioxidant found mainly in vegetable oil, nuts and oils, has been observed to significantly reduce the risk for PC among smokers in a Finnish intervention study (42). That study has shown that men receiving 50 mg/day of supplemental vitamin E (α-tocopherol) had a 30–40% reduction in PC incidence and mortality compared with men taking a placebo. Selenium is an essential micronutrient present mainly in grains, fish, and eggs. The level of selenium in the soil determines its level in the plants grown in that area. Therefore, any variation in the selenium levels of food may be largely derived from the levels of the geographic area in which they were grown. Selenium intake has been observed to predict a lower risk of PC in several large prospective studies, but this is not always the case (22,43). High vs. low selenium levels in nails or plasma resulted in a reduction of 50–65% in the risk of PC (44,45). In the randomized Nutrition Prevention of Cancer Trial study, men taking supplemental selenium had a 50% lower risk compared with the placebo group (46).

In recent years, a great deal of attention has been given to the so-called phytoestrogens. These phytochemicals with some estrogen-like activities are present in plant foods. Most frequently studied are soy foods, but, Westerners traditionally consume other plant foods containing so-called lignans (sources of which include flaxseed and rye), which are also ascribed estrogen-like and anticarcinogenic properties (47,48). In a recent large case-control study in Sweden, total or individual consumption of lignans or isoflavonoids was not associated with PC. However, high total consumption of foods rich in lignans and isoflavones was associated with moderate decrease in risk of PC (49).

There are several studies showing that fish consumption decreases PC incidence and mortality (22,24,50). The mechanism behind this observation might be linked to marine omega-3 fatty acids, a source of which is oily fish (salmon, mackerel, sardines, and herring). Fish is also an additional source of selenium and vitamin D and is also considered to have anticarcinogenic properties (51). However, it has to be noted that the main source of vitamin D remains exposure to ultraviolet light.

4.2. Breast Cancer

Migration studies suggest that lifestyle, aside from genetics, is a key factor in breast cancer risk. Breast cancer rates are rising globally in patterns that correspond with lifestyle changes. Belief such as fatty foods cause breast cancer (52) while consumption of vegetables and fruit reduce this risk have not confirmed (53). Instead, obesity and disordered energy balance are proving to be important risk factors (54). Indirect epidemiologic evidence suggests that diet in early life may matter most, possibly due to increased mammary sensibility to carcinogens (55). Adult diet composition may also play a role in breast neoplasia. Although dietary fat does not appear to influence breast cancer risk (52,56), carbohydrate quality intake may prove to be important. Even moderate alcohol consumption increases risk of breast cancer (57), yet this effect can be reduced by an adequate folate intake (58,59).

In the Pooling Project on Diet and Cancer analysis, which included over 7,000 cases of breast cancer, no association between total fat and risk of breast cancer was found (56). In recent analysis of the Nurses' Health Study (NHS), a cohort of over 120,000 nurses, longtime exposure to dietary fat and the effect of time latency were examined (60). In this study which included over 3,500 postmenopausal women, there was no association between total fat intake and breast cancer, even after considering various disease latencies up to 20 years. An association was observed only for a very low and very high intake of fat (below 20% and above 50% of energy from fat) and when tumor type was considered. Monounsaturated fat has been associated with lower breast cancer risk in some studies (61,62), whereas animal fat has been associated with higher risk (63). However, there was no association observed between poly- or mono-saturated fat and breast cancer incidence in the Pooling Project (52,56). Overall, substantial evidence demonstrates that adult consumption of fat does not increase the risk of breast cancer.

Carbohydrates and carbohydrate quality, as measured by glycemic index or glycemic load, have been positively associated with breast cancer risk in some case-control studies (64). Yet, no overall associations of carbohydrate or carbohydrate quality and breast cancer risk have been reported in prospective studies in adult diet. An inverse relationship of high fiber intake to postmenopausal breast cancer risk was noted in a Swedish prospective study (65), where the highest vs. the lowest quintile of fiber intake was associated with a significant 42% lower risk. However, in most other prospective studies the associations between dietary fiber and breast cancer were null (64).

Alcohol consumption increases risk of breast cancer in a dose-response manner; each additional 10 g of alcohol consumed daily corresponds to a 9% (95% confidence interval 4–13%) increase in breast cancer risk, according to the Pooling Project results (57). In an updated analysis of the Nurses' Health Study with over 5,300 cases, alcohol intake as low as half a drink daily was statistically significantly associated with breast cancer risk (66). This association was observed with a variety of alcoholic beverages and drinking patterns. Estrogen levels increase significantly with consumption of one to two alcoholic drinks daily (67), suggesting a potential mechanism through which alcohol may increase the risk of breast cancer. In a Swedish prospective cohort of over 1,200 cases of invasive breast cancer with known estrogen and progesterone receptor status, the association with alcohol seemed to be stronger for estrogen-positive breast cancer types (68). High intake of folic acid, which is involved in DNA-methylation and repair, has consistently been shown to minimize the excess risk of breast cancer associated with regular alcohol consumption (58). Analysis of plasma folic acid levels confirmed this mitigating effect, which is strongest in women who consume at least one drink daily (59). The public health implications of this positive association between alcohol consumption and breast cancer are complicated by the protective effect of moderate alcohol consumption on cardiovascular disease and the overall reduction in total mortality (69). Women who chose to consume alcohol regularly may benefit from a multivitamin containing folic acid to lessen the risk of breast cancer (58).

Neither fruit nor vegetable consumption in adulthood seems to protect against overall breast cancer. The Pooling Project analysis showed no effect of adult consumption of fruit and vegetable consumption on breast cancer incidence (53). This lack of association was recently confirmed in the EPIC cohort of ten European countries (70).

No association between total, red or white meat consumption, or dairy products and breast cancer was observed in the Pooling Project *(71)*. Both calcium and vitamin D were inversely related to risk of postmenopausal breast cancer; dietary calcium and other components of dairy products were inversely related to risk of postmenopausal breast cancer, especially among women with estrogen-positive tumors *(72)*. Dietary intake and plasma levels of vitamin D were associated with lower risk of breast cancer in observational studies *(73,74)*. In the Nurses' Health Study, dietary carotenoids and total vitamin A were associated with lower breast cancer risk only among premenopausal women, especially in those who had a family history of breast cancer *(75)*. However, no overall association between intake of carotenoids and breast cancer was shown in other prospective studies *(64)*. In analysis of the Nurses' Health Study cohort, a significant inverse association between high plasma levels of α-carotene, β-carotene, lutein and zeaxanthin, and total carotenoids and breast cancer risk was observed *(76)*. These data suggest that elevated serum carotenoids are associated with lower risk of breast cancer. Prospective studies have not found significant overall associations between vitamin E, vitamin C, or selenium and breast cancer *(64)*. Clarifying the role of diet in breast cancer etiology is important because there are few other factors to prevention. Obesity and disordered energy balance are proving to be important risk factors.

4.3. Colorectal Cancer

Colorectal cancer (CRC) is the third most common cancer among men and women combined in Sweden and the United States. Worldwide in 2002, approximately 1 million new cases of cancer were diagnosed (9.4% of new cases of cancer) and 529,000 individuals died from this malignancy *(77)*. Incidence rates vary approximately 25-fold around the world, with the highest rates in Japan, North America, and Europe. The international differences and trends together with data from migrant studies imply that environmental factors play an important role in the etiology of CRC. The 25-fold geographic variation may be explained in large part by different dietary and other environmental factors.

There is considerable evidence that high consumption of red meat and processed meat may increase the risk of CRC *(78)*. In a quantitative assessment of the association between red and processed meat consumption and CRC risk based on 15 prospective studies, there was an observed 28% increased risk in the highest relative to the lowest category of red meat consumption. Similarly, high vs. low processed meat consumption was associated with a 20% increase in CRC risk *(79)*. Dose-response meta-analysis showed a statistically significant 31% increased CRC risk associated with each 120 g/day increment for red meat consumption, and the statistically significant 11% increase in risk for each 30 g/day increment of processed meats *(79)*. The mechanisms behind these associations may involve a combination of factors such as the content of fat, protein, and heme iron, and/or meat preparation methods (for example, cooking in high temperature and preserving methods). The fat content of meat might influence the risk of CRC by increasing the production of secondary bile acids, which may promote colon carcinogenesis *(80)*. However, epidemiologic studies have generally not shown a relation between fat intake and risk of CRC *(81)*. Red meat contains higher amounts of heme iron than white meat (poultry and fish). Intake of heme iron was statistically significantly positively associated with the risk of CRC in an American prospective study *(82)* and in the Swedish Mammography Cohort *(83)*. Meta-analysis of prospective studies of poultry and chicken indicated a potential inverse association; comparing the highest to the lowest category of consumption a 12% decreased risk was indicated; there was no clear inverse association of CRC with fish consumption (84). The relationship between processed meat consumption and CRC may be partly due to N-nitroso-compounds (NOCs). An alternative mechanism through which red meat consumption might increase the risk of CRC is by increasing circulating insulin-like growth factor-1 levels. In a cross-sectional study of Swedish men, we found a statistically significant positive relation between red meat consumption and serum IGF-1; men in the highest quintile of red meat intake had 13% higher serum IGF-1 levels than men in the lowest quintile (29).

There is accumulating evidence that dairy products are associated with lower risk of colorectal cancer. Dairy products are the major source of calcium and dietary vitamin D in Sweden (85) and in the United States (86); milk products are fortified with vitamin D in these countries. Milk products also contain other potentially anticarcinogenic compounds, including conjugated linoleic acid (CLA) and sphingolipids (87,88). CLA has been shown to inhibit CRC cancerogenesis in animal models (89). In the Swedish Mammography Cohort, we observed statistically significant inverse association between intakes of CLA and high-fat dairy foods (the main source of CLA) and risk of CRC (90). The relationship between milk consumption and risk of CRC was examined in the Pooling Project of Prospective Studies on Diet and Cancer in which the primary data from ten cohort studies (in five countries) were pooled (91). The pooled results revealed a statistically significant inverse association between milk consumption and CRC (P trend < 0.001); compared with individuals in the lowest category of milk consumption (<70 g/day), the multivariate relative risk for those in the highest category (≥250 g/day) was statistically significantly 15% lower. In the Cohort of Swedish Men, not included in the Pooling Project, men in the highest category of milk consumption (≥1.5 glass/day) had a statistically significant 33% lower risk of CRC compared with those who consumed less than two glasses of milk per week (92). The inverse association between CRC and dairy products may be ascribed to calcium, vitamin D, CLA, sphingolipids, and other components of milk.

Studies that have examined circulating 25-hydroxy vitamin D [25(OH)D] serum concentrations and risk of colon and colorectal cancer have found reduced risk associated with higher vitamin D concentrations. Meta-analysis of these studies indicated that people in the highest category with the highest concentration of vitamin D had a significantly 54% lower risk of CRC in comparison to the lowest category (84). Meta-analysis of prospective studies based on intake of total vitamin D showed 21% statistically significantly decreased risk in those in the highest vs. the lowest category of intake (84).

Calcium has been hypothesized to reduce the risk of CRC by binding secondary bile acids and ionized fatty acids to form insoluble soaps in the colonic lumen, thereby diminishing the potentially proliferative stimulus of these compounds on colonic mucosa (93). Calcium may also directly influence the proliferative activity of the colonic mucosa and may also influence differentiation and apoptosis (94). Some clinical trials have shown that increased calcium intake could decrease colonic epithelial cell proliferation (95). Additionally, in randomized trials, calcium supplementation reduces the recurrence of colorectal adenoma (96,97) consistent with the role of calcium in the early stages of carcinogenesis. The totality of evidence from laboratory studies, observational epidemiological studies, and randomized trials of colorectal polyp recurrence supports the hypothesis that the high intake of calcium reduces the risk of CRC. In the Pooling Project of Prospective Studies of Diet and Cancer, where data from ten cohorts were analyzed together, the highest quintile when compared with the lowest quintile of dietary calcium intake was associated with a statistically significant 14% lower risk and total calcium intake (including calcium supplements) with a 22% lower risk (91). In the Cohort of Swedish Men (not included in the Pooling Project), men in the highest quartile (>1,445 mg calcium/day) compared with those in the lowest quartile (<956 mg/day) had a statistically significant 32% lower risk (92).

Fruits and vegetables, besides being a rich source of dietary fiber, carotenoids, certain vitamins (particularly folate and vitamin C), and magnesium contain numerous phytochemicals that may have anticarcinogenic properties. Although the majority of about 30 case-control studies have found inverse associations between fruit and/or vegetable consumption and CRC risk, findings from prospective cohort studies have been less consistent (35). In a meta-analysis (98), the estimated relative risk for 100 g/day increase in fruit consumption was decreased by 7% in case-control studies (statistically significant) and by 4% in cohort studies (not reaching significance). The corresponding risk for vegetable consumption was 13% in case-control studies (statistically significant) and 4% (not significant) in cohort studies. In summary, the hypothesis that high consumption of fruits and vegetables may reduce the risk of CRC has not been firmly established.

The idea that a high fiber diet might reduce the risk of CRC dates back to the early 1970s, when Burkit postulated that the low occurrence of CRC he observed in Southern Africa was related to high fiber intake (99). Although the fiber hypothesis gained support from a number of case-control studies from different countries, the findings of cohort studies of dietary fiber intake in relation to risk of CRC have been inconsistent (100). Findings from large prospective cohort studies provide some indications that dietary fiber intake might be related in some way to risk of colon or rectal neoplasia; however, results are not entirely consistent.

A meta-analysis of 12 case-control studies showed a statistically significant 28% reduction in risk of CRC for high vs. low coffee consumption (32). However, recent results from large prospective cohort studies have not supported an association with coffee consumption (101,102). In a meta-analysis of epidemiologic studies (13 case-control and seven cohort studies) of tea drinking, there was no association with black tea and a statistically significant 18% lower risk for green tea (based on four case-control and four cohort studies); however, that inverse association was limited only to case-control studies (103). The accumulated evidence does not support an association of coffee or tea with risk of colorectal cancer.

5. OBESITY, PHYSICAL ACTIVITY, AND CANCER

Obesity is increasing at an alarming rate in the US, Europe, and all over the world, and the increase in childhood obesity is particularly troublesome (104). Lifestyle factors including diet, eating habits, levels of physical activity as well as inactivity are often adopted during the early years of life. As childhood obesity is also strongly related to obesity in adulthood, the best time to address the problem is early in life. Maintaining normal weight is challenging nowadays. On the one hand, there is an abundance of energy-rich foods that are often poor in nutrients, such as different types of fat-rich and sugar-rich cakes and other sweets. On the other hand, there are decreasing needs and opportunities for physical activity both at work and at leisure time. Such simple activity as walking has been decreasing during the past several decades, in parallel with increasing modernization (Fig. 11a–b).

Even though people actually need less and less energy due to the increasing sedentary lifestyle, there has been a tendency for portion sizes to increase over time (105). The seriousness of these problems makes nutrition, physical inactivity, and obesity key priorities in the prevention of major chronic diseases including cancer.

In 2002, the IARC Prevention Report on Weight Control and Physical Activity concluded that obesity and lack of physical activity are major causes of cancer incidence and mortality (9). The accumulated evidence indicated that obesity was directly associated with risk of cancer at several organ sites including colon, breast (in postmenopausal women), endometrium, esophagus, and kidney (9). Furthermore, data from the American Cancer Society Cancer Prevention Study II, which followed more than 1 million men and women during 16 years, also showed direct associations between obesity and mortality from cancer of the prostate, pancreas, non-Hodgkin's lymphoma, and myeloma (106). The conclusion from this large prospective study was that 16–20% of cancer deaths among American women and 14% of cancer deaths among men are attributable to obesity (107).

The IARC Prevention Report from 2002 also stated that there was accumulated sufficient evidence to conclude that physical inactivity was linked to increased risk of breast and colon cancer (9). In a recent systematic review of 19 cohort studies and 29 case-control studies, it was reported that there was strong evidence for an inverse association between physical activity and postmenopausal breast cancer, but the evidence was much weaker for premenopausal breast cancer (108). In postmenopausal women, when comparing the highest with the lowest categories of physical activity, there were risk reductions ranging from 20 to 80%. In about half of the methodologically higher-quality studies, there was evidence for a dose-response relationship. Each additional 1 h of physical activity per week was associated with a 6% (95% confidence interval 3–8%) decrease in breast cancer risk. In a study of the California Teachers including over 110,000 women aged 20–79 years, strenuous long-term exercise activity was protective against invasive and in situ breast cancers. However, the protective effect was limited to estrogen receptor negative breast cancer (109).

We have recently reported that physical activity is also associated with decreased risk of endometrial cancer, especially among obese women (110). Interestingly, among diabetic women, who have two-fold increased risk, we observed that physical activity can reduce the risk to a similar level as among women without diabetes (111). The mechanisms by which physical activity may protect against breast and endometrial cancer may involve body size, which affects estrogen exposure in postmenopausal women (112), and serum hormone levels (113). Furthermore, physical activity may influence insulin sensitivity (114) and growth factors (115), as well as adiponectin (116). Adiponectin has been shown to be associated with decreased risk of breast (117), endometrial, and other cancers (118).

Convincing epidemiological data support the role of physical activity in reducing colon cancer risk (9,119). Meta-analysis of prospective studies (published through October 2006) on leisure time physical activity and risk of colon cancer has shown statistically significant 25% lower risk when comparing the highest to the lowest category (78). In contrast to colon cancer, there was no association between physical activity and risk of rectal cancer.

6. GUIDELINES FOR CANCER PREVENTION

6.1. American Cancer Society Guidelines on Diet and Physical Activity

The American Cancer Society (ACS) publishes nutrition and physical activity guidelines to serve as a foundation for its communication policy and community strategies and ultimately to affect dietary and physical activity patterns among Americans. These guidelines, published every 5 years, represent the most current scientific evidence related to dietary and activity patterns and cancer risk. The recent guidelines were updated in October 2006. They are consistent with guidelines from the American Heart Association *(120)* and the American Diabetes Association *(121)* for the prevention of coronary heart disease and diabetes, as well as for general health promotion, as defined by the Department of Health and Human Services' 2005 Dietary Guidelines for Americans *(122)*. In the ACS guidelines, it is very clearly stated that the most important modifiable determinants of cancer risk among those who do not use tobacco are weight control, healthy diet, and appropriate levels of physical activity. Evidence suggests that one third of cancers that occur in the USA each year can be attributed to diet and physical activity habits. Healthy behavior such as maintaining healthy weight, staying physically active throughout life, and consuming a healthy diet can substantially reduce one's lifetime risk of developing cancer *(10,13)*. The same behaviors are also associated with decreased risk of developing cardiovascular disease. Recent ACS guidelines for cancer prevention are presented in Table 1.

Table 1
American Cancer Society Guidelines on Nutrition and Physical Activity for Cancer Prevention, Updated in October 2006 *(123)*

Guidelines on nutrition and physical activity for cancer prevention
Maintain a healthy weight throughout life
Balance caloric intake with physical activity
Avoid excessive weight gain throughout the life cycle
Achieve and maintain a healthy weight if currently overweight or obese
Adopt a physically active lifestyle
Adults: engage in at least 30 min of moderate to vigorous physical activity, above usual activities, on 5 or more days of the week. Intentional physical activity is preferable for 45–60 min
Children and adolescents: engage in at least 60 min per day of moderate to vigorous physical activity at least 5 days per week
Consume a healthy diet with an emphasis on plant sources
Choose food and beverages in amounts that help achieve and maintain a healthy weight
Eat five or more servings of a variety of vegetables and fruits each day
Choose whole grains in preference to processed (refined) grains
Limit consumption of processed and red meats
If you drink alcoholic beverages, limit consumption
Drink no more than one drink per day for women and two per day for men

6.2. World Cancer Research Fund International Guidelines

The mission of the World Cancer Research Fund (WCRF) global network, an alliance of organizations dedicated to the prevention of cancer worldwide, is to raise awareness that the risk of cancer is reduced by healthy food and nutrition, physical activity, and weight management. WCRF supports research to develop and strengthen scientific knowledge of the relation of food and nutrition, physical activity, and weight management for cancer prevention.

The research and education programs of WCRF International and its national members are based on the conclusions and recommendations of the WCRF and American Institute for Cancer Research (AICR) Second Expert Report "Food, Nutrition, Physical Activity, and the Prevention of Cancer: a Global Perspective," which was published in November 2007 *(10)*. This report that summarized the accumulated knowledge on diet, physical activity, and cancer was distributed throughout the world and acclaimed as setting the agenda for the coming years on food, nutrition and lifestyle, and the prevention of cancer. Current recommendations in this Expert Report, based on meta-analysis and summaries of scientific articles, are presented in Table 2.

It is essential to understand that the evidence used to formulate the WCRF global networks health recommendations and research policy is based on the latest research investigation. It summarizes accumulated knowledge from about 10,000 scientific articles.

Table 2
World Cancer Research Fund and American Institute for Cancer Research, Guidelines for Cancer Prevention Through Diet and Physical Activity, 2007

Be as lean as possible within the normal range of body weight
Ensure that body weight through childhood and adolescent growth projects toward the lower end of the normal BMI range at age 21
Maintain body weight within the normal range from age 21
Avoid weight gain and increases in waist circumference throughout adulthood
Be physically active as a part of everyday life
Be moderately physically active, equivalent to brisk walking, for at least 30 min every day. As fitness improves, aim for 60 min or more of moderate, or for 30 min or more of vigorous, physical activity every day
Limit sedentary habits such as watching television
Limit consumption of energy-dense foods and avoid sugary drinks
Consume energy-dense foods sparingly
Avoid sugary drinks
Consume "fast foods" sparingly, if at all
Eat mostly foods of plant origin
Eat at least five portions/servings (at least 400 g or 14 oz) of a variety of nonstarchy vegetables and of fruits every day
Limit intake of red meat and avoid processed meat

(continued)

Table 2
(continued)

People who eat red meat from domesticated animals (beef, pork, lamb, goat) should
    consume less than 500 g (18 oz) a week, very little if any to be processed (meats
    preserved by smoking, curing or salting, or addition of chemical preservatives)
Limit alcoholic drinks
If alcoholic drinks are consumed, limit consumption to no more than two drinks a day for
    men and one drink a day for women
Limit consumption of salt and avoid mouldy cereals (grains) or pulses (legumes)
Avoid salt-preserved, salted or salty foods; preserve foods without using salt. Limit
    consumption of processed foods with added salt to ensure an intake of less than 6 g
    (2.4 g sodium) a day. Do not eat cereals (grains) or pulses (legumes) that have mold
Aim to meet nutritional needs through diet alone
Dietary supplements are not recommended for cancer prevention
Mothers should breastfeed; children should be breastfed
Aim to breastfeed infants exclusively up to 6 months and continue with complementary
    feeding thereafter
Cancer survivors should follow the recommendations for cancer prevention
All cancer survivors should receive nutritional care from an appropriately trained
    professional. If able to do so, and unless otherwise advised, aim to follow the
    recommendations for diet, healthy weight, and physical activity

7. MEDITERRANEAN DIET AND CANCER

Interestingly, many aspects in the guidelines on nutrition for cancer prevention are
very similar to dietary food patterns usually seen in Mediterranean basin countries, such
as Greece, Italy, Spain, and France. The term "Mediterranean diet" reflects the dietary
pattern characteristics of several Mediterranean countries during the early 1960s. Such
patterns defined in the early 1990s are composed of *(124)*:

- Abundant plant foods (vegetables, fruits, breads, other forms of cereals, beans, nuts, and seeds)
- Minimally processed, seasonally fresh, and locally grown foods
- Fresh fruits as typical daily dessert, and sweets based on nuts, olive oil, and concentrated
  sugars or honey consumed on feast days
- Olive oil as the principal source of dietary fat
- Dairy products (mainly cheese and yoghurt) consumed in low to moderate amounts
- Fewer than four eggs consumed per week
- Red meat consumed in low frequency and amounts
- Wine consumed in low to moderate amounts, generally with meals

Various aspects of the Mediterranean diet are considered favorable with regards to
cancer risk. Studies have suggested that the cancer-conferring benefits of this diet are
due to not only high consumption of fruits, vegetable, whole grains, and fish but also
olive oil *(125,126)*. The Greek variant of the Mediterranean diet is especially interesting
because Greeks have been in the area longer than other Mediterranean populations, and
the early studies that pointed to the beneficial effects of the Mediterranean diet were

largely based in Greece *(3)*. The diet of Crete is considered to represent the traditional diet of Greece prior to 1960 *(127)*. Overall, the traditional Mediterranean diet may be thought of as having eight components:

1. High monounsaturated/saturated fat ratio
2. Moderate ethanol consumption
3. High consumption of legumes
4. High consumption of grain products (particularly bread)
5. High consumption of fruits
6. High consumption of vegetables
7. Low consumption of meat and meat products
8. Moderate consumption of milk and dairy products

A diet that has all of the characteristics described above has a score of eight, whereas a diet with none of these characteristics should have a score of zero. It has been reported that death rates were lower and life expectancy was longer among people scoring high on this dietary pattern compared with those with low scores *(128,129)*.

In the Mediterranean diet, meals usually contain large quantities of whole-grain bread. Legumes and vegetables are consumed in large amounts in cooked dishes, soups, and salads are prepared with olive oil. Intake of milk is moderate, but consumption of cheese, and to a lesser extent yoghurt, is high; feta cheese is regularly added to most salads and vegetable stews. Meat, being expensive, used to be rarely consumed, whereas fish consumption was a function of proximity to the sea. Wine is consumed in moderation and almost always during meals *(130)*. These characteristics of the Mediterranean diet are still well reflected in the per capita availability of foods in Greece in 1990s as shown in Fig. 8a–d. The most pronounced differences in consumed food amounts between Greece and Sweden, USA, and Japan are observed for vegetables, fruits, and berries, pulses, and nuts.

In summary, present American and WCRF guidelines on healthy diet for cancer prevention are remarkably in line with the dietary profile of old Mediterranean traditions. A diet rich in plant foods and whole grain and low in foods of animal origin, accompanied by low to moderate alcohol consumption, should be actively promoted.

REFERENCES

1. WHO/IARC. World cancer report. Lyon: IARC Press, 2003.
2. Doll R, Peto R. The causes of cancer: quantitative estimates of avoidable risks of cancer in the United States today. J Natl Cancer Inst 1981;66:1191–308.
3. Trichopoulou A, Lagiou P, Kuper H, et al. Cancer and Mediterranean dietary traditions. Cancer Epidemiol Biomarkers Prev 2000;9:869–73.
4. Socialstyrelsen. http://www.socialstyrelsen.se, Prostate cancer mortality trends in Sweden, 2006.
5. WHO. Prevention of Cancer. Geneva: WHO, 1964.
6. Harvard Report on Cancer Prevention. Volume 1: Causes of human cancer. Cancer Causes Control 1996;7 Suppl 1:S3–59.
7. Colditz GA, Sellers TA, Trapido E. Epidemiology – identifying the causes and preventability of cancer? Nat Rev Cancer 2006;6:75–83.
8. Bergstrom A, Pisani P, Tenet V, et al. Overweight as an avoidable cause of cancer in Europe. Int J Cancer 2001;91:421–30.

9. Vainio H, Bianchini F. Weight control and physical activity. Lyon: IARC Press, 2002.

10. World Cancer Research Fund and American Institute for Cancer Research. Food, Nutrition and the Prevention of Cancer: A Global Perspective. Washington, DC: World Cancer Research Fund and American Institute for Cancer Research, 1997.

11. Lichtenstein P, Holm NV, Verkasalo PK, et al. Environmental and heritable factors in the causation of cancer–analyses of cohorts of twins from Sweden, Denmark, and Finland. N Engl J Med 2000;343:78–85.

12. Czene K, Lichtenstein P, Hemminki K. Environmental and heritable causes of cancer among 9.6 million individuals in the Swedish family-cancer database. Int J Cancer 2002;99:260–6.

13. Boyle P, Autier P, Bartelink H, et al. European code against cancer and scientific justification: third version (2003). Ann Oncol 2003;14:973–1005.

14. Larsson SC, Adami HO, Wolk A. Obesity, diabetes, and risk of cancer. In: Mantzoros CS, ed. Obesity and diabetes. Totowa: Humana Press, 2006.

15. WHO. WHO Global Infobase. Geneve: WHO, 2007.

16. Orsini N, Bellocco R, Bottai M, et al. Age and temporal trends of total physical activity among Swedish women. Med Sci Sports Exerc 2006;38:240–5.

17. Norman A, Bellocco R, Vaida F, et al. Age and temporal trends of total physical activity in Swedish men. Med Sci Sports Exerc 2003;35:617–22.

18. Statistics, Sweden. National Health Interview Survey, 2006.

19. Time trends in smoking in the USA, 1980–2005. Atlanta, GA: Center for Disease Control and Prevention, 2006.

20. WHO. Smoking in Greece and Japan. Geneva: WHO, 2006.

21. Hsing AW, Devesa SS. Trends and patterns of prostate cancer: what do they suggest? Epidemiol Rev 2001;23:3–13.

22. Wolk A. Diet, lifestyle and risk of prostate cancer. Acta Oncol 2005;44:277–81.

23. Rodriguez C, McCullough ML, Mondul AM, et al. Meat consumption among Black and White men and risk of prostate cancer in the Cancer Prevention Study II Nutrition Cohort. Cancer Epidemiol Biomarkers Prev 2006;15:211–6.

24. Chan JM, Gann PH, Giovannucci EL. Role of diet in prostate cancer development and progression. J Clin Oncol 2005;23:8152–60.

25. Stuart GR, Holcroft J, de Boer JG, et al. Prostate mutations in rats induced by the suspected human carcinogen 2-amino-1-methyl-6-phenylimidazo[4,5-b]pyridine. Cancer Res 2000;60:266–8.

26. Cross AJ, Peters U, Kirsh VA, et al. A prospective study of meat and meat mutagens and prostate cancer risk. Cancer Res 2005;65:11779–84.

27. Platz EA, Helzlsouer KJ. Selenium, zinc, and prostate cancer. Epidemiol Rev 2001;23:93–101.

28. Leitzmann MF, Stampfer MJ, Wu K, et al. Zinc supplement use and risk of prostate cancer. J Natl Cancer Inst 2003;95:1004–7.

29. Larsson SC, Wolk K, Brismar K, et al. Association of diet with serum insulin-like growth factor I in middle-aged and elderly men. Am J Clin Nutr 2005c;81:1163–7.

30. Renehan AG, Zwahlen M, Minder C, et al. Insulin-like growth factor (IGF)-I, IGF binding protein-3, and cancer risk: systematic review and meta-regression analysis. Lancet 2004;363:1346–53.

31. Giovannucci E, Rimm EB, Wolk A, et al. Calcium and fructose intake in relation to risk of prostate cancer. Cancer Res 1998;58:442–7.

32. Giovannucci E. Meta-analysis of coffee consumption and risk of colorectal cancer. Am J Epidemiol 1998;147:1043–52.

33. Holmes MD, Pollak MN, Willett WC, et al. Dietary correlates of plasma insulin-like growth factor I and insulin-like growth factor binding protein 3 concentrations. Cancer Epidemiol Biomarkers Prev 2002;11:852–61.

34. Thornburg T, Turner AR, Chen YQ, et al. Phytanic acid, AMACR and prostate cancer risk. Future Oncol 2002;2:213–23.

35. IARC. Fruit and vegetables. IARC handbooks of cancer prevention. Volume 8. Lyon: IARC Press, 2003.

36. Kristal AR, Schenk JM. Directions for future epidemiological research in lycopene and prostate cancer risk. J Nutr 2005;135:2037S–9S.

37. Etminan M, Takkouche B, Caamano-Isorna F. The role of tomato products and lycopene in the prevention of prostate cancer: a meta-analysis of observational studies. Cancer Epidemiol Biomarkers Prev 2004;13:340–5.

38. Key TJ, Allen N, Appleby P, et al. Fruits and vegetables and prostate cancer: no association among 1104 cases in a prospective study of 130544 men in the European Prospective Investigation into Cancer and Nutrition (EPIC). Int J Cancer 2004;109:119–24.

39. Giovannucci E, Rimm EB, Liu Y, et al. A prospective study of cruciferous vegetables and prostate cancer. Cancer Epidemiol Biomarkers Prev 2003;12:1403–9.

40. Garikapaty VP, Ashok BT, Tadi K, et al. Synthetic dimer of indole-3-carbinol: Second generation diet derived anti-cancer agent in hormone sensitive prostate cancer. Prostate 2006;66:453–62.

41. Hou Z, Lambert JD, Chin KV, et al. Effects of tea polyphenols on signal transduction pathways related to cancer chemoprevention. Mutat Res 2004;555:3–19.

42. Heinonen OP, Albanes D, Virtamo J, et al. Prostate cancer and supplementation with alpha-tocopherol and beta-carotene: incidence and mortality in a controlled trial. J Natl Cancer Inst 1998;90:440–6.

43. Shukla S, Gupta S. Dietary agents in the chemoprevention of prostate cancer. Nutr Cancer 2005;53:18–32.

44. Helzlsouer KJ, Huang HY, Alberg AJ, et al. Association between alpha-tocopherol, gamma-tocopherol, selenium, and subsequent prostate cancer. J Natl Cancer Inst 2000;92:2018–23.

45. Li H, Stampfer MJ, Giovannucci EL, et al. A prospective study of plasma selenium levels and prostate cancer risk. J Natl Cancer Inst 2004;96:696–703.

46. Duffield-Lillico AJ, Dalkin BL, Reid ME, et al. Selenium supplementation, baseline plasma selenium status and incidence of prostate cancer: an analysis of the complete treatment period of the Nutritional Prevention of Cancer Trial. BJU Int 2003;91:608–12.

47. McCann MJ, Gill CI, McGlynn H, et al. Role of mammalian lignans in the prevention and treatment of prostate cancer. Nutr Cancer 2005;52:1–14.

48. Wikstrom P, Bylund A, Zhang JX, et al. Rye bran diet increases epithelial cell apoptosis and decreases epithelial cell volume in TRAMP (transgenic adenocarcinoma of the mouse prostate) tumors. Nutr Cancer 2005;53:111–6.

49. Hedelin M, Klint A, Chang ET, et al. Dietary phytoestrogen, serum enterolactone and risk of prostate cancer: the cancer prostate sweden study (sweden). Cancer Causes Control 2006;17:169–80.

50. Terry P, Lichtenstein P, Feychting M, et al. Fatty fish consumption and risk of prostate cancer. Lancet 2001;357:1764–6.

51. Schwartz GG. Vitamin D and the epidemiology of prostate cancer. Semin Dial 2005;18:276–89.

52. Hunter DJ, Spiegelman D, Adami HO, et al. Cohort studies of fat intake and the risk of breast cancer– a pooled analysis. N Engl J Med 1996;334:356–61.

53. Smith-Warner SA, Spiegelman D, Yaun SS, et al. Intake of fruits and vegetables and risk of breast cancer: a pooled analysis of cohort studies. JAMA 2001;285:769–76.

54. van den Brandt PA, Spiegelman D, Yaun SS, et al. Pooled analysis of prospective cohort studies on height, weight, and breast cancer risk. Am J Epidemiol 2000;152:514–27.

55. Linos E, Holmes MD, Willett WC. Diet and breast cancer. Curr Oncol Rep 2007;9:31–41.

56. Smith-Warner SA, Spiegelman D, Adami HO, et al. Types of dietary fat and breast cancer: a pooled analysis of cohort studies. Int J Cancer 2001;92:767–74.

57. Smith-Warner SA, Spiegelman D, Yaun SS, et al. Alcohol and breast cancer in women: a pooled analysis of cohort studies. JAMA 1998;279:535–40.

58. Zhang S, Hunter DJ, Hankinson SE, et al. A prospective study of folate intake and the risk of breast cancer. JAMA 1999;281:1632–7.

59. Zhang SM, Willett WC, Selhub J, et al. Plasma folate, vitamin B6, vitamin B12, homocysteine, and risk of breast cancer. J Natl Cancer Inst 2003;95:373–80.

60. Kim EH, Willett WC, Colditz GA, et al. Dietary fat and risk of postmenopausal breast cancer in a 20-year follow-up. Am J Epidemiol 2006;164:990–7.

61. Wolk A, Bergstrom R, Hunter D, et al. A prospective study of association of monounsaturated fat and other types of fat with risk of breast cancer. Arch Intern Med 1998;158:41–5.

62. Voorrips LE, Brants HA, Kardinaal AF, et al. Intake of conjugated linoleic acid, fat, and other fatty acids in relation to postmenopausal breast cancer: the Netherlands Cohort Study on Diet and Cancer. Am J Clin Nutr 2002;76:873–82.

63. Cho E, Spiegelman D, Hunter DJ, et al. Premenopausal fat intake and risk of breast cancer. J Natl Cancer Inst 2003;95:1079–85.

64. Holmes MD, Willett WC. Does diet affect breast cancer risk? Breast Cancer Res 2004;6:170–8.

65. Mattisson I, Wirfalt E, Johansson U, et al. Intakes of plant foods, fibre and fat and risk of breast cancer– a prospective study in the Malmo Diet and Cancer Cohort. Br J Cancer 2004;90:122–7.

66. Chen WY, Willett, WC, Rossner, GA, et al. Moderate alcohol consumption and breast cancer risk (abstract). J Clin Oncol Proc ASCO 2005;23:515.

67. Reichman ME, Judd JT, Longcope C, et al. Effects of alcohol consumption on plasma and urinary hormone concentrations in premenopausal women. J Natl Cancer Inst 1993;85:722–7.

68. Suzuki R, Ye W, Rylander-Rudqvist T, et al. Alcohol and postmenopausal breast cancer risk defined by estrogen and progesterone receptor status: a prospective cohort study. J Natl Cancer Inst 2005;97:1601–8.

69. Fuchs CS, Stampfer MJ, Colditz GA, et al. Alcohol consumption and mortality among women. N Engl J Med 1995;332:1245–50.

70. van Gils CH, Peeters PH, Bueno-de-Mesquita HB, et al. Consumption of vegetables and fruits and risk of breast cancer. JAMA 2005;293:183–93.

71. Missmer SA, Smith-Warner SA, Spiegelman D, et al. Meat and dairy food consumption and breast cancer: a pooled analysis of cohort studies. Int J Epidemiol 2002;31:78–85.

72. McCullough ML, Rodriguez C, Diver WR, et al. Dairy, calcium, and vitamin D intake and postmenopausal breast cancer risk in the Cancer Prevention Study II Nutrition Cohort. Cancer Epidemiol Biomarkers Prev 2005;14:2898–904.

73. John EM, Schwartz GG, Dreon DM, et al. Vitamin D and breast cancer risk: the NHANES I Epidemiologic follow-up study, 1971–1975 to 1992. National Health and Nutrition Examination Survey. Cancer Epidemiol Biomarkers Prev 1999;8:399–406.

74. Bertone-Johnson ER, Chen WY, Holick MF, et al. Plasma 25-hydroxyvitamin D and 1,25-dihydroxy-vitamin D and risk of breast cancer. Cancer Epidemiol Biomarkers Prev 2005;14:1991–7.

75. Zhang S, Hunter DJ, Forman MR, et al. Dietary carotenoids and vitamins A, C, and E and risk of breast cancer. J Natl Cancer Inst 1999;91:547–56.

76. Tamimi RM, Hankinson SE, Campos H, et al. Plasma carotenoids, retinol, and tocopherols and risk of breast cancer. Am J Epidemiol 2005;161:153–60.

77. Parkin DM, Bray F, Ferlay J, et al. Global cancer statistics, 2002. CA Cancer J Clin 2005;55:74–108.

78. Larsson SC. Diet and gastrointestinal cancer – one-carbon metabolism and other aspects. Stockholm: Karolinska Institutet, 2006.

79. Larsson SC, Wolk A. Meat consumption and risk of colorectal cancer: a meta-analysis of prospective studies. Int J Cancer 2006a;119:2657–64.

80. Narisawa T, Magadia NE, Weisburger JH, et al. Promoting effect of bile acids on colon carcinogenesis after intrarectal instillation of N-methyl-N′-nitro-Nnitrosoguanidine in rats. J Natl Cancer Inst 1974;53:1093–7.

81. Giovannucci E, Goldin B. The role of fat, fatty acids, and total energy intake in the etiology of human colon cancer. Am J Clin Nutr 1997;66:1564S–71S.

82. Lee DH, Anderson KE, Harnack LJ, et al. Heme iron, zinc, alcohol consumption, and colon cancer: Iowa Women's Health Study. J Natl Cancer Inst 2004;96:403–7.

83. Larsson SC, Adami HO, Giovannucci E, et al. Heme iron, zinc, alcohol consumption, and risk of colon cancer. J Natl Cancer Inst 2005b;97:232–3.

84. Larsson SC. Diet and gastrointestinal cancer – one carbon metabolism and other aspects (PhD thesis) Stockholm: Karolinska Institutet, 2006.

85. Becker W, Pearson M. Riksmaten 1997–98. Dietary habits and nutrient intake in Sweden. The second national food consumption survey. Uppsala (Sweden): Livsmedelsverket, 2002.

86. Cotton PA, Subar AF, Friday JE, et al. Dietary sources of nutrients among US adults, 1994 to 1996. J Am Diet Assoc 2004;104:921–30.

87. Parodi PW. Cows' milk fat components as potential anticarcinogenic agents. J Nutr 1997;127:1055–60.

88. Molkentin J. Occurrence and biochemical characteristics of natural bioactive substances in bovine milk lipids. Br J Nutr 2000;84 Suppl 1:S47–53.

89. Kim KH, Park HS. Dietary supplementation of conjugated linoleic acid reduces colon tumor incidence in DMH-treated rats by increasing apoptosis with modulation of biomarkers. Nutrition 2003;19:772–7.

90. Larsson SC, Bergkvist L, Wolk A. High-fat dairy food and conjugated linoleic acid intakes in relation to colorectal cancer incidence in the Swedish Mammography Cohort. Am J Clin Nutr 2005d; 82:894–900.

91. Cho E, Smith-Warner SA, Spiegelman D, et al. Dairy foods, calcium, and colorectal cancer: a pooled analysis of 10 cohort studies. J Natl Cancer Inst 2004;96:1015–22.

92. Larsson SC, Bergkvist L, Ruteg rd J, et al. Calcium and dairy food intakes are inversely associated with colorectal cancer risk in the Cohort of Swedish Men. Am J Clin Nutr 2006;83:667–73.

93. Newmark HL, Wargovich MJ, Bruce WR. Colon cancer and dietary fat, phosphate, and calcium: a hypothesis. J Natl Cancer Inst 1984;72:1323–5.

94. Lamprecht SA, Lipkin M. Chemoprevention of colon cancer by calcium, vitamin D and folate: molecular mechanisms. Nat Rev Cancer 2003;3:601–14.

95. Lipkin M. Preclinical and early human studies of calcium and colon cancer prevention. Ann N Y Acad Sci 1999;889:120–7.

96. Baron JA, Beach M, Mandel JS, et al. Calcium supplements for the prevention of colorectal adenomas. Calcium Polyp Prevention Study Group. N Engl J Med 1999;340:101–7.

97. Bonithon-Kopp C, Kronborg O, Giacosa A, et al. Calcium and fibre supplementation in prevention of colorectal adenoma recurrence: a randomised intervention trial. European Cancer Prevention Organisation Study Group. Lancet 2000;356:1300–6.

98. Riboli E, Norat T. Epidemiologic evidence of the protective effect of fruit and vegetables on cancer risk. Am J Clin Nutr 2003;78:559S–69S.

99. Burkitt DP. Epidemiology of cancer of the colon and rectum. Cancer 1971;28:3–13.

100. Kushi LH, Meyer KA, Jacobs DR, Jr. Cereals, legumes, and chronic disease risk reduction: evidence from epidemiologic studies. Am J Clin Nutr 1999;70:451S–8S.

101. Michels KB, Willett WC, Fuchs CS, et al. Coffee, tea, and caffeine consumption and incidence of colon and rectal cancer. J Natl Cancer Inst 2005;97:282–92.

102. Larsson SC, Bergkvist L, Giovannucci E, et al. Coffee consumption and incidence of colorectal cancer in two prospective cohort studies of Swedish women and men. Am J Epidemiol 2006c;163:638–44.

103. Sun CL, Yuan JM, Koh WP, et al. Green tea, black tea and colorectal cancer risk: a meta-analysis of epidemiologic studies. Carcinogenesis 2006;27:1301–9.

104. Larsson SC, Wolk A. Epidemiology of obesity and diabetes, prevalence and trends. In: Mantzoros CS, ed. Obesity and diabetes. Boston: Humana, 2006:15–36.

105. Nestle M. Increasing portion sizes in American diets: more calories, more obesity. J Am Diet Assoc 2003;103:39–40.

106. Calle EE, Kaaks R. Overweight, obesity and cancer: epidemiological evidence and proposed mechanisms. Nat Rev Cancer 2004;4:579–91.

107. Calle EE, Rodriguez C, Walker-Thurmond K, et al. Overweight, obesity, and mortality from cancer in a prospectively studied cohort of U.S. adults. N Engl J Med 2003;348:1625–38.

108. Monninkhof EM, Elias SG, Vlems FA, et al. Physical activity and breast cancer: a systematic review. Epidemiology 2007;18:137–57.

109. Dallal C, Sullivan-Halley J, Ross R. Long-term recreational physical activity and risk of invasive and in situ breast cancer. Arch Intern Med 2007;167:408–15.

110. Friberg E, Mantzoros CS, Wolk A. Physical activity and risk of endometrial cancer: a population-based prospective cohort study. Cancer Epidemiol Biomarkers Prev 2006;15:2136–40.

111. Friberg E, Mantzoros CS, Wolk A. Diabetes and risk of endometrial cancer: a population-based prospective cohort study. Cancer Epidemiol Biomarkers Prev 2007;16:276–80.

112. Irwin ML, Yasui Y, Ulrich CM, et al. Effect of exercise on total and intra-abdominal body fat in post-menopausal women: a randomized controlled trial. JAMA 2003;289:323–30.

113. McTiernan A, Tworoger SS, Rajan KB, et al. Effect of exercise on serum androgens in postmenopausal women: a 12-month randomized clinical trial. Cancer Epidemiol Biomarkers Prev 2004;13:1099–105.

114. Goodyear LJ, Kahn BB. Exercise, glucose transport, and insulin sensitivity. Annu Rev Med 1998;49:235–61.

115. Gapstur SM, Kopp P, Chiu BC, et al. Longitudinal associations of age, anthropometric and lifestyle factors with serum total insulin-like growth factor-I and IGF binding protein-3 levels in Black and White men: the CARDIA Male Hormone Study. Cancer Epidemiol Biomarkers Prev 2004;13:2208–16.

116. Ring-Dimitriou S, Paulweber B, von Duvillard SP, et al. The effect of physical activity and physical fitness on plasma adiponectin in adults with predisposition to metabolic syndrome. Eur J Appl Physiol 2006;98:472–81.

117. Mantzoros C, Petridou E, Dessypris N, et al. Adiponectin and breast cancer risk. J Clin Endocrinol Metab 2004;89:1102–7.

118. Petridou E, Mantzoros C, Dessypris N, et al. Plasma adiponectin concentrations in relation to endometrial cancer: a case-control study in Greece. J Clin Endocrinol Metab 2003;88:993–7.

119. Samad AK, Taylor RS, Marshall T, et al. A meta-analysis of the association of physical activity with reduced risk of colorectal cancer. Colorectal Dis 2005;7:204–13.

120. Lichtenstein AH, Appel LJ, Brands M, et al. Summary of American Heart Association Diet and Lifestyle Recommendations revision 2006. Arterioscler Thromb Vasc Biol 2006;26:2186–91.

121. American Diabetes Association. ADA Dietary Guidelines. Alexandria, VA: ADA, 2006.

122. US Department of Health and Human Services and US Department of Agriculture. Dietary guidelines for Americans. Washington, DC: US Government Printing Office, US Department of Health and Human Services, US Department of Agriculture, 2005.

123. Kushi LH, Byers T, Doyle C, et al. American Cancer Society Guidelines on Nutrition and Physical Activity for cancer prevention: reducing the risk of cancer with healthy food choices and physical activity. CA Cancer J Clin 2006;56:254–81; quiz 313–4.

124. Serra-Majem L, Roman B, Estruch R. Scientific evidence of interventions using the Mediterranean diet: a systematic review. Nutr Rev 2006;64:S27–47.

125. Owen RW, Haubner R, Wurtele G, et al. Olives and olive oil in cancer prevention. Eur J Cancer Prev 2004;13:319–26.

126. Colomer R, Menendez JA. Mediterranean diet, olive oil and cancer. Clin Transl Oncol 2006;8:15–21.

127. Simopoulos AP. The traditional diet of Greece and cancer. Eur J Cancer Prev 2004;13:219–30.

128. Trichopoulou A. Traditional Mediterranean diet and longevity in the elderly: a review. Public Health Nutr 2004;7:943–7.

129. Trichopoulou A, Costacou T, Bamia C, et al. Adherence to a Mediterranean diet and survival in a Greek population. N Engl J Med 2003;348:2599–608.

130. Helsing E, Trichopoulou A. The Mediterranean diet and food culture: a symposium. Eur J Clin Nutr 1989;43:1–92.

IV Nutrition Recommendations

10 Food Guide Pyramids and the 2005 MyPyramid

Jessica Fargnoli and Christos S. Mantzoros

KEY POINTS

- In 1992, the USDA introduced the Food Guide Pyramid as a simple tool to aid the public in selecting and preparing the best foods for overall health and for prevention of chronic disease.
- The scientific community has been divided over the effectiveness and accuracy of the information relayed by the food pyramid.
- In response to evolving scientific concepts and evidence, the USDA released an updated Food Guide Pyramid, called MyPyramid, in 2005.
- The recommendations in the revised Food Pyramid and Dietary Guidelines are based on currently available scientific evidence, but some still doubt whether the new Pyramid includes enough valuable information to truly guide the public to a healthier lifestyle.

Key Words: USDA Food Pyramids, Nutrition recommendations

1. HISTORY OF THE DIETARY GUIDELINES AND THE FOOD PYRAMIDS

Since 1894, the United States Department of Agriculture (USDA) has been providing the public with food guidance based on scientific evidence of food's nutritional value. WO Atwater paved the way for the first USDA food guides with his research compiling food composition tables and determining nutritional requirements for the US population *(1)*. The USDA released the first official food guide in 1916. Developed by Caroline Hunt, a nutrition specialist at the USDA, the guide placed food into five groups: milk and meat, cereals, vegetables and fruits, fats and fat foods, and sugars and sugary foods *(2)*. Over time, food guides have been updated and revised as knowledge has changed, but the idea of selecting a variety of foods from different nutritional groups has been consistent since people usually eat a variety of foods. Among the most popular food guides was the "Basic Four." Released in 1956, this guide divided food into four categories:

From: *Nutrition and Health: Nutrition and Metabolism*
Edited by: C.S. Mantzoros, DOI: 10.1007/978-1-60327-453-1_10,
© Humana Press, a part of Springer Science + Business Media, LLC 2009

dairy, meat, grains, and fruit and vegetables. In 1979, a fifth group was added for fats, sweets, and alcohol *(2)*, and this is generally how food has been characterized by the USDA since then.

In response to the public's need for more comprehensive nutrition information, the USDA and DHHS released the first *Dietary Guidelines for Americans* booklet in1980. Developed to help individuals to choose and prepare foods for optimum health and prevention of chronic disease, this new food guide offered more detailed information about how to select the most nutritious foods and the harm caused by the least nutritious, along with recommendations on how to maintain a healthy body weight *(3)*. The first Dietary Guidelines encouraged consumption of a variety of foods, including starch and fiber, along with avoidance of fats, sugars, and sodium. It also recommended moderation of alcoholic beverages.

After implementation of the new dietary guidelines, it was found that consumers and some professionals were largely unaware of its existence. Many thought that the USDA was still using the "Basic Four" *(4)*. To remedy this, the USDA began research and development of a visual representation of the Dietary Guidelines in 1988. When designing the graph, the USDA stressed that it must convey variety, proportionality, moderation, and usability *(4)*. Many potential designs, such as shopping carts, circles, and funnel shapes, were tested for their ability to express these ideas. The pyramid and a bowl shape were most successful, but the pyramid was chosen for its edge in communicating the ideas of proportionality and moderation *(4)*. The resulting Food Guide Pyramid promoted a diet based heavily on bread, cereal, rice, and pasta (6–11 servings a day) and very low in fats and refined sugars *(5)*. It also recommended liberal consumption of fruits and vegetables, and two–three servings of meat and dairy a day. By this time, the differences between harmful saturated fats and beneficial unsaturated fats were well known. Despite this, the government largely considered the American public unable to distinguish between different types of fat *(6)*. Therefore, the Dietary Guidelines and corresponding Food Guide Pyramid offered no distinction between types of fat and promoted an overall low-fat diet in order to reduce consumption of saturated fats *(6)* (Fig. 1).

The release of the first Food Guide Pyramid was met with both support and criticism. For most, the largest inadequacy of the first Food Guide Pyramid was its simplicity. To many, it did not offer enough information to select the most nutritious foods within each food group. Some nutritional experts criticized its failure to distinguish between harmful animal fats and beneficial vegetable oils *(6–8)*, especially in light of the fact that the food guides of several nations, such as China, Australia, and Greece, address the use of different types of fat *(6)*. Others worried that the public would be confused because the Food Guide Pyramid did not make a distinction between red meat and other apparently healthier foods, such as poultry, fish, legumes, and eggs in the protein group *(8)*. The pyramid put an emphasis on consumption of breads, cereal products, and potatoes, though there was no evidence of a clear benefit from this *(8)*. Some thought it should be more specific about the consumption of whole grains leading to a decreased risk in heart disease rather than lumping all grains together in one recommendation *(8)*. The Pyramid was also criticized for lacking valuable information on physical activity and sodium and alcohol intake along with recommending confusing serving sizes that could lead to excess calorie consumption *(6)*. Perhaps the only recommendation of the Food Guide Pyramid not to be disputed was increased consumption of fruit and vegetables.

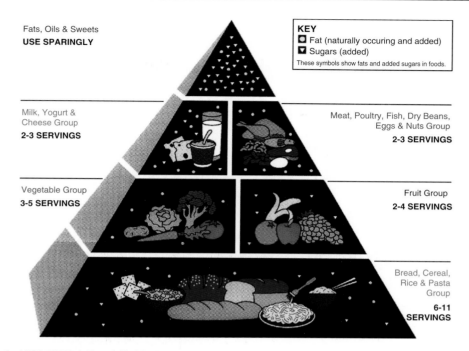

Fats, Oils & Sweets
USE SPARINGLY

KEY
☐ Fat (naturally occuring and added)
◧ Sugars (added)
These symbols show fats and added sugars in foods.

Milk, Yogurt &
Cheese Group
2-3 SERVINGS

Meat, Poultry, Fish, Dry Beans,
Eggs & Nuts Group
2-3 SERVINGS

Vegetable Group
3-5 SERVINGS

Fruit Group
2-4 SERVINGS

Bread, Cereal,
Rice & Pasta
Group
**6-11
SERVINGS**

Fig. 1. 1992 USDA Food Guide Pyramid.

Those who came to the Pyramid's defense proposed that its core recommendations of variety, proportionality, and moderation are valid and that the obesity epidemic is a result of the public's failure to follow these suggestions *(9)*. Despite the criticism, over a decade elapsed before the USDA released a revised version of the Food Guide Pyramid.

2. THE 2005 MYPYRAMID

In response to both widespread criticism and changing nutritional knowledge, the USDA released an updated version of the Food Guide Pyramid in 2005. As part of the revision it was renamed MyPyramid, to promote individuality in food choices, and was modernized with a companion website, http://www.mypyramid.gov. The new image itself contains very little information about each food group and no daily intake suggestions. It is intentionally vague, broadly representing the food groups and the recommendations of activity, moderation, personalization, proportionality, variety, and gradual improvement. The food groups are also now represented as vertical rather than horizontal bands on the pyramid. MyPyramid relies heavily on the website, MyPyramid. gov, and descriptive handouts to disseminate more detailed information about selecting foods and what quantities to eat. "Inside the Pyramid," on MyPyramid.gov, contains detailed explanations about each group of foods and offers information on how to choose the most healthful foods (Fig. 2).

In the information online, the 2005 Pyramid differentiates between different foods in the grain group, recommending that at least half of the public's grain intake should be from whole grains. Like the earlier version, this new pyramid also encourages a low-fat diet, but advises the public to choose healthier vegetable oils over solid animal fats.

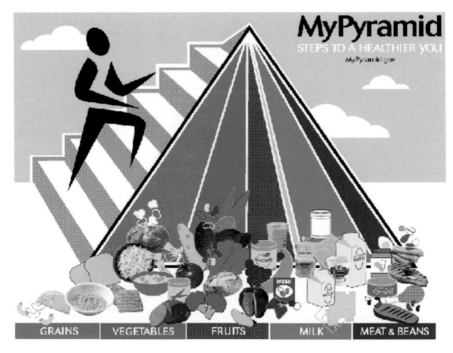

Fig. 2. 2005 MyPyramid (adapted from www.mypyramid.gov).

The 2005 Pyramid also offers more detailed recommendations in the meats and beans group, advocating for lean or low-fat meat choices and suggesting that fish, nuts, and seeds should be chosen over meat when possible. The revised Food Pyramid also improves upon its lack of information on physical activity and its previously confusing serving sizes. Exercise is now represented on the Pyramid and it recommends at least 30 min of physical activity a day. No longer does the Pyramid offer serving size suggestions for each group, instead the MyPyramid Plan on the MyPyramid.gov website calculates individualized serving needs based on gender, weight, age, and physical activity.

Another feature of MyPyramid.gov is the MyPyramidTracker. This online tool assesses the user's dietary and physical activity and calculates his or her energy balance. It allows each individual to track their own adherence to the Food Pyramid guidelines and adjust their intake accordingly.

Although the new, interactive Pyramid has addressed many of the problems of its predecessor, it has still been the subject of some criticism. MyPyramid.gov offers a wealth of educational materials, but it is not readily available to underprivileged populations who are at high risk for many chronic diseases *(10)*. Further research on the new Food Guide Pyramid should be conducted to determine if its recommendations are truly reaching the American public.

The USDA's Food Guide Pyramid has undergone tremendous revision and now offers much more detailed recommendations, which are very similar to those of other nations, such as Japan and Canada *(11)*. In the wake of the current obesity epidemic, it is essential that the American public stay informed and educated on which foods to choose, which to avoid, and what quantities they should eat. A graphic guide, such as the Food Guide

Pyramid, makes this information much more accessible. In addition, the features now offered on the corresponding MyPyramid.gov website should give users all of the tools needed to follow the USDA's Dietary Guidelines. The question that remains is whether the 2005 Food Guide Pyramid truly recommends the most effective diet for preventing chronic disease.

3. SCIENTIFIC EVIDENCE UNDERLYING THE CREATION OF MYPYRAMID

3.1. Ecological Studies

International comparisons have helped to shed light upon the effectiveness of various Food Pyramid recommendations in preventing chronic disease. Several studies comparing mortality and morbidity from coronary heart disease (CHD) among different countries have helped to elucidate the dietary factors involved. CHD mortality fell in USA and Australia in the 1960s, though it remained constant in England and Wales, which are comparable in demographics and quality of medical care (12). This drop in mortality was ultimately attributed to differences in fat consumption. Citizens of USA and Australia mostly switched from butter to margarine around 1960, and thus increased consumption of vegetable fat, while England and Wales did not begin the switch to margarine until 1973–1974 (12). In another study, a decline in mortality from heart disease in Poland in the 1990s was also related to a switch from animal to plant fats, along with increased fresh fruit and vegetable consumption (13). These findings, notwithstanding acknowledged limitations of ecological studies, support the beneficial nature of unsaturated plant fats over saturated animal fats.

In the Seven Countries Study, associations were found between the diets of certain regions and CHD. The two regions with diets lowest in saturated fat intake, Japan and the island of Crete in Greece, had the lowest mortality from ischemic heart disease. Concurrently, Finland had both the highest saturated fat intake and highest mortality from ischemic heart disease (14). Although the diets of the Japanese and Greeks in the study were both characterized by low saturated fat intake, the total fat intake of Greeks was over four times than that of the Japanese, mainly due to high consumption of olive oil (14). These findings led to many more investigations into the benefits of choosing vegetable oils over animal fats to prevent CHD.

Ecological studies have found several links between diet and various types of cancer too. Research comparing cancer incidence rates internationally found olive oil consumption to have a negative association with the development of colorectal cancer (15). Several studies have found a connection between high intake of dietary fat (particularly animal fat) and certain cancers, as well as an inverse association between fruit and vegetable intake and cancer risk (16–19). Importantly, many of the associations between diet and cancer risk seen in ecological studies have been found to be weak or nonexistent when analyzed in prospective cohort studies or clinical trials, underlying the main drawback of ecological studies, that is uncontrolled confounding.

3.2. Case-Control Studies

Many of the associations between dietary factors and chronic disease risk seen in ecological studies have also been validated by case-control studies. High-fat intake has been linked to various types of cancer, such as prostate, breast, and endometrial cancer *(20–22)*, along with higher risk of cardiovascular disease (CVD) *(23)*. Patients with severe nonalcoholic fatty liver disease (a condition related to the metabolic syndrome) had higher saturated fatty acid intakes (14% of daily energy) than age and BMI-matched controls (10% of daily energy) *(24)*.

In accordance with findings from previous ecological studies, a study based in Greece found that individuals with a closer adherence to Mediterranean diet were at decreased risk for acute CVD *(25)*. Higher consumption of vegetables has been connected to decreased risk of CVD *(23)*, and in several case-control studies, high fruit and vegetable intake has been linked to decreased risk of pancreatic, lung, breast, ovarian, and rectal cancer *(26–32)*. Risk for breast cancer and other cancers has been negatively associated with foods lower on the glycemic index, such as whole grains *(33)*. Research on the correlation between dairy and meat intake and various cancers has been inconclusive, showing positive and negative association with cancer risk depending on the type. With the possible exception of the dairy recommendations, the USDA's dietary guidelines seem to be consistent with most of these case-control studies.

3.3. Cohort Studies

Findings from cohort studies suggest that there is at least some relationship between adherence to the 1992 and 2005 Food Pyramid recommendations and reduced risk of chronic disease. Criticisms of the 1992 Food Guide Pyramid included whether it encouraged reasonable energy intake. A study of 4,994 men and women from the Third National Health and Nutrition Examination Survey found that participants who closely followed the 2005 Food Guide Pyramid consumed less calories than those who closely followed the 1992 Food Guide Pyramid guidelines *(34)*. Nutrient intakes were also improved for those who adhered to the 2005 Pyramid, with the exception of potassium and vitamin E. This information suggests that the 2005 Pyramid is improved in comparison to its earlier version in meeting nutritional needs while still constraining calories.

In 1995, the Healthy Eating Index (HEI) was designed to measure adherence to USDA's Dietary Guidelines, with higher scores corresponding to higher observance of the guidelines' recommendations *(35)*. This allowed researchers to begin assessing the effectiveness of the dietary guidelines in preventing chronic disease. Women among a cohort of the Nurses' Health study whose HEI scores adhered closely to the Dietary Guidelines were not found to be at significantly lower risk for overall chronic disease after a 12-year follow-up period *(36)*. They did, however, exhibit a small reduction in CVD risk. These findings were comparable with those from a cohort of men from the Health Professionals Follow-up Study, which found a weak inverse association between adherence to the Dietary Guidelines and overall risk for chronic disease *(37)*. Those men with the highest HEI score had a 28% lower risk of CVD, but no association was reported between HEI and cancer.

On the basis of these results, a new dietary index was developed called the Alternate Healthy Eating Index (AHEI), which was found it to be a more reliable predictor of chronic disease risk *(38)*. The predicted risk of CVD and overall chronic disease was lower for men and women with the highest AHEI scores. There was a much stronger inverse association between CVD and adherence to the Dietary Guidelines when using the AHEI *(38)*.

To examine the relationship between adherence to the 2005 Dietary Guidelines and insulin resistance, a study was conducted in the Framingham Offspring Cohort measuring the association between fasting insulin resistance and a diet consistent with the 2005 Dietary Guidelines. There was a positive association between women with a close adherence to the 2005 Dietary Guidelines and insulin sensitivity; however, no such association was found among men *(39)*. In prospective cohort studies, foods that are lower on the glycemic index improve insulin sensitivity and other risk factors for CVD *(40–42)*. The 2005 Pyramid currently recommends making half of all grains consumed whole grains, which are lower on the glycemic index. This may account for the increased insulin sensitivity seen in individuals who adhere to the 2005 Dietary Guidelines.

Little relationship has been found between following the Food Pyramid and cancer risk. Instead, some recent cohort studies have investigated the relationship between adherence to certain food groups and risk of cancer. Among prospective cohort studies, results are mixed on the relationship between consumption of dairy and certain cancers. An analysis of ten cohort studies found an association between high-milk and -calcium intake and reduced colorectal cancer risk *(43)*. Another prospective study among the Health Professionals Follow-up cohort found high-calcium intake to be associated with higher risk of advanced prostate cancer *(44)*. Further analyses of cohort studies found no association either way between breast and ovarian cancer and dairy intake *(45, 46)*. Thus, on the basis of current research, there seems to be little reason for the USDA to change their recommendations for three dairy servings per day until controlled trials are performed. Although ecological and case-control studies pointed to fruits and vegetables as important for cancer prevention, prospective cohort studies have shown little to no association between fruit and vegetable intake and cancer risk *(47–51)*. Although the latter study design offers the time sequence criterion for causality, neither one of these studies can prove causality. Thus, in order to truly determine the effectiveness of the Food Guide Pyramid and its corresponding food groups at reducing the risk of chronic disease, randomized trials must be performed.

3.4. Clinical Trials

The randomized trial is the only study design that can build on knowledge obtained and hypotheses generated by observational studies while at the same time is not plagued by the drawbacks of epidemiological studies. Few clinical trials to determine the Food Guide Pyramid's effectiveness at preventing chronic disease have been completed. One trial conducted among active-duty Air Force members in a 90-day fitness program found that a group receiving individualized counseling using the Food Guide Pyramid had significant reductions in cardiovascular risk factors and an improved response to exercise training *(52)*. Those using the Food Guide Pyramid experienced reduced energy from fat intake, BMI, total cholesterol levels, and LDL levels *(52)*.

There is little information deriving from clinical trials specifically on the Food Guide Pyramid's effectiveness in reducing chronic disease. In addition, several other diets have been shown to be beneficial, especially in reducing CVD outcomes, and may thus inform future dietary recommendations. A meta-analysis of 27 clinical trials suggests that replacing saturated fats with polyunsaturated fats is more beneficial than replacing them with either carbohydrates or monounsaturated fats *(53)*. In one trial, patients with a recent acute myocardial infarction (MI) were instructed to eat a low-fat diet, and an intervention group was also advised to eat more fruits, vegetables, nuts, and grain products. The early initiation of the intervention (within 72 h of MI) resulted in a significant decrease in cardiac events for the intervention group after a 1-year follow-up *(54)*. The group eating a diet high in fiber, vitamins, and minerals also resulted in significant decreases in blood lipoprotein levels and fasting blood glucose.

Another trial found that mortality was reduced by about 29% in a 2-year follow-up of patients recovering from an MI who increased their intake of fatty fish and fish oil *(55)*. In this same study, however, there was no evidence of benefit from increased fiber or decreased fat. Randomized trials have also shown that a diet high in monounsaturated fatty acids, such as those found in nuts, is more favorable than a low-fat diet, since it lowers LDL cholesterol but not HDL cholesterol *(56, 57)*. Diets that replace saturated fatty acids with polyunsaturated fatty acids can reduce LDL cholesterol by 9.8% *(58)*.

4. MEDITERRANEAN-TYPE DIET PYRAMID

Improved health outcomes have historically been associated with the diet followed by the Mediterranean region of the world. This diet pattern is generally defined by large intakes of whole grains and plant foods, olive oil as the major fat, low-to-moderate intakes of dairy, fish, and poultry, low intake of red meat, and low-to-moderate consumption of wine *(59)*. The Lyon Diet Heart Study performed a randomized trial to elucidate whether a Mediterranean-type diet might reduce the occurrence of cardiovascular outcomes in patients who have had an MI. After a 4-year follow-up, the final report confirmed the protective effects of the Mediterranean diet *(60)*. This diet may also be beneficial in prevention of the metabolic syndrome which is associated with type 2 diabetes and CVD *(61)*. Patients with the metabolic syndrome following a Mediterranean-style diet for 2 years benefited from a reduction in inflammatory markers, decreased insulin resistance, and improved endothelial function *(61)*. In addition, a Mediterranean-style diet has been shown to be associated with higher adherence rates than low-fat diets of the same calorie intake, resulting in healthier body weight *(62)*.

The benefits of the Mediterranean-type diet may be related to inclusion of whole grains over refined carbohydrates, moderate alcohol intake, as well as prudent use of nuts, especially walnuts. Several randomized trials have proven the benefits of whole grains in decreasing risk of heart disease, such as improving insulin sensitivity and lowering LDL cholesterol concentrations *(42)*. Moderate alcohol consumption has also been shown to improve insulin sensitivity, lower blood pressure, and reduce the risk of CVD, such as ischemic stroke *(63–66)*. A daily serving of 30 g of walnuts, which have higher polyunsaturated fat content than other nuts, increased HDL to total cholesterol ratio in patients with type 2 diabetes *(67)*. In addition, walnuts have been shown to improve endothelial function *(67, 68)*. We have recently shown that the combination of these food items in the context of the Mediterranean diet increases the circulating levels of adiponectin, an adipocyte secreted hormone which acts as an endogenous insulin sensitizer. Adiponectin can in turn improve insulin resistance, optimize glycemic control, and decrease lipid levels and inflammatory markers.

Clinical trials hoping to determine the effects of diet on cancer risk have been less conclusive. In the Women's Healthy Eating and Living randomized trial among women previously treated for breast cancer, an intervention group eating a diet low in fat and very high in vegetables, fruits, and fiber did not have a reduction in breast cancer events or mortality in a 7.3-year follow-up period *(69)*. Many of the dietary factors associated with cancer in case-control and observational ecological studies have not been replicated in controlled trials, making it difficult to make nutritional recommendations solely on the basis of cancer prevention. Obesity is a risk factor for many types of cancer, however, so diets effective in obesity prevention should be followed.

5. CONCLUSIONS

On the basis of current scientific evidence, the nutritional guidelines put forth by the USDA are reasonable for most healthy Americans. Several prospective cohort studies and one controlled trial have shown that closer adherence to the dietary guidelines provides at least some benefit in preventing chronic disease. However, more specificity is necessary so that the public may truly choose the healthiest foods from each food group. Importantly, more clinical trials are needed to conclusively demonstrate the efficacy and cost-effectiveness of not only the guidelines in general but also the individual recommendations more specifically.

Certain areas of uncertainty and/or areas where the recommendations of MyPyramid can be improved remain. MyPyramid's recommendation to make "half your grains whole" has been proposed to be a step in the right direction. On the basis of overwhelming scientific evidence on the benefits of choosing whole grains over refined carbohydrates in preventing type 2 diabetes and CVD and the readily available array of whole grain products now offered, it seems reasonable to recommend that Americans make all of their grains whole whenever possible for the optimum prevention of heart disease.

High fruit and vegetable intake does not seem to have the preventative powers for cancer that researchers once thought. Diets rich in fruits and vegetables still appear to be beneficial for the prevention of CVD and further investigations must be performed to determine which diets are most beneficial for cancer prevention. Fruits and vegetables are still a source of many essential vitamins and nutrients for overall health, however, and when added to a diet that previously lacked them, fruits and vegetables will likely take the place of other less nutritious foods. Further clinical trials are needed to fully substantiate these recommendations, though.

Although some associations have been made in cohort studies between dairy products and cancer risk, the relationship is still largely inconclusive. Given currently available evidence in conjunction with the beneficial effect of low-fat dairy products in obesity and metabolism, there seems to be no fault in recommending low-fat and fat-free dairy products at this time. Thus, future clinical trials must determine whether people at risk for certain cancers should be advised to lower dairy consumption, and controlled trials should be performed to determine what the effect of dairy products is on cancer outcomes as well as obesity, diabetes, and the metabolic syndrome.

Several authors have suggested that MyPyramid should be more authoritative in its advice on protein. Clinical evidence touts the benefits of fatty fish and nuts in the prevention of CVD, type 2 diabetes, and the metabolic syndrome. Since nuts, such as walnuts, are so useful in improving blood cholesterol profiles, it has been suggested that the USDA should recommend that one serving of protein a day be from nuts, and specifically walnuts, but again more clinical trials are also needed in this area. In a healthy diet, it is believed that red meat should be eaten very sparingly, and replaced by lean poultry and fish, as is done in the Mediterranean-type diet. In this area, it has been suggested that the Food Pyramid does not provide enough information to guide the public to the healthiest possible diet.

Clinical trials have consistently shown that a low-fat diet may not be as beneficial as a diet that replaces saturated fatty acids with mono- and polyunsaturated fatty acids. For example, the success of the Mediterranean diet in improving cardiovascular outcomes has been largely attributed to replacing animal fats with olive oil. In addition, diets, such as the Mediterranean, that replace saturated fats with these healthier fats are more palatable than low-fat diets and have higher adherence rates, resulting in more sustained weight loss and health benefits. After over a decade of advising Americans to avoid fat, several experts believe that the USDA needs to provide more information to change the public perception of fat *(6, 7)*. More detailed information, and thus more detailed clinical studies on the benefits of replacing animal fats and saturated fats with olive oil, monounsaturated fats, and polyunsaturated fats are clearly needed.

Last but not least, in a nation where over half of adults are overweight or obese, there is no question that authoritative dietary recommendations are necessary to educate Americans on the healthiest food choices. The USDA's dietary guidelines and corresponding Food Pyramids are useful in this regard, but several experts agree that these must be more discriminating in their advice on total energy intakes, grains, proteins, and fats based on current scientific evidence. Alternative pyramids have been proposed, such as Walter Willett's Healthy Eating Pyramid, that separate refined carbohydrates from whole grains and red meat and animal fats from leaner, more nutritious proteins.

Finally, another criticism by many experts is that the USDA's decision to put the more detailed information on each food group online fails to recognize the significant portion of the US population without home internet access. Without the additional information provided online, the 2005 pyramid is nothing more than a triangle that lists the different food groups, leaving no way for users to choose the healthiest foods in each group. A more effective way of distributing this information must be considered so that a large percentage of Americans, especially the underprivileged ones who tend to be more prone to consume a less healthy diet, are not left in the dark on the finer points of the USDA's nutritional guidelines.

In summary, although the 2005 MyPyramid appears to be a welcome advance in relation to previously available guidelines, much more is needed in terms of research to support dietary recommendations as well as public health efforts to best disseminate the message on a diet that can prevent and/or improve adverse health outcomes.

REFERENCES

1. Welsh S. Atwater to the present: evolution of nutrition education. J Nutr 1994; 124(9 Suppl):1799S–1807S.
2. Welsh S, Davis C, Shaw A. A brief history of Food Guides in the United States. Nutrition Today 1992; 6–11.
3. U.S. Department of Agriculture and U.S. Department of Health and Human Services. Nutrition and Your Health: Dietary Guidelines for Americans. 1980. Washington, DC, Home and Garden Bulletin.
4. Welsh S, Davis C, Shaw A. Development of the Food Guide Pyramid. Nutrition Today 1992; 12–23.
5. U.S. Department of Agriculture. The food guide pyramid. 1992. Washington, DC, Home and Garden Bulletin.
6. Gifford KD. Dietary fats, eating guides, and public policy: history, critique, and recommendations. Am J Med 2002; 113(Suppl 9B):89S–106S.

7. Willett WC. The dietary pyramid: does the foundation need repair. Am J Clin Nutr 1998; 68(2):218–219.

8. Willett WC, Stampfer MJ. Rebuilding the food pyramid. Sci Am 2003; 288(1):64–71.

9. Goldberg JP, Belury MA, Elam P et al. The obesity crisis: don't blame it on the pyramid. J Am Diet Assoc 2004; 104(7):1141–1147.

10. Johnston CS. Uncle Sam's diet sensation: MyPyramid – an overview and commentary. MedGenMed 2005; 7(3):78.

11. Murphy SP, Barr SI. Food guides reflect similarities and differences in dietary guidance in three countries (Japan, Canada, and the United States). Nutr Rev 2007; 65(4):141–148.

12. Hetzel BS, Charnock JS, Dwyer T, McLennan PL. Fall in coronary heart disease mortality in U.S.A. and Australia due to sudden death: evidence for the role of polyunsaturated fat. J Clin Epidemiol 1989; 42(9):885–893.

13. Zatonski WA, McMichael AJ, Powles JW. Ecological study of reasons for sharp decline in mortality from ischaemic heart disease in Poland since 1991. BMJ 1998; 316(7137):1047–1051.

14. Keys A. Coronary heart disease in seven countries. 1970. Nutrition 1997; 13(3):250–252.

15. Stoneham M, Goldacre M, Seagroatt V, Gill L. Olive oil, diet and colorectal cancer: an ecological study and a hypothesis. J Epidemiol Community Health 2000; 54(10):756–760.

16. Farchi S, Saba A, Turrini A, Forlani F, Pettinelli A, D'Amicis A. An ecological study of the correlation between diet and tumour mortality rates in Italy. Eur J Cancer Prev 1996; 5(2):113–120.

17. Sasaki S, Horacsek M, Kesteloot H. An ecological study of the relationship between dietary fat intake and breast cancer mortality. Prev Med 1993; 22(2):187–202.

18. Kneller RW, Guo WD, Hsing AW et al. Risk factors for stomach cancer in sixty-five Chinese counties. Cancer Epidemiol Biomarkers Prev 1992; 1(2):113–118.

19. Koo LC, Mang OW, Ho JH. An ecological study of trends in cancer incidence and dietary changes in Hong Kong. Nutr Cancer 1997; 28(3):289–301.

20. Kristal AR, Cohen JH, Qu P, Stanford JL. Associations of energy, fat, calcium, and vitamin D with prostate cancer risk. Cancer Epidemiol Biomarkers Prev 2002; 11(8):719–725.

21. Alothaimeen A, Ezzat A, Mohamed G, Muammar T, Al-Madouj A. Dietary fat and breast cancer in Saudi Arabia: a case-control study. East Mediterr Health J 2004; 10(6):879–886.

22. Dalvi TB, Canchola AJ, Horn-Ross PL. Dietary patterns, Mediterranean diet, and endometrial cancer risk. Cancer Causes Control 2007.

23. Zyriax BC, Boeing H, Windler E. Nutrition is a powerful independent risk factor for coronary heart disease in women – the CORA study: a population-based case-control study. Eur J Clin Nutr 2005; 59(10):1201–1207.

24. Musso G, Gambino R, De MF et al. Dietary habits and their relations to insulin resistance and postprandial lipemia in nonalcoholic steatohepatitis. Hepatology 2003; 37(4):909–916.

25. Panagiotakos DB, Pitsavos C, Matalas AL, Chrysohoou C, Stefanadis C. Geographical influences on the association between adherence to the Mediterranean diet and the prevalence of acute coronary syndromes, in Greece: the CARDIO2000 study. Int J Cardiol 2005; 100(1):135–142.

26. Chan JM, Wang F, Holly EA. Vegetable and fruit intake and pancreatic cancer in a population-based case-control study in the San Francisco bay area. Cancer Epidemiol Biomarkers Prev 2005; 14(9):2093–2097.

27. Galeone C, Negri E, Pelucchi C, La VC, Bosetti C, Hu J. Dietary intake of fruit and vegetable and lung cancer risk: a case-control study in Harbin, northeast China. Ann Oncol 2007; 18(2):388–392.

28. Malin AS, Qi D, Shu XO et al. Intake of fruits, vegetables and selected micronutrients in relation to the risk of breast cancer. Int J Cancer 2003; 105(3):413–418.

29. Pan SY, Ugnat AM, Mao Y, Wen SW, Johnson KC. A case-control study of diet and the risk of ovarian cancer. Cancer Epidemiol Biomarkers Prev 2004; 13(9):1521–1527.

30. Rylander R, Axelsson G. Lung cancer risks in relation to vegetable and fruit consumption and smoking. Int J Cancer 2006; 118(3):739–743.

31. Shannon J, Ray R, Wu C et al. Food and botanical groupings and risk of breast cancer: a case-control study in Shanghai, China. Cancer Epidemiol Biomarkers Prev 2005; 14(1):81–90.

32. Slattery ML, Curtin KP, Edwards SL, Schaffer DM. Plant foods, fiber, and rectal cancer. Am J Clin Nutr 2004; 79(2):274–281.

33. Augustin LS, Dal ML, La VC et al. Dietary glycemic index and glycemic load, and breast cancer risk: a case-control study. Ann Oncol 2001; 12(11):1533–1538.

34. Gao X, Wilde PE, Lichtenstein AH, Tucker KL. The 2005 USDA Food Guide Pyramid is associated with more adequate nutrient intakes within energy constraints than the 1992 Pyramid. J Nutr 2006; 136(5):1341–1346.
35. Kennedy ET, Ohls J, Carlson S, Fleming K. The Healthy Eating Index: design and applications. J Am Diet Assoc 1995; 95(10):1103–1108.
36. McCullough ML, Feskanich D, Stampfer MJ et al. Adherence to the Dietary Guidelines for Americans and risk of major chronic disease in women. Am J Clin Nutr 2000; 72(5):1214–1222.
37. McCullough ML, Feskanich D, Rimm EB et al. Adherence to the Dietary Guidelines for Americans and risk of major chronic disease in men. Am J Clin Nutr 2000; 72(5):1223–1231.
38. McCullough ML, Feskanich D, Stampfer MJ et al. Diet quality and major chronic disease risk in men and women: moving toward improved dietary guidance. Am J Clin Nutr 2002; 76(6):1261–1271.
39. Fogli-Cawley JJ, Dwyer JT, Saltzman E et al. The 2005 Dietary Guidelines for Americans and insulin resistance in the Framingham Offspring Cohort. Diabetes Care 2007; 30(4):817–822.
40. Liu S, Willett WC, Stampfer MJ et al. A prospective study of dietary glycemic load, carbohydrate intake, and risk of coronary heart disease in US women. Am J Clin Nutr 2000; 71(6):1455–1461.
41. Meyer KA, Kushi LH, Jacobs DR, Jr., Slavin J, Sellers TA, Folsom AR. Carbohydrates, dietary fiber, and incident type 2 diabetes in older women. Am J Clin Nutr 2000; 71(4):921–930.
42. Jenkins DJ, Kendall CW, Augustin LS et al. Glycemic index: overview of implications in health and disease. Am J Clin Nutr 2002; 76(1):266S–273S.
43. Cho E, Smith-Warner SA, Spiegelman D et al. Dairy foods, calcium, and colorectal cancer: a pooled analysis of 10 cohort studies. J Natl Cancer Inst 2004; 96(13):1015–1022.
44. Giovannucci E, Liu Y, Stampfer MJ, Willett WC. A prospective study of calcium intake and incident and fatal prostate cancer. Cancer Epidemiol Biomarkers Prev 2006; 15(2):203–210.
45. Genkinger JM, Hunter DJ, Spiegelman D et al. Dairy products and ovarian cancer: a pooled analysis of 12 cohort studies. Cancer Epidemiol Biomarkers Prev 2006; 15(2):364–372.
46. Moorman PG, Terry PD. Consumption of dairy products and the risk of breast cancer: a review of the literature. Am J Clin Nutr 2004; 80(1):5–14.
47. Feskanich D, Ziegler RG, Michaud DS et al. Prospective study of fruit and vegetable consumption and risk of lung cancer among men and women. J Natl Cancer Inst 2000; 92(22):1812–1823.
48. Hung HC, Joshipura KJ, Jiang R et al. Fruit and vegetable intake and risk of major chronic disease. J Natl Cancer Inst 2004; 96(21):1577–1584.
49. Smith-Warner SA, Spiegelman D, Yaun SS et al. Intake of fruits and vegetables and risk of breast cancer: a pooled analysis of cohort studies. JAMA 2001; 285(6):769–776.
50. Terry P, Giovannucci E, Michels KB et al. Fruit, vegetables, dietary fiber, and risk of colorectal cancer. J Natl Cancer Inst 2001; 93(7):525–533.
51. Voorrips LE, Goldbohm RA, van PG, Sturmans F, Hermus RJ, van den Brandt PA. Vegetable and fruit consumption and risks of colon and rectal cancer in a prospective cohort study: The Netherlands Cohort Study on Diet and Cancer. Am J Epidemiol 2000; 152(11):1081–1092.
52. Gambera PJ, Schneeman BO, Davis PA. Use of the Food Guide Pyramid and US Dietary Guidelines to improve dietary intake and reduce cardiovascular risk in active-duty Air Force members. J Am Diet Assoc 1995; 95(11):1268–1273.
53. Mensink RP, Katan MB. Effect of dietary fatty acids on serum lipids and lipoproteins. A meta-analysis of 27 trials. Arterioscler Thromb 1992; 12(8):911–919.
54. Singh RB, Rastogi SS, Verma R et al. Randomised controlled trial of cardioprotective diet in patients with recent acute myocardial infarction: results of one year follow up. BMJ 1992; 304(6833):1015–1019.
55. Burr ML, Fehily AM, Gilbert JF et al. Effects of changes in fat, fish, and fibre intakes on death and myocardial reinfarction: diet and reinfarction trial (DART). Lancet 1989; 2(8666):757–761.
56. Kris-Etherton PM, Pearson TA, Wan Y et al. High-monounsaturated fatty acid diets lower both plasma cholesterol and triacylglycerol concentrations. Am J Clin Nutr 1999; 70(6):1009–1015.
57. Rajaram S, Burke K, Connell B, Myint T, Sabate J. A monounsaturated fatty acid-rich pecan-enriched diet favorably alters the serum lipid profile of healthy men and women. J Nutr 2001; 131(9):2275–2279.
58. Heine RJ, Mulder C, Popp-Snijders C, van der Meer J, van der Veen EA. Linoleic-acid-enriched diet: long-term effects on serum lipoprotein and apolipoprotein concentrations and insulin sensitivity in noninsulin-dependent diabetic patients. Am J Clin Nutr 1989; 49(3):448–456.

59. Willett WC, Sacks F, Trichopoulou A et al. Mediterranean diet pyramid: a cultural model for healthy eating. Am J Clin Nutr 1995; 61(6):1402S–1406.

60. de LM, Salen P, Martin JL, Monjaud I, Delaye J, Mamelle N. Mediterranean diet, traditional risk factors, and the rate of cardiovascular complications after myocardial infarction: final report of the Lyon Diet Heart Study. Circulation 1999; 99(6):779–785.

61. Esposito K, Marfella R, Ciotola M et al. Effect of a Mediterranean-style diet on endothelial dysfunction and markers of vascular inflammation in the metabolic syndrome: a randomized trial. JAMA 2004; 292(12):1440–1446.

62. McManus K, Antinoro L, Sacks F. A randomized controlled trial of a moderate-fat, low-energy diet compared with a low fat, low-energy diet for weight loss in overweight adults. Int J Obes Relat Metab Disord 2001; 25(10):1503–1511.

63. Sierksma A, Patel H, Ouchi N et al. Effect of moderate alcohol consumption on adiponectin, tumor necrosis factor-alpha, and insulin sensitivity. Diabetes Care 2004; 27(1):184–189.

64. Thadhani R, Camargo CA, Jr., Stampfer MJ, Curhan GC, Willett WC, Rimm EB. Prospective study of moderate alcohol consumption and risk of hypertension in young women. Arch Intern Med 2002; 162(5):569–574.

65. Mezzano D, Leighton F, Martinez C et al. Complementary effects of Mediterranean diet and moderate red wine intake on haemostatic cardiovascular risk factors. Eur J Clin Nutr 2001; 55(6):444–451.

66. Elkind MS, Sciacca R, Boden-Albala B, Rundek T, Paik MC, Sacco RL. Moderate alcohol consumption reduces risk of ischemic stroke: the Northern Manhattan Study. Stroke 2006; 37(1):13–19.

67. Tapsell LC, Gillen LJ, Patch CS et al. Including walnuts in a low-fat/modified-fat diet improves HDL cholesterol-to-total cholesterol ratios in patients with type 2 diabetes. Diabetes Care 2004; 27(12):2777–2783.

68. Cortes B, Nunez I, Cofan M et al. Acute effects of high-fat meals enriched with walnuts or olive oil on postprandial endothelial function. J Am Coll Cardiol 2006; 48(8):1666–1671.

69. Pierce JP, Natarajan L, Caan BJ et al. Influence of a diet very high in vegetables, fruit, and fiber and low in fat on prognosis following treatment for breast cancer: the Women's Healthy Eating and Living (WHEL) randomized trial. JAMA 2007; 298(3):289–298.

11 Nutrition Recommendations for the General Population: Where Is the Science?

Walter C. Willett and Meir J. Stampfer

KEY POINTS

- During the 1990s dietary guidelines for the US and many other countries promoted a diet low in fat and high in "complex" carbohydrates.
- However, there was little evidence then that such a diet would promote health and reduce risk of chronic disease, and subsequent data have not supported benefits for cardiovascular disease, cancer, or weight control.
- Instead, the combination of controlled feeding studies of intermediate risk factors and prospective epidemiologic studies has indicated that the type of dietary fat and dietary carbohydrate have major impacts on risks of these diseases.
- Specifically, higher intake of *trans* fatty acids has adverse effects on blood lipids and inflammatory factors, and has also been associated with greater risks of coronary heart disease and type 2 diabetes.
- In contrast, both types of studies have indicated beneficial effects of unsaturated fats, especially polyunsaturated fats. The replacement of saturated fat with carbohydrates has little effect on the ratio of serum total to HDL cholesterol, and is minimally associated with risk of heart disease.
- Similarly, higher intake of refined starches and sugar, represented by dietary glycemic load, has adverse effects on blood lipids and inflammatory factors and is related to higher risks of coronary heart disease and type 2 diabetes.
- Conversely, higher consumption of whole grains is related to lower risks of these diseases.
- Regrettably, this evidence has yet to be translated clearly into dietary guidance for many populations.

Key Words: Diet, Dietary, Nutrition, Guidelines, Heart disease, Chronic disease

1. DIETARY GUIDANCE: WHERE IS THE SCIENCE?

In 1992, the United States Department of Agriculture (USDA) officially released its first Food Guide Pyramid, which was intended to help the American public make food choices that would maintain general good health and reduce risk of chronic disease (Fig. 1).

From: *Nutrition and Health: Nutrition and Metabolism*
Edited by: C.S. Mantzoros, DOI: 10.1007/978-1-60327-453-1_11,
© Humana Press, a part of Springer Science+Business Media, LLC 2009

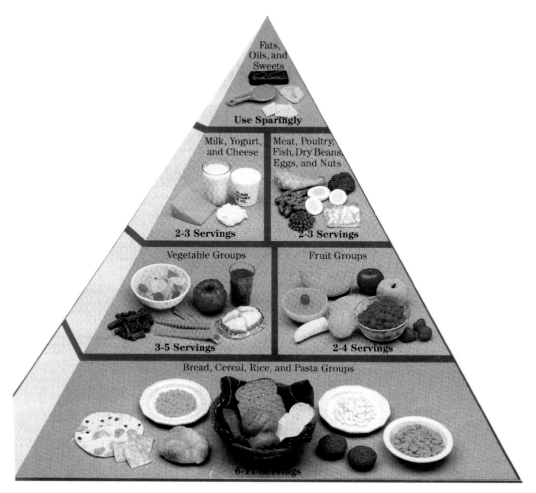

Fig. 1. USDA food pyramid.

Many other countries followed this lead; for example, the Iranian food guide pyramid was a direct translation. The core message of the USDA pyramid was resoundingly low fat: all fats and oils were to be consumed sparingly and, as replacement, "complex carbohydrates" were to be consumed in abundance, 6–11 servings a day. Generous amounts of vegetables (including more complex carbohydrates as potatoes), fruit, and dairy products were encouraged, and at least three servings per day from the "meat" group were advised, consisting of red meat, poultry, nuts, legumes, and eggs. Even at the time when the pyramid was first released, we had long known that some types of fat are essential, and that polyunsaturated fat could reduce plasma total cholesterol and incidence of coronary heart disease. In contrast, there was little evidence that high intake of starch is beneficial. Since 1992, evidence has continued to mount that the USDA pyramid provided misleading guidance to those seeking healthy food choices.

How did the pyramid go so wrong? Facing an epidemic of high cholesterol and coronary heart disease, and knowing that dietary saturated fats raise blood levels of cholesterol, policy makers sought to reduce dietary saturated fat. Apparently, however, it was considered too difficult to educate the public about the subtleties of types of fat. Instead, the thinking went, since saturated fat represented such a large fraction of dietary fat, if we advocate low fat, saturated fat intake would drop. Also, in the early 1980s, based largely on comparisons between countries, the belief developed that total fat in the diet was the primary factor underlying the high rates of breast, colon, and prostate cancer in Western counties. This led to a clear, simple message that fat is bad. Because protein in the diet is relatively constant (and often associated with saturated fat), the notion that fat is bad led to the corollary that carbohydrates are good, even without direct evidence. At the time the pyramid was developed, the typical US diet contained about 40% of calories from fat. It was thought that with a concerted campaign, we might have 30% as a reasonable goal. This led to the widespread adoption of 30% of calories from fat as a limit. The 30% limit became so entrenched in dietary guidelines in the US, and many other countries that even the sophisticated observer could be forgiven for thinking that there must be many studies showing that individuals with that level of fat intake enjoyed better health than those with higher levels. In fact, there were no such studies at all.

2. DIETARY FAT AND CORONARY HEART DISEASE

The concept that fat in general is to be avoided derives largely from observations that affluent Western countries have both high intakes of fat and high rates of coronary heart disease. However, this correlation was limited to saturated fat, and countries with high intake of monounsaturated fat tended to have lower rates. In the seminal study conducted by Keys and colleagues, the two regions with the lowest rates of heart disease were those following the traditional diets of Japan, with about 8–10% of calories from fat, and the traditional diet of Crete, with approximately 40% calories from fat (Fig. 2). International comparisons need to be interpreted cautiously, nevertheless, because many factors, such as smoking rates, physical inactivity, and adiposity, are also correlated with western affluence.

Evidence from early controlled feeding studies in the 1960s documented the adverse effects of saturated fat on total serum cholesterol levels, which are associated with higher risk of coronary heart disease, but also showed that polyunsaturated fat reduces serum cholesterol. Thus, dietary advice during the 1960s and 1970s emphasized replacement of saturated fat with polyunsaturated fat, not total fat reduction. The subsequent doubling of polyunsaturated fat consumption in the US probably contributed greatly to the halving of coronary heart disease rates in the US (1). For reasons described earlier, in the 1980s dietary advice subtly shifted to replacing fat in general with carbohydrate, which is the foundation of the USDA pyramid. The wisdom of this direction became questionable with the appreciation that total serum cholesterol can be subdivided: the LDL fraction increases but the HDL fraction reduces risk of coronary disease. More recently, serum triglyceride levels have also been associated with higher risk. Controlled feeding studies have shown that when saturated fat is replaced by carbohydrate, total and LDL cholesterol levels do fall, but HDL also falls proportionally, and triglyceride levels rise (2). Thus, the ratio of LDL or total cholesterol to HDL does not change, which would predict little reduction in heart disease risk. Replacing either poly or monounsaturated fat with carbo-hydrate would actually make the serum cholesterol ratio worse, but replacing saturated

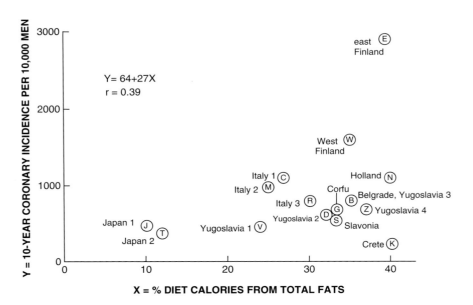

Ten-year incidence rate of coronary heart disease, by any diagnostic criterion,
plotted against the percentage of dietary calories supplied by total fats.
(Keys, 1980)

Fig. 2. Ten-year incidence of coronary heart disease, by any diagnostic criterion, plotted against the percentage of dietary calories supplied by total fats (Keys, 1980).

fat with either polyunsaturated or monounsaturated fat improves this ratio and would be expected to reduce heart disease. The relation of dietary fat to heart disease became more complicated with the appreciation that *trans*-unsaturated fatty acids (produced by the partial hydrogenation of liquid vegetable oils) have important biological effects. *Trans* fats have uniquely adverse characteristics because they raise serum LDL and triglycerides and reduce HDL *(3)*.

Although the effects of diet on blood cholesterol fractions and triglycerides are important, we now know that dietary factors can influence many other pathways that are important in the cause and prevention of coronary heart disease (Fig. 3, multiple pathways) *(4)*. For example, omega-3 fatty acids (from fish and some plant oils) can reduce the likelihood of ventricular fibrillation (and therefore sudden cardiac death), and there is now solid evidence that *trans* fats also increase inflammatory factors *(5,6)*, which appear to increase risks of cardiovascular disease and type 2 diabetes. Thus, it is also important to assess directly the relation of diet to heart disease incidence because this will integrate all the adverse and beneficial effects of a dietary factor. Ideally, studies of diet and heart disease would be conducted as trials in which individuals are randomly assigned to one diet or another and followed for many years. Because of practical constraints and cost, few such studies have been conducted, and most of these have been in patients with existing heart disease. Although limited, these studies have supported benefits of replacing saturated fat with polyunsaturated fat, but not with carbohydrate *(7)*. The best alternative is usually to conduct large prospective observational studies in which the diets of many persons are assessed periodically over time and participants are

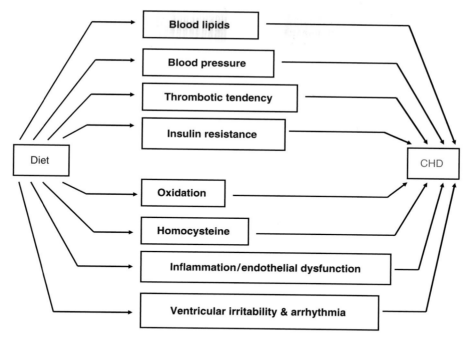

Fig. 3. Pathways leading from diet to incidence of coronary heart disease (CHD).

monitored for the development of heart disease and other conditions. In these studies, smoking, physical activity, and other potential risk factors can be measured and accounted for in the analysis. Thus, we have followed nearly 90,000 women who first completed detailed questionnaires on diet in 1980 and over 50,000 men who were enrolled in 1989. After adjusting for smoking, physical activity, and other recognized risk factors, we found strong relationships between type of dietary fat and risk of heart disease in the direction predicted by the controlled feeding studies. Specifically, compared with the same percentage of energy from carbohydrate, intake of *trans* fats was strongly associated with greater risk of coronary heart disease, saturated fat was only weakly related to risk, and both monounsaturated and polyunsaturated fats were associated with lower risk *(8)*. Because of the opposing relationships for specific types of fat, the percentage of calories from total fat was not associated with risk of heart disease. This adds further support to the conclusion of a report by the National Academy of Sciences in 1989 that total fat intake per se is not a determinant of coronary heart disease *(9)*. Although the relation of intake of *trans* fat to risk of coronary heart disease was initially controversial, this has been reproduced multiple times *(5)*.

3. DIETARY FAT AND CANCER

As for coronary heart disease, the belief that dietary fat is a major cause of cancer was derived largely from correlations among countries between per capita intake of total and animal fat and rates of cancers common in affluent countries, including cancers of the breast, colon, and prostate. However, in large prospective studies in which confounding variables could be better controlled, there has consistently been little relation between intakes of total and specific types of fat during mid life and risks of cancers of the breast and colon *(10)*. Data on diet and prostate cancer remain limited, but some studies have suggested positive associations with animal fat. Thus, it is reasonable to make decisions about dietary fat primarily on the basis of its effects on cardiovascular disease, not cancer.

4. DIETARY FAT AND BODY FAT

Excess body fat, including both mild overweight and obesity, is the most important nutritional problem in the US and an increasing number of countries, because it is a major risk factor for many diseases including type 2 diabetes, coronary heart disease, cancers of the breast, colon, kidney, esophagus, and endometrium, osteoarthritis, cataracts, and many other conditions. Dietary fat has been believed to be an important contributor to overweight because it contains more calories per gram and also it may be more efficiently stored as fat than carbohydrate. However, it is now clear that any differences in metabolic efficiency are not practically important and that the balance of total calories rather than just fat calories are important in weight control *(11)*. Thus, the critical issue is whether the fat composition of the diet influences our ability to control caloric intake, and theories abound why one diet should be better than another. Long-term empirical data are essential, but remarkably sparse. In randomized trials, individuals assigned to low fat diets often tend to loose a few pounds during the first months, but then regain their weight. In randomized trials lasting a year or longer, there has consistently been no greater weight loss with low fat diets *(11,12)*.

5. CARBOHYDRATES

Because adequate caloric intake is essential, a substantial reduction in dietary fat practically implies an increase in carbohydrate. Because of concerns about consumption of "empty calories" from sugar, high intake of "complex carbohydrates," mainly starch in the form of bread, rice, pasta and crackers, formed the base of the 1992 USDA pyramid. However, refined carbohydrates, such as white bread and white rice, are rapidly metabolized to simple sugars and cause a greater rise in blood glucose and insulin levels than grains that have not been milled into fine flour. In addition to producing a rapidly absorbed form of starch, the refining process also removes many vitamins and minerals and fiber. Indeed, potatoes raise blood sugar levels more rapidly than the same amount of calories from table sugar. The rapid rise in blood sugar stimulates insulin release, and a consequent sharp decline in blood sugar, sometimes even going below baseline. These sharp swings in glucose and insulin have deleterious metabolic consequences, raising triglycerides, and lowering HDL. The precipitous decline in glucose can also lead to more hunger after a carbohydrate rich meal, and may contribute to overeating and obesity. Thus, the concept of "complex carbohydrates" is not based on sound physiological principles. A different way to classify carbohydrates is by their propensity to raise blood sugar levels. Foods have a specific glycemic index, reflecting this propensity compared with a standard. The glycemic index depends not only on the chemical composition, but also on the physical form of the food *(13)*. The glycemic load takes into account both the glycemic index of the food, and the amount of carbohydrate. In our large prospective studies, we have found that high intake of starches from refined grains and potatoes (i.e., a high glycemic load) is associated with higher risk of type 2 diabetes and coronary heart disease, and that greater intake of cereal fiber is related to lower risk of these conditions (14,15).

As noted earlier, replacement of dietary fat with carbohydrate creates the adverse metabolic picture of low serum HDL and high triglycerides. Recent evidence also indicates that this adverse metabolic response to carbohydrate is substantially worse among persons who already have a greater degree of insulin resistance, mainly as the result of overweight and inactivity (16–19). This can account for the ability of traditional farmers in Asia and elsewhere, who have been extremely lean and active, to consume large amounts of carbohydrate without experiencing diabetes or heart disease, whereas the same diet in a more sedentary population can have deleterious effects.

6. FRUITS AND VEGETABLES

High intake of fruits and vegetables is perhaps the least controversial aspect of the dietary pyramid, and reduction in cancer risk has been a widely promoted benefit. However, most of the evidence for a cancer benefit has come from case–control studies, in which patients with cancer and selected control subjects are asked about their earlier diets. These retrospective studies are susceptible to numerous biases, and recent findings from large prospective studies have tended to show little relation between overall fruit and vegetable consumption and cancer incidence (20). Although some benefits probably exist for specific components of some fruits and vegetables and risks, the benefit of a general increase in fruit and vegetable consumption has probably been overstated. One component that does seem to be beneficial for reducing risk of colon and possibly other cancers is folic acid, but vitamin supplements and fortified foods are the major source of this vitamin in the US.

Although the benefits of fruits and vegetables for cancer prevention are probably small, substantial evidence from cohort studies indicates that higher intake will reduce risks of cardiovascular disease (20). This benefit is probably due to many constituents, but folic acid and potassium appear to be contributing factors. Inadequate folic acid is also responsible for higher risks of serious birth defects, and low intake of lutein, a pigment in green leafy vegetables, has been associated with greater risks of cataracts and degeneration of the retina. Thus, there are many reasons, besides being a primary source of many vitamins needed for good health, to consume the recommended five servings per day of fruits and vegetables, even if this has little impact on cancer risk. However, the inclusion of potatoes as a vegetable in the USDA pyramid had little justification as they are mainly consumed as a source of starch and do not contribute to the benefits seen for other vegetables. Not surprisingly, we have found that greater intake of potatoes was associated with higher risk of type 2 diabetes (21).

Low carbohydrate diets have been popular for weight control, although the long-term effects on weight are not clear, and concerns have been raised that these diets might increase risks of heart disease because they are often high in saturated fat and cholesterol. However, within the Nurses' Health Study (22) we found that low carbohydrate diets were not associated with risk of coronary heart disease, probably because the reduction in glycemic load balanced the higher intakes of saturated fat and cholesterol. When the sources of fat and protein were mainly from vegetable sources, we found that a reduced carbohydrate intake was associated with a lower risk of heart disease.

7. PROTEIN SOURCES

Although treated equally by the USDA pyramid, the health consequences of consuming red meat, poultry, fish, legumes, nuts, and eggs are quite different. High consumption of red meat has been associated with increased risk of coronary heart disease, probably because of its content of saturated fat and cholesterol, and higher risk of type 2 diabetes and cancers of the colon and possible prostate. The elevated risk of colon cancer does not seem to be due to the fat content of red meat; processed meats may be particularly related to this cancer. In contrast, the fat in poultry and fish is more unsaturated than that in red meat, and fish is an important source of the essential omega-3 fatty acids. Not surprisingly, we have seen that those who replace red meat with chicken and fish have a lower risk of coronary heart disease and colon cancer. Eggs are high in cholesterol, but consumption up to one per day does not appear to have adverse effects on heart disease risk (except among diabetics), probably because the effects of a slightly higher cholesterol level are counter balanced by other nutritional benefits. Many people have avoided nuts because of their high fat content, but the fat in nuts, including peanuts, is mainly unsaturated, and walnuts in particular are a good source of omega-3 fatty acids. In controlled feeding studies, nuts improve blood cholesterol fractions, and in multiple cohort studies those who consume more nuts have lower risks of heart disease. Thus, treating these various sources of proteins as equals fails to provide the public with information needed for healthy choices.

8. DAIRY FOODS

The USDA pyramid promoted high consumption of dairy products, which has usually been justified by their high content of calcium and the prevention of osteoporosis and fractures. Although the highest rates of fractures are found in countries with high dairy food consumption, large prospective studies have consistently not shown a lower risk of fractures among those with high intake of dairy products and thus more studies are needed (23). Calcium is an essential nutrient, but the US adequate intake of calcium for bone health (1,200 mg/day for persons over 50 years of age) has probably been overstated by reliance on short-term studies, whereas British and other EU countries' adequate intakes range between 700 and 800 mg/day. If a person needs more calcium, this can also be obtained at lower cost and without saturated fat or calories by taking a supplement. Several lines of evidence now suggest that low calcium intake can modestly increase risk of colon cancer (24), but most of the benefit of higher intake appears to be achieved by a good overall diet plus the equivalent of about one or two glasses of milk, or one or two portions of dairy products per day, which would correspond approximately to the UK definition of adequate intake of about 700 mg/day.

Higher than the recommended (see below) consumption of dairy products cannot a priori be assumed to be safe and effective because we are only now beginning to have the data to evaluate the consequences of high intake throughout life. In several studies, despite lower risk for colon cancer, men who consume high amounts of calcium or dairy products have experienced increased risk of prostate cancer (25) and in some cohort studies women with high intakes have had higher rates of ovarian cancer. Although fat was initially assumed to be the responsible factor, this has not been supported in more detailed analyses; high calcium intake itself seemed most clearly related to risk of prostate cancer. In contrast, low calcium intake is related to risk for colon cancer. The role of calcium, vitamin D, and dairy products in health and disease is thus an area in need of more research. At the moment, the authors consider it imprudent to recommend more than two servings per day.

9. THE OVERALL IMPACT OF FOLLOWING THE USDA FOOD PYRAMID

With strong support from many elements of the food industry, the USDA food guide pyramid became a highly recognized icon. Many studies have assessed how well its message was adopted by the American public, but few studies have evaluated the health of individuals who followed those guidelines, compared with others. Some benefits seem likely: by decreasing total fat intake consumption of saturated and *trans* fat will be reduced, and fruits and vegetables will be increased. However, the pyramid could also have led people to reduce desirable unsaturated fats and to increase consumption of refined starches, so that the benefits might be counterbalanced by harm.

To evaluate the overall impact of following the Pyramid message, we used the Healthy Eating Index (HEI), a score developed by the USDA, to measure adherence to the Pyramid and its accompanying dietary guidelines in federal nutrition programs. From the data collected in our large cohort studies, we calculated each participant's Healthy Eating Index score and then examined the relation of these scores to subsequent risk of major chronic disease, defined as any heart attack, stroke, cancer, or nontraumatic death from any cause *(25–27)*. In analyses adjusted only for age, women and men with the highest healthy eating index score did experience lower risks of major chronic disease. However, these individuals also smoked less, exercised more, and had generally healthier lifestyles; after adjusting for these variables, participants with the highest HEI scores did not experience significantly better overall health outcomes. This is consistent with a counterbalancing of benefits and harm from following the USDA pyramid, and a lost opportunity to improve health.

10. THE 2005 USDA MYPYRAMID AND AN ALTERNATIVE

Because the scientific evidence had become so discordant with the 1992 Food Guide Pyramid, in 2005 the USDA released a new graphic and corresponding Website called MyPyramid (http://www.mypyramid.gov/). An advantage of this new graphic is that the admonition to avoid dietary fat and eat large amounts of starch is no longer present. However, this new graphic consists of nothing more than colorful bands on a pyramid, and thus provides no dietary guidance at all. This represents a lost educational opportunity, but is consistent with the stated policy perspective of the USDA, which is that there is no such thing as a good for or a bad food, and that all foods can be part of a healthy diet.

Because of the serious deficiencies of the USDA pyramids, we have attempted to develop alternatives derived from the best available evidence. Thus our alternative Healthy Eating Pyramid (Fig. 4) emphasizes weight control, giving attention to calories from all sources, and regular physical activity; healthy fats and healthy forms of carbohydrate; an abundance of fruits and vegetables; healthy sources of protein, which can be consistent with either a vegetarian or omnivore diet; and suggests sparing use of red meat, butter, refined grain products, potatoes, and sugar. *Trans* fat does not appear because it has no

Healthy Eating Pyramid

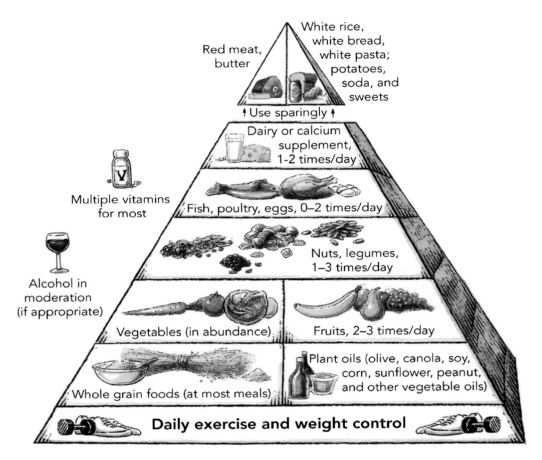

Fig. 4. Healthy eating pyramid.

place in an optimally healthy diet. A multiple vitamin is suggested for most people and moderate alcohol consumption is an option if not contraindicated. Data supporting the cardioprotective effects of moderate alcohol (in any form, wine, beer, or spirits) continues to accumulate. Policy makers are acutely aware of the risks entailed in promoting moderate alcohol consumption, so the pyramid is silent on this issue. Although clearly no alcohol is better than too much, a strong case can be made for including moderate consumption as part of a healthy diet for those without contraindications. One health risk associated with moderate consumption is an increase in breast cancer, but it appears this may be conteracted with adequate folate intake.

To evaluate the overall impact of this alternative approach to food choices on risk of chronic disease, we have created a revised dietary score based on our Healthy Eating pyramid *(28)*. Better adherence to this alternative index of healthy food choice was associated with lower risk of risk of major chronic disease in both men and women, but the benefits were due to reduced risk of cardiovascular disease, not cancer. Avoidance of overweight and regular physical activity, rather than specific food choices, is related to lower risk of many important cancers.

11. FUTURE NEEDS

Much research on the relation of diet to health remains; almost all aspects are in need of additional refinement and many uncertainties exist. Important topics include the role of dairy products, the effects on health of specific fruits and vegetables, the risks and benefits of vitamin supplements, and the effects of all aspects of diet during childhood and early adult life. The interaction of dietary factors with genetic predisposition is a topic of great interest, although its importance remains to be determined.

The amount of ongoing research on diet and health is massive, and this should provide improved and more specific dietary guidance in the future. It will be important to evaluate the validity of this information in relation to long-term health outcomes empirically. An additional challenge will be to convey this information to the public in a way that is strictly based on the best available scientific evidence. Agriculture is by far the largest and most powerful industry in the country, making it difficult for the Department of Agriculture to develop objective nutritional guidelines because of its dual role as an industry advocate and provider of guidance to consumers. Dietary guidance should be developed in a setting that is insulated from political and economic interests.

12. CONCLUSION

A wealth of research from many lines of investigation indicates that dietary choices have an important impact on our long-term health. However, the Department of Agriculture has provided poor guidance to persons seeking to maintain or improve their long-term health. Alternative national guidelines that emphasize healthy forms of carbohydrate, fats, and protein are needed.

REFERENCES

1. Hetzel BS, Charnock JS, Dwyer T, et al. Fall in coronary heart disease mortality in U.S.A. and Australia due to sudden death: evidence for the role of polyunsaturated fat. J Clin Epidemiol 1989;42:885–93.
2. Mensink RP, Katan MB. Effect of dietary fatty acids on serum lipids and lipoproteins: a meta-analysis of 27 trials. Arterioscler Thromb 1992;12:911–9.
3. Mensink RP, Zock PL, Kester AD, et al. Effects of dietary fatty acids and carbohydrates on the ratio of serum total to HDL cholesterol and on serum lipids and apolipoproteins: a meta-analysis of 60 controlled trials. Am J Clin Nutr 2003;77:1146–55.
4. Hu FB, Willett WC. Optimal diets for prevention of coronary heart disease. JAMA 2002;288:2569–78.
5. Mozaffarian D, Katan MB, Ascherio A, Stampfer MJ, et al. Trans fatty acids and cardiovascular disease. N Engl J Med 2006;354:1601–13.
6. Baer DJ, Judd JT, Clevidence BA, et al. Dietary fatty acids affect plasma markers of inflammation in healthy men fed controlled diets: a randomized crossover study. Am J Clin Nutr 2004;79:969–73.
7. Sacks FM, Katan MB. Randomized clinical trials on the effects of dietary fat and carbohydrate on plasma lipoproteins and cardiovascular disease. Am J Med 2002;113 Suppl 9B:13S–24.
8. Hu FB, Stampfer MJ, Manson JE, et al. Dietary fat intake and the risk of coronary heart disease in women. N Eng J Med 1997;337:1491–9.
9. National Research Council (U.S.), Committee on Diet and Health. Diet and health: implications for reducing chronic disease risk. Washington, DC: National Academy Press, 1989.

10. Kim EH, Willett WC, Colditz GA, et al. Dietary fat and risk of postmenopausal breast cancer in a 20-year follow-up. Am J Epidemiol 2006;164:990–7.

11. Willett WC, Leibel RL. Dietary fat is not a major determinant of body fat. Am J Med 2002;113 Suppl 9B:47S–59.

12. Dansinger ML, Gleason JA, Griffith JL, et al. Comparison of the Atkins, Ornish, Weight Watchers, and Zone diets for weight loss and heart disease risk reduction: a randomized trial. JAMA 2005;293:43–53.

13. Ludwig DS. The glycemic index – Physiological mechanisms relating to obesity, diabetes, and cardiovascular disease [Review]. JAMA 2002;287:2414–23.

14. Schulze MB, Liu S, Rimm EB, et al. Glycemic index, glycemic load, and dietary fiber intake and incidence of type 2 diabetes in younger and middle-aged women. Am J Clin Nutr 2004;80:348–56.

15. Liu S, Willett WC, Stampfer MJ, et al. A prospective study of dietary glycemic load, carbohydrate intake, and risk of coronary heart disease in US women. Am J Clin Nutr 2000;71:1455–61.

16. Jeppesen J, Schaaf P, Jones G, et al. Effects of low-fat, high-carbohydrate diets on risk factors for ischemic heart disease in postmenopausal women. Am J Clin Nutr 1997;65:1027–33.

17. Willett WC, Stampfer M, Chu N, et al. Assessment of questionnaire validity for measuring total fat intake using plasma lipid levels as criteria. Am J Epidemiol 2001;154:1107–12.

18. Liu S, Manson JE, Stampfer MJ, et al. Dietary glycemic load assessed by food frequency questionnaire in relation to plasma high-density lipoprotein cholesterol and fasting triglycerides among postmenopausal women. Am J Clin Nutr 2001;73:560–6.

19. Oh K, Hu FB, Cho E, et al. Carbohydrate intake, glycemic index, glycemic load, and dietary fiber in relation to risk of stroke in women. Am J Epidemiol 2005;161:161–9.

20. Hung HC, Joshipura KJ, Jiang R, et al. Fruit and vegetable intake and risk of major chronic disease. J Natl Cancer Inst 2004;96:1577–84.

21. Halton TL, Willett WC, Liu S, et al. Potato and french fry consumption and risk of type 2 diabetes in women. Am J Clin Nutr 2006;83:284–90.

22. Halton TL, Willett WC, Liu S, et al. Low-carbohydrate-diet score and the risk of coronary heart disease in women. N Engl J Med 2006;355:1991–2002.

23. Hegsted DM. Calcium and osteoporosis. J Nutr 1986;116:2316–19.

24. Cho E, Smith-Warner S, Spiegelman D, et al. Dairy foods and calcium and colorectal cancer: a pooled analysis of 10 cohort studies. J Natl Cancer Inst 2004; 96:1015–22

25. Giovannucci E, Liu Y, Stampfer MJ, et al. A prospective study of calcium intake and incident and fatal prostate cancer. Cancer Epidemiol Biomarkers Prev 2006;15:203–10.

26. McCullough ML, Feskanich D, Rimm EB, et al. Adherence to the Dietary Guidelines for Americans and risk of major chronic disease in men. Am J Clin Nutr 2000;72:1223–31.

27. McCullough ML, Feskanich D, Stampfer MJ, et al. Adherence to the Dietary Guidelines for Americans and risk of major chronic disease in women. Am J Clin Nutr 2000;72:1214–22.

28. McCullough ML, Feskanich D, Stampfer MJ, et al. Diet quality and major chronic disease risk in men and women: moving toward improved dietary guidance. Am J Clin Nutr 2002;76:1261–71.

12 Nutrition Recommendations and Interventions for Subjects with Cardiovascular Disease

Meropi Kontogianni, Mary Yannakoulia, Lauren Kuhn, Sunali Shah, Kristina Day, and Christos S. Mantzoros

KEY POINTS

- Diet influences cardiovascular health through a number of mechanisms.
- Nutrition recommendations are of major importance both in primary and secondary prevention of cardiovascular disease (CVD).
- A great body of research has examined the role of specific nutrients, including fat, carbohydrates, fiber, and alcohol, in reducing CVD risk.
- More recently the focus has shifted to the effect of food groups, such as fruits and vegetables, whole grains, and nuts and dairy products, and favorable dietary patterns that combine a variety of nutrients. In this perspective, a "prudent" dietary pattern, characterized by high intakes of fruits, vegetables, legumes, fish, poultry and wholegrain cereals, has been associated with significantly lower risks for CVD factors.
- Mediterranean dietary patterns, as well as the DASH (Dietary Approaches to Stop Hypertension) pattern, have been proven to exert significant cardioprotective effects in secondary prevention of CVD.
- Achieving and maintaining a healthy body weight change (as an initial goal to reduce body weight by ~10% from baseline), an active lifestyle (a minimum of 30 min of physical activity for most days of the week), and a balanced diet constitute the goals of the intensive counseling recommended for individuals with CVD.
- Effective interventions should combine nutrition education with behavior-oriented counseling to help patients acquire the skills, motivation, and support needed to alter their lifestyle patterns.

Key Words: Cardiovascular disease, Nutrition, Mediterranean diet, DASH diet

From: *Nutrition and Health: Nutrition and Metabolism*
Edited by: C.S. Mantzoros, DOI: 10.1007/978-1-60327-453-1_12,
© Humana Press, a part of Springer Science + Business Media, LLC 2009

1. INTRODUCTION: PREVENTION

Industrial and technological revolutions have resulted in dramatic shifts in the prevalence of several diseases over the last decades. Cardiovascular disease (CVD), in particular, has emerged as the dominant chronic disease in many parts of the world. Diet, tobacco smoking, physical inactivity, obesity, as well as hyperlipidemia, hypertension, and diabetes mellitus have contributed to the increasing morbidity and mortality from CVD. Thus, appropriate alterations of lifestyle and nutritional practices are of major importance in primary prevention of CVD. What a person routinely eats appears to play a central role in his or her long-term risk of CVD. Although much of the focus from the 1950s to the 1990s was on the contribution the diet made to blood levels of total cholesterol or low-density lipoprotein cholesterol (LDL-C), it has now been realized that this relationship is only one aspect of the diet's role in contributing to CVD risk. Diet is thought to influence coronary heart disease through a number of mechanisms, including abnormal lipid levels, raised blood pressure, thrombotic tendency, endothelial dysfunction, systemic inflammation, insulin resistance, altered cardiac rhythm, and elevated oxidative stress *(1)*.

Substantial research has examined the role of diet on CVD risk in terms of nutrients, food groups, or dietary patterns. On the one hand, nutrients including saturated fatty acids, *trans* fatty acids, and sodium have been proven to most significantly heighten CVD risk, resulting in detrimental increases in blood cholesterol levels and blood pressure. On the other hand, there are numerous beneficial nutrients including dietary fiber, various antioxidants (e.g., vitamins A, C and E), B vitamins (B_6, B_{12}, and niacin), folic acid, omega-3 fatty acids, monounsaturated fatty acids, calcium, and potassium. Food groups such as fruits, vegetables, low fat dairy products, nuts, whole-grain cereals, fatty fish, and olive oil have been linked to reduced CVD risk in many epidemiological studies *(2)*. Finally, studies examining the effect of the overall diet on CVD risk have revealed that adherence to a "prudent" dietary pattern (characterized by higher intake of fruits, vegetables, legumes, whole grains, poultry, and fish), to a DASH-style diet, or to the

Table 1
Major Dietary Recommendations for CVD Risk Prevention

Aim for balance between calorie intake and physical activity to achieve or maintain a
    healthy body weight. For overweight or obese subjects, a weight reduction program
    should be initiated
A wide variety of food items should be eaten
Consumption of a diet rich in vegetables and fruits, wholegrain cereals, and bread is
    recommended
Consumption of fish, especially oily fish, at least twice a week, lean meat and low fat dairy
    products should be emphasized
Limit saturated (animal) fat and partially hydrogenated fat intake by preferring the above-
    mentioned foods, as well as monounsaturated and polyunsaturated fats from vegetable
    and marine sources. Saturated fat should not exceed 10% of daily caloric intake
Reduction in beverage intake and in foods with added sugars is desirable
Foods should be prepared with little or no salt. Emphasis needs to be placed on fresh or fro-
    zen unsalted foods. Many processed and prepared foods, including bread are rich in salt
In case of habitual alcohol consumption, this should be done in moderation

traditional Mediterranean diet is associated with a lower risk of coronary heart disease and stroke and with greater life expectancy, independent of other lifestyle factors *(3–5)*. It should be noted, however, that evidence deriving from observational epidemiology studies has not always been confirmed by interventional trials.

According to the guidelines of the American Heart Association and the European Society of Cardiology, dietary changes constitute an integral part of cardiovascular risk management *(2,6)*. All individuals at high risk for CVD should be given professional and individualized advice on the food options that best reduce cardiovascular risk. A varied and energy-balanced regimen, together with regular exercise, is of critical importance for the preservation of cardiovascular health (Table 1). Moreover, intentional weight loss in obese patients can improve or prevent many of the obesity-related risk factors for CVD. It is now clear that body fat, and in particular intraabdominal visceral fat, is a metabolically active endocrine organ that is capable of synthesizing and releasing into the bloodstream an important array of peptide and non-peptide compounds that may play a role in cardiovascular homeostasis.

2. ASSESSMENT

The assessment and subsequent treatment of CVD begins with the identification of risk factors, particularly those that are nutrition-related. Careful and detailed assessment of nutritional status should focus on potential risk factors including diabetes, overweight/obesity, hypertension, and prothrombotic or proinflammatory states including elevated homocysteine levels, and should consider food choices, physical activity levels, and patients' readiness to change their habits toward a healthier pattern. Overweight is classified as a body mass index (BMI) of 25.0–29.9 kg/m^2. Class 1 obesity refers to a BMI of 30.0–34.9, class 2 obesity to a BMI of 35.0–39.9, and class 3, or extreme obesity, to a BMI of >40 kg/m^2*(7)*. A BMI of >30 kg/m^2 or >27 kg/m^2, along with comorbidities, calls for immediate initiation of weight management including pharmacological therapy. Weight management with life style modifications should also be considered for those subjects with BMI $\geq$ 25 kg/m^2. Moreover, the association between both increased waist circumference (WC) or waist to hip ratio (WHR) and greater risk of CVD development has been demonstrated in both cohort and case-control studies. Evidence from these sources shows WC to be a better marker of intraabdominal fat content than WHR. In the context of cardiovascular health, WC is shown to be an extremely useful marker of risk. Unlike BMI alone, WC is able to reflect visceral fat accumulation, which is associated with increased CVD risk and related metabolic risks to a greater extent than simply subcutaneous body fat alone. Larger WCs (>40 in. for men and > 35 in. for women) are closely linked to insulin resistance, sleep apnea, and inflammation, which are parti-cularly dangerous for the patient with coronary heart disease (CHD) *(7)*. Nutritional risk factors such as high intake of saturated fatty acids (SFA), trans fatty acids (TFA), cholesterol, and sodium as well as low intake of protective foods such as soluble fiber, fatty acids (including omega-3, or n-3) and a variety of fruits and vegetables should be thoroughly assessed through detailed diet histories *(1)*.

3. GOALS OF NUTRITION INTERVENTION

There is a wide variety of lifestyle and pharmacological treatments available for the prevention and treatment of CHD. The combination of nutrition management and behavioral modification with appropriate pharmacotherapy has been shown to be the

Table 2
Dietary Recommendations for Achieving Desirable Blood Lipid Profile and Especially LDL-C Levels *(8)*

Limit food items high in saturated fats

Replace saturated fats with lower-fat foods

Increase consumption of food items with unsaturated fat

Carefully monitor intake of food items high in cholesterol

Severely limit food items containing *trans* fatty acids

Increase food items rich in viscous fiber

Increase food items containing stanol/sterol esters (special margarines, fortified orange juice, special cocoa/chocolate bars)

In case of hypetriglyceridemia:

Limit dietary fat intake between 25 and 35% of total daily calories, as well as simple sugars and rapidly hydrolyzed starches, which have a greater glycemic effect than more complex carbohydrates

Limit excessive alcohol intake, which has a detrimental effect on triglycerides levels

There is accumulating evidence to support the beneficial influence of omega-3 fatty acids in the management of hypertriglyceridemia either through diet or supplements, but very high doses may be needed (see relevant chapter on pharmacotherapy)

Table 3
Therapeutic Lifestyle Changes for Patients with Already Established CVD *(9)*

Nutrient	Recommended Intake as percent of total calories
Total fat[a]	25–35%
Saturated fat	Less than 7%
Polyunsaturated fat	Up to 10%
Monounsaturated fat	Up to 20%
Carbohydrates[b]	50–60% of total calories
Protein[c]	~15%
Cholesterol	Less than 200 mg/day
Plant stanols/sterols	2 g/day
Increased soluble fiber	10–25 g/day
Total calories	Balance energy intake and expenditure to maintain desirable body weight and to prevent weight gain
Physical activity	Include enough moderate exercise to expend at least 200 kcal/day

[a]The 25–35% fat recommendation allows for increased intake of unsaturated fat in place of carbohydrates in people with the metabolic syndrome or diabetes.
[b]Carbohydrates should come mainly from foods rich in complex carbohydrates. These include grains (especially whole grains), fruits, and vegetables.
[c]Soy protein may be used as a replacement for some animal products.

most effective method of treatment. For patients with already-established CHD or dyslipidemia, it is recommended that dietary and lifestyle changes are made first, and pharmacologic treatment is added as needed *(8,9)*. Tables 2 and 3 summarize the dietary recommendations for patients with hyperlipidemia and already-established CHD, respectively. Pharmacotherapy is beyond the scope of this Chapter.

Dietary intervention by a registered dietitian, usually over the course of two to six sessions, has been shown to be most effective at helping patients achieve these goals. Nutrition therapy provided by a registered dietitian over a period of 6 weeks to 6 months can result in substantial changes in dietary habits. The first visit length is usually 45–90 min and subsequent visits should last between 30 and 60 min.

4. NUTRIENTS AND CVD

4.1. Fat

Reducing the total amount of fat in the diet has long been a method for decreasing the risk of CHD. Early studies also suggested that the type of fat might be more important than the total amount of fat in the diet. Two secondary prevention trials testing total fat reduction failed to find a significant reduction in serum cholesterol or CHD events *(10,11)*. Data from the largest analysis done in this area indicate that types of fats may play a more important role in CHD risk than total fat intake. The Nurses' Health Study revealed that higher intakes of TFA and, to a smaller extent SFA, are associated with increased risk. In contrast, higher intakes of nonhydrogenated polyunsaturated (PUFA) and monounsaturated fatty acids (MUFA) correlate with decreased risk *(12)*.

As shown in Table 3, total fat intake can cover up to 35% of total daily calories, as long as it comes mainly from MUFA. SFA should be limited to <7% of energy, TFA to <1% of energy, and dietary cholesterol to <200 mg/day. Evidence for the benefits of lowering dietary SFA was provided by the Seven Countries Study *(13)* in which regional differences in death from CHD were strongly correlated with SFA intake. Many population studies have since then provided evidence of associations between diets high in SFA and increased total cholesterol and LDL-C levels, as well as increased risk of both CHD and CVD *(14)*. When SFA were replaced by unsaturated fats, total plasma cholesterol was lowered *(15)*. Moreover, substituting PUFA for SFA does appear to be beneficial in lowering serum cholesterol and reducing cardiovascular mortality, as demonstrated by the Finnish Mental hospital Study, the Los Angeles Veteran Study, the Oslo Diet-Heart Study, and the MRC study *(1)*.

A recent study, known as The Omniheart Randomized Trial, evaluated the effects of three reduced SFA and dietary cholesterol diets that varied only in macronutrient content *(16)*. All three of the diets provided 6% of energy from SFA. Both the carbohydrate-rich and protein-rich diets provided 27% energy from total fat, although the content of the carbohydrate and protein varied. The carbohydrate-rich diet consisted of 58% from carbohydrate, whereas the protein-rich diet provided 25% of energy from protein. The third diet, the unsaturated fatty acid-rich diet, was higher in fat, providing 37% of energy from total fat (21% of which was MUFA). Both the protein and the unsaturated fatty acids-rich diet improved triglyceride levels statistically. The unsaturated fatty acids diet also improved high-density lipoprotein cholesterol (HDL-C) levels. These results suggest that partial substitution of carbohydrate for protein or unsaturated fatty acids

can favorably affect both blood triglycerides and HDL-C. Data from the Nurses Health
Study also suggest that the highest (5.7 g/day) vs. the lowest (2.4 g/day) quintile of TFA
intake is associated with an increase in CHD risk *(17)*. Other studies continue to emerge
that further bolster the argument to avoid *trans* fatty acids *(14)*.

The most commonly occurring MUFA in the diet is oleic acid (C18:1), which is abundant in olive and canola oils as well as in nuts. There has been continued debate over the
past several years on whether MUFA or PUFA should replace SFA in the diet. The early
metabolic studies by Mattson and Grundy *(18)* revealed that MUFA lowered LDL-C concentrations with no effect on HDL-C levels, whereas PUFA lowered both LDL-C and HDL-C
levels. Subsequent studies, even including metaanalyses, have suggested that the effects
of MUFA and PUFA on plasma lipoprotein profiles are similar *(15)*. Moreover, dietary fat
may influence the risk of CHD by altering the susceptibility of lipoproteins to oxidation.
Previous work has shown that, in the test tube, LDL-C particles enriched in MUFA are less
susceptible to oxidation than particles enriched in n-6 PUFA *(19)*. These results have also
been supported by a study that examined the oxidation of LDL-C from subjects consuming
diets enriched in olive oil (MUFA), rapeseed oil (MUFA plus n-3 PUFA), or sunflower
oil (n-6 PUFA) *(20)*. LDL-C oxidation was lowest in the olive oil group, intermediate in
the rapeseed oil group, and highest in the sunflower oil group. This indicated that MUFA
reduced LDL-C oxidation compared with n-6 PUFA. Also, when comparing MUFA and
PUFA, it may be important to distinguish between n-6 and n-3 PUFA. The potential health
benefits of n-3 PUFA are being presented in the supplements section.

Finally, epidemiological evidence and intervention studies clearly show that in humans
SFA significantly worsen insulin-resistance, while MUFA and PUFA improve it through
modifications of the composition of cell membranes. Shifting from SFA to MUFA intake can also affect blood pressure significantly, especially by reducing diastolic blood
pressure *(21)*.

Therefore, on the basis of current evidence, emanating mainly from observational
studies, patients should be encouraged to focus on replacing the main sources of SFA and
TFA. SFA are generally found in animal fats in foods such as meat and dairy. TFA are
generally produced by hydrogenation of vegetable oils and found in food items such as
bakery goods or fried foods. These foods should be replaced with foods high in MUFA
and PUFA, such as olive oil, nuts, seeds, and fish.

4.2. Protein

Protein does not directly affect serum LDL-C levels or other lipid profile components. By encouraging patients to replace some of their animal protein sources with
plant-based protein sources however, dietitians can indirectly address intake of total
dietary fat, particularly in the form of saturated fat. Plant sources of protein include
vegetables, legumes, whole-grains, and nuts. In addition, patients should be educated on
correct portion sizes of protein rich foods.

4.2.1. SOY PROTEIN

Epidemiological evidence from human subjects suggests that high soybean consumption, the main dietary source of isoflavones, may be cardioprotective. Existing data suggest that soybean food and soybean protein interventions may have a beneficial effect on

certain aspects of the lipoprotein profile, while there is limited data to support a lipid-lowering effect of isoflavone extracts. Available evidence in this area remains minimal however, and, at this time, the only potential link that has been suggested is between soy consumption and lowered LDL-C. No data have shown substantial benefits of soy protein consumption on HDL-C, total cholesterol, triglycerides, or lipoprotein(a). Data from in vitro and animal experiments are currently emerging and suggest that isoflavones may be cardioprotective by mechanisms independent of blood lipids, but these underlying mechanisms remain only partly understood. As a result, more recent research efforts have focused on the potential effects of phyto-oestrogens on blood pressure, in vivo measures of vascular function, such as flow-mediated dilation and novel biomarkers of CHD risk (i.e., inflammatory factors, coagulation, and fibrinolytic factors as well as markers of LDL-C oxidation). To date these studies have not been systematically reviewed. Data from human studies on the effects of soybean foods and soybean protein on blood pressure are equivocal, but it is clear that there is no evidence for an effect of isoflavone extracts on blood pressure. Moreover, although there is growing interest in the potential direct effects of isoflavones on the arterial wall, the available data from human studies are inconclusive (22).

Consumers should be advised that, although FDA issued a health claim in 1999 stating that 25 g/day soy protein was associated with reduced risk of CHD, the current body of research in this area does not appear to fully support this claim. Soy products such as tofu, soy butter, soy nuts, or some soy burgers may be beneficial to cardiovascular and overall health because of their high content of PUFA, fiber, vitamins, and minerals and low content of SFA. Therefore, using these and other soy foods to replace foods high in animal protein that contain saturated fat and cholesterol may confer benefits to cardiovascular health (23).

4.3. Carbohydrates

The relationship of carbohydrate dietary intake with CHD appears to be mediated by several, mainly indirect, mechanisms: contribution to total energy intake and effect on overweight and obesity, influence on central obesity, effects on plasma lipids (especially triglycerides), and effects on glycemic control. The balance between carbohydrates and fat as sources of energy as well as the fiber component of the diet are also areas of interest. In feeding experiments, an increase in dietary energy from carbohydrates is usually associated with a moderate increase in fasting plasma triglyceride levels in the first few weeks, but these return to near baseline levels in the following weeks (24).

The effect of a high-carbohydrate diet on HDL-C and thereby on the total to HDL cholesterol ratio, as well as on the particle size of LDL-C, are matters of scientific interest as is the influence on vascular function and subsequent risk of CHD. Diets high in carbohydrates appear to reduce HDL-C levels and increase the fraction of small dense LDL-C, both of which may adversely impact vascular disease. This dyslipidemic pattern is consistent with the elevation of plasma triglycerides. Currently, there is no clear evidence that the risk of CHD is independently altered by carbohydrate levels in the diet (25). On the contrary, postprandial hyperglycemia is increasingly recognized as an independent risk factor for cardiovascular disease. Glycemic "spikes" may adversely affect vascular structure and function via multiple mechanisms, including (acutely and/or chronically) oxidative stress, inflammation, low-density lipoprotein oxidation, protein glycation, and procoagulant activity. The glycemic index of foods might also be a determinant of the extent to which carbohydrates can influence the glycemic status. Low glycemic index diets in hyperlipidemic and type 2 diabetic subjects have been associated with significant reductions in LDL-C and triglycerides with no effect on HDL-C levels *(26,27)*.

In attempting to follow a low-fat diet, many patients erroneously substitute carbohydrates for SFA. Although this does generally reduce overall caloric intake, it does not effectively reduce cardiovascular risk. In fact, it can even exacerbate related metabolic risk factors, including insulin resistance, unless careful choices of low glycemic index foods are made.

4.4. Fiber

A diet that provides 25–30 g (or 10–13 g/1,000 Kcal) of total dietary fiber, including at least 7–13 g of soluble fiber, is a well tolerated and effective way to decrease lipid levels and CHD risk *(14)*. Foods rich in soluble fiber include oatmeal, oat bran, barley, fruits with skins intact, eggplant, Brussels sprouts, and ground flaxseed. Moreover, beans and legumes (such as black-eyed, soy, and kidney beans) are particularly good sources of fiber. Soluble fiber binds to LDL-C and carries it out of the body, improving the patient's overall lipid profile.

High fiber diets are also associated with other health benefits including improved glycemic control and reduced body weight due to increased satiety. Patients must be educated in reading food labels in order to better identify truly whole grains. The first ingredient reported on the labels must be a whole grain such as wheat, oats, or barley. Likewise, breads must list the first ingredient as "whole grain flour."

4.5. Alcohol

Several studies indicate that moderate drinking is associated with a decreased risk of CHD *(28)* but the exact mechanisms underlying risk reduction due to moderate alcohol consumption remain largely unknown. The beneficial effects of alcohol could be due to an increase in HDL-C cholesterol and apo A-1 and/or a modest improvement in hemostatic factors *(29)*. Alcohol may also be associated with lower LDL-C levels, but it is unclear whether this is independent of other dietary factors. A subset of heavier drinkers demonstrates a substantial increase in triglyceride levels, but this is infrequently seen with light/moderate drinking. Moreover, antithrombotic actions of alcohol could partially account for the lower CHD risk at very light drinking levels (e.g., several drinks per week) observed in several epidemiologic studies. During the last few years, both epidemiological and experimental studies have supported the hypothesis that, in addition to ethanol, certain substances in wine (especially red wine) have cardioprotective effects. The best studied of these substances are polyphenols, categorized as flavonoids [mainly flavonols (quercetin and myricetin), flavanols or flavan-3-ols (catechin and epicatechin), and the anthocyannins] and nonflavonoids [including the stilbenes (resveratrol), hydroxynnamates (caffeic, caftaric, and coutaric acids), and the hydroxybenzoates] *(30)*. Data suggest that ingestion of grape flavonoids is followed by a reduction in platelet activation *(31)*, inflammation and low-density lipoprotein oxidation *(32)*, improvement of endothelial function due to induction of nitric oxide release with the subsequent effect of vasorelaxation *(33)* and elevation in HDL-C levels *(34)*, but these data need to be confirmed and expanded.

It has been observed that the lipimic profile differs, among drinkers of different spirits, with wine drinkers having the most favorable CHD risk profile. Differences in drinking patterns among subjects consuming different beverage types could also play a role in terms of their effects on CHD risk factors. The question of whether the different risks and benefits associated with the different types of alcoholic beverages – beer, wine, and spirits – is still unresolved, but it seems likely that ethyl alcohol is one of the major factors lowering CHD risk *(35)*.

It has been shown in both the US National Alcohol Survey and a Finnish study that light to moderate drinkers who experienced occasional bouts of heavy drinking had a significantly higher mortality rate compared with those who had the same average intake *(36,37)*. A recent large study from Denmark also showed that, for the same average intake, binge drinkers had a higher all-cause mortality than steady drinkers *(38)*. Moreover, in a study of 11,511 cases of acute myocardial infarction or fatal CHD and 6,077 controls in New South Wales, Australia, it was shown that individuals who had a steady small intake of alcohol had lower odds for fatal CHD while those who had the same average intake, but consumed their alcohol once or twice per week, did not *(39)*. In the Health Professionals study, Mukamal et al. recently showed that cardioprotection seemed to be more strongly related to the frequency of intake rather than to the amount of alcohol ingested *(40)*. This study has very recently been followed by a more detailed description of the mediators of the effect of drinking pattern, namely HDL-C, hemoglobin A1c and fibrinogen, as responsible for 75–100% of the association observed *(41)*. In conclusion, these findings strongly suggest that drinking pattern – steady vs. binge drinking – plays a role in the apparent cardioprotective effect of alcohol. Finally, recent reports suggest that drinking during a meal, in a true Mediterranean diet pattern, is beneficial for both CHD and hypertension, while alcohol taken in between meals does not show any substantial benefit *(42,43)*.

Moderate drinking is defined as no more than one drink per day for women and no more than two drinks per day for men, ideally consumed with meals. A 12-ounce bottle of beer, a 4-ounce glass of wine, and a 1½ shot of 80-proof spirits all contain the same amount of alcohol (one half ounce) *(2)*. People who do not habitually consume alcohol are not advised to incorporate alcoholic drinks into their diets in order to reduce their CHD risk, and individuals who consume alcohol are advised to do so in moderation, as heavy consumption is associated with an increase in the prevalence of the metabolic syndrome, type 2 diabetes mellitus, stroke, peripheral arterial disease, and overall CHD *(44)*. It is also important for patients to remember to limit their intake of alcohol within a reasonable range to prevent weight gain, as alcohol supplies calories with limited nutritional benefits.

5. FOOD GROUPS AND CVD

5.1. Fruits and Vegetables

Although there has been a consensus that fruits and vegetables should be considered as cornerstones in a heart healthy diet, it is only recently that solid epidemiological evidence has linked these two food groups together. The largest relevant study has reported a significant inverse association between consumption of fruits and vegetables, particularly green leafy vegetables and vitamin C-rich fruits and vegetables, and risk of

CHD *(45)*. Every single serving per day of fruits and vegetables was associated with a 4% decrease in CHD risk. It is still unclear whether the fruits and vegetables themselves have cardioprotective features, or whether they simply displace from the diet other foods with harmful properties. Two examples of diet patterns that are consistent with the AHA guideline to increase fruits and vegetables are the DASH Diet and the TLC (Therapeutic Lifestyle Changes) Diet. Both recommend consumption of at least 8–10 servings of fruits and vegetables combined per day *(2)*. However, the biologic mechanisms whereby fruits and vegetables may exert their beneficial effects are not entirely clear and are likely to be numerous. Several nutrients and phytochemicals, including fiber, potassium, folate, lycopene, and polyphenols, could be independently or jointly responsible for the apparent reduction in CHD risk. Functional aspects of fruits and vegetables, such as their low dietary glycemic load and low energy density, may also play a significant role. Moreover, fruit and vegetable consumption has been positively associated with total adiponectin levels, an adipocytokine that has been shown to improve insulin action as well as glucose and lipid metabolism *(46)*. Additionally, consumption of fruits has been positively associated with high molecular weight adiponectin, the fraction of adiponectin that has been proposed to be more closely associated with insulin resistance and the presence of metabolic syndrome *(47)*. Although it is important to continue our quest for mechanistic insights, given the great potential shown in epidemiology studies, increased fruit and vegetable intake is recommended *(48)*. A variety of deep colored fruits and vegetables is recommended because of their high micronutrient content. Moreover, due to their significant nutrient density and fiber content, fruits and vegetables at the commencement and in between meals may play a role in inducing satiety, which would in turn reduce calorie intake and promote weight loss.

5.2. Whole Grains

Several epidemiological studies have reported that whole-grain intake is protective against CVD, diabetes, and obesity. Whole grains are concentrated sources of dietary fiber, resistant starch, and oligosaccharides, i.e. carbohydrates that escape digestion in the small intestine and are fermented in the gut, producing short chain fatty acids. Short-chain fatty acids lower colonic pH, serve as an energy source for the colonocytes, and may alter blood lipids. Moreover, whole grains are rich in antioxidants, including trace minerals and phenolic compounds, which have been linked to disease prevention. Finally, whole grains mediate insulin and glucose responses and also contain many other compounds, such as phytates, phyto-oestrogens (e.g., lignans), plant sterols/stanols, vitamins, and minerals that may protect against chronic diseases *(49)*. Recently, intake of whole grains has been associated with higher adiponectin levels. In a cross-sectional study of 220 apparently healthy adult Mediterranean women, it has been shown that adherence to a dietary pattern characterized by high intake of whole-grain cereals and low-fat dairy products, as well as low intake of refined cereals, was significantly and positively associated with adiponectin levels after controlling for potential confounders *(50)*. Moreover, intake of whole grains was associated with a reduced incidence of fatal and nonfatal CHD in many large prospective population studies *(51)*. These studies suggest a 20–30% reduced risk of CHD in persons with a daily intake of ≥3 servings of whole-grain food items.

Several RCTs examining the effect of whole grain consumption on CHD risk factors, such as blood lipids, hypertension, and insulin resistance, as well as on body weight and inflammatory markers, are currently in progress. Current guidelines for whole grain intake emanate mainly from epidemiological studies that cannot prove causality. The recommended amount of grain servings per day is 6–8 and the AHA recommends that at least half of these should come from whole grain sources (2). Servings size examples include one slice of wholemeal bread, 1 oz dry wholegrain cereal, and half cup cooked brown rice, wholegrain pasta or cereal.

5.3. Nuts

Nuts, which are naturally high in MUFA and PUFA, have been associated with LDL-C lowering effects and an overall improvement in lipid profiles (52). The species studied so far include walnuts, almonds, legume peanuts, macadamia nuts, pecans, and pistachio nuts. Collectively, clinical studies indicate that inclusion of nuts in a lipid-lowering diet has favorable effects, especially on LDL-C levels; however, existing studies do not provide unequivocal evidence of an additive effect of nuts to the effects of a low SFA diet per se. The fatty acid profile of nuts (high in unsaturated fatty acids and low in saturated fatty acids) lowers blood cholesterol by altering the fatty acid composition of the diet as a whole. Nuts are also a rich source of dietary fiber and micronutrients, such as phytosterols, arginine, potassium, copper, magnesium, selenium, and vitamin E (25). Frequent nut and seed consumption has been associated with lower levels of inflammatory markers (namely C-reactive protein and interleukin-6), lower levels of fibrinogen, and lower blood pressure (provided that they are unsalted) (53,54).

It must, however, be recognized that the high-fat content of nuts makes them high in calories too. Advice to include nuts in the diet must be tempered in accordance with the desired energy balance. Although further research is needed to characterize the independent protective effects of these food items against CHD and to identify the mechanisms of such protection, available evidence suggests that nuts should be recommended as part of an energy appropriate healthy diet, which is intended to reduce the risk of CHD. Federal guidelines recommend nut consumption in ¼ cup daily or up to 5 oz per week (55). Patients should be encouraged to focus on isocalorically substituting nuts for other foods in their diet to prevent excess calorie intake and subsequent weight gain.

5.4. Dairy Products

Dairy products, especially milk, have been considered as potential promoters of CHD because they are sources of cholesterol and SFA but the short-chain fatty acids and the long-chain stearic acid, which do not adversely affect cholesterol levels, are considerable parts of the SFA in milk fat. Milk intake is probably positively related to blood lipid levels, but the effect shown in many studies is either trivial or absent. In fact, milk supplementation led to a decrease in blood lipids in some studies, and it has also been suggested that milk and milk products may contain antiatherogenic bioactive substances to negate the effects of SFA and cholesterol (56). There is also growing evidence supporting a protective role of dairy consumption (especially low-fat); for example an inverse relationship has been observed between consumption of dairy products and the odds of having acute coronary syndrome (57). A dietary pattern that highlights the possible protective role of low-fat dairy products is the DASH diet. The DASH dietary pattern emphasizes fruits, vegetables, and low-fat dairy products and is reduced in saturated and total fats and cholesterol. This diet has been shown to lower blood pressure in men and women, those with or without hypertension, those who are young or old, and in African Americans and non-African Americans (58).

Calcium, bioactive peptides, and several as of yet unidentified components in whole milk may protect from hypertension. Folic acid, vitamins B_6 and B_{12} as well as other components may contribute to low homocysteine levels, while conjugated linoleic acid may have hypolipidemic and antioxidative (and thus antiatherogenic) effects (59). Additionally, hypocholesterolemic or hypotensive properties have been attributed to fermented dairy products (e.g., yogurt), although the existing data do not allow for definitive conclusions. It has also been proposed that different bacterial strains in fermented milk products have different cholesterol-reducing properties. Still, apparently a necessary condition is that the bacteria, called probiotic bacteria, are able to survive the gut and colonize the intestine (60). These data need to be confirmed by future studies.

6. WHOLE DIET APPROACH AND CVD

Although much of the research to date has focused on individual nutrients and their effect on CHD, broader research is now investigating the impact of diet as a whole. People consume meals consisting of several food items containing a broad combination of nutrients. Therefore, complicated or cumulative intercorrelations and interactions between nutrients and food groups should be studied. Rather than assessing single nutrients, foods, or food groups, it has been suggested that a holistic dietary approach, which examines the effect of dietary patterns in terms of chronic disease prevention and treatment, may be a more valuable approach to evaluate associations between diet and biological markers and/or disease outcomes (3).

6.1. "Prudent" vs. "Western" Dietary Patterns

The methodology for defining dietary patterns consists of three main approaches: analysis of dietary indices, cluster analysis, and factor analysis. The last two approaches often reveal a "prudent" dietary pattern, mainly characterized by higher intakes of fruits, vegetables, legumes, fish, poultry, and whole grains, and a "Western" dietary pattern, characterized by higher intakes of red and processed meats, sweets/desserts, French fries, and refined grains. Adherence to the "prudent" dietary pattern has been associated with significantly lower relative risks for CHD after adjustment for several factors known to affect CHD risk in men. Those at the highest quintile of adherence showed a 30% lower risk (61). The respective effect in women was 24% lower relative risk for CHD (62). Moreover, in the Health Professionals Follow-up Study, significant positive correlations between a "Western" dietary pattern and blood insulin, C-peptide, leptin, and homocysteine concentrations were observed. An inverse correlation with plasma folate concentrations was also noted. The "prudent" dietary pattern was positively correlated with plasma folate and inversely correlated with insulin and homocysteine concentrations (63). Adherence to the "prudent" pattern has also been inversely associated with plasma concentrations of CRP and E-selectin, after adjustment for age, body mass index, physical activity, smoking status, and alcohol consumption (64), as well as with lower risk for type II diabetes both in women (65) and men (66), with enhanced insulin sensitivity (67) and with stroke prevention (68).

6.2. Mediterranean Diet

The term "Mediterranean diet" has been widely used to describe the traditional dietary habits of people in Crete, South Italy, and other Mediterranean countries during the 1960s. It is schematically depicted as a food pyramid. This dietary pattern is characterized by plentiful plant foods (fruits, vegetables, breads, other forms of cereals, beans, nuts, and seeds), olive oil as the principal source of fat, moderate amounts of dairy products (mainly cheese and yogurt), low to moderate amounts of fish and poultry, red meat in low amounts and wine consumed in low to moderate quantities, usually with meals *(69)*. There are several beneficial nutrients that are abundant in the Mediterranean diet, such as MUFA, a balanced ratio of omega-6/omega-3 essential fatty acids, high amounts of fiber, antioxidants such as vitamins E and C, resveratrol, polyphenols, selenium, glutathione, and many others that are currently under investigation.

In a recent systematic review, Serra-Majem et al. reviewed and analyzed the experimental studies on Mediterranean diet and disease prevention *(70)*. Most of the clinical trials exploring the effect of Mediterranean diet on lipids levels found reductions in total and low-density lipoprotein cholesterol (LDL-C), triglycerides, apolipoprotein B, and very-low-density lipoprotein cholesterol, and an increase in HDL cholesterol. A decrease in the number of small LDL-C particles has also been observed in some studies. Endothelial function improved with the adoption of the Mediterranean diet, and endothelial dependent vasodilatation was increased by adding nuts to the Mediterranean diet. Insulin resistance and metabolic syndrome were reduced after shifting to a Mediterranean diet, but some studies showed no effects on insulin or glucose levels. Importantly, studies addressing secondary prevention of cardiovascular disease have shown a significantly reduced odds ratio for fatal myocardial infarction (between 0.25 and 0.7).

More specifically the results of three studies examining the effects of Mediterranean diet in the secondary prevention of CHD are of great interest. The Indo-Mediterranean diet Heart Study explored the cardioprotective effects of a Mediterranean style diet rich in α-linolenic acid vs. a Step I National Cholesterol Education Program (NCEP) prudent diet in 1,000 patients with angina pectoris, myocardial infarction, or surrogate risk factors for CHD *(71)*. Total cardiac end points were significantly fewer in the Mediterranean diet group compared with controls. Sudden cardiac deaths and nonfatal myocardial infarctions were also reduced. The investigators noted that in the Mediterranean diet group, patients with preexisting CHD had significantly greater benefits compared with such patients in the control group and concluded that an Indo-Mediterranean diet, rich in α-linolenic acid, might be more effective in primary and secondary prevention of CHD than the conventional step I NCEP prudent diet. Moreover, the Lyon Diet Heart Study, a randomized secondary prevention trial aimed at testing whether a Mediterranean-type diet may reduce the rate of recurrence after an initial myocardial infarction *(72)*, focused on cardiac death and nonfatal myocardial infarction, unstable angina, stroke, heart failure, and pulmonary or peripheral embolism. In the Mediterranean diet group, all the above-mentioned outcomes were significantly reduced compared with a prudent Western-type diet group during the 4 years of follow-up after the first infarction. Finally, the GISSI-Prevenzione clinical trial explored whether simple dietary advice to increase the consumption of Mediterranean foods, given in a clinical setting, leads to reduced mortality after a myocardial infarction *(73)*. When the range of observed scores of adherence to the Mediterranean-like dietary pattern was split into equal quartiles, the chance of death was decreased by 31%, 34%, and 49% for the second, third, and fourth quartiles, each compared with the first (depicting the least adherence), after adjustment for nondietary confounding variables. Overall, a 10% (one unit) increase in the dietary score reduced the risk of mortality by 15%. It has been concluded that patients with myocardial infarction can respond positively to simple dietary advice, and this can be expected to lead to a substantial reduction in the risk of early death. Regardless of any drug treatment prescribed, clinicians should routinely advise patients with myocardial infarction to increase the frequency of consumption of foods belonging to what is perceived as "Mediterranean diet."

6.3. DASH Diets

Dietary strategies to lower blood pressure play an important role in reducing overall CHD risk. The most well known controlled feeding study to test the dietary affects on hypertension is known as DASH (74). The results of the study clearly show that a diet high in fruits, vegetables, and low-fat dairy products, but low in saturated and total fat, reduces blood pressure in hypertensive and normotensive individuals (more so than the control diet). The composition of the DASH diet is 27% calories from total fat, 6% calories from SFA, 18% calories from protein, 55% calories from carbohydrate, 150 mg cholesterol and two levels of sodium intake – 2,400 or 1,500 mg. The calcium, magnesium and fiber content of the diet also stand out as high when compared with the typical American diet, with 1,250 mg calcium, 4,700 mg potassium, and 30 g fiber. The DASH diet was demonstrated to be effective as first-line therapy in individuals with stage I isolated systolic hypertension (i.e., with a systolic blood pressure of 140–159 mmHg and a diastolic blood pressure below 90 mmHg), with 78% of the persons on the DASH diet reducing their systolic blood pressure to <140 mmHg, in comparison to 24% in the control group (75). DASH has also be proven to be effective in lowering plasma levels of total and LDL-C but these changes were also accompanied by a reduction in HDL-C levels. While the Framingham risk score improved as a result of the impact on total and LDL-C as well as on blood pressure, the impact of the associated reduction in HDL-C needs to be assessed (76).

Furthermore, the PREMIER trial evaluated the effects of simultaneously implementing the DASH diet and established lifestyle recommendations for hypertension (weight loss, sodium reduction, increased physical activity, and limited alcohol intake) in free-living individuals. Participants in both intervention groups (established guidelines plus DASH vs. established guidelines) lost weight and reduced dietary sodium and fat intakes during the 18 months. In the established plus DASH group, participants made additional dietary changes, significantly increasing their intakes of fruits, vegetables, and dairy products and further reducing their intake of saturated and total fats. As a consequence, their hypertension status improved (77).

7. SUPPLEMENTS

7.1. Omega-3 Fatty Acids and Fish Oils

Fish oil, rich in omega-3 PUFA, is thought to contribute to the prevention or alleviation of many illnesses, though the most established benefits associated with fish oil are cardioprotective. Beneficial effects associated with fish oil include ameliorating arrhythmia, lowering serum triglycerides, decreasing thrombosis and inflammation, and improving endothelial function (78–80). The active ingredients are thought to be the long chain docosahexaenoic acids (DHA) and eicosapentaenoic acids (EPA). DHA and EPA rich oils are found in fatty fish such as salmon, mackerel, lake trout, herring, sardines, and albacore tuna. Currently, the AHA recommends consuming fatty fish at least twice a week (~8 oz per week). Eating more servings of fish per week is beneficial, but some fish, particularly tuna, may contain high amounts of contaminants such as methyl mercury. Sensitive subgroups of the population, primarily children and pregnant women, are advised by the FDA to avoid eating those fish with the potential for the highest level of mercury contamination (e.g., shark, swordfish, king mackerel, or tilefish), eat up to 12 oz (two average meals) per week of a variety of fish and shellfish that are lower in mercury (e.g., canned light tuna, salmon, pollock, catfish), and check local advisories about the safety of fish caught by family and friends in local lakes, rivers, and coastal areas (81). For those who are already diagnosed with heart disease, the AHA recommends taking 1,000 mg a day of DHA plus EPA from fish oil, preferably from fatty fish, but supplements can augment the amount taken in the diet and should be taken under the supervision of a doctor. Supplementation of 2,000–4,000 mg of DHA and EPA may also be beneficial for those who have hypertriglyceridemia (82). The FDA does not recommend taking more than 3,000 mg without consulting a physician due to risks that include bleeding associated with these supplements (see also chapter on hyperlipidemia).

α-Linolenic acid (ALA) is another form of omega-3 fatty acid derived from plant sources such as soybeans, flaxseed, and walnuts. ALA is a precursor molecule to EPA and DHA, and requires several metabolic steps before it can exert comparable benefits. Only 5–15% of ALA is converted into more active compounds, however, making it overall a less attractive source of long chain polyunsaturated fats. Trials, like the Lyon Diet Heart Study, which showed that ALA consumption in the context of a Mediterranean diet reduced total and cardiovascular mortality as well as nonfatal myocardial infraction, support the use of ALA and fish oil in the secondary prevention of CHD (1). However, at present, the body of research concerning the cardioprotective benefits of ALA is not conclusive.

7.2. Plant Sterols/Stanols

Plant sterols (β-sitosterol, campesterol, and stigmasterol) and their saturated derivatives, the stanols (sitostanol and campestanol), are the naturally occurring equivalents of the mammalian sterol cholesterol. Edible oils, seeds, and nuts have a high content of plant sterols. The Western diet contains about 100–300 mg/day of plant sterols and 20–50 mg/day of plant stanols (83). Because of their structural similarity to cholesterol, plant sterols and stanols can replace cholesterol in the human body; they decrease total cholesterol and LDL-C levels by reducing dietary and biliary cholesterol absorption via the displacement of cholesterol from micelles in the intestine. Plant sterols and stanols have been shown to lower LDL-C by 10–14% (84,85), but they do not alter HDL-C or triglyceride levels (86).

Available data indicate that the maximum effect of stanols/sterols is seen at an intake of at least 2 g/day (2) taken on a daily basis. In addition to plant sterol/stanol supplements, generally available in a soft gel capsule form, many products, including margarines, dairy products, cereals/cereal bars and beverages, now include stanols/sterols and are available in grocery stores. As with nuts, patients should be encouraged to substitute these foods for other isocaloric foods in their diet to prevent excess calorie intake and subsequent weight gain. Plant stanols/sterols are generally well tolerated with no adverse events. Some research indicates, however, that a decline in serum carotenoid and fat soluble vitamins levels may be brought on by consuming stanols/sterols (87). Thus, patients should be encouraged to consume foods that are high in carotenoids, including fruits and vegetables with deep colors of red, yellow, orange and green, such as carrots, kale, collard greens, tomatoes, sweet potatoes, peaches, and apricots.

7.3. Antioxidant Supplements and B Vitamins

Oxidative stress is a putative cause of atherosclerotic disease. Therefore, research has been directed toward the potential role of antioxidants in reducing CHD risk (9). At this time, however, there have been no clinical trials to strongly support the cardioprotective effects of antioxidants. Reports of the positive effects of antioxidants from foods and supplements on CHD have arisen from observational studies only. The most extensively studied antioxidants are vitamin C, E, β-carotene, coenzyme Q10, bioflavanoids, and selenium. For the time being, patients should not be encouraged to take in high levels of antioxidants in the form of supplements, due to available evidence from trials that they may, in fact, do more harm than good. β-Carotene supplementation has been associated with increased risk of lung cancer in smokers (88), whereas long-term vitamin E supplementation has been associated with increased risk for heart failure in patients with vascular disease or diabetes mellitus (89). Furthermore, a metaanalysis concluded that high doses of vitamin E may increase total mortality (90). It is therefore recommended that patients simply try to include in their diet more food sources of antioxidants, such as fruits, vegetables, and whole grains. Although antioxidant vitamins may theoretically be beneficial for reducing the risk of CHD, more conclusive data from large controlled clinical trials are clearly needed.

The current body of research on folate and other vitamins of the B complex is similarly inconclusive. There has been strong evidence showing a correlation between elevated homocysteine levels and CVD risk (91), but there is insufficient evidence to suggest that supplementation with folic acid, B_6, and B_{12} plays an important role in reduction of CVD risk. More research is necessary in this area before supplementation of these vitamins is recommended for CVD risk reduction.

8. ACHIEVING A HEALTHY BODY WEIGHT

Obesity is clearly a risk factor for CHD and has been consistently shown to influence several CHD factors, namely blood LDL-C, triglyceride, and HDL-C levels, hypertension, and insulin resistance (92). Weight gain prevention is obviously the most desirable method for avoiding the excess risk of CHD associated with obesity, but for the majority of CHD patients, weight gain has already occurred and weight reduction and/or maintenance becomes the greatest obstacle. For patients who are already overweight or obese, the initial goal of weight loss therapy is to reduce body weight by ~10% from baseline. If this goal is achieved, further weight loss can be attempted, as indicated through further evaluation. A reasonable time line for a 10% reduction in body weight is 6 months. For overweight patients with BMIs in the typical range of 25–35 kg/m^2, a decrease of 300–500 kcal/day will result in weight loss of about 0.5–1 lb/week and a 10% loss in 6 months. For more severely obese patients with BMIs > 35 kg/m^2, deficits of about 500–1,000 kcal/day will lead to weight loss of ~1–2 lbs/week and a 10% weight loss in 6 months *(7)*. Definitions of success for a weight management program are patient-specific. Reduction of risk factors, even if weight is not lost, is considered "success" from a health point of view. For patients unable to achieve significant weight reduction, prevention of further weight gain is an important goal; such patients may also be encouraged to participate in a weight management program. For patients resistant to weight reduction through dietary intervention alone, a concomitant pharmacotherapy and physical activity program may help to achieve the weight loss target, as indicated (see Chap. 16).

9. PHYSICAL ACTIVITY

Observational and randomized controlled clinical studies consistently show that physical activity is effective in both primary and secondary prevention of CHD. The effects of physical activity on CHD risk reduction are due, in part, to favorable effects on blood pressure, triglyceride levels, HDL-C levels, insulin sensitivity, glucose tolerance, and body weight. Physical activity and weight loss decrease LDL-C levels and lessen the reduction in HDL-C that often occurs with a diet that is low in total fat and SFA *(93)*.

The American College of Sports Medicine and the American Heart Association recommend that people should get a minimum of 30 min of moderate-intensity aerobic physical activity for 5 days each week or a minimum of 20 min of vigorous-intensity aerobic activity for 3 days each week *(94)*. Moderate physical activity is described as walking, climbing stairs, gardening, yard work, moderate-to-heavy housework, dancing, and exercise at home. Patients who stress that they are unable to find time for daily activity should be encouraged to accumulate exercise minutes in shorter bouts of 10 min at a time throughout the day to reach their 30 min goal. Although existing research evidence is not conclusive, a summary of the experimental findings suggests that moderate-intensity physical activity in shorter bouts (usually lasting 10 min) that is accumulated toward the 30-min minimum can be as effective as single, longer exercise sessions in reducing risk factors for chronic disease *(94)*. In patients with cardiovascular risk factors, individually tailored prescriptions must take into account the patient's main metabolic defect. To modify the lipid profile, exercise should be aerobic and of moderate intensity, with an energy expenditure greater than 300 kcal (equivalent to a weekly energy expenditure of at least 2,000 kcal). With regard to insulin sensitivity, power training is just as effective as aerobic exercise, and if the prime objective is to lose weight, prolonged, mild-intensity work should be performed daily if possible *(95)*.

Moreover, special care must be taken during the assessment of patients with chronic disease. Once the patient has been stabilized after an acute coronary event, physical activity, along with psychological support, educational and preventive strategies, should be included in rehabilitative therapy. It has been shown that to improve cardiovascular adaptability to effort, the intensity of physical exercise must be 60–75% VO$_2$max (determined during initial cardiopulmonary evaluation), which corresponds to a heart rate between 70 and 85% of that reached at the peak of exercise. Nevertheless, if the intensity of effort exceeds 80% of the maximum aerobic capacity, the risk of cardiovascular complications appears to outweigh the benefits *(95)*. Patients with CHD should be monitored closely during physiologic testing. The appraiser must have a clear understanding of the effects of the patient's clinical status and medications on the physiologic response to exercise.

Low-intensity exercise is generally better accepted by people naive to exercise training, those who are extremely deconditioned ("out of shape"), and older people. Low-intensity exercise may result in an improvement in health status with little or no change in physical fitness. Indeed, light or moderate activity is associated with a reduced risk of death from any cause among men with established CHD. Furthermore, regular walking or moderate to heavy gardening has been shown to be sufficient in achieving health benefits. Individuals with low baseline fitness levels can achieve significant improvements in physical fitness with a lower training intensity (e.g., 40–50% of heart rate reserve) than that needed by individuals with a higher baseline fitness level, whereas the latter would need a greater level of exercise intensity to achieve further improvements in fitness. Deconditioned individuals may improve their physical fitness with as little as two exercise sessions per week. Others have shown an improvement in aerobic fitness with exercise intensities as low as 30% of heart rate reserve in sedentary people. Long-term adherence to this form of exercise may be poor, however, and the risk of musculoskeletal injury high, especially in people unaccustomed to exercise (96).

10. NUTRITION COUNSELING AND ADHERENCE ISSUES IN PATIENTS WITH CVD

Implementation and maintenance of dietary and physical activity changes is of major importance. Evidence suggests that sustained improvements in diet composition require individualized and reinforced counseling in patients with CHD (97). Dietitians may be better able to help patients lower their total and LDL-C levels through nutrition counseling in the short to medium term (98,99). This may be due to the greater amount of time devoted to advising patients. Others have shown that the effects of a dietitian-based program for hyperlipidemia were additive to those observed after a physician-delivered intervention in the US healthcare system (100).

Individualized interventions based on the stages of change and behavioral techniques are more effective in inducing dietary changes and some improvements in CHD risk factors, compared with the more traditional methods of provision of information and exhortation (101–103). Still, corresponding changes in biochemical indexes are not always present. Stage-matched nutrition counseling promotes progress through stages of change (104) and future research should focus on feasible ways to keep patients in the postpreparation stage.

The U.S. Preventive Services Task Force recommends intensive behavioral dietary counseling for adult patients with hyperlipidemia and other known risk factors for cardiovascular disease, by primary care clinicians or by referral to other specialists and/or nutritionists/dietitians (105). Following these recommendations, effective interventions should combine nutrition education with behavior-oriented counseling to help patients acquire the skills, motivation, and support they need to alter their daily eating patterns and food preparation practices. Examples of behavior-oriented counseling interventions include teaching self-monitoring, helping patients to set their own goals and seek social support, providing guidance in shopping and food preparation, training patients to overcome everyday barriers in making appropriate food choices, and preventing relapse. In general, these interventions can be described with reference to the 5-A behavioral counseling framework (adapted from tobacco cessation interventions in clinical care) (106):

- *Assess*: Ask about dietary practices, behavioral health risks, and factors affecting choice of dietary change goals/methods.
- *Advise*: Provide clear, specific, and personalized advice on behavior change, including information about personal health, harms, and benefits.
- *Agree*: Collaboratively select appropriate treatment goals and methods based on the patient's interest in and willingness to change dietary and physical activity habits. The clinician employing an empathetic "partnership" approach emphasizes the patient's role in interpreting advice and explores, rather than prescribes, how to proceed best. Patient involvement in decision making about behavior change offers important benefits. Patients who are actively involved in healthcare decisions and engaged in a program have a greater sense of personal control; their choices are based on realistic expectations and patient values are promoted. Thus, resistance can be prevented.
- *Assist*: Using behavior change techniques helps the patient in achieving agreed-upon goals by acquiring the skills, self-efficacy, and social supports for behavior change.
- *Arrange*: Schedule follow-up contacts to provide ongoing assistance and to adjust the treatment plan as needed, including referral to more intensive or specialized treatment. As long-term efficacy of lifestyle interventions remains a challenge, some form of routine follow-up assessment and support through repeat visits, telephone calls, or other contact is generally deemed necessary to achieve long-term behavior change.

11. CONCLUSION

Nutrition intervention in CVD represents an evolving scientific area, which expands from the effects of single nutrients (e.g., fatty acids, fiber) to those of food groups (e.g., fruits, vegetables, whole grains) and dietary patterns. The latter, as a holistic approach, gains continuously more attention and has resulted in scientific data supporting the beneficial role of Mediterranean and DASH diets on CVD prevention and treatment. Furthermore, individuals with CVD should also be given individualized guidance to achieve a healthy body weight change (at a first stage to reduce their body weight by ~10% from baseline) and engage in a minimum of 30 min of moderate-intensity aerobic physical activity for 5 days a week. Nutrition and other health-related professionals should implement effective interventions combining education with behavior-oriented counseling, focusing on motivating and supporting patients to change their lifestyle habits.

REFERENCES

1. Hu FB, Willett WC. Optimal diets for prevention of coronary heart disease. JAMA 2002;288:2569–78.
2. Lichtenstein AH, Appel LJ, Brands M, et al.. Diet and lifestyle recommendations revision 2006: a scientific statement from the American Heart Association Nutrition Committee. Circulation 2006;114:82–96.
3. Hu FB. Dietary pattern analysis: a new direction in nutritional epidemiology. Curr Opin Lipidol 2002;13:3–9.
4. Fung TT, Chiuve SE, McCullough ML, Rexrode KM, Logroscino G, Hu FB. Adherence to a DASH-style diet and risk of coronary heart disease and stroke in women. Arch Intern Med 2008;168:713–20.
5. Trichopoulou A, Costacou T, Bamia C, Trichopoulos D. Adherence to a Mediterranean diet and survival in a Greek population. N Engl J Med 2003;348:2599–608.

6. Graham I, Atar D, Borch-Johnsen K, et al. European guidelines on cardiovascular disease prevention in clinical practice: executive summary. Fourth Joint Task Force of the European Society of Cardiology and other societies on cardiovascular disease prevention in clinical practice (constituted by representatives of nine societies and by invited experts). Eur J Cardiovasc Prev Rehabil 2007;14 Suppl 2:E1–40.

7. Clinical Guidelines on the Identification, Evaluation, and Treatment of Overweight and Obesity in Adults–The Evidence Report. National Institutes of Health. Obes Res 1998;6 Suppl 2:51S–209S.

8. Fletcher B, Berra K, Ades P, et al. Managing abnormal blood lipids: a collaborative approach. Circulation 2005;112:3184–209.

9. Executive Summary of The Third Report of The National Cholesterol Education Program (NCEP) Expert Panel on Detection, Evaluation, And Treatment of High Blood Cholesterol In Adults (Adult Treatment Panel III). JAMA 2001;285:2486–97.

10. Low-fat diet in myocardial infarction: A controlled trial. Lancet 1965;2:501–4.

11. Burr ML, Fehily AM, Gilbert JF, . Effects of changes in fat, fish, and fibre intakes on death and myocardial reinfarction: diet and reinfarction trial (DART). Lancet 1989;2:757–61.

12. Hu FB, Stampfer MJ, Manson JE, et al. Dietary fat intake and the risk of coronary heart disease in women. N Engl J Med 1997;337:1491–9.

13. Keys A. Coronary heart disease in seven countries. Circulation 1970;41:I1–198.

14. Van Horn L, McCoin M, Kris-Etherton PM, et al. The evidence for dietary prevention and treatment of cardiovascular disease. J Am Diet Assoc 2008;108:287–331.

15. Lada AT, Rudel LL. Dietary monounsaturated versus polyunsaturated fatty acids: which is really better for protection from coronary heart disease? Curr Opin Lipidol 2003;14:41–6.

16. Appel LJ, Sacks FM, Carey VJ, et al. Effects of protein, monounsaturated fat, and carbohydrate intake on blood pressure and serum lipids: results of the OmniHeart randomized trial. JAMA 2005;294:2455–64.

17. Willett WC, Stampfer MJ, Manson JE, . Intake of trans fatty acids and risk of coronary heart disease among women. Lancet 1993;341:581–5.

18. Mattson FH, Grundy SM. Comparison of effects of dietary saturated, monounsaturated, and polyunsaturated fatty acids on plasma lipids and lipoproteins in man. J Lipid Res 1985;26:194–202.

19. Perez-Jimenez F, Lopez-Miranda J, Mata P. Protective effect of dietary monounsaturated fat on arteriosclerosis: beyond cholesterol. Atherosclerosis 2002;163:385–98.

20. Kratz M, Cullen P, Kannenberg F, et al. Effects of dietary fatty acids on the composition and oxidizability of low-density lipoprotein. Eur J Clin Nutr 2002;56:72–81.

21. Riccardi G, Giacco R, Rivellese AA. Dietary fat, insulin sensitivity and the metabolic syndrome. Clin Nutr 2004;23:447–56.

22. Cassidy A, Albertazzi P, Lise Nielsen I, et al. Critical review of health effects of soyabean phytooestrogens in post-menopausal women. Proc Nutr Soc 2006;65:76–92.

23. Sacks FM, Lichtenstein A, Van Horn L, Harris W, Kris-Etherton P, Winston M. Soy protein, isoflavones, and cardiovascular health: an American Heart Association Science Advisory for professionals from the Nutrition Committee. Circulation 2006;113:1034–44.

24. Truswell AS. Food carbohydrates and plasma lipids–an update. Am J Clin Nutr 1994;59:710S–18S.

25. Srinath Reddy K, Katan MB. Diet, nutrition and the prevention of hypertension and cardiovascular diseases. Public Health Nutr 2004;7:167–86.

26. Jenkins DJ, Wolever TM, Kalmusky J, et al. Low-glycemic index diet in hyperlipidemia: use of traditional starchy foods. Am J Clin Nutr 1987;46:66–71.

27. Opperman AM, Venter CS, Oosthuizen W, Thompson RL, Vorster HH. Meta-analysis of the health effects of using the glycaemic index in meal-planning. Br J Nutr 2004;92:367–81.

28. Rotondo S, de Gaetano G. Protection from cardiovascular disease by wine and its derived products. Epidemiological evidence and biological mechanisms. World Rev Nutr Diet 2000;87:90–113.

29. Rimm EB, Williams P, Fosher K, Criqui M, Stampfer MJ. Moderate alcohol intake and lower risk of coronary heart disease: meta-analysis of effects on lipids and haemostatic factors. BMJ 1999;319:1523–8.

30. Waterhouse AL. Wine phenolics. Ann N Y Acad Sci 2002;957:21–36.

31. Pace-Asciak CR, Rounova O, Hahn SE, Diamandis EP, Goldberg DM. Wines and grape juices as modulators of platelet aggregation in healthy human subjects. Clin Chim Acta 1996;246:163–82.

32. Frankel EN, Kanner J, German JB, Parks E, Kinsella JE. Inhibition of oxidation of human low-density lipoprotein by phenolic substances in red wine. Lancet 1993;341:454–7.

33. Flesch M, Schwarz A, Bohm M. Effects of red and white wine on endothelium-dependent vasorelaxation of rat aorta and human coronary arteries. Am J Physiol 1998;275:H1183–90.

34. Perret B, Ruidavets JB, Vieu C, et al. Alcohol consumption is associated with enrichment of high-density lipoprotein particles in polyunsaturated lipids and increased cholesterol esterification rate. Alcohol Clin Exp Res 2002;26:1134–40.

35. Klatsky AL. Alcohol, cardiovascular diseases and diabetes mellitus. Pharmacol Res 2007;55:237–47.

36. Rehm J, Greenfield TK, Rogers JD. Average volume of alcohol consumption, patterns of drinking, and all-cause mortality: results from the US National Alcohol Survey. Am J Epidemiol 2001;153:64–71.

37. Laatikainen T, Manninen L, Poikolainen K, Vartiainen E. Increased mortality related to heavy alcohol intake pattern. J Epidemiol Community Health 2003;57:379–84.

38. Tolstrup JS, Jensen MK, Tjonneland A, Overvad K, Gronbaek M. Drinking pattern and mortality in middle-aged men and women. Addiction 2004;99:323–30.

39. McElduff P, Dobson AJ. How much alcohol and how often? Population based case-control study of alcohol consumption and risk of a major coronary event. BMJ 1997;314:1159–64.

40. Mukamal KJ, Conigrave KM, Mittleman MA, et al. Roles of drinking pattern and type of alcohol consumed in coronary heart disease in men. N Engl J Med 2003;348:109–18.

41. Mukamal KJ, Jensen MK, Gronbaek M, et al. Drinking frequency, mediating biomarkers, and risk of myocardial infarction in women and men. Circulation 2005;112:1406–13.

42. Dorn JM, Hovey K, Williams BA, et al. Alcohol drinking pattern and non-fatal myocardial infarction in women. Addiction 2007;102:730–9.

43. Stranges S, Wu T, Dorn JM, et al. Relationship of alcohol drinking pattern to risk of hypertension: a population-based study. Hypertension 2004;44:813–9.

44. Athyros VG, Liberopoulos EN, Mikhailidis DP, et al. Association of drinking pattern and alcohol beverage type with the prevalence of metabolic syndrome, diabetes, coronary heart disease, stroke, and peripheral arterial disease in a Mediterranean cohort. Angiology 2007;58:689–97.

45. Joshipura KJ, Hu FB, Manson JE, et al. The effect of fruit and vegetable intake on risk for coronary heart disease. Ann Intern Med 2001;134:1106–14.

46. Zyriax BC, Algenstaedt P, Hess UF, et al. Factors contributing to the risk of cardiovascular disease reflected by plasma adiponectin Data from the coronary risk factors for atherosclerosis in women (CORA) study. Atherosclerosis 2008;2:403–9.

47. Yannakoulia M, Yiannakouris N, Melistas L, et al. Dietary factors associated with plasma high molecular and total adiponectin levels in apparently healthy women. Eur J Endocrinol 2008;159:R5–10.

48. Bazzano LA, Serdula MK, Liu S. Dietary intake of fruits and vegetables and risk of cardiovascular disease. Curr Atheroscler Rep 2003;5:492–9.

49. Slavin J. Why whole grains are protective: biological mechanisms. Proc Nutr Soc 2003;62:129–34.

50. Yannakoulia M, Yiannakouris N, Melistas L, Kontogianni MD, Malagaris I, Mantzoros CS. A dietary pattern characterized by high consumption of whole-grain cereals and low-fat dairy products and low consumption of refined cereals is positively associated with plasma adiponectin levels in healthy women. Metabolism 2008;57:824–30.

51. Mellen PB, Walsh TF, Herrington DM. Whole grain intake and cardiovascular disease: a meta-analysis. Nutr Metab Cardiovasc Dis 2008;18:283–90.

52. Hu FB. The role of diet and lifestyle modifications in the statin era. J Am Diet Assoc 2005;105:1718–21.

53. Steffen LM, Kroenke CH, Yu X, et al. Associations of plant food, dairy product, and meat intakes with 15-y incidence of elevated blood pressure in young black and white adults: the Coronary Artery Risk Development in Young Adults (CARDIA) Study. Am J Clin Nutr 2005;82:1169–77; quiz 1363–4.

54. Jiang R, Jacobs DR, Jr., Mayer-Davis E, et al. Nut and seed consumption and inflammatory markers in the multi-ethnic study of atherosclerosis. Am J Epidemiol 2006;163:222–31.

55. Olendzki B, Speed C, Domino FJ. Nutritional assessment and counseling for prevention and treatment of cardiovascular disease. Am Fam Physician 2006;73:257–64.

56. St-Onge MP, Farnworth ER, Jones PJ. Consumption of fermented and nonfermented dairy products: effects on cholesterol concentrations and metabolism. Am J Clin Nutr 2000;71:674–81.

57. Kontogianni MD, Panagiotakos DB, Chrysohoou C, Pitsavos C, Stefanadis C. Modelling dairy intake on the development of acute coronary syndromes: the CARDIO2000 study. Eur J Cardiovasc Prev Rehabil 2006;13:791–7.

58. Svetkey LP, Simons-Morton D, Vollmer WM, . Effects of dietary patterns on blood pressure: sub-group analysis of the Dietary Approaches to Stop Hypertension (DASH) randomized clinical trial. Arch Intern Med 1999;159:285–93.

59. Pfeuffer M, Schrezenmeir J. Bioactive substances in milk with properties decreasing risk of cardiovascular diseases. Br J Nutr 2000;84 Suppl 1:S155–9.

60. Tholstrup T. Dairy products and cardiovascular disease. Curr Opin Lipidol 2006;17:1–10.

61. Hu FB, Rimm EB, Stampfer MJ, Ascherio A, Spiegelman D, Willett WC. Prospective study of major dietary patterns and risk of coronary heart disease in men. Am J Clin Nutr 2000;72:912–21.

62. Fung TT, Willett WC, Stampfer MJ, Manson JE, Hu FB. Dietary patterns and the risk of coronary heart disease in women. Arch Intern Med 2001;161:1857–62.

63. Fung TT, Rimm EB, Spiegelman D, et al. Association between dietary patterns and plasma biomarkers of obesity and cardiovascular disease risk. Am J Clin Nutr 2001;73:61–7.

64. Lopez-Garcia E, Schulze MB, Fung TT, et al. Major dietary patterns are related to plasma concentrations of markers of inflammation and endothelial dysfunction. Am J Clin Nutr 2004;80:1029–35.

65. Fung TT, Schulze M, Manson JE, Willett WC, Hu FB. Dietary patterns, meat intake, and the risk of type 2 diabetes in women. Arch Intern Med 2004;164:2235–40.

66. van Dam RM, Rimm EB, Willett WC, Stampfer MJ, Hu FB. Dietary patterns and risk for type 2 diabetes mellitus in U.S. men. Ann Intern Med 2002;136:201–9.

67. Villegas R, Salim A, Flynn A, Perry IJ. Prudent diet and the risk of insulin resistance. Nutr Metab Cardiovasc Dis 2004;14:334–43.

68. Ding EL, Mozaffarian D. Optimal dietary habits for the prevention of stroke. Semin Neurol 2006;26:11–23.

69. Willett WC, Sacks F, Trichopoulou A, et al. Mediterranean diet pyramid: a cultural model for healthy eating. Am J Clin Nutr 1995;61:1402S–6S.

70. Serra-Majem L, Roman B, Estruch R. Scientific evidence of interventions using the Mediterranean diet: a systematic review. Nutr Rev 2006;64:S27–47.

71. Singh RB, Dubnov G, Niaz MA, et al. Effect of an Indo-Mediterranean diet on progression of coronary artery disease in high risk patients (Indo-Mediterranean Diet Heart Study): a randomised single-blind trial. Lancet 2002;360:1455–61.

72. de Lorgeril M, Salen P, Martin JL, Monjaud I, Delaye J, Mamelle N. Mediterranean diet, traditional risk factors, and the rate of cardiovascular complications after myocardial infarction: final report of the Lyon Diet Heart Study. Circulation 1999;99:779–85.

73. Barzi F, Woodward M, Marfisi RM, Tavazzi L, Valagussa F, Marchioli R. Mediterranean diet and all-causes mortality after myocardial infarction: results from the GISSI-Prevenzione trial. Eur J Clin Nutr 2003;57:604–11.

74. Sacks FM, Obarzanek E, Windhauser MM, et al. Rationale and design of the Dietary Approaches to Stop Hypertension trial (DASH). A multicenter controlled-feeding study of dietary patterns to lower blood pressure. Ann Epidemiol 1995;5:108–18.

75. Moore TJ, Conlin PR, Ard J, Svetkey LP. DASH (Dietary Approaches to Stop Hypertension) diet is effective treatment for stage 1 isolated systolic hypertension. Hypertension 2001;38:155–8.

76. Obarzanek E, Sacks FM, Vollmer WM, et al. Effects on blood lipids of a blood pressure-lowering diet: the Dietary Approaches to Stop Hypertension (DASH) Trial. Am J Clin Nutr 2001;74:80–9.

77. Elmer PJ, Obarzanek E, Vollmer WM, et al. Effects of comprehensive lifestyle modification on diet, weight, physical fitness, and blood pressure control: 18-month results of a randomized trial. Ann Intern Med 2006;144:485–95.

78. Kris-Etherton PM, Harris WS, Appel LJ. Fish consumption, fish oil, omega-3 fatty acids, and cardiovascular disease. Circulation 2002;106:2747–57.

79. Kang JX, Leaf A. Antiarrhythmic effects of polyunsaturated fatty acids. Recent studies. Circulation 1996;94:1774–80.

80. Connor SL, Connor WE. Are fish oils beneficial in the prevention and treatment of coronary artery disease? Am J Clin Nutr 1997;66:1020S–31S.

81. US Department of Health and Human Services FaDA, Center for Food Safety and Applied Nutrition.. An important message for pregnant women and women of childbearing age who may become pregnant about the risk of mercury in fish, 2004.

82. Kris-Etherton PM, Harris WS, Appel LJ. Omega-3 fatty acids and cardiovascular disease: new recommendations from the American Heart Association. Arterioscler Thromb Vasc Biol 2003;23:151–2.

83. Devaraj S, Jialal I. The role of dietary supplementation with plant sterols and stanols in the prevention of cardiovascular disease. Nutr Rev 2006;64:348–54.

84. Plat J, Mensink RP. Plant stanol and sterol esters in the control of blood cholesterol levels: mechanism and safety aspects. Am J Cardiol 2005;96:15D–22D.

85. Grundy SM. Stanol esters as a component of maximal dietary therapy in the National Cholesterol Education Program Adult Treatment Panel III report. Am J Cardiol 2005;96:47D–50D.

86. Micallef MA, Garg ML. The lipid-lowering effects of phytosterols and (n-3) polyunsaturated fatty acids are synergistic and complementary in hyperlipidemic men and women. J Nutr 2008;138:1086–90.

87. Tuomilehto J, Tikkanen MJ, Hogstrom P, et al. Safety assessment of common foods enriched with natural nonesterified plant sterols. Eur J Clin Nutr 2008.

88. Albanes D, Heinonen OP, Taylor PR, et al. Alpha-tocopherol and beta-carotene supplements and lung cancer incidence in the alpha-tocopherol, beta-carotene cancer prevention study: effects of base-line characteristics and study compliance. J Natl Cancer Inst 1996;88:1560–70.

89. Lonn E, Bosch J, Yusuf S, et al. Effects of long-term vitamin E supplementation on cardiovascular events and cancer: a randomized controlled trial. JAMA 2005;293:1338–47.

90. Miller ER, 3rd, Pastor-Barriuso R, Dalal D, Riemersma RA, Appel LJ, Guallar E. Meta-analysis: high-dosage vitamin E supplementation may increase all-cause mortality. Ann Intern Med 2005;142:37–46.

91. Malinow MR, Bostom AG, Krauss RM. Homocyst(e)ine, diet, and cardiovascular diseases: a statement for healthcare professionals from the Nutrition Committee, American Heart Association. Circulation 1999;99:178–82.

92. Rashid MN, Fuentes F, Touchon RC, Wehner PS. Obesity and the risk for cardiovascular disease. Prev Cardiol 2003;6:42–7.

93. Thompson PD, Lim V. Physical Activity in the Prevention of Atherosclerotic Coronary Heart Disease. Curr Treat Options Cardiovasc Med 2003;5:279–85.

94. Haskell WL, Lee IM, Pate RR, et al. Physical activity and public health: updated recommendation for adults from the American College of Sports Medicine and the American Heart Association. Circulation 2007;116:1081–93.

95. Giada F, Biffi A, Agostoni P, et al. Exercise prescription for the prevention and treatment of cardiovascular diseases: part I. J Cardiovasc Med (Hagerstown) 2008;9:529–44.

96. Ignarro LJ, Balestrieri ML, Napoli C. Nutrition, physical activity, and cardiovascular disease: an update. Cardiovasc Res 2007;73:326–40.

97. Dalgard C, Thuroe A, Haastrup B, Haghfelt T, Stender S. Saturated fat intake is reduced in patients with ischemic heart disease 1 year after comprehensive counseling but not after brief counseling. J Am Diet Assoc 2001;101:1420–9.

98. Thompson RL, Summerbell CD, Hooper L, et al. Relative efficacy of differential methods of dietary advice: a systematic review. Am J Clin Nutr 2003;77:1052S–7S.

99. Henkin Y, Shai I, Zuk R, et al. Dietary treatment of hypercholesterolemia: do dietitians do it better? A randomized, controlled trial. Am J Med 2000;109:549–55.

100. Hebert JR, Ebbeling CB, Ockene IS, et al. A dietitian-delivered group nutrition program leads to reductions in dietary fat, serum cholesterol, and body weight: the Worcester Area Trial for Counseling in Hyperlipidemia (WATCH). J Am Diet Assoc 1999;99:544–52.

101. Steptoe A, Doherty S, Rink E, Kerry S, Kendrick T, Hilton S. Behavioural counselling in general practice for the promotion of healthy behaviour among adults at increased risk of coronary heart disease: randomised trial. BMJ 1999;319:943–7; discussion 947–8.

102. van der Veen J, Bakx C, van den Hoogen H, et al. Stage-matched nutrition guidance for patients at elevated risk for cardiovascular disease: a randomized intervention study in family practice. J Fam Pract 2002;51:751–8.

103. Timlin MT, Shores KV, Reicks M. Behavior change outcomes in an outpatient cardiac rehabilitation program. J Am Diet Assoc 2002;102:664–71.

104. Verheijden MW, Van der Veen JE, Bakx JC, et al. Stage-matched nutrition guidance: stages of change and fat consumption in Dutch patients at elevated cardiovascular risk. J Nutr Educ Behav 2004;36:228–37.

105. US Preventive Services Task Force. Behavioral counseling in primary care to promote a healthy diet: recommendations and rationale. Am J Prev Med 2003;24:93–100.

106. Whitlock EP, Orleans CT, Pender N, Allan J. Evaluating primary care behavioral counseling interventions: an evidence-based approach. Am J Prev Med 2002;22:267–84.

13 Medical Nutrition Therapy in the Treatment of Type 1 and Type 2 Diabetes

Olga Kordonouri, Caroline Apovian, Lauren Kuhn, Thomas Danne, and Christos S. Mantzoros

KEY POINTS

- Medical nutrition therapy (MNT), i.e., a goal-oriented approach in developing and in implementing a nutritional plan for the treatment of individuals with diabetes plays a central role in the care of their patients.
- More specifically, a well-designed nutritional plan is an essential component of the therapeutic regimen for all diabetics and should be designed in such a way that it should achieve the best long-term control of diabetes and its complications.
- There is growing evidence that MNT benefits patients with all forms of diabetes and, according to many, it is the single most important intervention for the prevention and probably treatment for type 2 diabetics, making it an essential part of diabetes self-management education.
- All members of the team involved in a diabetic patient's care should be involved in setting nutrition-related goals, but it is highly recommended that a registered dietitian who is trained in MNT for diabetics assumes the coordinating role in MNT education and management *(1)*.
- Achieving nutrition-related goals requires the efforts of a multidisciplinary team. Ultimately, the most important member of that team is the patient as she/he should be the primary decision maker during the process of implementing a lifestyle change.
- MNT plays an important role in three major areas of diabetes prevention and treatment: primary prevention, i.e., intervention(s) to prevent obesity and ensuing diabetes; secondary prevention, after diagnosis, to improve glycemic control and prevent diabetes related complications; and tertiary prevention to help prevent morbidity and mortality related to managing the complications of diabetes.

Key Words: Medical nutrition therapy, Diabetes Obesity

From: *Nutrition and Health: Nutrition and Metabolism*
Edited by: C.S. Mantzoros, DOI: 10.1007/978-1-60327-453-1_13,
© Humana Press, a part of Springer Science+Business Media, LLC 2009

1. TYPE 1 DIABETES

1.1. Nutrition and Causation of Type 1 Diabetes

Type 1 diabetes is an autoimmune disease with genetic and environmental factors influencing its development *(2)*. Prospective studies show that islet cell autoimmunity can begin early in life and that dietary factors can be possible triggers or protective factors. In particular, a short breastfeeding period and an early introduction of customary formulas based on cow's milk to infant's diet have been associated with an increased risk of diabetes in several ecological and epidemiological studies *(3–7)*. Although both animal and immunological studies in man further supported the cow's milk hypothesis *(8)*, the evidence cannot be regarded as fully conclusive so far. Two metaanalyses led to inconsistent results either ascribing the observed weak associations to causal relationships *(7)* or to methodological shortcomings of the studies *(9)*. In a recently published nationwide case–control study by Rosenbauer et al. *(10)* in Germany, short breastfeeding and early introduction of formula feeding (before vs. fifth month or later) were risk factors of the development of type 1 diabetes in preschool age children [adjusted odd ratios: 1.31 (1.01–1.69) and 1.34 (1.03–1.74), respectively]. In addition, late introduction of solid food (i.e., after the fourth month of age) was associated with reduced diabetes risk. Hopefully, in the near future, a worldwide, prospective, randomized, double-blinded intervention study (Trial to Reduce Diabetes in Genetically at Risk, TRIGR), including 2,160 newborns who carry high-risk HLA alleles and have first degree relative with type 1 diabetes will definitively answer the question of whether avoiding cow's milk protein in the first 6–8 months of life will reduce the appearance of multiple diabetes-related autoantibodies before the age of 6 years or the development of type 1 diabetes up to the age of 10 years *(11)*. The 6-year autoantibody results will be available in 2012 and the type 1 diabetes in 2016.

Early introduction of gluten, a wheat protein, in baby's diet is also thought to contribute as a trigger of the autoimmune process leading to destruction of pancreatic beta cells. In animal studies, elimination of this protein from the diet led to significant reduction of diabetes autoimmunity *(12)*. Since enteral permeability for macromolecules is increased during the first months of life, it is possible that early introduction of nutrients may lead to sensitization against several nutritional parameters. Increased enteral permeability has been already described in patients with type 1 diabetes *(13)*. Furthermore according to other theories, nutritional parameters like gliadin, a protein fraction of gluten, may elicit an inflammatory process in gut mucosa leading to an abnormal permeability and facilitating the exposure of the immune system to potential diabetogenic agents *(14)*. The effects of the elimination of gluten from the diet of children with a first degree relative with type 1 diabetes during the first year of life have been studied in an interventional prospective trial since 2001 *(15)*. Whether this intervention can postpone or even avoid the development of diabetes-related autoimmunity or even clinical diabetes in this population will be shown in the near future, since the first results of the BABYDIÄT Study are expected in 2008.

Vitamin D (1,25 dihydrocholecalciferol) has been discussed as a protective factor for the development of several diseases like type 1 diabetes, multiple sclerosis, rheumatic arthritis, hyperthyroidism, and Hashimoto thyroiditis *(16)* due to its immunomodulating action. Saggese et al. showed that vitamin D has an immunosuppressive action with in vitro suppression of proliferative T lymphocytes and influences on the production of cytokine profiles (17). The EURODIAB Trial showed that vitamin D supplementation during the first year of life was associated with reduced risk of type 1 diabetes (odds ratio [OR] 0.7, 95% confidence intervals [95%-CI] 0.5–0.9) (18). Hypponen et al. found that the incidence of type 1 diabetes was significantly lower among subjects who received a regular daily dose of 2,000 units of vitamin D compared with those without supplementation (OR 0.1, 95%-CI 0.03–0.5) (19). Vitamin D supplementation seems to be a promising prevention for beta cell autoimmunity, and relative vitamin D deficiency is now recognized as a pandemic. Some experts suggest that both children and adults should take 800–1,000 IU of vitamin D per day from dietary and supplementatal sources, if sunlight cannot provide adequate Vitamin D levels, but this remains to be conclusively demonstrated. In summary, these recommendations have not yet been recognized nationally or globally as yet (20).

Fish oil contains not only vitamin D but also polyunsaturated fatty acids (PUFA), particularly docosahexaenoic acid (DHA) and eicosapentaenoic acid (EPA). Long-chain n-3 fatty acids are incorporated into cell membranes and have antiinflammatory properties that may be relevant to the prevention of type 1 diabetes, such as decreased expression of HLA class II molecules on activated human monocytes (21) and reduced expression of interleukin 1β. These data suggest that the antiinflammatory n-3 fatty acids such as DHA and EPA may reduce the risk of disease development (22). The levels of vitamin D and PUFA in newborns depend on the nutritional state of the mother during gestation (23,24). In a Norwegian study, children from mothers with fish oil supplementation during pregnancy had a lower risk of type 1 diabetes (OR 0.3, 95%-CI 0.1–0.8) (25).

In summary, although there is promising evidence that nutrition in early stages of life may influence the initiation of beta cell autoimmunity in genetically predisposed individuals, there is currently no conclusive data allowing particular recommendations for nutritional interventions or vitamin supplementation to prevent the development of type 1 diabetes later in life. Until the results of the large prospective interventional studies are known, generally accepted guidelines for the nutrition of neonates and infants suggesting exclusive breastfeeding for the first 4–6 months of life are highly recommended.

1.2. Nutrition and Treatment in Type 1 Diabetes

The first nutrition priority for individuals requiring insulin therapy is to integrate an insulin regimen into their lifestyle. With the many insulin options now available, an appropriate insulin regimen can usually be developed to conform to an individual's preferred meal routine, food choices, and physical activity pattern.

1.2.1. NUTRITION OF CHILDREN AND ADOLESCENTS WITH TYPE 1 DIABETES

In general, the nutrition of children and adolescents with type 1 diabetes does not differ from that of their nondiabetic peers. Daily requirements of carbohydrates, fat, and proteins depend on age, gender, height, weight, levels of daily activity and particular living conditions such as climate and season. Energy and nutritional requirements including vitamins, minerals, and fluids show a higher inter and intraindividual variability in children and adolescents than in adults. Frequent change of energy and nutritional requirements accompanied by frequent changing of food types characterize the nutritional habits of young people. Personal preferences and different eating habits of the family serve to increase the variability of nutrition among young people with type 1 diabetes. Once overweight and/or obesity are absent, one can assume that the physiological regulation of appetite guarantees balanced nutritional and energy requirements of the growing child. For this reason, nutritional guidelines can only provide an orientation aid for pediatricians and pediatric diabetologists. Interestingly, the definition of overweight and obesity in childhood varies between the continents. Thus, in the US overweight and obesity are defined as body mass index (BMI) exceeding the 85th and 95th percentiles of the US CDC 2000 reference, in the UK the definitions use the 91st and 98th percentiles of the British 1990 reference, in Germany the 90th and 97th percentiles, respectively (26–28).

The oldest and simplest way to calculate energy needs (in kcal) of children is the one proposed by Priscilla White according to following formula (29):

$$\text{age (years)} \times 100 + 1{,}000 = \text{daily energy requirements (kcal)}.$$

The recommended amount of carbohydrates in daily energy intake varies worldwide. In some countries, it is between 60 and 70%, while in others, such as Europe, it is between 45 and 60%. The International Society for Pediatric and Adolescent Diabetes (ISPAD) recommends that carbohydrates should cover at least 50% of daily energy intake (Table 1) (30). Studies have shown that the higher the percentage of carbohydrates, the lower the consumption of fat.

Daily consumption of fiber is recommended to be around 14 g/1,000 kcal. In other words, for children older than 2 years, daily needs of fiber (in g) are equal with child's age (in years) plus five (31).

Fat consumption should not exceed 35% of daily energy intake in children older than 4 years. To prevent the development of cardiovascular diseases (CVDs) later in life, it is important to avoid triglycerides with saturated (animal fat) and *trans*-unsaturated fatty acids (cookies, chocolate, sweets). Otherwise, the consumption of polyunsaturated fatty acids (PUFA) of herbal or vegetarian origin or omega-3-fatty acids is recommended (Table 1) (31).

The calculation of daily protein needs depends on age, gender, and stage of the somatic development of the child. It varies between 1.2 and 0.8 g per kg body weight per day. This corresponds to 10–15% of the daily energy intake (Table 1) (31).

Table 1
Distribution of Elementary Nutrients in the Daily Energy Intake in Children and Adolescents *(30)*

Carbohydrates >50%
Prefer complex, non-affine, fiber-rich carbohydrates
Moderate saccharose intake
Fat 30–35%
Less than 10% saturated fatty acids
Less than 10% polyunsaturated fatty acids
More than 10% monounsaturated fatty acids
Protein 10–15%
Less protein with increasing age

Children and adolescents have higher daily fluid requirements compared with adults. Daily fluid intake corresponds to 10–15% of child's body weight, whereas this is only 2–4% in adults. Usually food items consumed by children are more rich in fluids than those of adults: solid foods contain ~60–70% water, fruits and vegetable almost 90%.

In summary, the following three rules for food consumption could benefit everybody in choosing healthy food for children and adolescents:

- Abundantly: fluids (possibly energy-free) and plant-based foods
- Moderately: animal products (fat reduced)
- Thriftily: food rich in fat and sugar

For the education of nonobese patients with type 1 diabetes, visual aids like the food guide pyramid by the US Health Department and Human Services are used (Fig. 1). Food guide pyramids (such as in Fig. 1 and/or the newer pyramids, see in appendix and at http://mypyramid.com) suggest optimal nutrition guidelines for each food category, using a mnemonic graphic of a pyramid with horizontal dividing lines to represent suggested percentages of the daily intake for each food group. For younger children, age-adjusted food pyramids such as the *aid infodienst*-pyramid are incorporated into their training programs (Fig. 2). This uses the traffic light system to indicate recommended consumption of nutrients (green = abundant, yellow = moderate, red = thriftily), modules of servings equal to child's hand size and the 6-5-4-3-2-1-rule *(32)*.

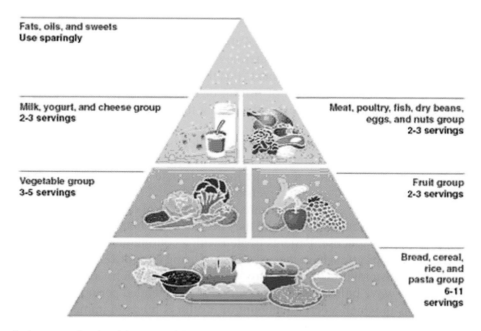

Fig. 1. A recent food guide pyramid by the US Health Department and Human Services. The food guide pyramids suggest optimal nutrition guidelines for each food category, per day, using a mnemonic graphic of a pyramid with horizontal dividing lines to represent suggested percentages of the daily diet for each food group. This food guide pyramid was recently replaced with the new food guide pyramid (see appendix and http://mypyramid.com).

Die 🔲🔲🔲-Ernährungspyramide
Gemüse plus

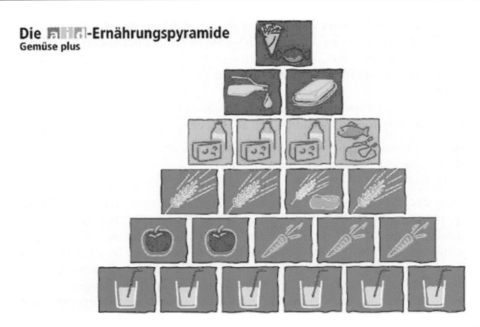

Fig. 2. German example of food pyramid for children using the traffic light system to indicate recommended consume of nutrients (*green* = abundant, *yellow* = moderate, *red* = thriftily), modules of servings equal to child's hand size and the 6-5-4-3-2-1-rule *(32)*. Copyright: aid infodienst.

1.3. Nutrition and Treatment of Type 1 Diabetes

For individuals receiving "conventional therapy," which is defined as prebreakfast and presupper injections of short and intermediate acting insulin, food should be kept consistent in terms of timing and amount. For those using "intensive therapy," which consists of three or more injections of insulin or use of an insulin pump, individuals should be taught to adjust their meal and snack at the times of insulin doses based on their total carbohydrate content.

Current knowledge about the content of carbohydrates in the daily nutrition of patients with type 1 diabetes suggests using different goals depending on the type of treatment. Patients treated with conventional therapy must calculate the amount of carbohydrate to avoid decreases of blood glucose levels after insulin injection. Patients treated with intensified insulin regimes should be aware of the amount of carbohydrate in their food in order to calculate the amount of insulin they need to avoid nonphysiological increases of postprandial blood glucose. Patients treated with a continuous subcutaneous insulin infusion (CSII) pump system have the possibility of using three different kinds of boluses to regulate their postprandial glycemic profiles: normal bolus delivering insulin rapidly as a shot, square-wave bolus delivering insulin for an extended period of time (h), and dual-wave bolus in which a certain amount of insulin is released immediately and the rest over an extended period of time *(33)*. Use of dual-wave bolus may be more effective than the use of a normal bolus to control postprandial glucose profile after meals rich in carbohydrates and fat *(33)*.

To achieve optimal glycemic profiles during conventional insulin treatment, food intake has to be distributed in frequent and small meals. A dietary plan consists mostly of three main meals (breakfast, lunch, and dinner), two snacks in between and one more before bedtime. During intensified insulin treatment with differentiated basal and prandial insulin substitution, however, patients are very flexible in their daily routine. They can decide when and how much they want to eat. The most important prerequisite is their ability to know and estimate the nutrient content of meals to calculate the amount of insulin they need for the planned meal.

Several methods can be used to estimate the nutrient content of meals, including carbohydrate counting, the exchange system, and experience-based estimation. The DAFNE (Dose Adjustment for Normal Eating) study demonstrated that patients can learn how to use glucose testing to better match insulin to carbohydrate intake (34,35). Improvement in HbA1c without a significant increase in severe hypoglycemia was demonstrated, as were positive effects on quality of life, satisfaction with treatment, and psychological well-being, even though increases in the number of insulin injections and blood glucose tests were necessary.

For planned exercise, reduction in insulin dosage is the preferred method to prevent hypoglycemia. For unplanned exercise, intake of additional carbohydrate is usually needed. Moderate-intensity exercise increases glucose utilization by 2–3 mg/kg/min above usual requirements (1). For that reason, high to normal levels of blood glucose between 150 and 180 mg/dL are the aim before physical activities. Patients on insulin treatment are educated to eat 10–15 g of carbohydrates before sports if blood glucose levels are below 150 mg/dL.

MNT has been reported to decrease HbA1c by ~1% in type 1 diabetic patients (36).

2. TYPE 2 DIABETES

2.1. Nutrition and Prevention of Type 2 Diabetes

For individuals at risk for diabetes or who have prediabetes, the goals of MNT are to decrease diabetes and CVD risk by encouraging moderate weight loss maintained by healthy food choices and physical activity (36). Evidence from epidemiologic studies suggests that certain individual foods and dietary patterns may help prevent type 2 diabetes. There is also accumulating evidence from clinical trials in favor of lifestyle changes that incorporate moderate weight loss and increasing leisure time physical activity. Use of certain medications could also achieve similar goals but use of medications for this purpose is not considered cost-effective and is not currently recommended.

Epidemiologic evidence suggests that certain dietary components and overall diet-quality may reduce the risk of developing type 2 diabetes. An evaluation of available observational studies found strong evidence that a diet high in soluble or insoluble fiber can reduce the risk of type 2 diabetes. Somewhat weaker evidence suggests an association between diets low in glycemic index and reduced risk of disease (37). Prospective cohort studies also suggest that diets higher in whole grains, cereal fiber, and magnesium may lower the risk of type 2 diabetes (38). Certain individual foods such as coffee (39,40) and nuts (41) have also been associated with reduced diabetes risk in cohort studies, while increased consumption of meat (42–44) and sugar-sweetened beverages (45) may increase the risk. Interestingly, our own studies have recently demonstrated that these beneficial diets also increase circulating levels of adiponectin, an adipocyte-secreted hormone and levels of which are a strong inverse predictor of insulin resistance and diabetes *(46–48)*. Prospective investigations also suggest that certain healthy dietary patterns may help prevent diabetes. In an analysis of 80,029 women from the Nurses' Health Study, those with the highest adherence to a healthy diet, as measured by the Alternative Healthy Eating Index, had lower risk of type 2 diabetes during 18 years of follow-up (RR = 0.64, 95% CI 0.58–0.71) *(49)*. Benefits of many individual dietary components in reducing the risk of diabetes have yet to be confirmed by interventional studies.

Prospective studies suggest that even modest sustained weight loss is associated with dramatically reduced risk of type 2 diabetes *(50,51)*. Leisure time physical activity has also been associated with lower risk of developing diabetes mellitus in cohort studies *(52–54)*, including moderate activities such as walking *(55)*. Recent interventional studies have sought to determine whether a combined program of moderate weight loss and physical activity can prevent type 2 diabetes among those at high risk. The Diabetes Prevention Program *(56)* randomized trial compared the effects of placebo, metformin, and intensive lifestyle intervention on prevention of type 2 diabetes in 3,234 subjects with impaired glucose tolerance. The goal of the lifestyle-modification intervention was to achieve 7% weight loss through a low-calorie, low-fat diet and to engage in at least 150 min of physical activity per week. After an average follow-up of 2.8 years, the incidence rate of diabetes was 11.0, 7.8, and 4.8 cases per 100 person-years in the placebo, metformin, and lifestyle groups, respectively. Incidence of type 2 diabetes was reduced by 58% in the lifestyle group and by 31% in the metformin group compared with placebo *(56)*. The Finnish Diabetes Prevention Study also found that a similar intensive lifestyle intervention involving dietary counseling and increased physical activity resulted in improved glucose levels, lipid markers, and BMI after 3 years compared with controls *(57)*. Extended follow-up of this study found that those who participated in the lifestyle intervention continued to have reduced risk of type 2 diabetes for years after the intervention ended *(58)*.

2.2. Nutrition and Treatment of Type 2 Diabetes

2.2.1. GOALS

There are several goals of MNT for individuals with diabetes, as recommended by the American Diabetes Association (ADA). The first goal is for the patient to achieve and maintain blood glucose levels in the normal range or as close to normal as is safely possible *(36)*. The ADA guidelines for normal blood glucose levels are as follows: Hemoglobin A1c (HbA1c) <6.5%, preprandial plasma glucose <110 mg/dL, and postprandial glucose <140 mg/dL. Another aim of MNT is to aid patients with diabetes in achieving and maintaining a lipid and lipoprotein profile that reduces their risk for vascular disease *(36)*. This includes the maintenance of optimal LDL-C levels, HDL-C levels, triglycerides, and total cholesterol. Effective MNT should also allow patients to achieve blood pressure levels in the normal range or as close to normal as is safely possible and to achieve a healthy BMI.

After diagnosis, medical nutrition therapists can use the initial consultation framework provided by the American Dietetic Associations Care Manual *(59)* in developing their initial care plan. Although every patient interaction will be different and the care plan will undoubtedly be tailored to reflect this, the framework can be helpful in providing consistency of care to all patients. When working with a patient who has been recently diagnosed with diabetes, the framework recommends educating the patient on basic nutrition, diabetes nutrition guidelines, and beginning strategies for altering eating patterns. Continuing self-management counseling includes both management skills and lifestyle changes. Flexibility in food planning should always be addressed. Topics emphasized or chosen are based on the following factors related to the individual *(59)*: choice, lifestyle, levels of nutrition knowledge, and experience in planning, purchasing, and preparing foods and meals. After the initial visit, it is important to establish a timeline for follow-up, which helps to identify expected outcomes (e.g., preprandial and postprandial blood glucose goals) and determine response to and effectiveness of nutritional care.

Patients with diabetes cannot rely on counting calories alone since carbohydrates are the major determinant of postprandial glucose levels. The amount of carbohydrate ingested is usually the primary determinant of postprandial response, but the type of carbohydrate can also have an effect. Patients may have the impression that there is a diabetic diet and that once type 2 diabetes is diagnosed all sugar(s) must be avoided. In reality, people with diabetes can eat the same foods as those who do not have the disease, but they must be sure to match insulin and insulin secretagogues to the carbohydrate content of their meals. Patients can be educated to do this in a variety of ways including the use of exchange lists and carbohydrate counting, the most widely used method. In educating a patient on carbohydrate counting, the first step is to teach the patient which foods contain carbohydrates (starches, fruits, starchy vegetables, milk, and sweets). For diabetes meal planning, one serving of a food with carbohydrates has about 15 g of carbohydrates. The number of grams of carbohydrates that a person can eat each day or at each meal is determined by factors such as the patient's weight, whether or not a calorie-restricted diet to induce weight loss is necessary, timing, and type of physical activity, and medications. For many adults, eating 3–5 servings of carbohydrate foods at each meal and one or two carbohydrate servings for each snack is effective. A meal plan that incorporates carbohydrate counting would highlight the number of servings to select per meal to avoid exceeding the amount of grams of carbohydrates per meal. This structure and consistency is a major tool in maintaining glucose control. Research has not demonstrated that one method of assessing the relationship between carbohydrate intake and blood glucose response is better than another. However, it is very important that individuals adhere to a system that they understand and which they can follow consistently – whether it is carbohydrate counting, the exchange system, or monitoring carbohydrate using experienced-based estimation.

In the US, the recommended daily allowance for carbohydrates is 130 g/day. Since there is no data regarding very low intake of carbohydrates specifically in patients with diabetes, diets restricting total carbohydrates to <130 g/day are not recommended in the management of diabetes. High-carbohydrate diets (55% of total energy from carbohydrates) increase postprandial plasma glucose, insulin, and triglycerides when compared with high-monounsaturated fat diets *(60)*, but diets restricting carbohydrates to <130 g/day have not been proven to be sustainable.

Individuals with diabetes should be encouraged to consume vegetables, fruits, legumes, and whole and minimally processed grains as their major source of carbohydrates. Refined carbohydrates or processed grains and starchy foods (especially pasta, white bread, low-fiber cereal, and white potatoes) are not recommended and should be consumed in limited quantities.

Current guidelines recommend at least 14 g/1,000 kcal of fiber per day for a healthy individual. For type 2 diabetics, available evidence suggests that consuming a high-fiber diet of at least 50 g of fiber per day leads to reduction in glycemia, hyperinsulinemia, and lipemia by slowing down the digestion of carbohydrates *(61)*. However, a goal of 50 g/day may not be realistic for the majority of the population due to barriers including taste and gastrointestinal side effects. These side effects can be diminished by increasing fiber in the diet gradually (~3–5 g/day) until the recommended goal is met and by increasing fluid intake. Increased fiber intake can be achieved by choosing a variety of fiber-containing foods such as legumes, fiber-rich cereals (>5 g fiber/serving), fruits, vegetables, and whole grain products, all of which provide vitamins, minerals, and other substances important for good health.

With respect to dietary fat, the primary goal for individuals with diabetes is to limit saturated fatty acids, *trans*-fatty acids, and cholesterol intake to reduce the risk for CVD. Saturated and *trans*-fatty acids are the principal dietary determinants of plasma LDL cholesterol. In nondiabetic individuals, reducing saturated and *trans*-fatty acids and cholesterol intakes decreases plasma total and LDL cholesterol *(62)*. Saturated and *trans*-fat should make up <10% *(59)* of caloric intake, but the most current recommendations state that <7% of the diet should consist of saturated fat alone *(36)*. Foods high in saturated fat, including beef, pork, lamb, and high fat dairy products (e.g., cream cheese, whole milk, or full fat cheese) are not recommended and should be consumed only in small amounts. Foods high in *trans*-fats (e.g., fast foods, commercially baked goods, some margarines) should also be avoided.

Fat restriction to <30% of the diet can decrease total and LDL cholesterol as well as obesity *(63,64)*. However, it is important to notice when patients consuming a low fat diet begin to supplement their diet with a greater proportion of carbohydrates. High carbohydrate intake leads to increased postprandial blood glucose and increased fasting triglycerides *(65)*. Because of these nuances, it is very important to individualize fat and carbohydrate intake for optimal results in a particular patient. If a low-fat diet is not producing desired outcomes, it may be necessary to shift ratios and evaluate caloric intake *(66)*.

Certain types of fat may have beneficial effects for individuals with diabetes. In those individuals who are already hyperlipidemic, studies have shown that mono and polyunsaturated fats have beneficial effects on lipid profiles *(67)*. Very-long-chain n-3 polyunsaturated fatty acid supplements have been shown to lower plasma triglyceride levels in individuals with type 2 diabetes who are hypertriglyceridemic. Although the accompanying small rise in plasma LDL cholesterol is of concern, an increase in HDL cholesterol may offset this concern *(68)*. Recommended fats such as olive oil and walnuts, which have high mono and polyunsaturated fats, should displace high saturated fat and *trans* fat-containing foods from the diet. Other recommended mono and polyunsaturated fats include canola oil, nuts/ seeds, and fish, particularly those high in omega-3 fatty acids. For instance, oily fish (e.g., salmon, herring, trout, sardines, fresh tuna) two times a week is an ample source of omega 3 fatty acids. More details about supplemental dose, if taken as a pill, can be found in the relevant chapter of this book.

Plant sterol and stanol esters block the intestinal absorption of dietary and biliary cholesterol. In the general public and in individuals with type 2 diabetes *(21)*, intake of 2 g/day plant sterols and stanols has been shown to lower plasma total and LDL cholesterol *(36)*.

Currently, there is a wide range of new food products that contain plant sterols. Because these are fats which carry 9 cal/g, it should be advised that, like mono and polyunsaturated fats, these should be avoided to prevent weight gain. Supplements are also available.

Individuals with diabetes have the same needs for protein as those who do not have diabetes. The Dietary Reference Intakes' acceptable macronutrient distribution range for protein is 10–35% of energy intake, with 15% being the average adult intake in the US and Canada (69). There are some special considerations related to protein for anyone that shows signs of kidney disease. Protein intake for those with renal problems will need to be modified. A diet that includes a lower amount of protein is recommended for these patients, but it is important to emphasize that protein does not need to be lowered to a point that may jeopardize the overall nutrition quality of their diet, and thus a nephrologist should be consulted before making any dietary changes. Although there is no evidence that strongly supports reduction of protein intake in diabetics without renal complications, studies have shown that in subjects with diabetes and microalbuminuria, reduction of protein intake to 0.8–1.0 g/kg/day decreased urinary albumin excretion rate and decreased rate of decline in glomerular filtration. This requires patients to limit meat, fish, and poultry intake to 3–5 oz/day, which may be difficult for some patients to achieve at first. Because individuals with diabetes are at an increased risk for cardiac disease, it is suggested that they first try to decrease protein in their diet from animal sources high in saturated fats. Favorable protein sources include fish, skinless poultry, nonfat or low-fat dairy, legumes, tofu, and tempeh. There is no evidence at this time to suggest that vegetable proteins have any nephrotoxic effects and these do not need to be limited.

High-protein diets are not recommended as a method for weight loss at this time. Although high protein diets may be effective at producing short-term weight loss results and improved blood glucose control, the long-term effects of protein intake >20% of calories on diabetes management and its complications, including effects on the kidneys, remain unknown.

Alternative sweeteners may be used to reduce sugar intake for diabetics. Sorbitol, mannitol, and fructose are commonly used sweeteners that have a lower glycemic effect than glucose or sucrose. However, they do contain the same amount of calories as glucose and sucrose (4 cal/g), a fact that is usually forgotten. Sorbitol and mannitol may cause bloating and diarrhea when >30 g/day are consumed (66). Though fructose produces a lower postprandial glucose response when it replaces sucrose or starch in the diet, there are concerns that it may adversely affect the lipid profile. Reduced calorie sweeteners approved by the FDA include sugar alcohols such as erythritol, isomalt, lactitol, maltitol, mannitol, sorbitol, xylitol, tagatose, and hydrogenated starch hydrolysates. Sugar alcohols contain about 2 cal/g. When calculating carbohydrate content of foods containing sugar alcohols, subtraction of half the sugar alcohol grams from total carbohydrate grams is appropriate. There is no evidence at this time to suggest that the amounts of sugar alcohols likely to be consumed will reduce glycemia, energy intake, or weight. The use of sugar alcohols appears to be safe; however, like sorbitol and mannitol, they may cause gastrointestinal upset. The FDA has approved five nonnutritive sweeteners for use in the US. These are acesulfame potassium, aspartame, neotame, saccharin, and sucralose, compounds that are 200 times sweeter than sugar, allowing their use in very small quantities. This makes them beneficial to diabetics because they add virtually no caloric or nutritional value to food (65). However, they may be used in foods that contain other sources of carbohydrates and calories such as ice cream, cookies, and puddings. Thus, not only the energy these compounds provide but total energy must be taken into account *(1)*.

Complete abstinence from alcohol is not necessary for diabetics. If alcohol is consumed, intake should be consistent with the 2005 USDA Dietary Guidelines for Americans, which recommend no more than one drink per day for women and two drinks per day for men. For education purposes, one alcohol containing beverage is defined as 12 oz beer, 5 oz wine, or 1.5 oz distilled spirits. Each contains >15 g alcohol. Alcohol itself has minimal effects on plasma glucose and serum insulin levels. However, when coingested with carbohydrates, blood glucose may rise. Diabetic patients should note that, when using insulin or insulin secretagogues, alcohol should be consumed with food to avoid hypoglycemia *(1,66)*. Alcohol should be avoided in patients with hypertriglyceridemia, however, because it causes increased elevation in postprandial triglyceride levels *(65)*.

Individuals with diabetes should be aware of the importance of acquiring daily vitamin and mineral requirements from natural food sources and a balanced diet. In select groups such as the elderly, pregnant, or lactating women, strict vegetarians, or those on calorie-restricted diets, a multivitamin supplement may be needed *(66)*. Uncontrolled diabetes is often associated with micronutrient deficiencies. With regard to antioxidants, there is no clear evidence that they improve glycemic control and long-term complications of diabetes. In contrast, there is some evidence of possible harm in taking high doses of antioxidant supplements such as vitamin E and carotene. Finally, there is no evidence at this time that antioxidant supplementation has any role in the prevention of CVD *(1)*.

Chromium, potassium, magnesium, and possibly zinc deficiency may aggravate carbohydrate intolerance. Serum levels of potassium and magnesium can be checked and should be replaced as needed, but there is no clear evidence that zinc or chromium replacement benefit those with diabetes, although definitive trials have yet to be performed. Thus, it is uncertain whether herbal or vitamin supplementation is beneficial to individuals with diabetes unless there is an established micronutrient deficiency. Because commercially available products are not standardized, vary in the content of active ingredients, and have the potential to interact with other medications, it is important that health care providers are aware of the use of these products by their diabetic patients. The following popular herbals have been shown to lower blood glucose (an effect which may potentially interact with blood glucose lowering medications): Ginseng (*Panax ginseng*); Fenugreek (*Trigonella foenum-graecum*); Bitter Melon (*Momordica charantia*); Garlic (*Allium sativum*). Their intake should also be taken under consideration by practicing physicians.

3. EXERCISE

3.1. Overview

Exercise increases both insulin sensitivity and uptake in skeletal muscle during and after activity. Exercise, unless otherwise contraindicated, should thus be included in all diabetic treatment regimens, whether the individual is overweight or of normal body weight, unless it is otherwise contraindicated. Exercise is the best predictor of sustained weight loss and, notably, it decreases central body fat (which is highly associated with insulin resistance and CVD). The greatest benefit that diabetics gain from regular exercise is reduction of cardiovascular risk factors including reduction in blood pressure, lowering very low density and low density lipoproteins as well as triglycerides, and improvement of the lipid profile. Exercise also raises high density lipoproteins.

Prolonged exercise can potentiate the effect of oral agents as well as the effect of insulin on blood glucose levels. It may also reduce hepatic glucose output and decrease both fasting and postprandial glycemia. Because its insulin sensitizing effects taper after 48 h, people should engage in at least 150 min/week of moderate-intensity aerobic physical activity 3–4 times weekly, without intervals of more than 48 h in between sessions. Resistance training is also effective in improving glycemia, and, in the absence of proliferative retinopathy, people with type 2 diabetes can be encouraged to perform resistance exercise three times a week.

However, if weight loss is the goal, it may be necessary to exercise 5–6 times per week. Individuals should gradually increase duration and intensity of exercise as is tolerable. Because of the hypoglycemic effects of exercise, patients should monitor their glucose and try to avoid hypoglycemia. With the introduction of regular exercise into the treatment regimen, patients will likely require less insulin and may reduce their need for oral agents.

Most patients can safely engage in light walking; however, it may be necessary to perform cardiac stress testing before patients can engage in regular strenuous exercise. A stress test is highly recommended for inactive people who are planning to start an exercise regimen above the age of 35 years. Strenuous exercise is contraindicated in individuals with significant diabetic complications including active proliferative retinopathy, neuropathy, and established significant CVD *(70,71)*.

Patients should be encouraged to choose their own modes of physical activity. Sustained interest in the exercise program is the key for long-term maintenance, and thus will have the greatest impact on achievement of weight, lipid profile and glycemic goals as well as prevention of complications of diabetes *(72)*. Precautions should be taken for patients taking agents such as adrenergic blocking agents, alcohol, or salicylates, which might make patients more susceptible to exercise-induced hypoglycemia.

4. CONCLUSION

In conclusion, MNT benefits patients with all forms of diabetes, and in the case of type 2 diabetes, it is the single most important intervention for prevention and treatment. Achieving the goals of MNT requires the efforts of a multidisciplinary team with expertise in behavioral techniques focusing on dietary change as well as exercise therapy. MNT goals should include attention to weight, lipid profile, and glycemic status to have its greatest impact on cardiovascular improvement.

REFERENCES

1. Bantle JP, Wylie-Rosett J, Albright AL et al. Nutrition recommendations and interventions for diabetes–2006: a position statement of the American Diabetes Association. Diabetes Care 2006; 29(9):2140–2157.
2. Soltesz G. Diabetes in the young: a paediatric and epidemiological perspective. Diabetologia 2003; 46(4):447–454.
3. Blom L, Dahlquist G, Nystrom L, Sandstrom A, Wall S. The Swedish childhood diabetes study–social and perinatal determinants for diabetes in childhood. Diabetologia 1989; 32(1):7–13.

4. Dahlquist G, Blom L, Lonnberg G. The Swedish Childhood Diabetes Study–a multivariate analysis of risk determinants for diabetes in different age groups. Diabetologia 1991; 34(10):757–762.

5. Virtanen SM, Rasanen L, Ylonen K et al. Early introduction of dairy products associated with increased risk of IDDM in Finnish children. The Childhood in Diabetes in Finland Study Group. Diabetes 1993; 42(12):1786–1790.

6. Kostraba JN, Cruickshanks KJ, Lawler-Heavner J et al. Early exposure to cow's milk and solid foods in infancy, genetic predisposition, and risk of IDDM. Diabetes 1993; 42(2):288–295.

7. Gerstein HC. Cow's milk exposure and type I diabetes mellitus. A critical overview of the clinical literature. Diabetes Care 1994; 17(1):13–19.

8. Harrison LC, Honeyman MC. Cow's milk and type 1 diabetes: the real debate is about mucosal immune function. Diabetes 1999; 48(8):1501–1507.

9. Norris JM, Scott FW. A meta-analysis of infant diet and insulin-dependent diabetes mellitus: do biases play a role?. Epidemiology 1996; 7(1):87–92.

10. Rosenbauer J, Herzig P, Kaiser P, Giani G. Early nutrition and risk of Type 1 diabetes mellitus–a nation-wide case-control study in preschool children. Exp Clin Endocrinol Diabetes 2007; 115(8):502–508.

11. TRIGR Study Group. Study design of the Trial to Reduce IDDM in the Genetically at Risk (TRIGR). Pediatr Diabetes 2007; 8(3):117–137.

12. Norris JM, Barriga K, Klingensmith G et al. Timing of initial cereal exposure in infancy and risk of islet autoimmunity. JAMA 2003; 290(13):1713–1720.

13. Couper JJ, Steele C, Beresford S et al. Lack of association between duration of breast-feeding or introduction of cow's milk and development of islet autoimmunity. Diabetes 1999; 48(11):2145–2149.

14. Akerblom HK, Virtanen SM, Ilonen J et al. Dietary manipulation of beta cell autoimmunity in infants at increased risk of type 1 diabetes: a pilot study. Diabetologia 2005; 48(5):829–837.

15. Ziegler AG, Schmid S, Huber D, Hummel M, Bonifacio E. Early infant feeding and risk of developing type 1 diabetes-associated autoantibodies. JAMA 2003; 290(13):1721–1728.

16. Arnson Y, Amital H, Shoenfeld Y. Vitamin D and autoimmunity: new aetiological and therapeutic considerations. Ann Rheum Dis 2007; 66(9):1137–1142.

17. Saggese G, Federico G, Balestri M, Toniolo A. Calcitriol inhibits the PHA-induced production of IL-2 and IFN-gamma and the proliferation of human peripheral blood leukocytes while enhancing the surface expression of HLA class II molecules. J Endocrinol Invest 1989; 12(5):329–335.

18. Vitamin D supplement in early childhood and risk for Type I (insulin-dependent) diabetes mellitus. The EURODIAB Substudy 2 Study Group. Diabetologia 1999; 42(1):51–54.

19. Hypponen E, Laara E, Reunanen A, Jarvelin MR, Virtanen SM. Intake of vitamin D and risk of type 1 diabetes: a birth-cohort study. Lancet 2001; 358(9292):1500–1503.

20. Holick MF, Chen TC. Vitamin D deficiency: a worldwide problem with health consequences. Am J Clin Nutr 2008; 87(4):1080S–1086S.

21. Lee YM, Haastert B, Scherbaum W, Hauner H. A phytosterol-enriched spread improves the lipid profile of subjects with type 2 diabetes mellitus–a randomized controlled trial under free-living conditions. Eur J Nutr 2003; 42(2):111–117.

22. Stene LC, Joner G. Use of cod liver oil during the first year of life is associated with lower risk of childhood-onset type 1 diabetes: a large, population-based, case-control study. Am J Clin Nutr 2003; 78(6):1128–1134.

23. Nettleton JA. Are n-3 fatty acids essential nutrients for fetal and infant development? J Am Diet Assoc 1993; 93(1):58–64.

24. Delvin EE, Salle BL, Glorieux FH, Adeleine P, David LS. Vitamin D supplementation during pregnancy: effect on neonatal calcium homeostasis. J Pediatr 1986; 109(2):328–334.

25. Stene LC, Ulriksen J, Magnus P, Joner G. Use of cod liver oil during pregnancy associated with lower risk of Type I diabetes in the offspring. Diabetologia 2000; 43(9):1093–1098.

26. Krebs NF, Jacobson MS. Prevention of pediatric overweight and obesity. Pediatrics 2003; 112(2):424–430.

27. Hall DM, Cole TJWhat use is the BMI?. Arch Dis Child 2006; 91(4):283–286.

28. Reinehr T, de SG, Toschke AM, Andler W. Comparison of metabolic syndrome prevalence using eight different definitions: a critical approach. Arch Dis Child 2007; 92(12):1067–1072.

29. White P, Graham CA. The child with diabetes. In: Marble A, White P, Bradley RF, Krall LP, editors. Joslin's Diabetes mellitus. Philadelphia: Lea & Febinger; 1971, p. 339ff.

30. ISPAD Guidelines 2000. Zeist Netherlands: Medforum; 2000.

31. Gidding SS, Dennison BA, Birch LL et al. Dietary recommendations for children and adolescents: a guide for practitioners: consensus statement from the American Heart Association. Circulation 2005; 112(13):2061–2075.

32. aid infodienst e.V. Die aid-Ernahrungspyramide: Richtig essen lehren und lernen. Bonn: 2003.

33. Chase HP, Saib SZ, MacKenzie T, Hansen MM, Garg SK. Post-prandial glucose excursions following four methods of bolus insulin administration in subjects with type 1 diabetes. Diabet Med 2002; 19(4):317–321.

34. DAFNE Study Group. Training in flexible, intensive insulin management to enable dietary freedom in people with type 1 diabetes: dose adjustment for normal eating (DAFNE) randomised controlled trial. BMJ 2002; 325(7367):746.

35. Knowles J, Waller H, Eiser C et al. The development of an innovative education curriculum for 11–16 yr old children with type 1 diabetes mellitus (T1DM). Pediatr Diabetes 2006; 7(6):322–328.

36. Bantle JP, Wylie-Rosett J, Albright AL et al. Nutrition recommendations and interventions for diabetes: a position statement of the American Diabetes Association. Diabetes Care 2008; 31 Suppl 1:S61–S78.

37. Riccardi G, Rivellese AA, Giacco R. Role of glycemic index and glycemic load in the healthy state, in prediabetes, and in diabetes. Am J Clin Nutr 2008; 87(1):269S–274S.

38. Schulze MB, Hu FB Primary prevention of diabetes: what can be done and how much can be prevented?. Annu Rev Public Health 2005; 26:445–467.

39. Rosengren A, Dotevall A, Wilhelmsen L, Thelle D, Johansson S. Coffee and incidence of diabetes in Swedish women: a prospective 18-year follow-up study. J Intern Med 2004; 255(1):89–95.

40. Salazar-Martinez E, Willett WC, Ascherio A et al. Coffee consumption and risk for type 2 diabetes mellitus. Ann Intern Med 2004; 140(1):1–8.

41. Jiang R, Manson JE, Stampfer MJ, Liu S, Willett WC, Hu FB. Nut and peanut butter consumption and risk of type 2 diabetes in women. JAMA 2002; 288(20):2554–2560.

42. Fung TT, Schulze M, Manson JE, Willett WC, Hu FB. Dietary patterns, meat intake, and the risk of type 2 diabetes in women. Arch Intern Med 2004; 164(20):2235–2240.

43. Schulze MB, Manson JE, Willett WC, Hu FB. Processed meat intake and incidence of Type 2 diabetes in younger and middle-aged women. Diabetologia 2003; 46(11):1465–1473.

44. Song Y, Manson JE, Buring JE, Liu S. A prospective study of red meat consumption and type 2 diabetes in middle-aged and elderly women: the women's health study. Diabetes Care 2004; 27(9):2108–2115.

45. Schulze MB, Manson JE, Ludwig DS et al. Sugar-sweetened beverages, weight gain, and incidence of type 2 diabetes in young and middle-aged women. JAMA 2004; 292(8):927–934.

46. Mantzoros CS, Williams CJ, Manson JE, Meigs JB, Hu FB. Adherence to the Mediterranean dietary pattern is positively associated with plasma adiponectin concentrations in diabetic women. Am J Clin Nutr 2006; 84(2):328–335.

47. Qi L, Meigs JB, Liu S, Manson JE, Mantzoros C, Hu FB. Dietary fibers and glycemic load, obesity, and plasma adiponectin levels in women with type 2 diabetes. Diabetes Care 2006; 29(7):1501–1505.

48. Yannakoulia M, Yiannakouris N, Melistas L, Kontogianni MD, Malagaris I, Mantzoros CS. A dietary pattern characterized by high consumption of whole-grain cereals and low-fat dairy products and low consumption of refined cereals is positively associated with plasma adiponectin levels in healthy women. Metabolism 2008; 57(6):824–830.

49. Fung TT, McCullough M, van Dam RM, Hu FB. A prospective study of overall diet quality and risk of type 2 diabetes in women. Diabetes Care 2007; 30(7):1753–1757.

50. Resnick HE, Valsania P, Halter JB, Lin X. Relation of weight gain and weight loss on subsequent diabetes risk in overweight adults. J Epidemiol Community Health 2000; 54(8):596–602.

51. Moore LL, Visioni AJ, Wilson PW, D'Agostino RB, Finkle WD, Ellison RC, Can sustained weight loss in overweight individuals reduce the risk of diabetes mellitus?. Epidemiology 2000; 11(3):269–273.

52. Manson JE, Nathan DM, Krolewski AS, Stampfer MJ, Willett WC, Hennekens CH. A prospective study of exercise and incidence of diabetes among US male physicians. JAMA 1992; 268(1):63–67.

53. Manson JE, Rimm EB, Stampfer MJ et al. Physical activity and incidence of non-insulin-dependent diabetes mellitus in women. Lancet 1991; 338(8770):774–778.

54. Helmrich SP, Ragland DR, Leung RW, Paffenbarger RS, Jr. Physical activity and reduced occurrence of non-insulin-dependent diabetes mellitus. N Engl J Med 1991; 325(3):147–152.

55. Hu FB, Sigal RJ, Rich-Edwards JW et al. Walking compared with vigorous physical activity and risk of type 2 diabetes in women: a prospective study. JAMA 1999; 282(15):1433–1439.

56. Knowler WC, Barrett-Connor E, Fowler SE et al. Reduction in the incidence of type 2 diabetes with lifestyle intervention or metformin. N Engl J Med 2002; 346(6):393–403.

57. Lindstrom J, Louheranta A, Mannelin M et al. The Finnish Diabetes Prevention Study (DPS): lifestyle intervention and 3-year results on diet and physical activity. Diabetes Care 2003; 26(12):3230–3236.

58. Lindstrom J, Ilanne-Parikka P, Peltonen M et al. Sustained reduction in the incidence of type 2 diabetes by lifestyle intervention: follow-up of the Finnish Diabetes Prevention Study. Lancet 2006; 368(9548):1673–1679.

59. ADA. American Dietetic Association Care Manual; 2008.

60. Garg A, Bantle JP, Henry RR et al. Effects of varying carbohydrate content of diet in patients with non-insulin-dependent diabetes mellitus. JAMA 1994; 271(18):1421–1428.

61. Chandalia M, Garg A, Lutjohann D, von BK, Grundy SM, Brinkley LJ. Beneficial effects of high dietary fiber intake in patients with type 2 diabetes mellitus. N Engl J Med 2000; 342(19):1392–1398.

62. Schaefer EJ. Lipoproteins, nutrition, and heart disease. Am J Clin Nutr 2002; 75(2):191–212.

63. Ornish D, Scherwitz LW, Billings JH et al. Intensive lifestyle changes for reversal of coronary heart disease. JAMA 1998; 280(23):2001–2007.

64. Elmer PJ, Obarzanek E, Vollmer WM et al. Effects of comprehensive lifestyle modification on diet, weight, physical fitness, and blood pressure control: 18-month results of a randomized trial. Ann Intern Med 2006; 144(7):485–495.

65. Lau SH, editor. Nutrition. In: Medica Management of Non-Insulin-Dependent (Type II) Diabetes. 3 ed. Alexandria, VA: ADA; 1994, p. 45–67.

66. Franz MJ. Medical nutrition therapy. In: Davidson MB, editor. Diabetes mellitus Diagnosis and Treatment. 4 ed. Philadelphia, PA: WB Saunders; 1998, p. 45–79.

67. Lada AT, Rudel LL. Dietary monounsaturated versus polyunsaturated fatty acids: which is really better for protection from coronary heart disease? Curr Opin Lipidol 2003; 14(1):41–46.

68. West SG, Hecker KD, Mustad VA et al. Acute effects of monounsaturated fatty acids with and without omega-3 fatty acids on vascular reactivity in individuals with type 2 diabetes. Diabetologia 2005; 48(1):113–122.

69. Institute of Medicine. Dietary Reference Intakes: Energy, Carbohydrate, Fiber, Fat, Fatty Acids, Cholesterol, Protein and Amino Acids. Washington DC: Academies; 2002.

70. Albers AR, Krichavsky MZ, Balady GJ. Stress testing in patients with diabetes mellitus: diagnostic and prognostic value. Circulation 2006; 113(4):583–592.

71. ADA. Standards of medical care in diabetes. Diabetes Care 2005; 28 Suppl 1:S4–S36.

72. Lau SH. Exercise. In: Lau SH, editor. Medical Management of Non-Insulin-Dependent(Type II) Diabetes. 3 ed. Alexandria, VA: ADA; 1994, p. 36–39.

V

CLINICAL ASSESSMENT AND MANAGEMENT

14 Mediterranean Diet in Disease Prevention: Current Perspectives

Jessica Fargnoli, Yoon Kim, and Christos S. Mantzoros

KEY POINTS

- Populations living around the Mediterranean Sea experience increased longevity and reduced risk of cardiovascular diseases and cancers in relation to populations living in other regions of the world.
- Much of this health benefit has been attributed to the traditional dietary patterns of the inhabitants of the Mediterranean basin.
- The traditional Mediterranean dietary pattern is often characterized by high consumption of plant foods such as vegetables, fruits, legumes, and whole grains; use of olive oil as the primary source of fat; moderate intake of fish, poultry, dairy, and alcohol; and low consumption of red meat.
- Results from ecological, case–control, and cohort studies have suggested that consumption of a diet similar to a traditional Mediterranean dietary pattern may reduce the risk of chronic diseases such as the metabolic syndrome, type 2 diabetes, cardiovascular disease, and many cancers.
- Present scientific knowledge suggests that this dietary pattern may have more health benefits than other currently used diets for the prevention of several chronic diseases.

Key Words: Mediterranean diet, Metabolic syndrome, Diabetes, Cardiovascular disease, Cancer

1. INTRODUCTION

The "Mediterranean Diet" has been the focus of countless books, weight loss programs, and research investigations, steadily rising in popularity since its benefits were first noticed. In the 1950s, the scientific community began to observe that populations in the Mediterranean basin were far less susceptible to chronic diseases, such as cardiovascular disease (CVD), than populations in more westernized countries (1). These findings were certainly not due to an advantage in medical care. In fact, at that time socioeconomic indicators in many Mediterranean countries were lower when compared with more westernized countries (2). What, then, was responsible for these health

From: *Nutrition and Health: Nutrition and Metabolism*
Edited by: C.S. Mantzoros, DOI: 10.1007/978-1-60327-453-1_14,
© Humana Press, a part of Springer Science+Business Media, LLC 2009

benefits? The aspect of the Mediterranean lifestyle that the scientific community quickly focused on was the diet these populations consumed. This was largely due to information garnered from a groundbreaking cohort study undertaken by Ancel Keys. The Seven Countries Study began in 1958 and collected information on diet, lifestyle, and chronic disease in middle-aged men in the countries of Japan, Italy, Greece, the Netherlands, Finland, Yugoslavia, and the United States. This ecologic study was the first study to bring to light the mortality benefit enjoyed by the populations living in the Mediterranean basin *(1)* by demonstrating that inhabitants of Greece and southern Italy were less likely to develop cardiovascular disease compared with inhabitants of countries with a more westernized diet. This health benefit was thus linked to foods that abounded in the Mediterranean region at this time such as whole grains, legumes, a variety of fresh local and wild vegetables, seasonal fruits, seafood and fish, nuts, yogurt, wine, and perhaps most importantly, extra virgin olive oil.

2. WHAT CONSTITUTES A MEDITERRANEAN DIET?

Broadly defined, the Mediterranean Diet is the traditional dietary pattern of the population living in the olive-growing regions of the Mediterranean basin in the late 1950s and early 1960s. This may be misleading however, because there are many olive-growing countries in the Mediterranean region, with variations in culture and dietary patterns between them. This region spans southern Europe, northern Africa, and the Middle East, but research has focused mainly on the diets in the European countries of Spain, Greece, Italy, and France. However, dietary patterns are not uniform even among the European countries. For instance, a traditional Greek Mediterranean diet may include total fat intake of up to 40% of daily energy, depending on the region, while a traditional Italian Mediterranean diet is defined by a much lower total fat intake, less than 30% of daily energy *(3,4)*. The diet of Mediterranean Italy is characterized by higher intake of complex carbohydrates, mostly due to pasta consumption, while the diet of Spain is defined by a higher intake of fish *(5)*. Though there is variation among dietary patterns, the central characteristic of Mediterranean cuisine is high olive oil consumption. A rich source of monounsaturated fat, olive oil has been widely studied for its health benefits. In addition to its own beneficial properties, olive oil may encourage higher consumption of vegetables and legumes. Since olive oil is the major source of fat in most traditional Mediterranean cooking, the resulting diets are very low in saturated fat, as low as 8% of daily energy intake in the areas where Keys first noticed the health benefit *(1)*. Likely as a result of its use of olive oil, the entire Mediterranean region has higher ratios of monounsaturated fatty acid (MUFA) intake to saturated fatty acid (SFA) intake than other regions of the world *(5)*. Many have attributed the lower risk of CVD in the Mediterranean region to this aspect of the diet. Furthermore, it appears that the percentage of total fat in the diet is not as significant as the ratio of poly and monounsaturated fat to saturated and *trans*-fat for CVD prevention *(6)*. Dietary recommendations in the USA and elsewhere were strongly influenced by this discovery, and as saturated fat was replaced with polyunsaturated fat over the next 25 years, CVD rates declined by about 50% in the USA, the UK, and Australia *(7)*. Emphasis has also been placed on the increased consumption of vegetables and fish and the decreased consumption of meat in the Mediterranean region. The area's reduced cancer and CVD rates have been partially attributed to the high intake of fruits and vegetables *(8,9)* and the low intake of red meat

(5,10). Moreover, diets high in fish and n-3 fatty acids have been shown to be beneficial for the prevention of cardiovascular disease *(10)*. Research increasingly points to the Mediterranean dietary pattern as a possible explanation for the longevity of populations living in this area; however, other aspects of the relaxed Mediterranean lifestyle such as the after-lunch siesta and the presence of strong social networks cannot be ignored as potential contributors to good health and long life *(11)*.

3. DEFINING THE MEDITERRANEAN DIET

Initial public health efforts led to more research into the beneficial effects of the Mediterranean diet as a whole, and thus a need for a better definition of the dietary pattern emerged. At the International Conference on the Diets of the Mediterranean in 1993, the Mediterranean diet was defined as a dietary pattern composed of: abundant plant foods; minimally processed, seasonally fresh, and locally grown foods; fresh fruits as the typical daily dessert with sweets based on nuts, olive oil, and concentrated sugars or honey consumed during feast days; olive oil as the principal source of added fat; dairy products (mainly cheese and yogurt) consumed in low to moderate amounts; fewer than four eggs consumed per week; red meat consumed in low frequency amounts; and wine consumed in low to moderate amounts generally with meals *(12)*.

This definition was expanded upon in 1995 when a group of Harvard-led scientists created a Mediterranean dietary pyramid (Fig. 1) *(12)* consisting of (a) daily consumption: of nonrefined cereals and products (whole grain bread, pasta, brown rice, etc.), vegetables (2–3 servings/day), fruits (6 servings/day), olive oil (as the main added lipid) and dairy products (1–2 servings/day); (b) weekly consumption: of fish (4–5 servings/week), poultry (3–4 servings/week), olives, pulses, and nuts (3 servings/week), potatoes, eggs and sweets (3–4 servings/week); and (c) monthly consumption: of red meat and meat products (4–5 servings/month). It is also characterized by moderate consumption of wine (1–2 glasses/day) and high monounsaturated: saturated fat ratio (>2). Similar recommendations are included in a Greek Column Food Guide, created to take the Greek culture into account *(13)*.

In addition, many Mediterranean diet scores have been developed for investigational purposes. Trichopoulou et al. developed the Mediterranean Diet Score (MDS), which measures individuals' adherence to a traditional Greek-style Mediterranean diet pattern. It is scored in terms of eight components: (1) high ratio of monounsaturated to saturated fats; (2) moderate alcohol consumption; (3) high consumption of legumes; (4) high consumption of cereals; *(5)* high consumption of fruits; *(6)* high consumption of vegetables; *(7)* low consumption of meat and meat products; (8) low consumption of milk and dairy products *(14)*. Panagiotakos et al. also developed a diet score used to measure subjects' adherence to a Greek Mediterranean-type diet *(15–17)*. The MedDietScore is based on 11 components of the Mediterranean diet (nonrefined cereals, fruits, vegetables, potatoes, legumes, olive oil, fish, red meat, poultry, full fat dairy products, and alcohol) *(18,19)*. For each component, an individual is assigned a score from 0 to 5 based on their level of consumption; however, red meat, poultry, and full fat dairy products are scored on a reverse scale since they deviate from the Mediterranean diet. These are added together to create a Mediterranean diet scale from 0 to 55, with the highest score corresponding to the closest adherence to the dietary pattern. Alternatively, the Mediterranean Adequacy Index (MAI) is associated with individuals' adherence to

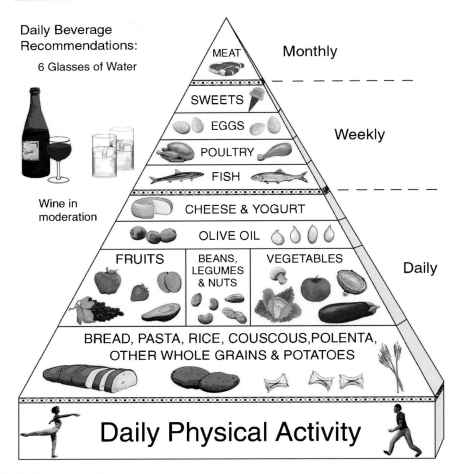

Fig. 1. Mediterranean diet pyramid.

a traditional Italian-style Mediterranean dietary pattern *(20)*. It uses as its reference the diet of Nicotera, Italy, in the 1960s, which was one of the rural areas studied in Keys' Seven Countries Study. The MAI is calculated by dividing the sum of the percentage of total energy from typical Mediterranean food groups (bread, cereals, legumes, potatoes, vegetables, fruit, fish, vegetable oils, and red wine) by the sum of the percentage of total energy from nontypical Mediterranean food groups (milk, cheese, meat, eggs, animal fats and margarines, cakes, pies, and cookies, and sugar) *(21)*. Of the three, the MAI has not been as widely studied. Several other measures of Mediterranean diet adherence exist and have been used in investigations *(22)*. Thus far, the scientific community has not defined one universal Mediterranean diet pattern, which may have ramifications when it comes to the generalizablility and comparability of investigational studies.

Unfortunately, as research has begun to uncover the benefits of a traditional Mediterranean diet, the diet of the Mediterranean region has progressively become more westernized since the 1960s. For example, three of the rural Italian towns, which were part of Keys' Seven Countries Study, now seem to be following a diet much more similar to the average Western diet than a traditional Mediterranean diet. When studied in the 1990s, the inhabitants of Nicotera, Crevalcore, and Montegiorgio were consuming much higher amounts of animal foods, cakes, cookies, and sweet beverages than at the commencement of the Seven Countries Study (23,24). As obesity rises to epidemic proportions and the dietary patterns of many cultures are increasingly westernized, research into the health benefits of a traditional Mediterranean diet becomes ever more necessary. The following chapter will discuss the current body of scientific evidence on the Mediterranean dietary pattern as a whole and its implications for the prevention of chronic disease, as well as the public health importance of further clinical research into the effects of this diet. Though sample sizes vary and different definitions of the Mediterranean diet have been implemented, the evidence consistently demonstrates the benefits of the Mediterranean dietary pattern on the metabolic syndrome and type 2 diabetes, cardiovascular disease and its risk factors, certain types of cancer, and overall mortality.

4. MEDITERRANEAN DIET AND CARDIOVASCULAR DISEASE

Attention was first drawn to the diet of the Mediterranean through anecdotal evidence about the significantly decreased prevalence of cardiovascular disease (CVD) in the region (25). The Seven Countries Study went on to demonstrate the reduced risk of CVD in the Mediterranean region, particularly in Crete, Greece (1). This led to further research into the cardio-protective effects of a diet high in unsaturated fat and low in saturated fat, as previously discussed. Similarly, other areas of the Mediterranean have also been shown to have cardiac benefits as well. For example, studies of middle-aged men in Finland, the Netherlands, and Italy have demonstrated that death rates from coronary heart disease are much lower in Italy (26).

Cross-sectional associations between Mediterranean diet and CVD risk factors have also been studied. A higher Mediterranean Diet Score has been associated with reduction in blood pressure (27) and an inverse relationship has been found between increased MedDietScore and hypercholesterolemia (28).

In general, case–control studies have confirmed and expanded upon links between CVD risk and the Mediterranean diet seen in population-based and cross-sectional research. A number of case-control studies on the Mediterranean diet have found positive effects on cardiovascular disease and cardiovascular risk factors including lipid profile, blood pressure, BMI, and inflammatory markers. The multi-center case-control CARDIO2000 study has shown inverse associations between adherence to a Mediterranean-type diet and risk of cardiovascular disease (29–33) and more specifically risk of developing nonfatal acute coronary syndromes. Participants were recruited from all parts of Greece and 848 hospitalized patients with a first event of an acute coronary syndrome were enrolled and compared with 1,078 people without any evidence of cardiovascular disease. Among a sample of 661 patients with a first event of myocardial infarction or unstable angina and 661 matched controls, adherence to a Mediterranean-type diet was associated with a 16% reduction in risk of developing acute coronary syndromes, even when controlling for exercise, smoking status, and various other cardiovascular risk factors (29). Adherence to the diet was also associated with reduced risk of diabetes mellitus and hypertension. Various substudies of the CARDIO2000 have found relationships between the Mediterranean diet and CVD among high-risk groups. Hypercholesterolemic patients following a Mediterranean-type diet in conjunction with statin treatment experienced an additional reduction in CVD risk of 43% *(30)*. In addition, CVD risk was lowered by 7–17% among controlled and uncontrolled hypertensive patients with a high adherence to a Mediterranean-type diet *(31)*. With the addition of moderate leisure-time physical activity, risk of CVD was reduced even further, by 11–25% *(32)*. Results from the CARDIO2000 were also promising for patients with the metabolic syndrome. Adoption of the Mediterranean diet by these subjects in this subgroup was associated with a 35% decline in risk for an acute coronary event, after adjusting for various potential confounders *(33)*. Results from the CARDIO2000 suggest that consuming a traditional Mediterranean diet could be invaluable for the prevention of CVD, even among high-risk groups.

In a case–control study conducted by Martinez-Gonzalez et al. in Spain, higher adherence to a Mediterranean-type diet led to a lower odds ratio of myocardial infarction among 171 patients compared with matched controls *(34)*. This relationship remained after adjustment for the main CVD risk factors.

The cardiovascular benefits of adhering to a Mediterranean dietary pattern have been affirmed by several prospective studies. Based on these studies, the Mediterranean diet may be advantageous for the primary and secondary prevention of CVD as well as the curbing of typical CVD risk factors. Recently, prospective analyses of the EPIC (European Prospective Investigation into Cancer and Nutrition) cohort in Greece have provided a wealth of information on a Mediterranean-type diet's effects on CVD prevention. This study was conducted in 22 research centers in ten European countries and was coordinated by the International Agency for Research on Cancer (IARC). A cohort of over 22,000 Greeks between the ages of 20 and 86 was recruited during a 5-year period (1994–1999). In this cohort, an inverse association between higher MDS scores and death due to coronary heart disease was shown. Better adherence to the Mediterranean diet conferred up to a 25% reduction in total mortality and 35% reduction in coronary heart disease mortality over a median 44 months of follow-up *(35)*. Additionally, Trichopoulou and colleagues showed an inverse association between greater adherence to the Mediterranean diet and death among persons with prevalent coronary heart disease in a Greek cohort *(36)*. Better adherence to the diet conferred up to a 27% reduction in total mortality. Associations between individual food groups corresponding to the Mediterranean diet and mortality were not significant, however.

Information from clinical trials has provided further evidence for the Mediterranean dietary pattern's cardiovascular benefits. First, a number of small, short-term interventional studies have examined the effect of the Mediterranean diet on the lipid profile. According to a recent review, Mediterranean-type diets, often being compared with a prudent Western diet as recommended by the American Heart Association, have been shown to lower VLDL, LDL, and triglycerides more than control diets *(37)*. Consuming a Mediterranean-type diet may lower total cholesterol by as much as 7.4% with an average decrease across studies of 2.7%. Among these studies, reductions in LDL cholesterol levels of up to 10.4% have been seen, with an average reduction of 4.0% across studies. Decreases in VLDL levels of as much as 35% have been seen as well, with an average decrease across studies of 17.5%. There is also a benefit for plasma triglyceride levels, which have been lowered by as much as 31.6% in intervention groups and an average of 10.2% among all the studies looked at. Moreover, studies looking at apolipoprotein B levels showed a decrease of 5.1% at most and on average a decrease of 3.7%. However, few studies have shown improvement in HDL levels among subjects following a Mediterranean-type diet. At best, the Mediterranean diet has been shown to increase HDL levels by 9.6%, but most interventions have shown no beneficial effect of the diet on HDL levels *(37)*.

The Mediterranean Diet, Cardiovascular Risks, and Gene Polymorphisms (Medi-RIVAGE) study also found promising results when looking at the Mediterranean diet's effects on traditional CVD risk factors *(38)*. Two hundred and twelve volunteers were randomized to either a Mediterranean-type diet or a low-fat American Heart Association type diet and followed for 3 months. The intervention group had an increased intake of fruit, vegetables, legumes, olive oil, nuts, and fish, along with a reduced intake of other vegetable oils, dairy products, and meat. Furthermore, this group had decreased glycemia, insulinemia, and HOMA scores after 3 months. Another interesting finding from this study was that subjects randomized to the Mediterranean diet group were more likely to remain in the study and had better compliance than subjects randomized to the low-fat diet group.

Results from clinical trials have also been promising concerning the primary and secondary prevention of CVD. The Prevención con Dieta Mediterránea (PREDIMED) Study, a large randomized trial in Spain, is currently investigating the effects of two different types of Mediterranean diet on CVD prevention *(39)*. Over 700 patients with at least one cardiac risk factor have been randomized to either an American Heart Association recommended low-fat diet, a Mediterranean-style diet supplemented with virgin olive oil, or a Mediterranean-style diet supplemented with mixed nuts. Follow-up is ongoing, but after 3 months, participants in both Mediterranean diet groups exhibited a reduction in hypertension, improvement in lipid panels, and hyperglycemia when compared with the low-fat diet group. The mean changes in the Mediterranean diet with olive oil group and the Mediterranean diet with nuts group were 0.39 mmol/L (95% CI, 0.70–0.07 mmol/L) and 0.30 mmol/L (CI, 0.58–0.01 mmol/L) for plasma glucose levels, respectively; 5.9 mmHg (CI, 8.7–3.1 mm Hg) and 7.1 mm Hg (CI, 10.0–4.1 mmHg) for systolic blood pressure, respectively; and 0.38 (CI, 0.55–0.22) and 0.26 (CI, 0.42–0.10) for the cholesterol-high-density lipoprotein cholesterol ratio, respectively. The Mediterranean diet with olive oil also reduced C-reactive protein levels by 0.54 mg/L (CI, 1.04–0.03 mg/L) compared with the low-fat diet. Initial results from this intervention suggest that consuming a Mediterranean-type diet may be beneficial for the primary prevention of CVD.

The Lyon Heart Study, a randomized trial, examined the effects of following a Mediterranean-type diet on overall survival and cardiovascular disease among patients with a history of myocardial infarction and found that a Mediterranean diet can be beneficial in secondary prevention of CVD. Participants followed either a cardio-protective Mediterranean-type diet or a control diet close to the step 1 American Heart Association prudent diet. Adherence was high, and those following the Mediterranean-type diet had significantly higher intakes of fruits, vegetables, and cereals, providing them with larger amounts of fiber and vitamin C *(40)*. In addition, the intakes of cholesterol and saturated and polyunsaturated fats were lower and those of oleic acid and omega-3 fatty acids were higher in subjects on the Mediterranean diet. After 2 years of follow-up, recurrent myocardial infarction, all other cardiovascular events, and cardiac and total death were reduced significantly by over 70% when compared with the control group *(11)*. At 4 years of follow-up, a significantly reduced risk of cardiovascular events was sustained in the Mediterranean diet group *(41)*. These results, which need to be confirmed, indicate that the Mediterranean diet may be more effective for the prevention of coronary heart disease than the diet recommended by the American Heart Association *(42,43)*.

5. MEDITERRANEAN DIET, THE METABOLIC SYNDROME, AND TYPE 2 DIABETES

A diet rich in traditional Mediterranean foods may also help prevent incidence of the metabolic syndrome and type 2 diabetes, which are both major public health concerns. Observational studies have shown that the prevalence of the metabolic syndrome is lower in the Mediterranean region than in other regions of the world *(15)*. The ATTICA study, which was conducted in Greece from 2001 to 2002, reported that the prevalence of the metabolic syndrome was 19.9% in this area *(15)*. This is lower than the prevalence of the syndrome in the US according to the National Health and Nutritional Exam Survey conducted in 1999–2000, which reported a prevalence of 26.7% *(44)*. After controlling for a number of demographic, lifestyle, and inflammatory markers, the investigators found the prevalence of the metabolic syndrome in subjects of the ATTICA study who adopted the Mediterranean diet to be 16.6%. This gave an absolute risk reduction of 3.3% and an odds ratio of 0.81. Higher adherence to a Mediterranean-type diet was also linked cross-sectionally to 7% lower blood glucose, 5% lower insulin levels, and a 15% lower HOMA-IR score in nondiabetics *(17)*. Furthermore, results from the ATTICA survey in Greece revealed a relationship between the MedDietScore and type 2 diabetes. A ten-unit increase in MedDietScore was associated with a 21% lower odds of type 2 diabetes cross-sectionally *(45)*.

Many of the cross-sectional relationships between the Mediterranean dietary pattern, the metabolic syndrome, and type 2 diabetes have been supported by prospective studies. An investigation conducted in the SUN cohort found Mediterranean diet to be inversely associated with the incidence of metabolic syndrome *(46)*. Participants who had higher adherence to the Mediterranean diet had a significantly lower cumulative incidence of metabolic syndrome after a 6-year follow-up, even after adjustment for other risk factors.

The beneficial properties attributed to a Mediterranean diet may also help prevent type 2 diabetes. A prospective study conducted in Italy examined incidence of type 2 diabetes and impaired fasting glucose in patients with recent myocardial infarction. Closer adherence to a Mediterranean-type diet was significantly associated with a 35% lower risk of developing type 2 diabetes after a mean 3.2 years of follow-up *(47)*. This remained true even after adjustment for other risk factors. Grains, nuts, and legumes were not included in the diet score used in this study, however, so it may not be a true indicator of the effects of the Mediterranean diet.

One potential mechanism underlying the Mediterranean diet's beneficial effects on insulin resistance may be through changes in adiponectin, and endogenous insulin sensitizer. In a prospective study conducted among diabetic women, subjects with the highest average 10-year adherence to the Mediterranean diet had 23% higher median circulating plasma adiponectin concentrations *(48)*, even after adjustment for anthropometric, lifestyle, and medical history variables.

Several clinical trials have been conducted to further explore the effects of a Mediterranean dietary pattern in patients with the metabolic syndrome and type 2 diabetes. Adherence to a Mediterranean-type diet has been found to improve the metabolic profile in patients with the metabolic syndrome. Esposito et al. *(49)* conducted an interventional study in patients with metabolic syndrome to evaluate the effect of a Mediterranean-style diet on endothelial function and vascular inflammation. Intervention patients were advised to consume at least 250–300 g of fruits, 125–150 g of vegetables, and 25–50 g of walnuts per day; in addition, they were also encouraged to consume 400 g of whole grains (legumes, rice, maize, and wheat) daily and to increase their consumption of olive oil. The control group followed a low-fat prudent diet. After 2 years, patients in the intervention group had significant decreases in body weight; body mass index; waist circumference; HOMA score; blood pressure; levels of glucose, insulin, total cholesterol, and triglycerides; and a significant increase in levels of high-density lipoprotein cholesterol, all of which were greater than those recorded in the control group. Consumption of a Mediterranean-style diet by patients with the metabolic syndrome was associated with improvement of endothelial function and a significant reduction of markers of systemic vascular inflammation. Moreover, participants who followed the active intervention diet showed a reduction in the number of the components of the syndrome, such that the overall prevalence of the metabolic syndrome was reduced by approximately one half. Because data were adjusted for changes in body weight, the overall reduction in the prevalence of the metabolic syndrome after the intervention is likely to represent a conservative measure. Despite a robust inverse association between the overall Mediterranean-diet score and mortality, no appreciable associations were seen for most of the individual dietary components, which would suggest that the cumulative effects (synergistic or interactive) of multiple dietary components maybe substantial. In other words, the effect of the Mediterranean dietary pattern appears to be more than the sum of its parts.

Individuals with diabetes are at a much higher risk for CVD than those without diabetes. In a randomized clinical trial, investigators sought to determine if an intensive lifestyle intervention, called the Mediterranean Lifestyle Program (MLP), could reduce CVD risk factors in postmenopausal women with type 2 diabetes *(50)*. Two hundred and seventy-nine patients were randomized either to usual care or the MLP intervention group, which included a Mediterranean-style diet, exercise, stress management, smoking cessation, and support groups. Mediterranean diet advice included increasing intake of bread, root vegetables, green vegetables, legumes, and fish; replacing red meat with poultry; eating fruit every day; and substituting olive oil and canola oil for butter and cream. Results were modest, but the intervention group had a significant reduction in HbA1c, plasma fatty acids, and BMI when compared with the reference group, after 6 months. This suggests that a Mediterranean-type diet in combination with other lifestyle interventions may be beneficial for women with type 2 diabetes, but further trials with longer follow-up periods should be conducted.

6. MEDITERRANEAN DIET AND CANCER

Ecological comparisons imply that a traditional Mediterranean diet may also have a role in the prevention of certain cancers. Incidence of cancer has been found to be lower in Mediterranean countries than Scandinavian countries, the UK, and the US *(5)*. This is largely due to a decreased incidence of large bowel, pancreas, breast, endometrium, and prostate cancers. Epidemiological studies have linked many of these cancer types to low consumption of fruits and vegetables and high consumption of meat, provoking many to hypothesize that the Mediterranean basin's lower cancer rates may be due to nutritional factors. However, observational studies on the Mediterranean diet and its effect on cancer have produced conflicting results.

Studies of a relation between the Mediterranean dietary pattern and cancer risk are much scarcer than those showing a relation with CVD risk factors. However, in a composite of three case-control studies conducted in Italy, Bosetti et al. demonstrated a negative relationship between the Mediterranean diet score and cancers of the oral cavity and pharynx, esophagus, and larynx (51). Though few cancer case-control studies have looked specifically at relationships with the Mediterranean diet, components and characteristics of this dietary pattern have been widely studied. In 2000, Trichopoulou et al. conducted a review of case–control studies on diet and cancers of the stomach, large bowel, pancreas, breast, endometrium, and prostate (5). Six of the eight component characteristics of the Mediterranean diet, as defined earlier by Trichopoulou's MDS, were inversely associated with at least one of the six types of cancer. Dairy products, however, exhibited a weakly positive association with cancers of the large bowel and prostate, while alcohol appeared to be positively associated with both stomach and breast cancer.

A few clinical trials have provided promising evidence linking the Mediterranean diet to decreased risk of certain cancers. To assess the Mediterranean diet's effect on cancer prevention, the Mediet Project, conducted in Palermo, Sicily, sought to investigate the relationship between a traditional Mediterranean dietary pattern and breast cancer risk factors. Healthy postmenopausal women were randomized either to a control group, which was instructed to increase their consumption of fruits and vegetables, or an intervention group, which was instructed to follow a traditional Sicilian Mediterranean diet and received weekly cooking courses on this topic. After 1 year, compliance was over 80% in both groups and among women who adopted the Mediterranean diet there was a trend toward weight loss and reduction in cholesterol levels (52). The intervention group experienced a significant decrease in total estrogen levels, which could possibly account for decreased breast cancer risk in women who adhere to a traditional Mediterranean diet (53). The increase in antioxidants and flavenoids consumed due to large fruit and vegetable intake and the consumption of wild greens have been proposed as potential reasons for beneficial health effects of the Mediterranean diet on cancer (5).

The Lyon Heart Study, in addition to cardiovascular outcomes, also examined the effects of following a Mediterranean-type diet on cancer morbidity and mortality (40). Findings from this study were impressive with regard to cancer prevention. After adjustment for age, sex, smoking, leukocyte count, cholesterol level, and aspirin use, the reduction of risk in experimental subjects compared with control subjects was 56% for total deaths, 61% for newly diagnosed cancers, and 56% for the combination of deaths and newly diagnosed cancers, after 4 years of follow-up (40). Further clinical trials are necessary to confirm whether consuming a Mediterranean-type diet can prevent cancer.

7. MEDITERRANEAN DIET AND OBESITY

Several investigators have raised the hypothesis that the high-fat nature of some Mediterranean diet patterns might lead to weight gain and obesity *(4)*. Several studies seem to refute this. A cross-sectional analysis of the Greek population sample enrolled in the EPIC cohort found no relationship between the Mediterranean diet and BMI or waist to hip ratio *(54)*. Conversely, two cross-sectional analyses of cohorts in Europe found an inverse association between adherence to a Mediterranean-type dietary pattern and obesity *(16,55)*. Prospective studies have also demonstrated mixed results in regards to the Mediterranean diet and obesity. Subjects in the SUN cohort in Spain who closely followed a Mediterranean dietary pattern gained less weight over 28 months of follow-up than those who did not *(56)*; however, this relationship was not statistically significant after adjustment for other lifestyle factors. Nevertheless, subjects in the Spanish segment of the EPIC cohort who had high Mediterranean Diet Scores had a significantly reduced incidence of obesity after a 3 year follow-up period *(57)*. Evidence from epidemiological studies does not consistently demonstrate an inverse relationship between adherence to Mediterranean diet and obesity, but these studies do not suggest that following this dietary pattern could lead to weight gain and obesity.

Although there is conflicting observational evidence concerning the Mediterranean diet's effects on obesity, a randomized controlled trial conducted in the United States demonstrated that a moderate-fat intake Mediterranean-type diet may lead to weight loss through advantages in participation and adherence when compared with currently prescribed low-fat diets *(58)*. One hundred and one overweight adults were randomized to an energy-controlled diet containing either 35% energy from fat or 20% energy from fat. After 18 months, the moderate-fat intervention group exhibited a mean decrease in body weight of 4.1 kg, BMI of 1.6 kg/m^2, and waist circumference of 6.9 cm, while the low-fat group had mean increases in all three categories. Participants were much more likely to adhere to the moderate-fat diet; 54% were still participating after 18 months compared with 20% in the low-fat group. These results provide promising evidence for the benefit of a moderate-fat Mediterranean-type diet over a currently prescribed low-fat diet, both for weight-loss and ease of observance. Further clinical research is warranted to determine whether Mediterranean-type diets may be effective interventions for weight loss and prevention of obesity.

8. MEDITERRANEAN DIET AND OVERALL MORTALITY

As noted earlier, Keys with his "Seven countries study" was the first to identify that there was a statistically significant difference in the mortality of the population living in the Mediterranean basin. This was confirmed by WHO mortality statistics from 1960 to 1990, which also demonstrated the increased longevity of people living in this region *(59)*.

Mortality benefits of the Mediterranean diet were also seen in a cohort of elderly Europeans from the HALE (Healthy Ageing: a Longitudinal study in Europe) project, where higher scores on both the MDS and the MAI correlated with reduced all-causes mortality *(21)*. Further analysis showed that higher MDS scores were associated with a 50% lower rate of all causes and cause-specific mortality after a 10-year follow up *(60)*.

These findings seem to substantiate Keys' hypothesis that the mortality benefit that the Seven Countries Study saw in the Mediterranean region could be due to diet.

Promising results regarding the effects of Mediterranean-type diets on mortality outside of the Mediterranean region have been reported as well. In another analysis of the EPIC cohort, investigators wanted to see if the Mediterranean diet, as modified so that it could be applied across Europe, would still be associated with increased survival. In this modified Mediterranean diet score, unsaturated fats were substituted for monounsaturated fats. Even with this modification, an increase in Mediterranean diet score was associated with lower overall mortality (61). Investigators conducting a cohort study in Australia also sought to determine whether the benefits of the Mediterranean diet could apply across different populations. In their study, higher Mediterranean diet score was associated with longevity regardless of ethnicity (62). Another study conducted in Australia, the Melbourne Collaborative Cohort Study, investigated cardiovascular mortality in relation to a Mediterranean dietary factor characterized by frequent consumption of foods such as garlic, cucumber, olive oil, salad greens, legumes, feta and ricotta cheeses, olives, steamed fish, and boiled chicken (63). Subjects who had the most frequent consumption of foods from this Mediterranean diet factor had a 30% reduced risk of death from CVD when compared with those with the lowest intake of Mediterranean-type foods. This association was significant even after adjusting for country of origin, lifestyle factors, and CVD risk factors. These studies suggest that the cardio-protective effects of the Mediterranean diet are not limited to populations in the Mediterranean region of the world.

9. CONCLUSIONS

Without the advantage of superior health care and despite higher prevalence of cigarette smoking, the mortality of the people of the Mediterranean region used to be lower than that of other regions of the world. Current evidence suggests that this mortality benefit could at least in part be due to the dietary pattern of the population living in the region. Numerous studies have shown that the Mediterranean dietary pattern has beneficial effects on lipid panel, inflammatory markers, insulin resistance, and certain cancers, but most of these studies have been short-term observational studies. As evidence from observational studies accumulates and more interest in this diet and its beneficial effects is demonstrated, more informative studies are being conducted.

Weaknesses in the studies that have been done up to this point include inconsistencies in the definition of the Mediterranean diet. Few studies have controlled for adherence to a predefined score or pattern, and thus, it is difficult to evaluate study results without controlling for adherence. Finally, although several investigators have created validated Mediterranean diet scores as a tool for assessment of adherence to the diet, available scores differ from each other and thus results reported in various studies may not be directly comparable.

We believe that further randomized clinical trials with long-term clinical outcome data are needed in all areas including the role of the Mediterranean diet in the primary prevention of cardiovascular and other chronic diseases. On one hand, without long-term clinical outcome studies, it is difficult to assess accurately the morbidity and mortality benefits of the Mediterranean diet. On the other hand, there is substantial accumulating evidence supporting the beneficial effects of the Mediterranean diet on the secondary prevention of cardiovascular disease on the basis of published prospective cohort studies and randomized trials. Significantly, there is a paucity of studies on the beneficial effects of the Mediterranean diet on cancer despite some preliminary data that the diet may reduce incidence of colorectal, breast, prostate, pancreas, and endometrial cancers. Clinical studies on the use of a Mediterranean dietary pattern as an intervention for both the primary and secondary prevention of malignancies would be of value.

There is short-term data in support of lifestyle changes toward adoption of the Mediterranean dietary pattern. In many randomized trials, Mediterranean-type diets seem to be easier to adhere to than the currently prescribed Prudent diet. Given its general acceptability by patients, along with available evidence from studies on the Mediterranean diet's benefits, it might be argued that the NCEP ATP III recommendations for Therapeutic Lifestyle Changes should shift toward adoption of the Mediterranean dietary pattern. Such translation of available evidence into clinical recommendations could provide a more straightforward approach to a healthier diet for the general population, would be generally less confusing, and might eventually improve compliance. Some experts also contend that promoting increased fruit and vegetable intake in the context of a Mediterranean dietary pattern might be more appealing to the public than campaigns such as the 5-a-day program *(64)* by potentially focusing on the aesthetic and enjoyable nature of foods eaten in the context of a traditional Mediterranean diet.

The potential role of the Mediterranean diet and thus relevant studies on the effects of consuming a traditional Mediterranean diet are of major public health importance because of the increasing prevalence of dyslipidemia, the metabolic syndrome, cardiovascular disease, and cancer worldwide. Without overlooking other important aspects of the Mediterranean lifestyle, including the relaxed lifestyle and strong social bonds, based on current evidence, the health benefits noticed in the Mediterranean region do seem to be at least partially attributable to this dietary pattern, which patients seem to be able to adopt with relative ease. Since adoption of a Mediterranean-style diet would be a fairly low cost intervention that might have major preventative health benefits and reduce the risk of chronic diseases in many different populations, further research is warranted to determine whether dietary recommendations for the prevention of chronic disease should be based on the traditional diet of the Mediterranean region, as initial evidence suggests.

REFERENCES

1. Keys A. Coronary heart disease in seven countries. 1970. Nutrition 1997; 13(3):250–252.
2. Nestle M. Mediterranean diets: historical and research overview. Am J Clin Nutr 1995; 61(6 Suppl):1313S–1320S.
3. Ferro-Luzzi A, Branca F. Mediterranean diet, Italian-style: prototype of a healthy diet. Am J Clin Nutr 1995; 61(6 Suppl):1338S–1345S.
4. Ferro-Luzzi A, James WP, Kafatos A. The high-fat Greek diet: a recipe for all? Eur J Clin Nutr 2002; 56(9):796–809.
5. Trichopoulou A, Lagiou P, Kuper H, Trichopoulos D. Cancer and Mediterranean dietary traditions. Cancer Epidemiol Biomarkers Prev 2000; 9(9):869–873.
6. Panagiotakos DB, Polychronopoulos E. The role of Mediterranean diet in the epidemiology of metabolic syndrome; converting epidemiology to clinical practice. Lipids Health Dis 2005; 4(1):7.
7. Willett WC. The Mediterranean diet: science and practice. Public Health Nutr 2006; 9(1A):105–110.

8. Tavani A, La VC. Fruit and vegetable consumption and cancer risk in a Mediterranean population. Am J Clin Nutr 1995; 61(6 Suppl):1374S–1377S.

9. Kushi LH, Lenart EB, Willett WC. Health implications of Mediterranean diets in light of contemporary knowledge. 1. Plant foods and dairy products. Am J Clin Nutr 1995; 61(6):1407S–1415S.

10. Kushi LH, Lenart EB, Willett WC. Health implications of Mediterranean diets in light of contemporary knowledge. 2. Meat, wine, fats, and oils. Am J Clin Nutr 1995; 61(6):1416S–1427S.

11. Renaud S, de LM, Delaye J et al. Cretan Mediterranean diet for prevention of coronary heart disease. Am J Clin Nutr 1995; 61(6 Suppl):1360S–1367S.

12. Willett WC, Sacks F, Trichopoulou A et al. Mediterranean diet pyramid: a cultural model for healthy eating. Am J Clin Nutr 1995; 61(6):1402S–1406S.

13. Simopoulos AP. The Mediterranean food guide: Greek column rather than Egyptian pyramid. Nutr Today 1995; 30:54–61.

14. Trichopoulou A, Kouris-Blazos A, Wahlqvist ML et al. Diet and overall survival in elderly people. BMJ 1995; 311(7018):1457–1460.

15. Panagiotakos DB, Pitsavos C, Chrysohoou C et al. Impact of lifestyle habits on the prevalence of the metabolic syndrome among Greek adults from the ATTICA study. Am Heart J 2004; 147(1):106–112.

16. Panagiotakos DB, Chrysohoou C, Pitsavos C, Stefanadis C. Association between the prevalence of obesity and adherence to the Mediterranean diet: the ATTICA study. Nutrition 2006; 22(5):449–456.

17. Panagiotakos DB, Tzima N, Pitsavos C et al. The association between adherence to the Mediterranean diet and fasting indices of glucose homoeostasis: the ATTICA Study. J Am Coll Nutr 2007; 26(1):32–38.

18. Panagiotakos DB, Pitsavos C, Stefanadis C. Dietary patterns: a Mediterranean diet score and its relation to clinical and biological markers of cardiovascular disease risk. Nutr Metab Cardiovasc Dis 2006; 16(8):559–568.

19. Panagiotakos DB, Pitsavos C, Arvaniti F, Stefanadis C. Adherence to the Mediterranean food pattern predicts the prevalence of hypertension, hypercholesterolemia, diabetes and obesity, among healthy adults; the accuracy of the MedDietScore. Prev Med 2007; 44(4):335–340.

20. Alberti-Fidanza A, Fidanza F. Mediterranean adequacy index of Italian diets. Public Health Nutr 2004; 7(7):937–941.

21. Knoops KT, Groot de LC, Fidanza F, Alberti-Fidanza A, Kromhout D, van Staveren WA. Comparison of three different dietary scores in relation to 10-year mortality in elderly European subjects: the HALE project. Eur J Clin Nutr 2006; 60(6):746–755.

22. Waijers PM, Feskens EJ, Ocke MC. A critical review of predefined diet quality scores. Br J Nutr 2007; 97(2):219–231.

23. De LA, Alberti A, Andreoli A, Iacopino L, Serrano P, Perriello G. Food habits in a southern Italian town (Nicotera) in 1960 and 1996: still a reference Italian Mediterranean diet?. Diabetes Nutr Metab 2001; 14(3):121–125.

24. Alberti-Fidanza A, Fidanza F, Chiuchiu MP, Verducci G, Fruttini D. Dietary studies on two rural italian population groups of the Seven Countries Study. 3. Trend of food and nutrient intake from 1960 to 1991. Eur J Clin Nutr 1999; 53(11):854–860.

25. Keys A. Mediterranean diet and public health: personal reflections. Am J Clin Nutr 1995; 61(6 Suppl):1321S–1323S.

26. Menotti A, Keys A, Kromhout D et al. Twenty-five-year mortality from coronary heart disease and its prediction in five cohorts of middle-aged men in Finland, The Netherlands, and Italy. Prev Med 1990; 19(3):270–278.

27. Psaltopoulou T, Naska A, Orfanos P, Trichopoulos D, Mountokalakis T, Trichopoulou A. Olive oil, the Mediterranean diet, and arterial blood pressure: the Greek European Prospective Investigation into Cancer and Nutrition (EPIC) study. Am J Clin Nutr 2004; 80(4):1012–1018.

28. Polychronopoulos E, Panagiotakos DB, Polystipioti A. Diet, lifestyle factors and hypercholesterolemia in elderly men and women from Cyprus. Lipids Health Dis 2005; 4:17.

29. Panagiotakos DB, Pitsavos C, Chrysohoou C, Stefanadis C, Toutouzas P. The role of traditional mediterranean type of diet and lifestyle, in the development of acute coronary syndromes: preliminary results from CARDIO 2000 study. Cent Eur J Public Health 2002; 10(1–2):11–15.

30. Pitsavos C, Panagiotakos DB, Chrysohoou C et al. The effect of Mediterranean diet on the risk of the development of acute coronary syndromes in hypercholesterolemic people: a case-control study (CARDIO2000). Coron Artery Dis 2002; 13(5):295–300.
31. Panagiotakos DB, Chrysohoou C, Pitsavos C et al. The association of Mediterranean diet with lower risk of acute coronary syndromes in hypertensive subjects. Int J Cardiol 2002; 82(2):141–147.
32. Pitsavos C, Panagiotakos DB, Chrysohoou C et al. The effect of the combination of Mediterranean diet and leisure time physical activity on the risk of developing acute coronary syndromes, in hypertensive subjects. J Hum Hypertens 2002; 16(7):517–524.
33. Pitsavos C, Panagiotakos DB, Chrysohoou C et al. The adoption of Mediterranean diet attenuates the development of acute coronary syndromes in people with the metabolic syndrome. Nutr J 2003; 2:1.
34. Martinez-Gonzalez MA, Fernandez-Jarne E, Serrano-Martinez M, Marti A, Martinez JA, Martin-Moreno JM. Mediterranean diet and reduction in the risk of a first acute myocardial infarction: an operational healthy dietary score. Eur J Nutr 2002; 41(4):153–160.
35. Trichopoulou A, Costacou T, Bamia C, Trichopoulos D. Adherence to a Mediterranean diet and survival in a Greek population. N Engl J Med 2003; 348(26):2599–2608.
36. Trichopoulou A, Bamia C, Trichopoulos D. Mediterranean diet and survival among patients with coronary heart disease in Greece. Arch Intern Med 2005; 165(8):929–935.
37. Serra-Majem L, Roman B, Estruch R. Scientific evidence of interventions using the Mediterranean diet: a systematic review. Nutr Rev 2006; 64(2 Pt 2):S27–S47.
38. Vincent-Baudry S, Defoort C, Gerber M et al. The Medi-RIVAGE study: reduction of cardiovascular disease risk factors after a 3-mo intervention with a Mediterranean-type diet or a low-fat diet. Am J Clin Nutr 2005; 82(5):964–971.
39. Estruch R, Martinez-Gonzalez MA, Corella D et al. Effects of a Mediterranean-style diet on cardiovascular risk factors: a randomized trial. Ann Intern Med 2006; 145(1):1–11.
40. de Lorgeril M, Salen P, Martin JL, Monjaud I, Boucher P, Mamelle N. Mediterranean dietary pattern in a randomized trial: prolonged survival and possible reduced cancer rate. Arch Intern Med 1998; 158(11):1181–1187.
41. de Lorgeril M, Salen P, Martin JL, Monjaud I, Delaye J, Mamelle N. Mediterranean diet, traditional risk factors, and the rate of cardiovascular complications after myocardial infarction: final report of the Lyon Diet Heart Study. Circulation 1999; 99(6):779–785.
42. Simopoulos AP. The Mediterranean diets: what is so special about the diet of Greece? The scientific evidence. J Nutr 2001; 131(11 Suppl):3065S–3073S.
43. Zarraga IG, Schwarz ER. Impact of dietary patterns and interventions on cardiovascular health. Circulation 2006; 114(9):961–973.
44. Ford ES, Giles WH, Mokdad AH. Increasing prevalence of the metabolic syndrome among U.S. adults. Diabetes Care 2004; 27(10):2444–2449.
45. Panagiotakos DB, Pitsavos C, Chrysohoou C, Stefanadis C. The epidemiology of Type 2 diabetes mellitus in Greek adults: the ATTICA study. Diabet Med 2005; 22(11):1581–1588.
46. Tortosa A, Bes-Rastrollo M, Sanchez-Villegas A, Basterra-Gortari FJ, Nunez-Cordoba JM, Martinez-Gonzalez MA. Mediterranean diet inversely associated with the incidence of metabolic syndrome: the SUN Prospective Cohort. Diabetes Care 2007; 30(11): 2957–2959.
47. Mozaffarian D, Marfisi R, Levantesi G et al. Incidence of new-onset diabetes and impaired fasting glucose in patients with recent myocardial infarction and the effect of clinical and lifestyle risk factors. Lancet 2007; 370(9588):667–675.
48. Mantzoros CS, Williams CJ, Manson JE, Meigs JB, Hu FB. Adherence to the Mediterranean dietary pattern is positively associated with plasma adiponectin concentrations in diabetic women. Am J Clin Nutr 2006; 84(2):328–335.
49. Esposito K, Marfella R, Ciotola M et al. Effect of a mediterranean-style diet on endothelial dysfunction and markers of vascular inflammation in the metabolic syndrome: a randomized trial. JAMA 2004; 292(12):1440–1446.
50. Toobert DJ, Glasgow RE, Strycker LA et al. Biologic and quality-of-life outcomes from the Mediterranean Lifestyle Program: a randomized clinical trial. Diabetes Care 2003; 26(8):2288–2293.
51. Bosetti C, Gallus S, Trichopoulou A et al. Influence of the Mediterranean diet on the risk of cancers of the upper aerodigestive tract. Cancer Epidemiol Biomarkers Prev 2003; 12(10):1091–1094.

52. Castagnetta L, Granata OM, Cusimano R et al. The Mediet project. Ann N Y Acad Sci 2002; 963:282–289.
53. Carruba G, Granata OM, Pala V et al. A traditional Mediterranean diet decreases endogenous estrogens in healthy postmenopausal women. Nutr Cancer 2006; 56(2):253–259.
54. Trichopoulou A, Naska A, Orfanos P, Trichopoulos D. Mediterranean diet in relation to body mass index and waist-to-hip ratio: the Greek European Prospective Investigation into Cancer and Nutrition Study. Am J Clin Nutr 2005; 82(5):935–940.
55. Schroder H, Marrugat J, Vila J, Covas MI, Elosua R. Adherence to the traditional mediterranean diet is inversely associated with body mass index and obesity in a spanish population. J Nutr 2004; 134(12):3355–3361.
56. Sanchez-Villegas A, Bes-Rastrollo M, Martinez-Gonzalez MA, Serra-Majem L. Adherence to a Mediterranean dietary pattern and weight gain in a follow-up study: the SUN cohort. Int J Obes (Lond) 2006; 30(2):350–358.
57. Mendez MA, Popkin BM, Jakszyn P et al. Adherence to a Mediterranean diet is associated with reduced 3-year incidence of obesity. J Nutr 2006; 136(11):2934–2938.
58. McManus K, Antinoro L, Sacks F. A randomized controlled trial of a moderate-fat, low-energy diet compared with a low fat, low-energy diet for weight loss in overweight adults. Int J Obes Relat Metab Disord 2001; 25(10):1503–1511.
59. Trichopoulou A, Vasilopoulou E. Mediterranean diet and longevity. Br J Nutr 2000; 84(Suppl 2):S205–S209.
60. Knoops KT, de Groot LC, Kromhout D et al. Mediterranean diet, lifestyle factors, and 10-year mortality in elderly European men and women: the HALE project. JAMA 2004; 292(12):1433–1439.
61. Trichopoulou A, Orfanos P, Norat T et al. Modified Mediterranean diet and survival: EPIC-elderly prospective cohort study. BMJ 2005; 330(7498):991.
62. Kouris-Blazos A, Gnardellis C, Wahlqvist ML, Trichopoulos D, Lukito W, Trichopoulou A. Are the advantages of the Mediterranean diet transferable to other populations? A cohort study in Melbourne, Australia. Br J Nutr 1999; 82(1):57–61.
63. Harriss LR, English DR, Powles J et al. Dietary patterns and cardiovascular mortality in the Melbourne Collaborative Cohort Study. Am J Clin Nutr 2007; 86(1):221–229.
64. Heimendinger J, Van Duyn MA. Dietary behavior change: the challenge of recasting the role of fruit and vegetables in the American diet. Am J Clin Nutr 1995; 61(6 Suppl):1397S–1401S.

15 Lifestyle and Pharmacology Approaches for the Treatment of Hypertension and Hyperlipidemia

Peter Oettgen

KEY POINTS

- Hypertension and hyperlipidemia are two of the most common risk factors for cardiovascular disease, and are often present in individuals with the metabolic syndrome and/or diabetes mellitus.
- Lifestyle modifications including regular exercise and alterations in diet can help to minimize or eliminate the need for medication.
- Emerging evidence suggests that important structural changes in the blood vessels, or vascular remodeling, can often predate the onset of overt hypertension.
- In this chapter, the epidemiology, pathogenesis, and approaches toward treating these cardiovascular risk factors are reviewed.

Key Words: Hypertension, Hypertriglyceridemia, Hypercholesterolemia

1. INTRODUCTION

Cardiovascular disease remains the number one cause of morbidity and mortality in the United States *(1)*. There are approximately 13 million Americans with known coronary heart disease. Of these, 7.1 million individuals have sustained a myocardial infarction, 4.9 million suffer from congestive heart failure, and 5.4 million have had a stroke. Two of the most common risk factors for the development of coronary heart disease are hypertension and hyperlipidemia. Despite the fact that hypertension and dyslipidemia are well-known risk factors, they continue to be highly prevalent and under-treated. Approximately 27% of adults in the United States have hypertension and 31% have borderline hypertension *(2)*. On the basis of data from the National Health and Nutrition Examination Survey (NHANES), approximately 50% of Americans have total cholesterol levels that are greater than or equal to 200 mg/dl, and 17% have levels greater than 240 mg/dl. Of those patients with hypercholesterolemia,

From: *Nutrition and Health: Nutrition and Metabolism*
Edited by: C.S. Mantzoros, DOI: 10.1007/978-1-60327-453-1_15,
© Humana Press, a part of Springer Science + Business Media, LLC 2009

69.5% had had their cholesterol levels checked, 35% were aware that they had hyper-cholesterolemia, 12% were being treated, and only 5.4% with hypercholesterolemia were being adequately treated *(3)*. Lifestyle modifications including exercise and dietary changes can significantly impact blood pressure levels, and in some cases prevent the onset of hypertension. Lifestyle changes can similarly have favorable effects on hyperlipidemias, including hypercholesterolemia and hypertriglycerdemia. Although many patients may ultimately require medications for adequate control of their blood pressure or lipids, lifestyle modifications can often decrease the amount of medications that are needed. The purpose of this review is to discuss current life-style and pharmacological approaches in the management of hypertension and dys-lipidemia.

2. LIFESTYLE MODIFICATIONS FOR THE TREATMENT OF HYPERTENSION

For patients with hypertension, small reductions in blood pressure can be associated with significant decreases in morbidity and mortality from cardiovascular disease. For every 3 mmHg reduction in blood pressure, there is an associated 8% reduction in stroke rate and 5% reduction in CHD mortality. There are a variety of lifestyle modifications that are associated with reductions in blood pressure *(4)*. A 5 kg reduction in weight is associated with an average 4.4 mmHg reduction in systolic blood pressure and 3.6 mmHg reduction in diastolic blood pressure *(4)*. Modest reductions in weight can pre-vent the conversion of prehypertension to hypertension, and can also prevent further increases in blood pressure in patients with known hypertension (Fig. 1).

A variety of dietary interventions have been shown to lead to reductions in blood pressure. The so-called "DASH" diet (Dietary Approaches to Stop Hypertension) consists of a diet rich in fruits and vegetables, whole grains, poultry, fish, low-fat dairy products, nuts, reduced red meat, sweets, and sugar containing beverages. Adherence to the DASH diet is associated with an average reduction of 5.5 mmHg in the systolic blood pressure and a 3.0 mmHg reduction in the diastolic blood pres-sure *(5)*. A low salt diet (1.8 g of sodium per day) leads to an average reduction of 5.0 mmHg in the systolic blood pressure and a 2.7 mmHg reduction in the diastolic blood pressure in hypertensive patients *(5)*. It has been suggested that salt sensitivity is related to underlying kidney disease. In general, the effects of sodium restriction are greater for blacks, middle-aged and older persons, and individuals with preex-isting diabetes or kidney disease *(6)*. Other dietary modifications that can result in improvements in blood pressure include an increase in potassium intake, consump-tion of fish oils and fiber, and decreased consumption of alcohol. A Mediterranean diet has been shown to lower blood pressure in hypertensive patients. The average reduction for patients on this diet is a decrease in the systolic blood pressure by 6–7% *(7)*. Vegetarian diets are also generally associated with reductions in blood pressure. The combined effects of weight loss, increased physical activity, and the DASH diet were recently evaluated in the PREMIER trial *(6)*. In hypertenstive patients, this combined approach led to an average 14.2% reduction in systolic and 7.4% reduction in diastolic blood pressure.

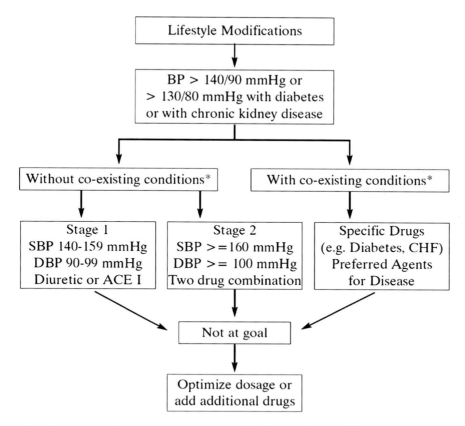

Fig. 1. Algorithm for treating hypertension. *Asterisk*: Coexisting conditions refer to those conditions where a particular antihypertensive medication may be preferred drug to treat the condition compared to other antihypertensive agents; *ACE* angiotensin converting enzyme, *SBP* systolic blood pressure, *DBP* diastolic blood pressure, *CHF* congestive heart failure.

3. DRUG TREATMENT FOR PATIENTS WITH HYPERTENSION

For many patients, lifestyle modifications may lead to significant reductions in blood pressure. However, these reductions may not be sufficient to lead to normal blood pressure levels, so that the use of medications may be necessary. There are several different classes of medications (Table 1). General approaches toward deciding when to initiate drug therapy are shown in Fig. 1. For patients who have other diseases or conditions, certain types of antihypertensive medications may be preferred. For example, for patients with diabetes mellitus, the use of angiotensin converting enzyme (ACE) inhibitors has been shown to be particularly useful in limiting the onset and progression of proteinuria related to kidney dysfunction *(8)*. Similarly, for patients with congestive heart failure, the use of ACE inhibitors and beta blockers has also shown to have therapeutic benefits over the other antihypertensive agents *(8)*. In many cases, two or more medications may be required to treat hypertension adequately. For those patients with particular rapid onset of hypertension, or lability in the blood pressure, evaluation for potential secondary causes such as renal artery stenosis, pheochromocytoma, or hyperthyroidism may be warranted.

Table 1
Classes of Antihypertensive Medications

Diuretics (thiazides, loop diuretics, potassium sparing diuretics)
Beta blockers
Calcium channel blockers
Angiotensin converting enzyme inhibitors
Angiotensin II receptor blockers
Aldosterone receptor blockers
Alpha blockers
Direct vasodilators

4. VASCULAR REMODELING IN PATIENTS WITH HYPERTENSION

The onset of hypertension is associated with significant structural changes in the architecture of the blood vessel wall. These changes include an increase in the thickness of the blood vessel wall, because of hypertrophy of the vascular smooth muscles cells in the medial layer. Abnormalities in the endothelium also occur at an early stage and are associated with altered vascular reactivity. Over time the influx of inflammatory cells leads to structural changes in the vessel including further increases in the thickness of the vessel and perivascular fibrosis. These changes in vessel architecture are often present when hypertension is first detected. Significant increases in carotid medial intimal thickness were detected by ultrasound in 28% of children with newly diagnosed hypertension *(9)*. With respect to vascular remodeling, all antihypertensive medications may not be the same. In the recently published LIFE trial in which the ACE inhibitor Losartan was compared with the beta blocker Atenelol, partial reversal in medial thickness of the blood vessels was observed in patients treated with Losartan but not with Atenelol *(10)*. This translated into an improved outcome for patients treated with Losartan. Because vascular remodeling may occur prior to the onset of overt hypertension, there has been some interest in determining whether patients with prehypertension should be treated more aggressively. The recently published TROPHY trial randomized patients with prehypertension to receive either a low dose of the angiotensin receptor blocker Candesartan or placebo *(11)*. After 2 years of treatment, the medication was stopped and patients were followed for an additional 2 years. At 2 and 4 years, the number of patients with hypertension remained significantly greater in those who had not been initially treated with the angiotensin receptor blocker. These studies suggest that in addition to measuring blood pressure, optimal management of patients with hypertension, or who are at risk for developing hypertension may eventually benefit from noninvasive assessment of vascular remodeling using ultrasound or magnetic resonance imaging to monitor the efficacy of treatment beyond just blood pressure control. However, additional studies are needed to further define the utility of using these modalities with respect to determining outcomes and to also define how frequently these noninvasive methods should be used to monitor the effectiveness of therapy.

5. LIFESTYLE MODIFICATIONS FOR PATIENTS WITH HYPERLIPIDEMIAS

General recommendation regarding lifestyle and diet were recently released from the American Heart Association Nutrition Committee *(12)*. Lifestyle modifications can lead to significant improvements in serum lipid levels in patients with hyperlipidemia. The cornerstone of lifestyle changes for patients with hyperlipidemia is the diet. Several different types of dietary changes promote significant changes in serum lipids. The diet should be rich in fruits and vegetables, including whole grains, and high fiber foods. The consumption of fish, particularly oily fish, is recommended at least twice a week; alternatively, the regular consumption of omega-3 fatty acids can be recommended. It is suggested that the consumption of saturated fatty acids should be restricted less than 7% of the diet, with less than 1% intake of *trans* hydrogenated fatty acids. The consumption of cholesterol should be limited to less than 300 mg/day. The intake of simple sugars and salt should be minimized, and alcohol should be consumed in moderation. Physical activity has also been shown to improve blood lipid levels. An overall goal of 30 min/day of aerobic exercise is suggested as a minimum. To promote weight loss, closer to 60 min/day may be needed. Although there has been considerable interest in the use of additional nutritional supplements, the AHA Nutritional Committee did not feel that supplementation of the diet with antioxidants, folate, B vitamins, soy protein, or dietary flavenoids led to proven benefits. Supplementation of the diet with fish oils, up to 1 g/day was considered reasonable, and consumption of plant stanols or sterols could lead to LDL reductions of up to 15% when consumed in quantities of 2 g/day.

6. ASSESSING CARDIOVASCULAR RISK IN PATIENTS WITH HYPERCHOLESTEROLEMIA

Although hypercholesterolemia is a well-known risk factor for the development of coronary heart disease and other vascular diseases, the cholesterol level alone is not a very good predictor of who will go on to develop vascular disease *(13)*. Data from the Framingham Heart Study supports that there is considerable overlap in the cholesterol levels for patients that went on to develop heart disease and those that did not *(14)*. As a result of these findings, the so-called "Framingham Risk Score" was developed to promote better risk assessment of those patients at low, intermediate, and high risk for developing coronary heart disease within the next 10 years. This risk assessment tool was adopted as part of the latest recommendations of the National Cholesterol Education Panel (NCEP) or Adult Treatment Panel III (ATP III) *(15)*. Points are assigned based on age and gender for total cholesterol, HDL cholesterol, smoking, and blood pressure to come up with a total point score. This point score can be used to predict the 10-year likelihood of developing coronary artery disease (CAD). Patients are considered at low risk if their 10-year likelihood of developing CAD is less than 10%, in the intermediate range if the likelihood was 10–20%, and high risk if the likelihood is greater than 20%. Patients in the high-risk group are also considered a "coronary heart disease equivalent" because their risk of having a future cardiovascular event is similar to patients with known heart disease.

7. HYPERTRIGLYCERIDEMIA AS A RISK FACTOR FOR HEART DISEASE

Several recent studies have supported the importance of hypertriglyceridemia as a risk factor for coronary heart disease. In the latest ATP III guidelines, the cutoff for a normal triglyceride level has been reduced to 150 mg/dl, with a borderline level being between 150 and 200 mg/dl, and a high level above 200 mg/dl *(15)*. Data from the Framingham Heart Study supports a linear relationship between the triglyceride levels and the relative risk of developing coronary heart disease *(16)*. This is particularly true for women, where the relative risk is approximately fourfold higher for women with triglyceride levels of 400 mg/dl, or higher, compared with those with normal levels, whereas the relative risk for men is about twofold greater. Similar findings were observed in the Prospective Cardiovascular Munster (PROCAM) study *(17)*.

Hypertriglycerdemia is associated with other abnormalities that promote and increase risk for cardiovascular disease. Elevated triglyceride levels are associated with increased clotting factors, including factor VIIc, plasminogen activator inhibitor one (PAI-1) *(18,19)*. Hypertriglyceridemia is also seen in patients with abnormalities in carbohydrate metabolism, particularly those patients with diabetes mellitus *(20)*.

Several studies support a synergistic increase in risk associated with the combination of hypertriglyceridemia and hypercholesterolemia. In the Paris Prospective Study, for example, those patients with a combination of hypercholesterolemia and hypertriglyceridemia had a fivefold increase in annual mortality from CHD compared with those with normal triglycerides and normal cholesterol levels, whereas those with isolated hypertriglyceridemia or hypercholesterolemia had a twofold increase in annual CHD mortality rates *(21)*. Similar findings were observed in the Helsinki Heart Study. Those patients with elevated triglyceride levels and an elevated LDL/HDL cholesterol ratio in the placebo arm had about a fivefold greater incidence of cardiac events than those receiving gemfibrozil or those with normal triglycerides and a normal LDL/HDL cholesterol ratio *(22)*. One of the principle reasons for the synergistic increase in risk in patients with the combination of hypercholesterolemia and hypertriglyceridemia may relate to LDL particle size. In patients with hypercholesterolemia, as triglycerides increase, there is a shift in LDL particle size from the large, type A particle, to the smaller denser, type B particles. Small dense LDL particles are more easily oxidized, taken up into the vessel wall, and therefore more likely to promote atherosclerosis *(22)*. A similar relationship exists between HDL and LDL cholesterol particle size. Patients with diminished HDL levels have smaller, denser LDL particle size. Patients with diabetes mellitus or insulin resistance often have associated hypertriglyceridemia, low HDL, and small dense LDL particles. The mechanism by which triglyceride rich particles lead to small dense LDL particles has recently been determined. Cholesterol ester transport protein (CETP) is an enzyme that promotes the exchange of triglycerides for cholesterol esters. In patients with hypertriglyceridemia, CETP promotes a reduction in the cholesterol ester content of LDL particles in exchange for triglycerides *(23)*. Further modification by hepatic lipase promotes the removal of the triglycerides and formation of the small dense LDL particles.

8. TREATMENT FOR PATIENTS WITH HYPERTRIGLYCERIDEMIA

Initial treatment for patients with hypertriglyceridemia should focus on lifestyle modifications. In particular, a reduction in the intake of simple and complex carbohydrates can lead to substantial reduction in triglyceride levels. Many patients with hypertriglyceridemia

Table 2
Categories of Lipid Lowering Medications

HMG-CoA reductase inhibitors (statins, lower LDL)
Cholesterol absorption inhibitors (resins, ezetimibe, lower LDL)
Nicotinic acid (lowers triglycerides, LDL, and raise HDL)
Fibric acid deriviatives (lower triglycerides)
Fish oil supplements (lower triglycerides, LDL)

are overweight or have diabetes mellitus. Weight reduction and tight control of underlying diabetes can also lead to improvement in triglyceride levels. Alcohol intake should be minimized. For patients with persistent hypertiglyceridemia despite lifestyle modifications, several types of medications or dietary supplements can be used. Fish oil supplements can lower triglycerides. Up to 4 g/day can be used to lower triglycerides. The average reduction in triglycerides associated with this intake of fish oils is 25–30% *(24)*. There is also an associated increase of 5–10% in LDL cholesterol, and 1–3% increase in HDL cholesterol. In addition, two medications can lower triglycerides as well. The fibric acid derivatives are particularly useful for lowering triglycerides (Table 2). Two fibric agents currently used include fenofibrate and gemfibrozil. For some patients who have a mixed dylipidemia may require combination therapy. The use of gemfibrozil is generally contraindicated in combination with the HMG-CoA reductase inhibitors (statins), because of a marked increase in the incidence of myositis. In contrast, the combination of fenofibrate with a statin is generally well tolerated. Nicotinic acid or niacin can also be used, but it may be more difficult for patients to tolerate this medication due to associated flushing.

9. AGGRESSIVE LDL LOWERING IN PATIENTS WITH ACUTE CORONARY SYNDROMES

Several recent studies have been conducted supporting an aggressive approach to lipid lowering therapy in patients with established coronary heart disease. The MIRACL trial was the first to evaluate aggressive lipid management in patients hospitalized with acute coronary syndromes *(25)*. In this trial, 3,086 patients were randomized to diet or the maximal dose of the lipid lowering medication atorvastatin (80 mg) within 96 h of admission for unstable angina or a non Q-wave myocardial infarction. After just 16 weeks follow-up, there was a statistically significant reduction in cardiac events in those patients receiving atorvastatin. Over the same time period, there was also a 50% reduction in incidence of stroke among those patients treated with atorvastatin. A more recent trial, the PROVE IT trial, demonstrated that improved outcomes in patients with acute coronary syndromes are related to the intensity of statin therapy *(26)*. In this trial, patients were randomized to receive either moderate intensity therapy with 40 mg of Pravastatin, vs. high dose therapy with 80 mg of Atorvastatin. As a result of the more aggressive therapy, there was a significant reduction in cardiovascular events at 2 years. Two additional studies have also demonstrated the benefits of cholesterol lowering in high-risk patients, despite normal cholesterol levels. In the lipid lowering arm of the ASCOT trial, a study in high risk patients with hypertension but normal cholesterol levels, administration of statin resulted in improved outcomes *(27)*. Similarly in the

CARDS trial, when patients with diabetes mellitus with normal cholesterol levels were treated with statin, it resulted in improved outcomes *(28)*.

10. PLAQUE STABILIZATION AND REGRESSION OF ATHEROSCLEROTIC LESIONS WITH LIPID LOWERING THERAPY

There has been considerable interest in identifying better ways to prevent the progression of coronary heart disease and promote plaque stabilization. Two recent studies using intravascular ultrasound support the importance of aggressive lipid management in patients with established coronary heart disease. In the REVERSAL study, patients with known coronary heart disease were randomized to moderate cholesterol lowering receiving 40 mg of Pravastatin vs. high dose statin therapy with 80 mg of Atorvastatin *(29)*. After 18 months, there was a 2.7% increase in plaque size among patients taking Pravastatin, whereas there was a 0.4% reduction in plaque size among patients receiving Atorvastatin. In the ASTER-OID trial, patients with established coronary artery disease were treated with 40 mg of the statin Crestor *(30)*. After 18 months of therapy, there was an average reduction in lesion size of 6.8%. These studies strongly support the concept that aggressive cholesterol lowering in patients with known atherosclerosis is associated with regression of plaque size and may thereby promote plaque stabilization. Future prospective studies are needed to evaluate whether these favorable changes in atherosclerotic plaque composition translate into significant improvements in cardiovascular events for all patients with known atherosclerosis, other than those with acute coronary syndromes.

11. SUMMARY

Hypertension and hyperlipidemia are two of the most common modifiable risk factors for cardiovascular disease. Lifestyle modifications can have a significant impact on lowering blood pressure levels for patients with hypertension and lipid levels for patients with hyperlipidemia. In many cases, patients with borderline hyperlipidemia and hypertension can be treated with lifestyle modifications alone. With advancing age however, optimal treatment may require the use of medications. Optimization of treatment in patients with hyperlipidemia and hypertension is associated with significant reductions in the morbidity and mortality associated with cardiovascular disease.

REFERENCES

1. Thom T., Haase N., Rosamond W., et al. Heart disease and stroke statistics-2006 update: a report from the American Heart Association Statistics Committee and Stroke Statistics Subcommittee. Circulation 2006;113:e85–e151.
2. Wang Y., Wang Q.J. The prevalence of prehypertension and hypertension among US adults according to the new joint national committee guidelines: new challenges of the old problem. Arch Intern Med 2004;164:2126–2134.
3. Ford E.S., Mokdad A.H., Giles W.H., Mensah G.A. Serum total cholesterol concentrations and awareness, treatment, and control of hypercholesterolemia among US adults: findings from the National Health and Nutrition Examination Survey, 1999 to 2000. Circulation 2003;107:2185–2189.
4. Stamler R. Implications of the INTERSALT study. Hypertension 1991;17:I16–I20.

5. Sacks, F.M., Svetkey, L.P., Vollmer, W.M., et al. Effects on blood pressure of reduced dietary sodium and the Dietary Approaches to Stop Hypertension (DASH) diet. DASH-Sodium Collaborative Research Group. N Engl J Med 2001;344:3–10.

6. Appel L.J., Champagne C.M., Harsha D.W., et al. Effects of comprehensive lifestyle modification on blood pressure control: main results of the PREMIER clinical trial. JAMA 2003;289:2083–2093.

7. Estruch R., Martinez-Gonzalez M.A., Corella, D., et al. Effects of a Mediterranean-style diet on cardiovascular risk factors: a randomized trial. Ann Intern Med 2006;145:1–11.

8. Chobanian A.V., Bakris G.L., Black H.R., et al. Seventh report of the Joint National Committee on Prevention, Detection, Evaluation, and Treatment of High Blood Pressure. Hypertension 2003;42:1206–1252.

9. Sorof J.M., Alexandrov A.V., Cardwell G., et al. Carotid artery intimal-medial thickness and left ventricular hypertrophy in children with elevated blood pressure. Pediatrics 2003;111:61–66.

10. Franklin S.S., Wachtell K., Papademetriou V., et al. Cardiovascular morbidity and mortality in hypertensive patients with lower versus higher risk: a LIFE substudy. Hypertension 2005;46:492–499.

11. Julius S., Nesbitt S.D., Egan B.M., et al. Feasibility of treating prehypertension with an angiotensin-receptor blocker. N Engl J Med 2006;354:1685–1697.

12. Lichtenstein A.H., Appel L.J., Brands M., et al. Diet and lifestyle recommendations revision 2006: a scientific statement from the American Heart Association Nutrition Committee. Circulation 2006;114:82–96.

13. Klag M.J., Ford D.E., Mead L.A., et al. Serum cholesterol in young men and subsequent cardiovascular disease. N Engl J Med 1993;328:313–318.

14. Castelli W.P. Epidemiology of coronary heart disease: the Framingham study. Am J Med 1984;76:4–12.

15. Expert Panel on Detection, Evaluation, and Treatment of High Blood Cholesterol in Adults. Executive Summary of The Third Report of The National Cholesterol Education Program (NCEP) Expert Panel on Detection, Evaluation, And Treatment of High Blood Cholesterol In Adults (Adult Treatment Panel III). JAMA 2001;285:2486–2497.

16. Castelli W.P. Cholesterol and lipids in the risk of coronary artery disease-the Framingham Heart Study. Can J Cardiol 1988;4 Suppl A:5A–10A.

17. Assmann G., Schulte H. Role of triglycerides in coronary artery disease: lessons from the Prospective Cardiovascular Munster Study. Am J Cardiol 1992;70:10H–13H.

18. Mussoni L., Mannucci L., Sirtori M., et al. Hypertriglyceridemia and regulation of fibrinolytic activity. Arterioscler Thromb 1992;12:19–27.

19. Carvalho de Sousa J., Bruckert E., Giral P., et al. Coagulation factor VII and plasma triglycerides. Decreased catabolism as a possible mechanism of factor VII hyperactivity. Haemostasis 1989;19:125–130.

20. Reaven G.M., Lerner R.L., Stern M.P., et al. Role of insulin in endogenous hypertriglyceridemia. J Clin Invest 1967;46:1756–1767.

21. Fontbonne A., Eschwege E., Cambien F., et al. Hypertriglyceridaemia as a risk factor of coronary heart disease mortality in subjects with impaired glucose tolerance or diabetes. Results from the 11-year follow-up of the Paris Prospective Study. Diabetologia 1989;32:300–304.

22. Manninen V., Tenkanen L., Koskinen P., et al. Joint effects of serum triglyceride and LDL cholesterol and HDL cholesterol concentrations on coronary heart disease risk in the Helsinki Heart Study. Implications for treatment. Circulation 1992;85:37–45.

23. Sandhofer A., Kaser S., Ritsch A., et al. Cholesteryl ester transfer protein in metabolic syndrome. Obesity (Silver Spring) 2006;14:812–818.

24. Kris-Etherton P.M., Harris W.S., Appel L.J. Fish consumption, fish oil, omega-3 fatty acids, and cardiovascular disease. Circulation 2002;106:2747–2757.

25. Schwartz G.G., Olsson A.G., Ezekowitz M.D., et al. Effects of atorvastatin on early recurrent ischemic events in acute coronary syndromes: the MIRACL study: a randomized controlled trial. JAMA 2001;285:1711–1718.

26. Cannon C.P., Braunwald E., McCabe C.H., et al. Intensive versus moderate lipid lowering with statins after acute coronary syndromes. N Engl J Med 2004;350:1495–1504.

27. Sever P.S., Dahlof B., Poulter N.R., et al. Prevention of coronary and stroke events with atorvastatin in hypertensive patients who have average or lower-than-average cholesterol concentrations, in the

Anglo-Scandinavian Cardiac Outcomes Trial–Lipid Lowering Arm (ASCOT-LLA): a multicentre randomised controlled trial. Lancet 2003;361:1149–1158.

28. Colhoun H.M., Betteridge D.J., Durrington P.N., et al. Primary prevention of cardiovascular disease with atorvastatin in type 2 diabetes in the Collaborative Atorvastatin Diabetes Study (CARDS): multi-centre randomised placebo-controlled trial. Lancet 2004;364:685–696.

29. Nissen S.E., Tuzcu E.M., Schoenhagen P., et al. Effect of intensive compared with moderate lipid-lowering therapy on progression of coronary atherosclerosis: a randomized controlled trial. JAMA 2004;291:1071–1080.

30. Nissen S.E., Nicholls S.J., Sipahi I., et al. Effect of very high-intensity statin therapy on regression of coronary atherosclerosis: the ASTEROID trial. JAMA 2006;295:1556–1565.

16 Diagnosis, Evaluation, and Medical Management of Obesity and Diabetes

Jean L. Chan and Christos S. Mantzoros

Key Points

- Obesity, diabetes, and the metabolic syndrome have become world-wide health problems of epidemic proportions with important health consequences.
- These closely related conditions have become the "plague" of the modern era, and measures on a global public health scale will be needed to stem the tide.
- This chapter focuses first on diagnostic criteria and then on lifestyle modification and medical management of the individual patient with these disorders.

Key Words: Obesity, Diabetes, Metabolic syndrome

1. INTRODUCTION

Obesity, diabetes, and the metabolic syndrome have become world-wide health problems of epidemic proportions with important health consequences. Although initially considered mainly a disease of affluent developed nations, the rates of obesity and diabetes are increasing at a staggering pace in developing countries as well *(1)*. These closely related conditions have become the "plague" of the modern era, and measures on a global public health scale will be needed to stem the tide. We will focus in this chapter first on diagnostic criteria and then on lifestyle modification and medical management of the individual patient with these disorders.

2. OBESITY

2.1. Diagnosis of Obesity

Obesity is a condition characterized by an excess of body fat. Criteria for defining obesity are necessarily somewhat arbitrary, but a body mass index (BMI) greater than 30 kg/m^2 is commonly accepted as diagnostic of obesity. Importantly, obesity should be distinguished from simply an increase in body weight, which may be observed in individuals who are very muscular and thus have a higher BMI based on muscle mass.

From: *Nutrition and Health: Nutrition and Metabolism*
Edited by: C.S. Mantzoros, DOI: 10.1007/978-1-60327-453-1_16,
© Humana Press, a part of Springer Science + Business Media, LLC 2009

2.1.1. Ideal Body Weight: Formulas and Tables

The definition of obesity as a state of excess body fat implicitly raises the question of what the most optimal or ideal body weight is. Unfortunately, there is little consensus on what exactly constitutes the ideal body weight and/or which formula or height-weight table is the most accurate. Historically, ideal body weight has been defined as the weight associated with the lowest mortality according to insurance actuarial data. The Metropolitan Life Insurance tables (see Chap. 19) have been among the most commonly used for this purpose, but have certain limitations, including a potentially skewed socioeconomic representation, lack of breakdown by age or race, a bias toward healthy subjects, and a decrease in accuracy at extremes of height. On a practical level, Metropolitan Life Insurance tables may be difficult to use as ideal weight ranges are categorized by frame size, whose measurement is not well-defined. There have been several formulas for calculating ideal body weight, including equations developed by Broca, Devine, Robinson, Miller, and Hamwi/Hammond (see Chap. 19). A recent comparison of these formulas and height–weight tables showed that most formulas and tables predicted an ideal body weight within a range corresponding to a BMI between 20 and 25 kg/m^2 *(2)*.

2.1.2. Body Mass Index

For practical purposes, BMI remains the most clinically useful method for classifying obesity, with widely accepted normative ranges for normal weight (BMI 18.5–25 kg/m^2), overweight (BMI > 25 and <30 kg/m^2), obese (BMI 30–40 kg/m^2), and severely obese (BMI > 40 kg/m^2) (see Chap. 19). BMI is calculated as body weight (in kilograms) divided by height (in meters) squared, or body weight (in pounds) times 704 divided by height (in inches) squared (see also Chap. 19 for nomograms and tables). BMI correlates well with directly measured body fat, and large-scale epidemiological studies have demonstrated that the inflection point at which mortality rates start to rise more sharply corresponds to a BMI of about 30 kg/m^2 *(3)*. In children, BMI must be standardized for age due to changes in body composition during growth (see Chap. 6 for discussion of childhood obesity). As noted earlier, the use of BMI has certain caveats. Specifically, BMI may overestimate obesity in muscular individuals and underestimate obesity in elderly or other individuals who have lost muscle mass.

2.1.3. Abdominal Obesity

It is well recognized that abdominal (android or central) obesity is associated with more metabolic complications than obesity that is predominantly peripheral (gynecoid) in distribution. Abdominal obesity is a marker for visceral adiposity, and visceral adiposity correlates highly with insulin resistance as assessed by glucose disposal during an euglycemic insulin clamp whereas subcutaneous adipose tissue does not *(4)*. Assessment of abdominal obesity can be performed with a simple measure of waist circumference (preferred) or alternatively by measuring the waist-to-hip ratio (WHR). Circumference at the waist is usually measured at the midpoint between the lower border of the rib cage and the top of the iliac crest or at the point of maximum circumference. According to the Expert Panel on the Identification, Evaluation, and Treatment of Overweight and Obesity in Adults convened by the National Heart, Lung, and Blood Institute and the National Institute of Diabetes and Digestive and Kidney Diseases, a waist circumference >102 cm (40 in.) or WHR > 0.95 in men or a waist circumference >88 cm (35 in.) or WHR > 0.85

in women is indicative of abdominal obesity *(5)*. This Expert Panel suggests that disease risk is elevated to the next higher category in individuals with a BMI range of 25–35 kg/m^2 if they have waist circumference greater than 102 cm for men or 88 cm for women (i.e. from "increased" disease risk to "high" for BMI 25.0–29.9 kg/m^2 and from "high" to "very high" for BMI 30.0–34.9) *(5)*. Individuals with BMI of 35.0–39.9 or ≥40 kg/m^2 have very high or extremely high risk, respectively, regardless of waist circumference since a BMI of ≥35 kg/m^2 is usually associated with this degree of abdominal obesity (see Chap. 19).

In a large study of over 9,000 adults in the third National Health and Nutrition Survey (NHANES), information on waist circumference did not offer much additional clinical utility in assessing the need for treatment; specifically >98% of patients received the same treatment recommendations based on their BMI and cardiovascular risk factors *(6)*. However, more recent data from almost 6,000 adults in the 1999–2004 NHANES indicates that waist circumference remained a significant predictor of diabetes even after adjusting for BMI and other cardiovascular risk factors *(7)*. In addition, measurement of waist circumference may be useful in certain situations (e.g., in certain ethnic populations such as Asians in whom normative BMI ranges may not apply as well because of higher percentage body fat at a given BMI compared with other ethnic groups *(8)* and whose metabolic risk may start to increase at a BMI ranging from 22 to 25 kg/m^2) *(9)*. Individuals with high waist circumference (as defined earlier) have been shown to have a greater likelihood of having hypertension, diabetes, and dyslipidemia after adjusting for potential confounding variables, even within normal-weight and overweight categories *(10)*. Thus, the finding of abdominal obesity may heighten awareness of and decision to screen for these related metabolic abnormalities.

2.1.4. OTHER MEASURES OF BODY FAT

Multiple methods exist to directly measure body fat, including densitometry by underwater weighing (considered the "gold standard"), total body water estimates using tritiated or deuterated water, total body potassium measurements, electrical impedance, CT, or MRI, but are primarily limited to research use because of expense and/or requirement for specialized equipment or materials. Body fat can also be indirectly estimated from anthropometry by measurement of skin-fold thicknesses at certain sites (e.g., biceps, triceps, subscapular, suprailiac) using calibrated calipers. Tables for converting the measured thicknesses to percent body fat are available (see Chap. 19). Although noninvasive and potentially easy to perform in clinical practice, anthropometry measurements are limited by the need for training to obtain accurate results, the assessment at only a few sites that may not reflect total adiposity due to differences in fat distribution, and the lack of well-established normative criteria for defining obesity based on this technique.

2.2. Screening for Obesity

The US Preventive Services Task Force (USPSTF) has conducted an extensive survey of the medical literature to determine the effectiveness of screening for and treating adult patients for obesity *(11)*. Although there were no large trials evaluating the efficacy of mass screening for obesity on which to base recommendations for screening, the USPSTF concluded that BMI is the easiest method for screening based on ease of use, reliability, and close correlation with body fat. In addition, counseling and pharmacotherapy were found to produce a modest weight loss of approximately 3–5 kg over at least 6–12 months, which improved clinical outcomes such as blood pressure, lipid levels, and glucose metabolism. Counseling for diet and activity was most effective when intensive (person-to-person contact more frequent than once per month for the first 3 months) and when combined with behavior therapy *(11)*.

2.3. Evaluation

2.3.1. HISTORY

The evaluation of the obese patient begins with a detailed history and examination to investigate for any potential secondary underlying causes, particularly treatable or reversible causes, as well as to develop an appropriate and comprehensive plan for evaluation and management. Although the vast majority of obese patients have simple "garden-variety" obesity related to the combined influences of over-nutrition and inadequate physical activity in the setting of predisposing genetic factors, weight gain can occur in the setting of certain endocrine disorders, hypothalamic disease, or a number of commonly used medications (primarily psychoactive/neurologic and hormonal/endocrine) (Table 1). Endocrine disorders that may be associated with weight gain include thyroid disease (typically hypothyroidism, but occasionally hyperthyroidism due to the accompanying hyperphagia), Cushing's syndrome, polycystic ovary syndrome (in women), hypogonadism (men), GH deficiency, and insulinoma. Patients are often concerned that a "slow-down" in their "metabolism" has contributed to weight gain, and it is important to exclude such potential contributing factors, although the new diagnosis of these conditions based only on weight gain in the absence of suggestive symptoms and signs is not common. Research in recent years has started to shed insight into the complex hypothalamic pathways of energy regulation and resulted in the identification of certain rare monogenic causes of obesity, such as deficiency of leptin, leptin receptor, proopiomelanocortin, melanocortin-4 receptor, prohormone convertase-1 *(12)* (discussed in detail in Chap. 2). Although defects at a single gene are a rare cause of obesity, and only a handful of such subjects with some of these defects have been identified around the world, it has been estimated that pathogenic mutations at the leptin receptor gene accounts for about 3% of individuals with very severe, early-onset obesity *(13)* and mutations at the melanocortin-4 receptor gene for around 6% of those with severe obesity starting in childhood *(14)*. However, these are also enriched databases of severe childhood obesity, and the estimated prevalence of single gene mutations from these studies may not be directly applicable to the general population. In addition, there are about 30 genetic disorders in which obesity is an accompanying feature, which are often associated with mental retardation, dysmorphic features, and organ-specific developmental abnormalities (Table 1). Future research in this area may soon help to elucidate additional genetic factors that predispose toward obesity in the appropriate environmental context (see Chap. 2).

In addition to identifying potential secondary causes of obesity that may explain weight gain and/or be amenable to treatment, it is instructive to identify certain key factors in the history, including age of onset of obesity, weight at age 18, history of weight gain, and previous weight loss attempts. The development of obesity at an early age can have ominous implications, as obesity markedly decreases life expectancy, particularly

Table 1
Etiology of Obesity or Conditions Associated with Weight Gain or Obesity

Simple obesity	*Drug-induced*
Dietary and/or sedentary lifestyle with predisposing genetic background	Neuroleptics (thioridazine, olanzapine, clozapine, risperidone, quetiapine)
Endocrine	Antidepressants
Polycystic ovary syndrome (women)	Tricyclics (amitriptyline, nortiptyline, imipramine)
Hypogonadism (men)	α-2 Antagonist (mitrazapine)
Hypothyroidsim	Selective serotonin reuptake inhibitors (paroxetine)
Hyperthyroidism	Antihistamines (cyproheptidine)
Cushings' syndrome	Lithium
Insulinoma	Antiepileptics (valproate, gabapentin, carbamazpine)
Growth hormone deficiency	Diabetes treatment
Hypothalamic	Insulin
Injuries	Sulfonylureas
Infections	Thiazolidinediones
Tumors	Others
Infiltrative diseases	Hormonal contraceptives
Miscellaneous	Corticosteroids
Smoking cessation	Progestational agents
	Antihistamines
	β-Blockers (propranolol), α-blockers (terazosin)

Examples of genetic disorders in which obesity is a feature (additional major features in parentheses)

Monogenic disorders [gene locus] (severe, early-onset obesity and hyperphagia)
  Leptin [7q31.3] (also abnormal immune function and hypogonadism)
  Leptin receptor [1q31] (also hypogonadism, hypothalamic hypothyroidism, mild growth delay)
  Melanocortin-4 receptor [18q22] (also increased lean body mass, bone mineral density, and growth)
  Pro-opiomelanocortin (POMC) [2p23.3] (also adrenal crisis in infancy, pale skin, red hair)
  Prohormone convertase-1 deficiency [5q15-q21] (also hypogonadism, hypocortisolemia)
  Single-minded homolog 1 (SIM1) [6q16.3-q21]
  Neurotropic tyrosine kinase receptor type 2 (NTRK2) [9q22.1]
  Corticotropin-releasing hormone receptor 1 (CRHR1) [17q12-q22]
  G-Protein-coupled receptor 24 (GPR24) [22q13.3]
  Melanocortin-3-receptor (MC3R) [20q13.2]
Genetic syndromes
  Albright hereditary osteodystrophy (short stature, round facies, brachydactyly, ectopic soft tissue ossification, resistance to several hormones including parathyroid hormone)
  Alström (diabetes mellitus, insulin resistance, neurosensory deficits; subset with dilated cardiomyopathy, hepatic dysfunction, hypothyroidism, male hypogonadism, short stature, mild to moderate developmental delay)

(continued)

Table 1
(continued)

Bardet–Biedl (mental retardation, dysmorphic extremities, retinal dystrophy or pigmentary retinopathy, hypogonadism or hypogenitalism [male], renal abnormalities)

Borjeson-Forssman-Lehmann (mental retardation, epilepsy, hypogonadism, gynecomastia)

Carpenter (mental retardation, male hypogonadism, acrocephaly, polydactyly, syndactyly)

Cohen (mental retardation, microcephaly, characteristic facial features, progressive retinochoroidal dystrophy)

Fragile X (mental retardation, macroorchidism, large ears, macrocephaly, prominent jaw, high-pitched speech)

Prader–Willi (diminished fetal activity, hypotonia, mental retardation, short stature, central hypogonadism)

Ulnar–Mammary (developmental abnormalities in limbs, teeth, hair, apocrine glands, and genitalia)

WAGR (Wilms tumor, anorexia, ambiguous genitalia, mental retardation)

in younger adults less than 40. This is likely due to the longer duration during which comorbid conditions can have their toll *(15)*. Ascertaining the weight at age 18 can not only provide a useful reference point for interpreting subsequent weight gain, but data from large cohort studies such as the Nurses' Health Study in women *(16)* and the Health Professional Study in men *(17)* have shown that weight gain increases the risk of diabetes and cardiovascular disease. Specifically, there was a 1.9 times increased relative risk of developing diabetes in women who had gained 5.0–7.9 kg from age 18 *(18)*. It is also important to understand the pace of weight gain, e.g., a relatively sudden weight gain suggestive of an underlying cause or a gradual weight gain over the years usually reflecting chronic imbalances in energy intake versus expenditure. In women, a history of weight changes around pregnancy may be helpful as weight gain over the years often occurs in the setting of a failure to return to prepregnancy weight. Finally, an understanding of previous attempts at weight loss may help in the design and implementation of a more effective weight loss program.

It is important to obtain an assessment of the patient's current dietary habits and level of physical activity. Although formal evaluation by a nutritionist to determine precise caloric intake on which to base specific recommendations for dietary changes is highly recommended, even a cursory review of the patient's typical diet may reveal areas amenable to improvement, such as large portion sizes, high-fat foods, high-sugar sodas, or unhealthy snacking habits. Similarly, an assessment of the patient's activity habits provides a starting point for making recommendations on exercise. Comorbidites that may affect the patient's ability to exercise (e.g., cardiac or pulmonary disease, arthritis, etc.) should be taken into consideration. Other relevant aspects of the history include history of smoking, excess alcohol intake, general medical history (particularly for obesity-related conditions), family history of obesity, and/or related disorders (particularly diabetes and cardiovascular disease), and relevant factors in the social history such as sedentary occupation, frequent work-related travel, and night work.

2.3.2. PHYSICAL EXAMINATION

The initial clinical examination should include measurement of weight, height, waist circumference (as indicated), and blood pressure; assessment of obesity distribution (android or gynecoid); evaluation for secondary causes of weight gain (such as goiter, delayed reflexes, edema for hypothyroidism; central fat accumulation, proximal myopathy, dark striae, or ecchymoses for Cushing's; hirsutism or other signs of androgen excess in women for polycystic ovary syndrome); or associated metabolic abnormalities (such as acanthosis nigricans for underlying insulin resistance).

2.3.3. LABORATORY EVALUATION

Laboratory testing is usually relatively limited and focuses on the potential metabolic abnormalities, including fasting plasma glucose (or oral glucose tolerance test if suspicion for impaired glucose regulation is high), full lipid panel, and liver function tests (for evidence of steatohepatitis). Evaluation for potential underlying causes of obesity is guided by the clinical suspicion, e.g., thyroid function tests, assessment for adrenal overactivity for Cushing's, androgens and gonadotropin levels for PCOS, sleep apnea studies, etc. If suspicion for a genetic cause of obesity is present (e.g., severe early-onset obesity and/ or characteristic features), then more specialized testing can be considered.

2.4. Risk Assessment and Goals of Therapy

As noted earlier, the NHBLI/NIDDK Expert panel suggests adjusting the disease risk associated with obesity based on a high waist circumference *(5)*. Bray et al. has also suggested a method for adjusting the BMI and reclassifying risk based on factors including weight gain since age 18, triglycerides, HDL, waist circumference, blood pressure, presence of sleep apnea, and level of physical activity *(19)*. Further recommendations for lifestyle, medication, or surgical intervention would depend on this risk-adjusted BMI.

In general, lifestyle modification (diet and exercise) is recommended for all individuals with a BMI > 25 kg/m^2. Patients with a BMI of >30 or >27 kg/m^2 with comorbidities (such as diabetes, dyslipidemia, hypertension, cardiovascular disease, sleep apnea) are eligible for pharmacotherapy. For severely obese patients with BMI of >40 or >35 kg/m^2 with serious comorbidities and acceptable operative risks who have failed previous weight loss attempts, consideration can be given to bariatric surgery (see Chap. 17 for more detailed discussion of this topic) since this approach is the only method currently available that has been shown to result in substantial and sustained losses of weight in the morbidly obese.

The treatment of obesity may have multiple goals, depending on the patient's degree of obesity, level of risk, and commitment to therapeutic intervention. From a public health standpoint, the prevention of the weight gain that often occurs after age 18 may represent an enormous achievement in improving the metabolic, cardiovascular, and other risks that accompany obesity. A weight gain of just 1–2 pounds per year is an almost imperceptible rate of change to most people but can amount to a total weight gain of over 30 pounds by the time an individual reaches 50 years of age. Gradual weight gain on this order of magnitude can be explained by an extra energy intake of less than 50 kcal/day, and the 90th percentile for weight gain in a population can be explained by an excess of just 100 kcal/day *(20)*. Fortunately, the body has remarkable homeostatic mechanisms for regulating weight to account for potential large day-to-day fluctuations in energy intake versus expenditure.

Most obese individuals, however, have far more ambitious goals than merely the prevention of weight gain. It is important for physicians to have a good understanding of what a patient hopes to achieve from a weight loss program and also to convey the typical efficacy of treatment as patients' expectations are often unrealistic. Although individual responses to weight loss programs can vary substantially, currently available medications typically produce an average weight loss of ~3–5 kg over 6–12 months *(21)*. This amount of weight loss may not achieve the cosmetic goals that the patient desires, but even a modest weight loss of 5–10% of baseline body weight can be associated with substantial metabolic improvements in blood pressure, lipid levels, and/or glucose regulation *(22)*. Thus, a weight loss goal of 5–10% from baseline over 6 months is reasonable and amounts to a half-pound to 1 pound per week for a 100-kg person.

Finally, just as important, and perhaps even more important, than the attainment of weight loss is the long-term maintenance of weight loss and prevention of weight regain. This is particularly true since the typical obese patient who seeks help from the medical profession has usually tried multiple weight-loss strategies in the past with some initial success but subsequent recidivism. In states of insufficient food availability, the ability of the body to maintain weight clearly conveys survival advantage, but this same ability becomes detrimental in an environment of affluence. Complex and redundant systems exist to tightly defend body weight, and multiple compensatory mechanisms quickly become operational once weight loss starts to occur. In addition, once weight is lost, an individual's total energy requirement (including resting metabolic rate, the thermic effect of food, and energy cost of physical activity) declines – a concept termed the "energy gap" by Hill and Wyatt *(20)*. Thus, patients who are successful at weight loss may find that they must adjust their dietary and activity habits indefinitely to maintain the lost weight.

2.5. Behavior Modification

One of the major difficulties in the treatment of obesity is that lifestyle modification represents a central and pivotal component of the overall approach, but modifying one's diet and activity is not only difficult, requiring a concerted effort and decision to change potentially deeply engrained habits, but is also tied to multiple social and other economic factors (e.g., whether a person has the time and/or money that may be required to promote more healthy eating habits and exercise patterns, whether there is an adequate support network available, etc.). Thus, key to a successful weight management program is assessing readiness to change and facilitating behavior change. This involves several important components, including self-monitoring (keeping track of energy ingested and activity performed), modification of the environment (including physical environment, e.g. to keep healthy foods at home, and thinking patterns, to avoid tempting circumstances and to set clear, specific, and attainable short-term goals), self-efficacy or a positive and optimistic attitude that focuses on success rather than failure, and social supports from the family and physician (see Chap. 19) *(23)*.

2.6. Nutrition

There have been many different types of diets advocated to promote weight loss. In general, the over-riding principle in achieving weight loss is the institution of an energy deficit diet, generally in combination with exercise. No adult studied by direct calorimetry has needed less than 1,200 kcal/day to maintain body weight *(24)*, which implies that actually following a diet of less than this should induce weight loss. More drastic diets including very low calorie diets (VLCD) (400–600 kcal) and low calorie diets (800–1,000 kcal) have been used, but the safety of VLCD has been questioned due to the predisposition to cardiac arrhythmias *(25)*. Thus, these diets should only be undertaken under the supervision of a physician. In addition, such stringent diets are difficult to maintain for a prolonged period of time. Formal consultation with a nutritionist is helpful not only for obtaining a more accurate assessment of a patient's dietary intake (e.g. based on a detailed 3-day food record), but also for making specific recommendations to modify the diet. In general, a safe and reasonable initial strategy is a 500–1,000 kcal deficit diet, i.e. 500–1,000 kcal less than the patient's typical diet.

2.6.1. Low-Fat Diets

There has also been much debate, substantial press coverage in the popular media, and many clinical trials conducted to determine the importance of dietary composition in weight-loss diets. Traditionally, low-fat diets have been promoted as the preferred approach to achieve weight loss, since fat is more energy-dense, high-fat foods may be more palatable, and there exists a notion that dietary fat is positively associated with body fat. Although a small amount of weight loss may be observed in individuals randomized to a low-fat diet in short-term trials, trends in the US demonstrating an increase in obesity despite a substantial decrease in the percentage of fat in the diet suggest otherwise *(26)*. A metaanalysis of more long-term studies lasting for 1 year or more shows that reducing fat consumption to 18–40% of dietary intake has minimal effects on body weight *(26)*. Similarly, a large randomized interventional study (the Women's Health Initiative Dietary Modification Trial) that reduced fat intake to 20% of total in one group with an average follow-up of 7.5 years showed no difference in weight loss between the intervention group and controls who followed their usual diet *(27)* (also discussed in detail in Chap. 7). In this trial, dietary fat restriction did not have a significant effect on incidence of cardiovascular disease during this time frame of follow-up.

2.6.2. Low Glycemic-Index Diets

It has been suggested that decreased fat consumption may lead to compensatory increases in carbohydrate consumption, particularly refined carbohydrates that may have detrimental effects on weight loss and metabolic status. Specifically, foods containing refined carbohydrates are more rapidly digestible and elicit marked fluctuations in glucose and insulin levels, which can stimulate hunger and inhibit fat oxidation *(28)*. Since carbohydrates differ in their ability to stimulate glucose and insulin release, the notion of glycemic index has developed to quantify this and is defined as the incremental area under the glucose response curve after a standard amount of carbohydrate from a test food relative to that of a control food (white bread or glucose) (see Chap. 21) *(28)*. Glycemic load is the weighted average glycemic index of individual foods multiplied by the percentage of dietary energy as carbohydrate; thus, foods such as potatoes and carrots may have similar high glycemic indexes, but those with a greater percentage of carbohydrate (e.g., potatoes) have a higher glycemic load. A recent 12-week randomized trial of 129 overweight or obese young adults demonstrated that individuals assigned to a low glycemic index diet were twice as likely to achieve weight loss of 5% or more compared with those on a traditional high-carbohydrate diet and that reduced glycemic load diet was associated with 80% more fat loss compared with a conventional low-fat diet *(29)*. In a smaller but longer-term study of 23 obese young adults, those assigned to an ad libitum consumption of low glycemic index foods over 12 months lost a similar amount of weight compared with a control group receiving an energy and fat-restricted diet, but showed greater improvements in triglycerol and PAI-1 levels *(30)*. Larger and more long-term studies are needed to determine the efficacy of diets based on low glycemic index foods, particularly when controlled for total energy content, on weight loss and other metabolic parameters.

2.6.3. Low-Carbohydrate Diets

In recent years, the proverbial pendulum swung to the other extreme with a great interest in very low carbohydrate diets, some with ad libitum fat and protein intake, since replacement of fat with carbohydrates in traditional low-fat diets may contribute to an adverse metabolic profile (e.g., rapid conversion of refined carbohydrates to simple sugars and stimulation of high insulin levels). The Atkins diet *(31)* is the prototype "low carb" diet, and the South Beach diet *(32)* is an example of a more moderate version (see Chap. 19). A recent metaanalysis of five clinical trials comparing low-carbohydrate versus low-fat diets of at least 6 months duration found that although individuals lost more weight at 6 months on the low-carbohydrate diet (5.3 kg compared with 1.4 kg), this difference was no longer significant by 12 months *(33)*. Although low-carbohydrate diets resulted in a more favorable triglyceride and HDL profile, low-fat diets had better effects on total cholesterol and LDL. The greater initial weight loss observed on low-carbohydrate diets may be related to changes in total body water as glycogen stores are mobilized and increased circulating ketone bodies are renally cleared *(34)*. In addition, total calorie intake on low-carbohydrate diets is lower, which may result from greater satiety during a ketotic state as well as limited food choice on such diets. Regardless, the difficulty with chronically adhering to a strict low carbohydrate diet is evidenced by the lack of difference in weight loss during more prolonged follow-up. A recent randomized trial that compared the effect of four popular weight-loss diets – Atkins (low carbohydrate), Zone (macronutrient balance), Weight Watchers (calorie restriction), and Ornish (low fat) diets – in 160 overweight or obese adults found a modest amount of weight loss (2.1–3.3 kg) at 1 year with favorable effects on the LDL to HDL ratio, but an overall low dietary adherence *(35)*. Importantly, in the National Weight control Registry (an observational study of individuals who had maintained a weight loss of at least 30 pounds for 1 year), those who were successful at long-term weight maintenance continued to consume a low-energy, low-fat diet *(36)*.

2.6.4. Mediterranean Diets

The Mediterranean diet has long been touted for its health benefits, including greater longevity and quality of life based mainly on epidemiological studies. This diet encourages the moderate consumption of fat (~40% of calories), mainly from foods high in monounsaturated fatty acids, as well as fruits, vegetables, tree nuts, legumes, whole grains, fish, and moderate consumption of alcohol, as shown in Chap. 14. Studies evaluating the effect of Mediterranean diets on weight loss and cardiovascular risk factors are discussed in greater detail in Chap. 14. Importantly, although these diets contain higher amounts of fat than traditional low-fat diets (but mainly from unsaturated "good" fat), there was no increase in body weight. Those assigned to a Mediterranean-style diet either lost more weight *(37)* or had no difference in weight *(38)* compared with those taking a traditional low-fat diet in randomized studies. Because this type of diet as well as other diets not described in detail herein, such as the Paleolithic diet *(39,40)*, diets with a high Alternate Healthy Eating Index score *(41,42)*, and the Dietary Approaches to Stop Hypertension (DASH) diet *(43)*, encourages the consumption of a variety of healthy and palatable foods, they may promote greater long-term adherence.

2.7. Exercise

Although exercise is a critical component of a successful weight loss program in addition to having cardiovascular benefits, the amount of weight loss achieved through exercise alone without caloric restriction tends to be quite small, on the order of 1–2 kg *(44,45)*. Exercise added to a dietary program can produce a 20% greater initial weight loss (13 kg vs. 9.9 kg) and a 20% greater sustained weight loss at 1 year compared with diet alone (6.7 kg vs. 4.5 kg) based on a metaanalysis of six studies ranging from 10 to 52 weeks *(46)*, although the effect of exercise and diet compared with diet alone may be more modest in other studies *(45)*. Importantly, increased levels of physical activity can be beneficial at all levels of adiposity, although it does not eliminate the increased risk of mortality associated with obesity *(47)*.

Even though the effect of exercise on weight loss is small, exercise may offer other important benefits, including favoring a body composition higher in fat-free mass and a higher resting metabolic rate that can provide an advantage in maintaining weight loss. In fact, a major rationale for incorporating exercise into a weight loss program is that a high level of physical activity is an important predictor for successful long-term maintenance of lost weight. This is supported by data from the National Weight Control Registry (NWCR), a prospective observational study started in 1993 of individuals who had maintained a weight loss of at least 30 pounds for 1 year, currently with over 6,000 registrants *(20)*. Participants in the NWCR who were successful in long-term maintenance of weight loss reported expending ~2,800 kcal/week. Others have shown that maintaining a physical activity level equivalent to ~80 min per day of moderate-intensity physical activity (e.g., brisk walking) or ~35 min per day of vigorous activity (e.g., jogging) decreases the risk of weight regain *(48,49)*. On the basis of these and other studies, there is good consensus that ~2,500–2,800 kcal/week (equivalent to 60–90 min of moderate-intensity physical activity) is necessary to prevent weight regain *(50)*.

Although it may be difficult and impractical for the typical overweight or obese person who follows a sedentary lifestyle to achieve this level of activity right away, a reasonable recommendation is to start with 30–45 min of moderate-intensity physical activity 3–5 days per week and encourage the establishment of a regular exercise routine. Ideally, this can ultimately be increased to at least 60 min per day of physical activity most if not all days of the week.

2.8. Medications

Medications may be a useful adjunct to lifestyle modification, mainly by helping to reinforce the intention to restrict food intake. There are currently two agents approved in the US for the long-term treatment of obesity (sibutramine and orlistat) – and another one previously approved in Europe that never receive approval in the US due to concerns of

Table 2
Medications for the Treatment of Obesity

Agents (trade name)	Mechanism of action	Available doses	
Approved for long-term use			
Orlistat (Xenical®)	Pancreatic lipase inhibitor	120 mg	120 mg three times daily
Sibutramine (Meridia®, Reductil®)	Norepinephrine and serotonin reuptake inhibitor	5, 10, 15 mg	10–15 mg once daily
Rimonabant (Acomplia®)[a]	Antagonist of CB1 endocannabinoid receptor	5, 20 mg	20 mg once daily
Approved for short-term use			
Diethylpropion (Tenuate®, Tenuate Dospan®)	Centrally acting sympathomimetic	25 mg	25 mg three times daily
		75 mg	75 mg once daily
Phentermine (Adipex®, Ionamin®)	Centrally acting sympathomimetic	37.5 mg	37.5 mg once daily
		15, 30 mg	15–30 mg once daily
Benzphetamine (Didrex®)	Centrally acting sympathomimetic	50 mg	25–50 mg three times daily
Phendimetrazine (Bontril®, Prelu-2®)	Centrally acting sympathomimetic	35 mg	17.5–70 mg three times daily
		105 mg	105 mg once daily

[a] Originally approved in Europe, but later withdrawn from the market, never approved in US.

psychiatric side effects (rimonabant) (Table 2). Several medications are approved for the short-term (up to 12 weeks) treatment of obesity, including diethylpropion, phentermine, benzphetamine, and phendimetrazine (Table 2). In addition, there are medications approved for the treatment of other conditions that have also been found to have beneficial effects on weight loss and medications studied for the treatment of obesity, which will be discussed briefly herein.

There are several important points to convey to patients when discussing the use of medications for the treatment of obesity. First, currently available medications produce on an average a placebo-corrected weight loss of about 3–5 kg at 1 year (or total weight loss of about 8 kg). Although individual patients may fare better than the average, certainly the efficacy of currently available medications is not ideal, and this is an area of intense ongoing research with multiple agents in the development pipeline (see below). Second, although data up to 2 years is available for sibutramine and up to 4 years for orlistat, the long-term safety of these medications has not been clearly established. Studies to date with these medications have not demonstrated serious side effects on the scale of the valvular heart disease problems observed with fenfluramine, which resulted in that medication's withdrawal from the market. However, these medications are not approved beyond 2 years, and experience with use for more than 2–4 years is lacking. Third, based on their mechanism of action and the chronic nature of the condition they are treating, it is reasonable to expect that weight may be regained once these medications are discontinued, unless substantial and permanent lifestyle modifications have been instituted to maintain weight loss. Thus, these medications represent only a temporary solution. Finally, these medications can have potential undesirable and/or clinically relevant side effects, as discussed later. Long-term effects of pharmacotherapy are discussed in detail in Chap. 18.

2.8.1. MEDICATIONS APPROVED FOR OBESITY

Sibutramine (Meridia®), an inhibitor of norepinephrine and serotonin reuptake, acts to suppress appetite and (in animals) to increase thermogenesis. In metaanalyses of studies of at least 44–54 weeks duration (at a dose of 10–15 mg/day), sibutramine was associated with an average weight loss of 4.2 *(51)* to 4.5 kg *(21)*. Importantly, most studies incorporated dietary intervention and excluded patients with known cardiovascular disease. In a 2-year trial in which 605 obese patients were treated with sibutramine 10 mg for 6 months, with subsequent randomization of those losing at least 5% body weight to either sibutramine or placebo for another 18 months, 43% maintained >80% of their weight loss at 2 years compared with 16% on placebo *(52)*. Sibutramine is available in 5, 10, and 15 mg tablets, with a usual initial starting dose of 10 mg and titration up accordingly. Because of sibutramine's known side effects to modestly increase heart rate and blood pressure, these parameters should be monitored after initiation of therapy. Sibutramine is contraindicated in patients receiving monoamine oxidase inhibitors or serotonergic agents or those with coronary artery disease, congestive heart failure, poorly controlled hypertension, arrhythmias, stroke, or severe liver failure. The initial weight loss can predict long-term response, e.g. 49% of patients losing greater than 2 kg in the first 4 weeks lost >10% body weight at 12 months compared with less than 20% of those with less initial weight loss *(53)*. Thus, patients who fail to lose at least 4 pounds after 4–8 weeks of treatment can be considered "treatment failures," and the medication should be stopped at that time.

Orlistat (Xenical®), a lipase inhibitor, acts to inhibit ~30% of fat absorption and thus prevent a portion of energy ingested from being absorbed. Many weight-loss trials using orlistat have been conducted, and metaanalyses of studies (all of which used dietary intervention) have found an average placebo-corrected weight loss of 2.9 kg at 1 year *(21,51)* and a similar amount at 2 years (3.2 kg greater than placebo) *(54)*. Orlistat as an adjunct to lifestyle modification has also been studied up to 4 years in the context of a randomized placebo-controlled trial in obese patients with normal or impaired glucose tolerance to determine whether a weight-reducing agent would decrease the risk of diabetes. This demonstrated a placebo-corrected weight loss of 2.4 kg (5.4 kg vs. 3.0 kg with placebo) as well as a 37.3% relative risk reduction in the development of diabetes *(55)*. Orlistat is dosed at 120 mg three times daily with meals and can be omitted if a meal is skipped or contains minimal fat. A low-dose (60 mg) formulation (*Alli®*) has been approved for over-the-counter sale. Because less than 1% of an oral dose of orlistat is absorbed systemically, it is relatively safe with few contraindications to use except chronic malabsorption and cholestasis. However, side effects related to its mechanism of action (including diarrhea, flatulence, fecal soilage) are relatively common (15–30%), although usually mild and tend to improve after several weeks. Because the absorption of fat-soluble vitamins is decreased, it is recommended that a multivitamin be administered with orlistat, and levels of fat-soluble vitamins (A, D, E, and beta-carotene) may need to be monitored. Similar to sibutramine, the amount of initial weight loss predicts the long-term response, and a similar guideline can be used for identifying non-responders.

Rimonabant (Accomplia®) is an antiobesity medication with a novel mechanism of action as a selective antagonist of the CB1 cannabinoid receptor, which received approval in Europe in 2006. The appetite-stimulating effects of marijuana (*cannabis sativa*) has long been known, and endogenous cannabinoid receptors were discovered in the early 1990s. The endocannabinoid system includes two major receptors (CB1 and CB2), and the CB1 receptor is a G-protein coupled receptor extensively expressed in the central nervous system, including areas involved in the regulation of food intake. CB1-knockout mice are lean and resistant to diet-induced obesity *(56)*. Four major randomized placebo-controlled studies have been conducted using rimonabant at 5 and 20 mg daily doses – RIO (Rimonabant In Obesity)-Europe *(57)*, RIA-North America *(58)*, RIO-Lipids *(59)*, and RIO-Diabetes *(60)* with over 6,600 subjects studied total. These studies have shown a 1-year placebo-corrected weight loss ranging from 3.9 to 5.4 kg (total weight loss: 5.3–6.9 kg) at the 20 mg dose with a much smaller effect at the 5 mg dose (placebo-corrected: 0.9–1.6 kg, total: 2.3–3.4 kg). Rimonabant had beneficial effects on waist circumference and metabolic parameters, including HDL and triglyceride levels, with no or minimal effects on LDL or blood pressure. Follow-up rates ranged from 53 to 66%, and the adverse effects (most commonly nausea, dizziness, and depression) resulted in 13–16% of patients discontinuing treatment, 6–7% due to psychiatric disorders. Patients with significant psychiatric disorders were excluded, potentially making the estimates of psychiatric side effects more conservative, and rimonabant did not receive approval by the US Food and Drug Administration mainly due to these concerns. Due to long-term safety concerns, rimonabant was subsequently withdrawn from all markets in 2008.

Phentermine (Adipex®, Ionamin®) and *diethylpropion (Tenuate®)* are sympathomimetic agents approved as short-term aids to weight loss. Studies using these medications have ranged from 2 to 24 weeks for phentermine and 6 to 52 weeks for diethylpropion. Placebo-corrected weight loss associated with these medications averaged around 3.0–3.6 kg, at doses of 15–30 mg for phentermine and 75 mg for diethylpropion *(61)*. Although there have been no major side effects causally related to these medications, there is a lack of long-term studies, and side effects are typical of those sympathomimetics (i.e., restlessness, dizziness, insomnia, palpitations, tachycardia, elevated blood pressure). These medications are limited by the development of tolerance, and weight regain is common after discontinuation of their use.

2.8.2. MEDICATIONS APPROVED FOR OTHER INDICATIONS

There are several medications approved for other uses, mainly psychiatric and neurologic, that have been found to be associated with weight loss. *Fluoxetine (Prozac®)* is a selective serotonin reuptake inhibitor that has been shown to cause weight loss ranging from 0.9 to 9.1 kg at 6 months in seven studies (six of which were significant), but at 12 months only three of six studies found statistically significant weight loss ranging from 0.5 to 14.5 kg relative to placebo *(21)*. Notably, the dose used for weight loss (60 mg) was considerably higher than that used for depression (20 mg). *Bupropion (Wellbutrin®, Zyban®)* is an antidepressant of the aminoketone class that is chemically unrelated to other antidepressants and is also approved for use in smoking cessation. Three studies reporting at least 6 months (and up to 12 months in one study) of treatment found an average weight loss of 2.8 kg with bupropion at 400 mg/day relative to placebo *(62–64)*. *Topiramate (Topamax®)* is an anticonvulsant approved for refractory seizures with an unknown mechanism of action to induce weight loss. Six studies reporting 6-month weight loss outcomes found an average percentage weight loss of 6.5% compared with placebo (absolute weight loss not reported) at doses ranging from 96 to 192 mg/day *(21)*. All of the findings were statistically significant but with considerable variation in magnitude. *Zonisamide (Zonegran®)* is another anticonvulsant used for the treatment of partial seizures that causes weight loss likely due to its serotonergic and dopaminergic activity. One randomized placebo-controlled weight loss trial has been conducted using this agent and found a placebo-corrected weight loss of 5% (6% vs. 1% in placebo) in 60 obese patients after 16 weeks at a dose starting at 100 mg that was titrated up to 600 mg *(65)*. *Sertraline (Zoloft®)* has also been studied in a weight-maintenance trial but showed no statistically significant findings compared with placebo *(66)*.

Ciliary neurotrophic factor (CNTF, Axokine®) is an endogenous neuroprotective factor, initially studied for the treatment of amyotrophic lateral sclerosis and incidentally found to induce anorexia and weight loss. The mechanism for weight loss appears to be through activation of hypothalamic leptin-like signaling pathways that bypassed leptin resistance in animal models of obesity *(67)*. In a 12-week, dose-ranging, randomized clinical trial, CNTF was administered by once daily subcutaneous injection at doses of 0.3, 1.0, or 2.0 µg/kg to 173 obese individuals in conjunction with a 500 kcal/day deficit diet resulting in a weight loss of 1.5, 4.1, and 3.4 kg, respectively, versus a gain of 0.1 kg for placebo *(68)*. CNTF was fairly well tolerated, although there was a high incidence of adverse effects (78–93%) with the most frequent being mild injection site reactions that was dose-related (34.4% at 0.3 µg/kg, 39.5% at 1 µg/kg, and 63.6% at 2 µg/kg). Unfortunately, the development of neutralizing antibodies appears to limit CNTF's efficacy. In summary, although several medications not specifically designed to treat obesity have been found to have some beneficial effects to induce weight loss, the findings from controlled studies have shown variable results. If patients require medications for the treatment of conditions such as depression or seizures, the judicious selection of these agents may be advantageous, but otherwise should be used prudently given the potential for side effects.

2.8.3. Agents in Development

Although currently available antiobesity agents are in general not as efficacious as would be desired, it is important to remind patients that drug development in this area is at an early phase and there is intense, active research to map the complex and redundant pathways that underlie weight regulation and to develop new medications. Discussion of all the targets currently being evaluated is beyond the scope of this work and has recently been summarized *(69)*, but agents currently in clinical development include other CB1 receptor antagonists (e.g., CP-945,598 (Pfizer)), CB1 receptor inverse agonists (taranabant (Merck)), other lipase inhibitors (including Cetilistat (Alizyme)), selective 5-HT$_{2C}$ receptor agonists (including APD356 (Arena Pharmaceuticals) and WAY-163909 (Wyeth)), a combined low-dose phentermine and topiramate agent (Qnexa (Vivus)), a combined bupropion and naltrexone agent (Contrave (Orexigen)), an orally available lipolytic domain of human growth hormone (AOD9604 (Metabolic Pharmaceuticals)), and gastrointestinal hormones and/or their analogues including peptide YY_{3-36} (Amylin Pharmaceuticals), a synthetic analogue of peptide YY and pancreatic polypeptide (TM30338 (7TM Pharma)), a synthetic analogue of amylin approved for use in diabetes (pramlintide, alone or in combination with leptin or peptide YY_{3-36} (Amylin Pharmaceuticals)), and a glucagon-like peptide-1 (GLP-1) agonist approved for use in diabetes (exenatide or Byetta® (Amylin/Lilly)).

3. METABOLIC SYNDROME

The metabolic syndrome (also known as syndrome X or the insulin resistance syndrome) is a clinical syndrome characterized by the clustering of metabolically related cardiovascular risk factors. It is not clear whether a single unifying mechanism causes the metabolic syndrome, although recent work in a mouse model that lacks the insulin receptor only in the liver has shed some insight into this. The presence of insulin resistance in the liver is sufficient to cause dyslipidemia and atherosclerosis, suggesting that hepatic insulin resistance may play a key role in the development of the metabolic syndrome *(70)*. The core components of the metabolic syndrome include obesity, insulin resistance, dyslipidemia, and hypertension, although the exact definition has varied in the past, depending on the criteria used by various scientific organizations including the National Cholesterol Education Program – Third Adult Treatment Panel (NCEP ATP III), the World Health Organization (WHO), European Group for the Study of Insulin Resistance (EGIR), International Diabetes Foundation (IDF), and American Association of Clinical Endocrinologists (AACE).

3.1. Definitions

In 1999, the *World Health Organization* formulated a working guideline for the metabolic syndrome, based on the assumption that insulin resistance is a key feature *(71)*. It thus required a diagnosis of glucose intolerance, diabetes, and/or insulin resistance *plus* two or more of the following:

- Obesity: waist to hip ratio >0.90 (men) or >0.85 (women) and/or BMI > 30 kg/m²
- Elevated blood pressure: systolic ≥140 mmHg, diastolic ≥90 mmHg
- Elevated triglycerides ≥150 mg/dL (1.7 mmol/L)
- Low HDL cholesterol <35 mg/dL (0.9 mmol/L) in men or <39 mg/dL (1.0 mmol/L) in women
- Microalbuminuira: urinary albumin excretion rate ≥20 µg/min or albumin:creatinine ratio ≥30 mg/g

Some controversies raised by this definition include the practical measurement of insulin resistance, the inclusion of microalbuminuria, and the most appropriate assessment of obesity.

The *European Group for the Study of Insulin Resistance* subsequently modified this slightly to use a simpler surrogate of insulin resistance (fasting insulin levels) and to substitute impaired fasting glucose for impaired glucose tolerance (thus obviating the need for an oral glucose tolerance test) *(72)*. Thus, metabolic syndrome was defined as hyperinsulinemia (top 25% of fasting insulin values among individuals without diabetes) plus two of the following:

- Obesity: waist circumference ≥94 cm (men) or ≥80 cm (women)
- Elevated blood pressure: systolic ≥140 mmHg, diastolic ≥90 mmHg or on treatment

- Elevated triglycerides >178 mg/dL (2.0 mmol/L) or on treatment
- Low HDL cholesterol <39 mg/dL (1.0 mmol/L) or on treatment
- Elevated fasting plasma glucose >110 mg/dL (6.1 mmol/L) but not meeting criteria for diabetes

The *NCEP ATIP III* definition of the metabolic syndrome was proposed in 2001 as part of a program to provide education on decreasing cardiovascular risk factors such as hypertension *(73)* and has some important differences from the WHO and EGIR definitions. Specifically, insulin resistance was not considered a key and required component of the syndrome, and equal weight was placed on each of the other components. Thus, an individual could have metabolic syndrome based on having three or more of the following five risk factors:

- Obesity: waist circumference >102 cm (men) or >88 cm (women)
- Elevated blood pressure: systolic ≥130 mmHg, diastolic ≥85 mmHg
- Elevated triglycerides ≥150 mg/dL (1.7 mmol/L)
- Low HDL cholesterol <40 mg/dL (1.03 mmol/L) in men or <50 mg/dL (1.29 mmol/L) in women
- Elevated fasting plasma glucose ≥100 mg/dL (5.6 mmol/L)

The *American Association of Clinical Endocrinologists* has also issued a position statement on what they term the "insulin resistance syndrome" *(74)*. Several of the same factors as proposed by the other organizations are identified as abnormalities of the syndrome, but the exact diagnosis is left up to clinical judgment. Factors to consider include overweight or obesity (BMI ≥ 25 kg/m^2), family history of type 2 diabetes, polycystic ovary syndrome, sedentary lifestyle, advancing age, and ethnicity. Other components of the insulin resistance syndrome include:

- Elevated blood pressure: systolic >130 mmHg, diastolic >85 mmHg
- Elevated triglycerides ≥150 mg/dL (1.7 mmol/L)
- Low HDL cholesterol <40 mg/dL (1.03 mmol/L) in men or <50 mg/dL (1.29 mmol/L) in women
- Elevated fasting plasma glucose of 110–125 mg/dL (6.1–6.9 mmol/L) or 2-h post-glucose challenge 140–200 mg/dL (7.8–11.1 mmol/L)

Thus, it was clear that the scientific organizations agreed on most of the key components of the metabolic syndrome, with differing views on the relative importance of some components compared with others and on exact cut-offs and/or best assessment of some components. Given the need for one simple definition and diagnostic tool that was convenient to use in clinical practice and could be used around the world, the IDF convened a workshop in 2004 with participants from each of the five continents as well as from the WHO and NCEP ATP III organizations to establish a simple, unified definition for the metabolic syndrome *(75)*. Criteria for the *new International Diabetes Foundation* metabolic syndrome include:

- Central obesity: based on ethnicity-specific waist circumference

	Male (cm)	*Female (cm)*
Europids	≥94	≥80
South Asians, Chinese	≥90	≥80
Japanese	≥85	≥90

Sub-Saharan Africans, Eastern Mediterranean, and Middle East should use European recommendations, and ethnic South and Central Americans should use South Asian recommendations until more specific data become available.

PLUS any two of the following four factors:

- Elevated blood pressure: systolic ≥130 or diastolic ≥85 mmHg (or treatment of previously diagnosed hypertension)
- Elevated triglycerides ≥150 mg/dL (1.7 mmol/L) or specific treatment
- Low HDL cholesterol <40 mg/dL (1.03 mmol/L) in men and <50 mg/dL (1.29 mmol/L) in women or specific treatment
- Elevated fasting plasma glucose ≥100 mg/dL (5.6 mmol/L) (or previously diagnosed type 2 diabetes)

Other parameters that may be related to the metabolic syndrome and that require further research include: abnormal body fat distribution, atherogenic dyslipidemia such as Apo B or small LDL particles, impaired glucose tolerance, insulin resistance (other than elevated fasting glucose), vascular dysregulation such as endothelial dysfunction or microalbuminuria, proinflammatory state, prothrombotic factors, and hormonal factors such as the pituitary-adrenal axis *(75)*.

3.2. Management

Since the main concern with the metabolic syndrome is the associated increased cardiovascular risk, management is primarily directed toward addressing the specific factors that increase risk of cardiovascular disease. The National Cholesterol Education Program (NCEP) has recommended that reducing cardiovascular risk should focus first on lowering LDL, since multiple clinical trials have demonstrated the benefits of lowering LDL on morbidity and mortality, and secondarily on the metabolic syndrome since this constellation of risk factors enhances cardiovascular risk at any given LDL level *(73)*. First-line intervention for the metabolic syndrome involves lifestyle change, which includes weight control and increased physical activity, since these will effectively reduce all of the risk factors associated with the syndrome. Secondary analysis of the Finnish Diabetes Prevention Study found that overweight individuals with impaired glucose tolerance assigned to an individualized lifestyle intervention group had a significant reduction in the prevalence of metabolic syndrome and abdominal obesity (odds ratio 0.62 and 0.48, respectively) compared with the standard care control group *(76)*. Thus, it is clear that lifestyle modification is a critical component of the management plan for individuals with the metabolic syndrome and that long-term adherence to these lifestyle changes is important for the successful management of this chronic condition. The role of diet and exercise with specific attention to long-term adherence are reviewed further in Chap. 8. Similarly, the management of hypertension and dyslipidemia (elevated triglycerides and low HDL) is discussed in greater detail in Chap. 12. It is important to note that some disparities may exist in the guidelines to treat dyslipidemia according to classification by metabolic syndrome versus other criteria such as the Framingham risk score *(77)*. Finally, there have been a few large-scale trials that have addressed the issue of impaired fasting glucose or impaired glucose tolerance associated with the metabolic syndrome since it is well known that individuals with these conditions are at higher risk for developing type 2 diabetes mellitus. The Finnish Diabetes Prevention Study that followed more than 500 overweight individuals with impaired glucose tolerance over an average of ~3 years found that lifestyle intervention (through diet and exercise with a mean weight loss of 3.5 kg at 2 years) reduced the risk of diabetes by 58% *(78)*. The Diabetes Prevention Program, which randomized over 3,200 individuals with impaired fasting glucose or impaired glucose tolerance to placebo, metformin, or lifestyle modification with an average follow-up of almost 3 years, found a similar reduction in incidence of diabetes with lifestyle modification (58% compared to placebo) *(22)*. Importantly, lifestyle change was nearly twice as effective as metformin in reducing the incidence of diabetes (31% compared with placebo) *(22)*. Thus, it is recommended for individuals at high risk for developing diabetes to achieve moderate weight loss (7% of body weight) and regular physical activity (150 min per week), using dietary strategies that include reduced caloric and/or fat intake, to prevent the development of diabetes *(79)*.

4. DIABETES

4.1. Terminology and Classification

Diabetes mellitus (DM) is a heterogeneous group of metabolic diseases characterized by abnormal carbohydrate, fat, and protein metabolism resulting in hyperglycemia, which is related to a relative or absolute deficiency of insulin. Marked hyperglycemia can cause symptoms of increased thirst, increased urination, and/or blurry vision. Acute, life-threatening consequences can include ketoacidosis or nonketotic hyperosmolar syndrome, and chronic hyperglycemia results in long-term complications, including microvascular (affecting the eyes, kidneys, and nerves) and macrovascular (causing cardiovascular disease). The severity of the metabolic abnormality can progress, regress, or remain stable depending on the underlying disease process and treatment.

Previously used terms that are no longer in favor include insulin-dependent diabetes (IDDM), non-insulin-dependent diabetes (NIDDM), juvenile-onset diabetes, and maturity-onset diabetes. This reflects the recognition that diabetes can have a variable age at presentation as well as the lack of accuracy of descriptions based on treatment modality. Instead, the recommended terms are type 1 and type 2 diabetes to reflect the etiology of the condition, i.e., absolute insulin deficiency due most commonly to autoimmune destruction of β-cells (type 1 DM) or relative insulin deficiency usually associated with insulin resistance (type 2 DM) (see Chap. 20). Diabetes can also occur due to specific genetic defects, diseases of the exocrine pancreas, in association with other endocrine diseases or genetic syndromes, or due to other insults to the pancreatic β-cell, such as drugs, chemicals, or infections (see Chap. 20). Gestational diabetes is classified separately and is diagnosed based on different diagnostic criteria.

Conditions of abnormal glucose regulation not meeting criteria for diabetes (i.e., "pre-diabetes") are also now recognized, including impaired fasting glucose (IFG) and impaired glucose tolerance (IGT). Importantly, both conditions are associated with a higher risk of progression to type 2 DM, and IGT has also been associated with cardiovascular mortality. The DECODE (Diabetes Epidemiology: Collaborative analysis Of Diagnostic criteria in Europe) study composed of 13 prospective European cohorts (with over 18,000 men and over 7,000 women) found an independent relationship between 2-h glucose following an oral glucose tolerance test (OGTT) and all-cause mortality, even after adjustment for fasting plasma glucose *(80)*. The Funagata diabetes prevalence study conducted in an agricultural area of Japan from 1990 to 1992 followed over 2,500 individuals for 7 years and found that IGT but not IFG was a risk factor for cardiovascular mortality (81). Individuals with pre-diabetes should be monitored for the development of diabetes on an annual basis (79).

4.2. Diagnostic Tests and Criteria

A random plasma glucose level is easily obtained and can be useful in the symptomatic patient with severe hyperglycemia (plasma glucose >200 mg/dL or 11.1 mmol/L) but is not always diagnostic. Fasting plasma glucose (FPG) levels performed after an overnight fast of at least 8 h is much more useful and the preferred diagnostic test because of ease of use, patient acceptability, and lower cost.

An oral glucose tolerance test (OGTT) is performed with the administration of a standardized glucose load of 75 g in 300 mL of water that is consumed within 5 min. The amount for children is 1.75 g of glucose per kg of ideal body weight. Previously, blood samples were obtained at baseline and every 30 min for 2 h, but only the baseline and 2 h time points are required for diagnosis. Insulin levels do not need to be measured as they provide little diagnostic utility and are mainly used for research purposes. For 3 days preceding the OGTT, the patient's diet should include at least 150–200 g of carbohydrate daily to optimize insulin secretion. The OGTT is more sensitive and modestly more specific than FPG for diagnosis, but not indicated for routine use except in pregnancy. The test has also been shown to have overall poor reproducibility (only ~60% in one study) (82).

Glycosylated hemoglobin (HbA1c) represents hemoglobin components formed nonenzymatically from hemoglobin and glucose, and thus reflects the average circulating glucose level over the preceding 3–4 months, which is the average erythrocyte life span. The advantages of this test include its good reproducibility and correlation with glycemic markers such as postprandial glucose, and the direct correlation with the likelihood of developing diabetes-related complications (83,84). In this regard, HbA1c is extremely useful for the monitoring of glycemic control, including response to therapy. Although it has been proposed as a potentially useful screening test (85–87), with a value of over 2 standard deviations above the mean (6.1%) showing high specificity in the third NHANES study (86), HbA1c is currently not recommended for use as a diagnostic (or screening) test (88). Potential disadvantages of the test include lack of standardization of assays, limited sensitivity for mild hyperglycemia, limited use in conditions associated with decreased erythrocyte survival (such as anemia and hemoglobinopathies), potential interference of the assay by substances such as alcohol, opiates, lead, and salicylates, lack of availability in some countries, and lack of correlation with fasting plasma glucose. Importantly, ~60% of individuals diagnosed with diabetes based on fasting plasma glucose had normal HbA1c (89).

Normal ranges of fasting plasma glucose and 2-h glucose following a standard 75-g OGTT and criteria for defining IFG, IGT, and DM are summarized in Table 3. In the absence of unequivocal hyperglycemia, any of the criteria for diabetes should be confirmed on a subsequent day. If the FPG is <126 mg/dL, but suspicion is high for diabetes, an OGTT should be performed, but otherwise the American Diabetes Association (ADA) does not recommend the routine use of OGTT except for gestational DM (88). The World Health Organization (WHO) uses similar definitions, but considers the use of OGTT in those with IFG (90).

Table 3
Medical Evaluation of Patients with Type 2 Diabetes

Medical history
- Age and characteristics of onset of diabetes (e.g., routine laboratory evaluation, symptoms)
- Review of previous treatments (lifestyle modification, medications, insulin)
- Previous glycemic control (including HbA1C levels)
- Self blood glucose monitoring: frequency, timing, blood glucose patterns
- Meal plan and eating patterns, prior nutritional evaluation, and weight history
- Physical activity and exercise patterns
- Current treatment of diabetes, including medications and patient's use of data
- Hypoglycemic episodes: frequency, severity, cause, associated symptoms
- History of diabetes-related complications
  - Microvascular: eye, kidney, nerve
  - Macrovascular: cardiovascular disease, peripheral arterial disease
  - Other: sexual dysfunction, autonomic dysfunction

Physical examination – full physical exam with special attention to:
- Blood pressure measurement (orthostatics if indicated)
- Fundoscopic examination
- Thyroid palpation
- Skin examination for acanthosis nigricans or lipodystrophy at insulin injection sites
- Vascular examination
- Foot examination for skin integrity, bony deformities, nail pathology, including: vascular assessment (palpation of dorsalis pedis and posterior tibial pulses) and neurological assessment (proprioception, vibration, monofilament sensation, reflexes)

Laboratory evaluation
- HbA1c
- Fasting lipid profile, including LDL and HDL cholesterol and triglycerides
- Liver function tests, thyroid-stimulating hormone
- Serum creatinine and calculated glomerular filtration rate
- Urine for albumin to creatinine ratio

Referrals
- Diabetes educator (if not provided by physician or staff)
- Nutritionist for medical nutrition therapy
- Ophthalmologist for dilated eye exam
- Podiatrist for foot complications
- Nephrologist for stage 3 or worse chronic kidney disease
- Vascular specialist if evidence of vascular disease

HbA1c Hemoglobin A1c.

Gestational diabetes (GDM) is defined as glucose intolerance that is first recognized during pregnancy, regardless of whether the patient requires therapy or the condition persists after pregnancy. Because of the known adverse effects of hyperglycemia on the fetus, early diagnosis and intervention is important to reduce morbidity and mortality. Risk assessment for GDM should be undertaken at the first prenatal visit. Although screening for GDM was previously recommended for all pregnancies, and some still advocate universal screening, this approach may not be cost effective. Thus, the ADA does not recommend screening low-risk individuals who meet all of the following criteria: less than 25 years of age, normal body weight, no family history of diabetes in a first-degree relative, no history of abnormal glucose tolerance or poor obstetrical outcome, and not a member of an ethnic or racial group with high diabetes prevalence (e.g., Hispanic American, Native American, Asian American, African American, or Pacific Islander) *(88)*. Those at high risk of GDM (severe obesity, prior history of GDM or delivery of a large for gestational age infant, glycosuria, diagnosis of polycystic ovary syndrome, or strong family history of diabetes) should be tested as soon as possible, and if negative initially, retested at 24–28 weeks (see Chap. 20). Otherwise, those at average risk should undergo testing at 24–28 weeks. A two-step approach involves an initial screening with a 50-g glucose load, and if the 1-h glucose value is >140 mg/dL (7.8 mmol/L), then a confirmatory OGTT performed with a 100-g load on a separate day (see Table 3 for diagnostic values, also Chap. 20). Women with GDM should be screened for diabetes 6 to 12-weeks postpartum *(79)*. In high-risk patients or populations, proceeding directly to the diagnostic OGTT may be more cost-effective.

4.3. Screening for Type 2 DM

Screening individuals for diabetes should be distinguished from diagnostic testing in those exhibiting signs or symptoms of the disorder. Hyperglycemia may be minimally symptomatic in the beginning, and it has been estimated that diabetes may be present for as many as 9–12 years prior to clinical diagnosis *(91)*. Screening of the population at large is not recommended because of the uncertainty of follow-up and potential for efforts to not to be well-targeted. The US Preventive Services Task Force finds insufficient evidence to recommend for or against routine screening of asymptomatic adults, but good evidence to support screening adults with hypertension or hyperlipidemia *(92)*. However, the ADA recommends that screening for diabetes be considered in individuals ≥45 years of age, particularly those with BMI ≥25 kg/m^2, with repeat screening at 3-year intervals if testing is normal initially, as well as in those younger than 45 if additional risk factors are present (see Chap. 20) *(79)*. Either FPG or 75-g OGTT can be used, with an OGTT considered in patients with IFG. The American Association of Clinical Endocrinologists (AACE) recommends screening individuals at age 30 if they have risk factors (as above) using a 2-h OGTT as the most sensitive method *(93)*.

4.4. Evaluation and Goals of Therapy for Type 2 DM

The initial evaluation of a patient with diabetes should include a comprehensive review of their medical history (with a focus on prior diagnosis of diabetes, glycemic control, treatments, and related conditions), physical examination with attention to potential neurologic and vascular complications, and laboratory testing to establish baseline glycemic control and screen for coexisting cardiovascular risk factors and/or complications (e.g., lipid levels, renal function, etc.) (Tables 4 and 5).

The ADA has suggested the following target goals for glycemic control: HbA1c < 7.0%, pre-prandial plasma glucose of 70–130 mg/dL (3.9–7.2 mmol/L), and post-prandial plasma glucose (measured 1–2 h after the beginning of the meal <180 mg/dL (<10.0 mmol/L)) *(79)*. AACE recommends more stringent guidelines: HbA1c < 6.5%, fasting or pre-prandial glucose <110 mg/dL, and 2-h post-prandial <140 mg/dL *(94)*. These are general guidelines and may need to be individualized for the specific patient to a

Table 4
Diagnostic Tests of Type 2 Diabetes and Impaired Glucose Regulation: Impaired Fasting Glucose, Impaired Glucose Tolerance, or Diabetes

Category	Fasting plasma glucose[a]	2-h Plasma glucose[b]
Normal	<100 mg/dL (<5.6 mmol/L)	<140 mg/dL (<7.8 mmol/L)
Impaired fasting glucose	100–125 mg/dL (5.6–6.9 mmol/L)	–
Impaired glucose tolerance	–	140–199 mg/dL (7.8–11.0 mmol/L)
Diabetes[c]	≥126 mg/dL (≥7.0 mmol/L)	≥200 mg/dL (≥11.1 mmol/L)

[a]After an overnight fast of at least 8 h.
[b]After a standard 75-g oral glucose tolerance test (75 g in 300 ml water consumed within 5 min) and after an unrestricted diet with ≥150 g of carbohydrate daily for at least 3 days prior to test.
[c]Diabetes can also be diagnosed on the basis of symptoms of diabetes (polyuria, polydipsia, weight loss, visual blurring) plus a random plasma glucose ≥200 mg/dL (11.1 mmol/L). In the absence of unequivocal hyperglycemia, any criteria for diabetes should be confirmed on a subsequent day.

Table 5
Diagnostic Tests of Type 2 Diabetes and Impaired Glucose Regulation: Gestational Diabetes

	Two or more abnormal values for a positive diagnosis			
	Fasting	1 h	2 h	3 h
100-g Glucose tolerance test[a]	≥95 mg/dL (≥5.3 mmol/L)	≥180 mg/dL (≥10.0 mmol/L)	≥155 mg/dL (≥8.6 mmol/L)	≥140 mg/dL (≥7.8 mmol/L)
75-g Glucose tolerance test[a]	≥95 mg/dL (≥5.3 mmol/L)	≥180 mg/dL (≥10.0 mmol/L)	≥155 mg/dL (≥8.6 mmol/L)	

[a]After an overnight fast of at least 8 h and after an unrestricted diet with ≥150 g of carbohydrate daily for at least 3 days prior to test.

HbA1c as close to normal as possible without substantial hypoglycemia. Findings from the UKPDS on the relationship between HbA1c and microvascular and macrovascular complications showed no evidence for a lower threshold of HbA1c at which these risks plateau *(95)*. Conversely, patients with limited life expectancy, severe hypoglycemia, or comorbid conditions adversely affected by hypoglycemia may warrant more liberal glycemic targets.

4.5. Overall Management of Type 2 DM

Since diabetes is a chronic disease whose course is heavily influenced by lifestyle factors and thus requires a great deal of management by the patient on a day-to-day basis, self-management education is a critical component of the overall approach. In this context, it is important to assess a patient's psychological and social status to identify potential impediments to an effective management program, such as cognitive impairment, depression, eating disorders, and/or lack of social support or financial resources. A key aspect of this is self-monitoring of blood glucose (SMBG) to provide real-time feedback to the patient on the need for adjustments in diet, exercise, and medications, particularly insulin therapy, and for determining whether symptoms are due to hypoglycemia or hyperglycemia. The optimal timing and frequency should be tailored to the individual patient's needs but should be performed in patients receiving insulin (three or more times daily in those on multiple daily injections). Measurement of postprandial as well as fasting or premeal blood glucose levels provides useful information.

HbA1c measurement should be performed at least twice per year in patients who have stable glycemic control and are meeting treatment goals, and more frequently (once every 3 months) in those who are not meeting glycemic goals and/or who are having changes in therapy.

The comprehensive discussion of the management of diabetes-related complications is beyond the scope of this chapter and are summarized briefly from reference *(79)* herein. The management of hypertension and hyperlipidemia is discussed in greater detail in Chap. 15.

- The target goal for blood pressure is systolic <130 mmHg and diastolic <80 mmHg. All patients with diabetes and hypertension (systolic ≥ 140 mmHg and diastolic ≥90 mmHg) should be treated with either an ACE inhibitor or angiotensin receptor blocker, in addition to lifestyle therapy. If needed, a thiazide diuretic can be used in those with an estimated glomerular filtration rate (GFR) ≥50 mL/min per 1.73 m^2, and a loop diuretic in those with GFR < 50 mL/min per 1.73 m^2. Additional therapy should include drugs demonstrated to reduce cardiovascular events in patients with diabetes such as β-blockers and calcium channel blockers.

- Lipid levels should be tested at least annually, with goals of LDL <100 mg/dL (2.6 mmol/L) in patients without overt cardiovascular disease (<70 mg/dL (1.8 mmol/L) can be considered in those with overt cardiovascular disease), triglyceride <150 mg/dL (1.7 mmol/L), and HDL >40 mg/dL (1.0 mmol/L) in men and >50 mg/dL (1.3 mmol/L) in women. All patients with diabetes over age 40 who have one or more other cardiovascular risk factors and those with overt cardiovascular disease should receive statin therapy to achieve an LDL reduction of 30–40% regardless of baseline LDL.

- Aspirin therapy (75–162 mg/day) should be used as primary prevention in those with type 2 diabetes and increased cardiovascular risk (over age 40 or additional risk factors such as family history of cardiovascular disease, hypertension, smoking, dyslipidemia, albuminuria) and as secondary prevention in those with diabetes and a history of cardiovascular disease.

- All patients should be advised to stop smoking.

- Cardiac stress testing is indicated for those with typical or atypical cardiac systems and an abnormal resting electrocardiogram; a history of peripheral or carotid occlusive disease; or sedentary lifestyle, age greater than 35, and plans to begin a vigorous exercise program.

- Measure serum creatinine (to estimate GFR) and test for microalbuminuria annually. Stages of chronic kidney disease (CKD) are classified as follows based on GFR (in mL/min per 1.73 m^2 body surface area): ≥90 – stage 1; 60–89 (mildly decreased) – stage 2; 30–59 (moderately decreased) – stage 3; 15–29 (severely decreased) – stage 4; <15 or dialysis (kidney failure) – stage 5. Consider referral to a nephrologist in stage 3 or worse CKD or with difficulty managing hypertension or hyperkalemia. Microalbuminuria is a urine albumin of 30–299 µg/mg creatinine and macroalbuminuria is ≥ 300 µg/mg creatinine, based on at least two of three spot urine specimens being abnormal over a 3- to 6-month period. ACE inhibitors and ARBs in patients with type 2 DM, hypertension, and microalbuminuria delay the progression to macroalbuminuria, and ARBs in patients with type 2 DM, hypertension, macroalbuminuria, and renal insufficiency delay the progression of nephropathy.

- Refer patients to an ophthalmologist for a dilated and comprehensive eye examination at the time of diagnosis of diabetes and annually thereafter. Less frequent exams can be considered in the setting of a normal eye exam. Women with type 2 DM (but not GDM) who are pregnant should have an eye exam in the first trimester with close monitoring throughout pregnancy and for 1-year postpartum.
- Screen patients for distal polyneuropathy at diagnosis and at least annually thereafter using clinical tests such as pinprick, temperature, vibration, and 10-g monofilament pressure (at the distal plantar aspect of both great toes) sensation and ankle reflexes. Assess for symptoms of autonomic neuropathy at diagnosis based on resting tachycardia, exercise intolerance, orthostatic hypotension, constipation, gastroparesis, bladder or sexual dysfunction, or erratic glucose control.
- Perform a comprehensive foot examination at least annually, including assessment of neuropathy as above, peripheral vascular disease (pedal pulses), skin integrity including evidence of increased pressure or tissue damage, bony deformities, and/or severe nail pathology. Provide education on foot self-care, and refer patients who smoke or have prior foot complications to a foot care specialist and those who have claudication or evidence of peripheral vascular disease for further vascular assessment.

4.6. Nutrition and Exercise

Obesity plays an important role in the development of diabetes and also complicates the management of diabetes by increasing insulin resistance. Patients with type 2 diabetes who are obese can have substantial metabolic benefits from even a modest ~5–10% loss of body weight. In fact, a recent randomized controlled trial that assigned patients with type 2 diabetes to either lifestyle modification with a focus on weight loss or laparoscopic adjustable gastric banding to achieve weight loss found that individuals randomized to surgical therapy who lost an average of 20.7% of their body weight were more likely to achieve remission of their diabetes than those assigned to conventional therapy who lost 1.7% of their weight at 2 years *(96)*.

In general, the same principles for diet and exercise as discussed above apply as for the obese patient without diabetes. The American College of Physicians suggests recommending frequent small meals to add in weight loss and using the following starting formula for basing calorie recommendations in patients with diabetes: 10 cal per pound of body weight, plus 20% for sedentary patients, 33% for those who have light physical activity, 50% for moderately active patients, and 75% for those who are very active *(97)*. We will discuss herein a few guidelines for the patient with type 2 DM. More specific recommendations are found in Chap. 13, based on the recent ADA consensus statement *(98)*.

There is no single best diet for patients with diabetes or specific macronutrient distribution that is most optimal. Even though it may seem logical to limit carbohydrates to control glucose, low-carbohydrate diets (i.e., less than 130 g of total carbohydrates per day) are generally not recommended because carbohydrate-containing foods are an important source of energy, fiber, and micronutrients. Limiting the amount of carbohydrate at a single meal to a reasonable amount with attention to the type and quality of carbohydrate (e.g., carbohydrates such as whole grains are preferred to simple or refined carbohydrates) is helpful to avoid exacerbating postprandial hyperglycemia. A recent metaanalysis of randomized controlled trials using low glycemic index diets in patients with diabetes found a modest but potentially clinically use overall reduction in HbA1c by 0.4% compared with high glycemic index diets *(99)*. Saturated fats should be limited to less than 7% of total calories and intake of *trans* fat minimized since these are the two main dietary determinants of LDL, and cholesterol should be limited to less than 200 mg/day. The usual amount of protein intake is ~15–20% of the diet, and there is no evidence indicating that this should be altered in patients with diabetes. However, since the ingestion of protein can stimulate insulin without increasing glucose, protein should not be used to treat or prevent hypoglycemia.

Exercise is not only important in weight loss, particularly the maintenance of lost weight as discussed above, but in patients with diabetes, it has the additional benefit of improving insulin resistance and therefore blood glucose levels, cardiovascular risk factors, and overall sense of well-being. A metaanalysis of randomized controlled studies that used structured exercise interventions for at least 8 weeks found a lower HbA1c (by 0.66%) in exercise groups compared with controls that appeared to be independent of changes in body weight *(100)*. Aerobic exercise is usually recommended but resistance exercise (e.g., weight lifting or exercises using weight machines) is also useful. Supervised high-intensity resistance training 3 days per week for ~45 min per session has been shown to improve HbA1c by 0.6% *(101)* to 1.1% *(102)* independent of changes in body weight, although improvements in glycemic control were not maintained by a home-based resistance program following the supervised training *(103)*. Patients who can exercise can be recommended to begin about 15 min of low-impact aerobic exercise and gradually increasing to 30–45 min of moderate-intensity (50–70% of maximal heart rate) physical activity most (ideally all) days of the week. However, before a vigorous exercise regimen is instituted, patients should be evaluated for potential contraindications (e.g., active cardiovascular disease, uncontrolled hypertension, proliferative, or severe nonproliferative retinopathy) or factors that may predispose them to injury (such as peripheral or autonomic neuropathy). In addition, patients who are on insulin or insulin secretagogues should be advised to check their blood glucose before exercise and have a carbohydrate snack if glucose levels are less than 100 mg/dL (5.6 mmol/L) before exercise to avoid hypoglycemia.

4.7. Oral Medications and Other Agents

There are now several classes of oral anti-hyperglycemic medications and other agents available for the treatment of diabetes (either alone or in combination with other agents) (Table 6):

4.7.1. SULFONYLUREAS

Available agents include *glimepiride (Amaryl®), glipizide (Glucotrol®, Glucotrol XL®), glyburide (Micronase®, Diaβeta®, Glynase®)*. These stimulate insulin secretion through activation of a potassium channel on the pancreatic β-cell. They may be used as monotherapy or in combination with other oral agents and may be most useful in thinner patients with greater relative insulin deficiency. Potential side effects include hypoglycemia, hypersensitivity, and weight gain.

4.7.2. BIGUANIDES

Available agents include *metformin (Glucophage®, Glucophage XR®)*. Metformin acts to improve insulin sensitivity primarily by decreasing hepatic glucose production and secondarily by enhancing peripheral insulin sensitivity in the muscle. It can be used as

Table 6

Medications for the Treatment of Type 2 Diabetes

Class Agents (trade name)	Year of introduction or approval	Mechanism of action	HbA1c reduction (%)	Available doses	Daily dose	Doses per day
Biguanide						
Metformin (Glucophage®, Glucophage XR®)	1957 1995	Decreases hepatic glucose production	1.5	500, 850, 1,000 mg 500, 750, 1,000 mg	500–2,550 mg 500–2,000 mg	2–3 1
Sulfonylureas						
Glyburide (Micronase®, Diaβeta®)	1946	Stimulates insulin secretion	1.5	1.25, 2.5, 5 mg	2.5–20 mg	1–2
Glyburide micronized (Glynase®)				3, 6 mg	3–12 mg	1–2
Glimepiride (Amaryl®)				1, 2, 4 mg	1–8 mg	1
Glipizide (Glucotrol®)				5, 10 mg	2.5–40 mg	1–2
Glipizide-CR (Glucotrol XL®)				2.5, 5, 10 mg	2.5–20 mg	1
Thiazolidinediones						
Rosiglitazone (Avandia®)	1999	Enhances tissue sensitivity to insulin through activation of intracellular PPAR-γ receptors	1–1.5	2, 4, 8 mg	2–8 mg	1–2
Pioglitazone (Actos®)				15, 30, 45 mg	15–45 mg	1
α-Glucosidase inhibitors						
Acarbose (Precose®)	1995	Inhibits α-glucosidase enzymes in the small intestine, slowing digestion of carbohydrates and glucose absorption	0.5–1	25, 50, 100 mg	75–300 mg	3
Miglitol (Glyset®)				25, 50, 100 mg	75–300 mg	3
Non-sulfonylurea Secretagogues						
Repaglinide (Prandin®)	1997	Stimulates release of insulin in response to a meal	1–1.5	0.5, 1, 2 mg	0.5–16 mg	2–4
Nateglinide (Starlix®)				60, 120 mg	120–360 mg	3

(continued)

Table 6
(continued)

Class Agents (trade name)	Year of introduction or approval	Mechanism of action	HbA1c reduction (%)	Available doses	Daily dose	Doses per day
DPP-IV Inhibitors						
Sitagliptin (Januvia®)	2006	Inhibits dipeptidyl-peptidase-IV enzymes that degrade incretin hormones (GLP-1, GIP) that stimulate insulin secretion in response to a meal	0.8–0.9%	25, 50, 100 mg	25–100 mg	1
GLP-1 Analogues						
Exenatide (Byetta®)	2005	Analogue of GLP-1, which stimulates insulin secretion in response to a meal	1.1	5, 10 μg, s.c.	10–20 μg	2
Amylin analogues						
Pramlinitide (Symlin®)	2005	Synthetic amylin hormone, which is secreted with insulin and contributes to postprandial glucose control	0.6	60, 120 μg, s.c.	180–360 μg	3

CR controlled-release; PPAR-γ peroxisome proliferator-activated receptor-γ; GLP-1 glucagon-like peptide 1; GIP glucose-dependent insulinotropic peptide; s.c. subcutaneous.

monotherapy or in combination with other oral agents or insulin. Metformin is the first-line treatment in the overweight or obese patient with type 2 DM because of its efficacy and tendency to cause no weight gain or to induce mild weight loss. It is contraindicated in patients prone to develop metabolic acidosis (such as renal dysfunction, liver failure, congestive heart failure, major surgery, dye procedures, sepsis, alcoholism). Main side effects are gastrointestinal (nausea, anorexia, diarrhea) and tend to subside with treatment.

4.7.3. THIAZOLIDINEDIONES

Available agents include *rosiglitazone (Avandia®)* and *pioglitazone (Actos®)* (troglitazone has been withdrawn from the market). These are insulin sensitizers that activate intracellular peroxisome proliferator-activated receptor-γ (PPAR-γ) receptors found primarily in adipose tissue and alter transcription of proteins involved in insulin resistance. They can be used as monotherapy or in combination with sulfonylureas, metformin, or insulin. Contraindications include active liver disease (alanine transaminase (ALT) >2.5 times the upper limit of normal). Main side effects include weight gain and edema. Transaminase levels should be checked prior to therapy and monitored every 2 months for the first 12 months and periodically thereafter with discontinuation if ALT is >2.5–3 times the upper limit of normal on two separate occasions. Recent metaanalyses have raised, but not fully substantiated, concern for increased cardiovascular risk (including myocardial infarction) associated with the use of rosiglitazone *(104,105)*, although another metaanalysis found no increased cardiovascular mortality *(106)*, and interim analysis from an ongoing clinical trial designed to address cardiovascular outcomes with rosiglitazone was inconclusive with respect to myocardial infarction *(107)*. Metaanalyses evaluating cardiovascular risk associated with pioglitazone have shown no increased risk *(106)* or a protective effect *(108)*. Regardless, both agents are clearly associated with an approximately twofold increased risk of fluid retention and congestive heart failure *(106,107)*. Because of these findings, the FDA has added a "black box" warning to the prescribing information for TZDs. Both TZDs have also been associated with increased risk of osteoporosis and peripheral fractures (distal upper or lower extremity), especially in women *(109)*. Development of selective PPAR-γ modulators (such as INT-131 (InteKrin, Inc.)), which appear to have improved efficacy and/or safety profiles, is currently underway.

4.7.4. NON-SULFONYLUREA SECRETAGOGUES ("GLINIDES")

Available agents include *repaglinide (Prandin®)* and *nateglinide (Starlix®)*. These stimulate acute insulin secretion in response to nutrient ingestion by binding to a pancreatic β-cell site distinct from the sulfonylurea binding site and have a greater effect on postprandial rather than fasting glucose. They can be used as monotherapy or in combination with metformin or a TZD. Contraindications include type 1 diabetes or diabetic ketoacidosis. Similar to the sulfonylureas, they can cause weight gain and hypoglycemia, although they may be a useful option in patients with irregular meal schedules since they are taken with meals but omitted when a meal is skipped, which reduces the risk of hypoglycemia. These agents can also be used safely in renal impairment.

4.7.5. α-GLUCOSIDASE INHIBITORS

Available agents include *acarbose (Precose®)* and *miglitol (Glyset®)*. These medications slow the digestion of carbohydrates and thus delay glucose absorption and reduce postprandial hyperglycemia. They have modest effects on HbA1c and fasting glucose and can be used as monotherapy (mainly in patients with HbA1c < 7%) or in combination with sulfonylureas or metformin (acarbose) or insulin (acarbose). Contraindications include major gastrointestinal disorders, and the major side effects that can lead to a high rate of discontinuation are gastrointestinal including flatulence and bloating due to increased delivery of carbohydrates to the distal intestine. They may be useful in patients in whom postprandial hyperglycemia is the main problem.

4.7.6. DPP-IV Inhibitors

Available agents include *sitagliptin (Januvia®)* and, in Europe, *vildagliptin (Galvus®)*. Other agents in development include saxagliptin (Bristol Myers Squibb) and alogliptin (Takeda). This is a new class of medications that enhance the action of incretins, hormones such as glucagon-like peptide-1 (GLP-1) and glucose-dependent insulinotropic peptide (GIP) which are released in response to a meal and stimulate insulin secretion and suppress glucagon release in a glucose-dependent manner, delay gastric emptying, and increase satiety. GLP-1 and GIP are rapidly degraded by dipeptidyl peptidase-4 (DPP-IV) enzymes, and DPP-IV inhibitors act to prolong the activity of these hormones. Sitagliptin was approved in 2006 for use as monotherapy or in combination with metformin or TZDs. As monotherapy, it produces placebo-corrected improvements in HbA1c of 0.8–0.9% *(110)* and produced an additional lowering of ~0.7% when added to metformin *(111)* or pioglitazone *(112)*.

4.7.7. GLP-1 Analogues

Exenatide or synthetic exendin 4 (Byetta®) is an analogue of GLP-1 derived from lizard venom that shares about 50% sequence homology to the native hormone but has a longer circulating half-life due to greater resistance to DPP-IV enzymes. It is approved for use with sulfonylureas and/or metformin but currently not with other antihyperglycemic agents or insulin. Exenatide is administered as a subcutaneous injection at a dose of 5 µg twice daily within 60 min before the morning and evening meal, which can be titrated up to 10 µg twice daily after 1 month. Patients on sulfonylureas may require a decrease in their sulfonylurea dose to avoid hypoglycemia but no adjustment of metformin is necessary. It should not be used in those with severe renal impairment or severe gastrointestinal disease, since its use is commonly associated with gastrointestinal side effects such as nausea, vomiting, and diarrhea, which may subside with treatment. HbA1c improved by 1.1% at 6 months, with a reduction in body weight of 2.3 kg *(113)*. A pancreatitis caution has been added to the prescribing information for exenatide based on the recent report of 30 cases of pancreatitis in patients taking exenatide, 27 of whom had at least one other risk factor for acute pancreatitis (gallstones, severe hypertriglyceridemia, alcohol). It is recommended that patients receive prompt medical attention if they develop severe, persistent, and unexplained abdominal pain while taking exenatide. A long-acting form of exenatide (exenatide LAR (Amylin, Inc.)), which can be administered once weekly, as well as modified GLP-1 analogues and GLP-1 linked to molecules that prolong its half-life are currently under development.

Amylin (Pramlinitide (Symlin®)) is a synthetic form of the hormone amylin, which is cosecreted from pancreatic β-cells along with insulin and contributes to postprandial glucose control. It is approved for use in patients with type 2 diabetes on mealtime insulin, with or without a sulfonylurea and/or metformin, when glycemic control is inadequate.

Amylin is administered as a subcutaneous injection at a dose of 60 μg before each major meal, which can be increased up to 120 μg if nausea does not occur after 3–7 days, in patients with type 2 DM. Patients may need to reduce their dose of short-acting prandial insulin by ~50% to avoid hypoglycemia and should not mix insulin with amylin since this can alter the pharmacokinetics of amylin. It is contraindicated in patients with gastroparesis or hypoglycemic unawareness, and main side effects are gastrointestinal (nausea, vomiting, abdominal pain) and headache. HbA1c improved by ~0.6% at 1 year, with a reduction in body weight of ~1.5 kg *(114,115)*.

4.8. Insulin

Although insulin resistance plays a major role in the pathophysiology of type 2 DM, insulin therapy remains an integral component of the therapeutic regimen for these patients. Insulin is typically viewed as a treatment of last resort, but initial therapy with insulin should be considered in those presenting with severe symptoms and/or evidence of ketoacidosis, in pregnant patients or those planning to become pregnant soon, in patients with comorbid conditions that make the use of oral agents difficult (e.g., renal or hepatic disease, myocardial infarction, etc.), and in those who are not meeting glycemic goals on two oral agents. The normal physiology of insulin is a basal level of secretion at all times to regulate hepatic glucose production overnight and between meals, with a burst of release at mealtime to inhibit hepatic glucose production, promote glucose disposal, and thus maintain glucose levels in a normal range. We classify the currently available insulins into basal, prandial, or combination (premixed) below. Importantly, several new insulin analogues with more physiologic profiles and/or easier methods of administration have become available in recent years.

4.8.1. BASAL INSULIN

Available agents include *NPH (Humulin N or Novolin N), insulin detemir (Levemir®), insulin glargine (Lantus®)*. Previously available agents include Lente and ultralente, which were not used as commonly due to variable absorption and erratic therapeutic outcomes and have been recently discontinued. *NPH* is an intermediate-acting insulin with an onset of action between 2 and 4 h, which typically requires twice daily administration for 24-h basal coverage. *Insulin detemir* is an insulin analogue soluble at neutral pH that binds to albumin through its fatty acid chain and provides stable levels of free insulin. It has a duration of action of approximately 20 h and is thus administered twice daily in most patients. *Insulin glargine* is an insulin analogue with reduced solubility at a physiologic pH, which forms microprecipitates in subcutaneous tissue following injection, thus delaying systemic absorption. It has a gradual and relatively constant release pattern over 24 h, reaching a plateau at about 4–6 h, without a pronounced peak and can be administered once daily (ideally at approximately the same time each day). Both detemir and glargine have more stable and less variable pharmacokinetic profiles compared with NPH.

4.8.2. PRANDIAL INSULIN

Available agents include *regular insulin (Humulin R®or Novolin R®), insulin lispro (Humalog®), insulin aspart (Novolog®), insulin glulisin (Apidra®)*. Regular insulin peaks approximately 2–4 h after administration with a duration of action about 4–6 h. More rapid-acting formulations involving modifications to the insulin molecule have been developed (*lispro, aspart, glulisin*) that have a shorter time to peak action (half hour to 2 h) and duration of action (3–5 h), which more closely mimics normal meal-time physiology. Because their pharmacokinetic profiles have less intraindividual variability and reduce early postprandial hyperglycemia and late postprandial hypoglycemia compared with regular insulin, they are generally preferred for prandial use. *Inhaled insulin (Exubera®)* was approved by the FDA in 2006, but withdrawn from the market by the manufacturer in 2007 for financial reasons due to lack of widespread adoption and use.

4.8.3. COMBINATION

Available agents include *70/30 Humulin®* or *Novolin®* (70% NPH and 30% regular), *50/50 Humulin®* (50% NPH and 50% regular), *75/25 Humalog®* (75% neutral protamine lispro (NPL) and 25% lispro), *50/50 Humalog®* (50% NPL and 50% lispro), *70/30 Novolog Neutral®* (70% protamine aspart, 30% aspart). These premixed insulin formulations containing both prandial and basal insulin can provide more flexibility and convenience for patients by eliminating the need for self-mixing, simplifying the insulin regimen, and reducing the number of daily injections. However, they do not allow the dose of each component to be adjusted separately.

4.9. Treatment Approach

Although lifestyle intervention with medical nutrition therapy and exercise forms the cornerstone of therapy of type 2 diabetes and should remain an integral component, many patients eventually require pharmacologic therapy. A consensus statement from the ADA and the European Association for the Study of Diabetes (EASD) in 2006 suggested metformin as the first-line pharmacologic therapy in the absence of contraindications, based on its demonstrated efficacy (improvement in HbA1c by ~1.5% as monotherapy), weight-neutral profile, general tolerability, and low cost (Fig. 1) (*117*). Therapy can be initiated at a dose of 500 mg once or twice per day with meals, and increased to 850 or 1,000 mg before breakfast and dinner after a week if no gastrointestinal side effects occur. If HbA1c remains ≥7%, then a second agent should be added within 2–3 months, which could include insulin, a sulfonylurea, or a TZD (*117*). This consensus algorithm was updated in 2008 to reflect the concerns related to potential increased cardiovascular risk and fractures associated with TZDs (*118*). The availability of the DPP-IV inhibitors provides another option for a second agent in patients whose HbA1c is close to target and/or in whom hypoglycemia and/or weight gain are an important consideration. Exenatide is also an option for those in whom weight gain and/or titration of insulin doses are a concern. Glinides and α-glucosidase inhibitors could be considered in patients close to goal and have the advantage of having a short duration of action in those with erratic eating schedules or being weight neutral, respectively.

In patients presenting with more severe hyperglycemia, consideration can be given to initial combination treatment with metformin and a sulfonylurea, which can achieve greater glycemic control compared with either agent alone (*119*). If therapy with two agents does not achieve target HbA1c goals, the ADA/EASD suggests starting or intensifying (e.g., adding prandial coverage) insulin treatment. If the HbA1c is close to target and/or the patient is resistant to starting insulin, an alternative option is to add a third oral agent. The addition of a TZD (rosiglitazone) to patients suboptimally control-

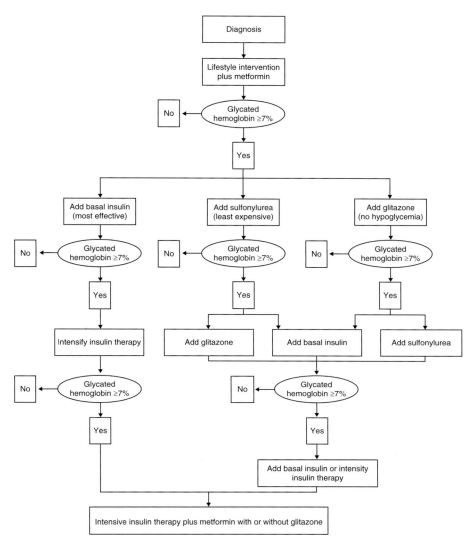

Fig. 1. Algorithm for the medical management of patients with type 2 diabetes. Practitioners should reinforce lifestyle interventions with patients at every visit. Hemoglobin A1c levels should be checked every 3 months until the level is under 7%; after that, levels should be checked at least every 6 months. "No" indicates that no change in pharmacologic intervention is indicated. Used by permission from *(116)*.

led with a sulfonylurea and metformin resulted in the further lowering of HbA1c by 1% *(120)*; however, triple oral therapy has been shown to be equivalent in efficacy to insulin 70/30 and metformin but less cost-effective and with a lower rate of adherence *(121)*. Once patients require prandial insulin, oral secretagogues can be discontinued but insulin sensitizers should be continued. Pramlintide is an option for patients on meal-time insulin and may improve glycemic control and/or reduce insulin requirements while tending to induce a small amount of weight loss. Combination therapy with insulin and metformin or insulin and a TZD are effective, although the latter may be associated with more edema and weight gain.

For initiation of insulin therapy, typically the simplest way to start is with a single bedtime injection of a long-acting insulin (such as NPH or glargine) to reduce elevated fasting blood glucose levels. A starting dose of ~10 units or 0.1 units/kg can be used. Fasting blood glucose should be monitored, and the dose of bedtime insulin adjusted every 3–5 days to achieve target levels (usually <120 mg/dL (6.6 mmol/L)), provided that nocturnal hypoglycemia does not occur. The dose can be increased by 2 units for every 20 mg/dL (1.1 mmol/L) of fasting blood glucose over 120 mg/dL. Once fasting glucose levels are in range, postprandial glucose levels should also be monitored if HbA1c levels are not at goal. If postprandial glucose levels are consistently higher than goal despite a reasonable meal plan, prandial insulin therapy with a rapid-acting insulin should be initiated. The initial starting dose can be 2–4 units with titration up accordingly. As noted previously, the use of premixed insulins may provide more convenience and decrease the number of injections, but there is greater flexibility with dose adjustment if the long-acting and prandial insulins are administered separately.

5. SUMMARY

Obesity, diabetes, and their accompanying metabolic abnormalities represent major public health problems in the modern era, and efforts on a global level are needed to address this important issue. Overnutrition and inadequate physical activity in the appropriate genetic background account in large part for the epidemic of these conditions, and lifestyle modification is a critical component of the treatment approach. Fortunately, intense research into the pathophysiology of these conditions is shedding light on the complex mechanisms underlying the regulation of body weight and metabolism. Correspondingly, there is great interest in the development of new therapeutic agents with novel mechanisms of action for the treatment of obesity and diabetes, as evidenced by the recent approval of several new medications for these conditions. Hopefully, the concerted efforts of public health policy to improve nutritional guidelines and promote increased activity will align with those of medical research to develop more targeted and rational approaches to therapy that will lead to a fitter and healthier population.

REFERENCES

1. Caballero B. Introduction. Symposium: obesity in developing countries: biological and ecological factors. J Nutr 2001; 131(3):866S–870S.
2. Shah B, Sucher K, Hollenbeck CB. Comparison of ideal body weight equations and published height-weight tables with body mass index tables for healthy adults in the United States. Nutr Clin Pract 2006; 21(3):312–319.
3. Calle EE, Thun MJ, Petrelli JM, Rodriguez C, Heath CW, Jr. Body-mass index and mortality in a prospective cohort of U.S. adults. N Engl J Med 1999; 341(15):1097–1105.
4. Banerji MA, Lebowitz J, Chaiken RL, Gordon D, Kral JG, Lebovitz HE. Relationship of visceral adipose tissue and glucose disposal is independent of sex in black NIDDM subjects. Am J Physiol 1997; 273(2 Pt 1):E425–E432.
5. Executive summary of the clinical guidelines on the identification, evaluation, and treatment of overweight and obesity in adults. Arch Intern Med 1998; 158(17):1855–1867.

6. Kiernan M, Winkleby MA. Identifying patients for weight-loss treatment: an empirical evaluation of the NHLBI obesity education initiative expert panel treatment recommendations. Arch Intern Med 2000; 160(14):2169–2176.

7. Janiszewski DA, Janssen I, Ross R. Does waist circumference predict diabetes and cardiovascular disease beyond commonly evaluated cardiometabolic risk factors?. Diabetes Care 2007; 30(12):3105–3109.

8. Gallagher D, Heymsfield SB, Heo M, Jebb SA, Murgatroyd PR, Sakamoto Y. Healthy percentage body fat ranges: an approach for developing guidelines based on body mass index. Am J Clin Nutr 2000; 72(3):694–701.

9. WHO Expert Consultation. Appropriate body-mass index for Asian populations and its implications for policy and intervention strategies. Lancet 2004; 363(9403):157–163.

10. Janssen I, Katzmarzyk PT, Ross R. Body mass index, waist circumference, and health risk: evidence in support of current National Institutes of Health guidelines. Arch Intern Med 2002; 162(18):2074–2079.

11. McTigue KM, Harris R, Hemphill B, et al. Screening and interventions for obesity in adults: summary of the evidence for the U.S. Preventive Services Task Force. Ann Intern Med 2003; 139(11):933–949.

12. Farooqi IS, O'Rahilly S. Monogenic obesity in humans. Annu Rev Med 2005; 56:443–458.

13. Farooqi IS, Wangensteen T, Collins S, et al. Clinical and molecular genetic spectrum of congenital deficiency of the leptin receptor. N Engl J Med 2007; 356(3):237–247.

14. Farooqi IS, Keogh JM, Yeo GS, Lank EJ, Cheetham T, O'Rahilly S. Clinical spectrum of obesity and mutations in the melanocortin 4 receptor gene. N Engl J Med 2003; 348(12):1085–1095.

15. Fontaine KR, Redden DT, Wang C, Westfall AO, Allison DB. Years of life lost due to obesity. JAMA 2003; 289(2):187–193.

16. Willett WC, Manson JE, Stampfer MJ, et al. Weight, weight change, and coronary heart disease in women. Risk within the 'normal' weight range. JAMA 1995; 273(6):461–465.

17. Chan JM, Rimm EB, Colditz GA, Stampfer MJ, Willett WC. Obesity, fat distribution, and weight gain as risk factors for clinical diabetes in men. Diabetes Care 1994; 17(9):961–969.

18. Colditz GA, Willett WC, Rotnitzky A, Manson JE. Weight gain as a risk factor for clinical diabetes mellitus in women. Ann Intern Med 1995; 122(7):481–486.

19. Bray GA, Ryan DH. Medical approaches to treatment of the obese patient. In: Mantzoros C.S., editor. *Obesity and Diabetes*. Totowa: Humana; 2006, pp. 457–469.

20. Hill JO. Understanding and addressing the epidemic of obesity: an energy balance perspective. Endocr Rev 2006; 27(7):750–761.

21. Li Z, Maglione M, Tu W, et al. Meta-analysis: pharmacologic treatment of obesity. Ann Intern Med 2005; 142(7):532–546.

22. Knowler WC, Barrett-Connor E, Fowler SE, et al. Reduction in the incidence of type 2 diabetes with lifestyle intervention or metformin. N Engl J Med 2002; 346(6):393–403.

23. Thompson WG, Cook DA, Clark MM, Bardia A, Levine JA. Treatment of obesity. Mayo Clin Proc 2007; 82(1):93–101.

24. Bray GA, Gray DS. Treatment of obesity: an overview. Diabetes Metab Rev 1988; 4(7):653–679.

25. Lantigua RA, Amatruda JM, Biddle TL, Forbes GB, Lockwood DH. Cardiac arrhythmias associated with a liquid protein diet for the treatment of obesity. N Engl J Med 1980; 303(13):735–738.

26. Willett WC. Dietary fat plays a major role in obesity: no. Obes Rev 2002; 3(2):59–68.

27. Howard BV, Van HL, Hsia J, et al. Low-fat dietary pattern and risk of cardiovascular disease: the Women's Health Initiative Randomized Controlled Dietary Modification Trial. JAMA 2006; 295(6):655–666.

28. Ludwig DS. The glycemic index: physiological mechanisms relating to obesity, diabetes, and cardio-vascular disease. JAMA 2002; 287(18):2414–2423.

29. Millan-Price J, Petocz P, Atkinson F, et al. Comparison of 4 diets of varying glycemic load on weight loss and cardiovascular risk reduction in overweight and obese young adults: a randomized controlled trial. Arch Intern Med 2006; 166(14):1466–1475.

30. Ebbeling CB, Leidig MM, Sinclair KB, Seger-Shippee LG, Feldman HA, Ludwig DS. Effects of an ad libitum low-glycemic load diet on cardiovascular disease risk factors in obese young adults. Am J Clin Nutr 2005; 81(5):976–982.

31. Atkins R. *Dr. Atkins' New Diet Revolution*. New York: Avon Books, 1998.

32. Agatston A. *The South Beach Diet: The Delicious, Doctor-Designed, Foolproof Plan for Fast and Healthy Weight Loss*. New York: Random House, 2003.

33. Nordmann AJ, Nordmann A, Briel M, et al. Effects of low-carbohydrate vs low-fat diets on weight loss and cardiovascular risk factors: a meta-analysis of randomized controlled trials. Arch Intern Med 2006; 166(3):285–293.

34. Denke MA. Metabolic effects of high-protein, low-carbohydrate diets. Am J Cardiol 2001; 88(1):59–61.

35. Dansinger ML, Gleason JA, Griffith JL, Selker HP, Schaefer EJ. Comparison of the Atkins, Ornish, Weight Watchers, and Zone diets for weight loss and heart disease risk reduction: a randomized trial. JAMA 2005; 293(1):43–53.

36. Shick SM, Wing RR, Klem ML, McGuire MT, Hill JO, Seagle H. Persons successful at long-term weight loss and maintenance continue to consume a low-energy, low-fat diet. J Am Diet Assoc 1998; 98(4):408–413.

37. Esposito K, Marfella R, Ciotola M, et al. Effect of a mediterranean-style diet on endothelial dysfunction and markers of vascular inflammation in the metabolic syndrome: a randomized trial. JAMA 2004; 292(12):1440–1446.

38. Estruch R, Martinez-Gonzalez MA, et al. Corella D, . Effects of a Mediterranean-style diet on cardiovascular risk factors: a randomized trial. Ann Intern Med 2006; 145(1):1–11.

39. Osterdahl M, Kocturk T, Koochek A, Wandell PE. Effects of a short-term intervention with a paleolithic diet in healthy volunteers. Eur J Clin Nutr 2008; 62(5):682–685.

40. Lindeberg S, Jonsson T, Granfeldt Y, et al. A Palaeolithic diet improves glucose tolerance more than a Mediterranean-like diet in individuals with ischaemic heart disease. Diabetologia 2007; 50(9):1795–1807.

41. McCullough ML, Feskanich D, Stampfer MJ, et al. Diet quality and major chronic disease risk in men and women: moving toward improved dietary guidance. Am J Clin Nutr 2002; 76(6):1261–1271.

42. Fung TT, McCullough M, van Dam RM, Hu FB. A prospective study of overall diet quality and risk of type 2 diabetes in women. Diabetes Care 2007; 30(7):1753–1757.

43. Azadbakht L, Mirmiran P, Esmaillzadeh A, Azizi T, Azizi F. Beneficial effects of a Dietary Approaches to Stop Hypertension eating plan on features of the metabolic syndrome. Diabetes Care 2005; 28(12):2823–2831.

44. Garrow JS, Summerbell CD. Meta-analysis: effect of exercise, with or without dieting, on the body composition of overweight subjects. Eur J Clin Nutr 1995; 49(1):1–10.

45. Wing RR. Physical activity in the treatment of the adulthood overweight and obesity: current evidence and research issues. Med Sci Sports Exerc 1999; 31(11 Suppl):S547–S552.

46. Curioni CC, Lourenco PM. Long-term weight loss after diet and exercise: a systematic review. Int J Obes (Lond) 2005; 29(10):1168–1174.

47. Hu FB, Willett WC, Li T, Stampfer MJ, Colditz GA, Manson JE. Adiposity as compared with physical activity in predicting mortality among women. N Engl J Med 2004; 351(26):2694–2703.

48. Schoeller DA, Shay K, Kushner RF. How much physical activity is needed to minimize weight gain in previously obese women?. Am J Clin Nutr 1997; 66(3):551–556.

49. Weinsier RL, Hunter GR, Desmond RA, Byrne NM, Zuckerman PA, Darnell BE. Free-living activity energy expenditure in women successful and unsuccessful at maintaining a normal body weight. Am J Clin Nutr 2002; 75(3):499–504.

50. Saris WH, Blair SN, van Baak MA, et al. How much physical activity is enough to prevent unhealthy weight gain? Outcome of the IASO 1st Stock Conference and consensus statement. Obes Rev 2003; 4(2):101–114.

51. Rucker D, Padwal R, Li SK, Curioni C, Lau DC. Long term pharmacotherapy for obesity and overweight: updated meta-analysis. BMJ 2007; 335(7631):1194–1199.

52. James WP, Astrup A, Finer N, et al. Effect of sibutramine on weight maintenance after weight loss: a randomised trial. STORM Study Group. Sibutramine Trial of Obesity Reduction and Maintenance. Lancet 2000; 356(9248):2119–2125.

53. Bray GA, Blackburn GL, et al. Ferguson JM, . Sibutramine produces dose-related weight loss. Obes Res 1999; 7(2):189–198.

54. O'Meara S, Riemsma R, Shirran L, Mather L, ter Riet G. A systematic review of the clinical effectiveness of orlistat used for the management of obesity. Obes Rev 2004; 5(1):51–68.

55. Torgerson JS, Hauptman J, Boldrin MN, Sjostrom L. XENical in the prevention of diabetes in obese subjects (XENDOS) study: a randomized study of orlistat as an adjunct to lifestyle changes for the prevention of type 2 diabetes in obese patients. Diabetes Care 2004; 27(1):155–161.

56. Ravinet TC, Delgorge C, Menet C, Arnone M, Soubrie P. CB1 cannabinoid receptor knockout in mice leads to leanness, resistance to diet-induced obesity and enhanced leptin sensitivity. Int J Obes Relat Metab Disord 2004; 28(4):640–648.

57. Van Gaal LF, Rissanen AM, Scheen AJ, Ziegler O, Rossner S. Effects of the cannabinoid-1 receptor blocker rimonabant on weight reduction and cardiovascular risk factors in overweight patients: 1-year experience from the RIO-Europe study. Lancet 2005; 365(9468):1389–1397.

58. Pi-Sunyer FX, Aronne LJ, Heshmati HM, Devin J, Rosenstock J. Effect of rimonabant, a cannabinoid-1 receptor blocker, on weight and cardiometabolic risk factors in overweight or obese patients: RIO-North America: a randomized controlled trial. JAMA 2006; 295(7):761–775.

59. Despres JP, Golay A, Sjostrom L. Effects of rimonabant on metabolic risk factors in overweight patients with dyslipidemia. N Engl J Med 2005; 353(20):2121–2134.

60. Scheen AJ, Finer N, Hollander P, Jensen MD, Van Gaal LF. Efficacy and tolerability of rimonabant in overweight or obese patients with type 2 diabetes: a randomised controlled study. Lancet 2006; 368(9548):1660–1672.

61. Haddock CK, Poston WS, Dill PL, Foreyt JP, Ericsson M. Pharmacotherapy for obesity: a quantitative analysis of four decades of published randomized clinical trials. Int J Obes Relat Metab Disord 2002; 26(2):262–273.

62. Anderson JW, Greenway FL, Fujioka K, Gadde KM, McKenney J, O'Neil PM. Bupropion SR enhances weight loss: a 48-week double-blind, placebo-controlled trial. Obes Res 2002; 10(7):633–641.

63. Croft H, Houser TL, Jamerson BD, et al. Effect on body weight of bupropion sustained-release in patients with major depression treated for 52 weeks. Clin Ther 2002; 24(4):662–672.

64. Jain AK, Kaplan RA, Gadde KM, Bupropion SR vs. placebo for weight loss in obese patients with depressive symptoms. Obes Res 2002; 10(10):1049–1056.

65. Gadde KM, Franciscy DM, Wagner HR, Krishnan KR. Zonisamide for weight loss in obese adults: a randomized controlled trial. JAMA 2003; 289(14):1820–1825.

66. Wadden TA, Bartlett SJ, Foster GD, et al. Sertraline and relapse prevention training following treatment by very-low-calorie diet: a controlled clinical trial. Obes Res 1995; 3(6):549–557.

67. Lambert PD, Anderson KD, Sleeman MW, et al. Ciliary neurotrophic factor activates leptin-like pathways and reduces body fat, without cachexia or rebound weight gain, even in leptin-resistant obesity. Proc Natl Acad Sci U S A 2001; 98(8):4652–4657.

68. Ettinger MP, Littlejohn TW, Schwartz SL, et al. Recombinant variant of ciliary neurotrophic factor for weight loss in obese adults: a randomized, dose-ranging study. JAMA 2003; 289(14):1826–1832.

69. Cooke D, Bloom S. The obesity pipeline: current strategies in the development of anti-obesity drugs. Nat Rev Drug Discov 2006; 5(11):919–931.

70. Biddinger SB, Hernandez-Ono A, Rask-Madsen C, et al. Hepatic insulin resistance is sufficient to produce dyslipidemia and susceptibility to atherosclerosis. Cell Metab 2008; 7(2):125–134.

71. World Health Organization. *Definition, Diagnosis and Classification of Diabetes Mellitus and Its Complications. Report of a WHO Consultation.* Geneva: World Health Organization, 1999.

72. Balkau B, Charles MA. Comment on the provisional report from the WHO consultation. European Group for the Study of Insulin Resistance (EGIR). Diabet Med 1999; 16(5):442–443.

73. Expert Panel on Detection, Evaluation, and Treatment of High Blood Cholesterol in Adults. Executive Summary of The Third Report of The National Cholesterol Education Program (NCEP) Expert Panel on Detection, Evaluation, and Treatment of High Blood Cholesterol in Adults (Adult Treatment Panel III). JAMA 2001; 285(19):2486–2497.

74. Einhorn D, Reaven GM, Cobin RH, et al. American College of Endocrinology position statement on the insulin resistance syndrome. Endocr Pract 2003; 9(3):237–252.

75. Alberti KG, Zimmet P, Shaw J. Metabolic syndrome – a new world-wide definition. A Consensus Statement from the International Diabetes Federation. Diabet Med 2006; 23(5):469–480.

76. Ilanne-Parikka P, Eriksson JG, Lindstrom J, et al. Effect of lifestyle intervention on the occurrence of metabolic syndrome and its components in the Finnish Diabetes Prevention Study. Diabetes Care 2008; 31(4):805–807.

77. Aguilar-Salinas CA, Mehta R, Rojas R, Gomez-Perez FJ, Olaiz G, Rull JA. Management of the metabolic syndrome as a strategy for preventing the macrovascular complications of type 2 diabetes: controversial issues. Curr Diabetes Rev 2005; 1(2):145–158.

78. Tuomilehto J, Lindstrom J, Eriksson JG, et al. Prevention of type 2 diabetes mellitus by changes in lifestyle among subjects with impaired glucose tolerance. N Engl J Med 2001; 344(18): 1343–1350.

79. American Diabetes Association. Standards of medical care in diabetes - 2008. Diabetes Care 2008; 31(Suppl 1):S12–S54.

80. Glucose tolerance and mortality: comparison of WHO and American Diabetes Association diagnostic criteria. The DECODE study group. European Diabetes Epidemiology Group. Diabetes Epidemiology: Collaborative analysis of Diagnostic criteria in Europe. Lancet 1999; 354(9179): 617–621.

81. Tominaga M, Eguchi H, Manaka H, Igarashi K, Kato T, Sekikawa A. Impaired glucose tolerance is a risk factor for cardiovascular disease, but not impaired fasting glucose. The Funagata Diabetes Study. Diabetes Care 1999; 22(6):920–924.

82. Ko GT, Chan JC, Woo J, et al. The reproducibility and usefulness of the oral glucose tolerance test in screening for diabetes and other cardiovascular risk factors. Ann Clin Biochem 1998; 35 (Pt 1):62–67.

83. The effect of intensive treatment of diabetes on the development and progression of long-term complications in insulin-dependent diabetes mellitus. The Diabetes Control and Complications Trial Research Group. N Engl J Med 1993; 329(14):977–986.

84. Intensive blood-glucose control with sulphonylureas or insulin compared with conventional treatment and risk of complications in patients with type 2 diabetes (UKPDS 33). UK Prospective Diabetes Study (UKPDS) Group. Lancet 1998; 352(9131):837–853.

85. Tsuji I, Nakamoto K, Hasegawa T, et al. Receiver operating characteristic analysis on fasting plasma glucose, HbA1c, and fructosamine on diabetes screening. Diabetes Care 1991; 14(11):1075–1077.

86. Rohlfing CL, Little RR, Wiedmeyer HM, et al. Use of GHb (HbA1c) in screening for undiagnosed diabetes in the U.S. population. Diabetes Care 2000; 23(2):187–191.

87. Barr RG, Nathan DM, Meigs JB, Singer DE. Tests of glycemia for the diagnosis of type 2 diabetes mellitus. Ann Intern Med 2002; 137(4):263–272.

88. American Diabetes Association. Diagnosis and classification of diabetes mellitus. Diabetes Care 2007; 30(Suppl 1):S42–S47.

89. Davidson MB, Schriger DL, Peters AL, Lorber B. Relationship between fasting plasma glucose and glycosylated hemoglobin: potential for false-positive diagnoses of type 2 diabetes using new diagnostic criteria. JAMA 1999; 281(13):1203–1210.

90. Alberti KG, Zimmet PZ. Definition, diagnosis and classification of diabetes mellitus and its complications. Part 1: diagnosis and classification of diabetes mellitus provisional report of a WHO consultation. Diabet Med 1998; 15(7):539–553.

91. Harris MI, Klein R, Welborn TA, Knuiman MW. Onset of NIDDM occurs at least 4–7 yr before clinical diagnosis. Diabetes Care 1992; 15(7):815–819.

92. U.S. Preventive Services Task Force. Screening for type 2 diabetes mellitus in adults: recommendations and rationale. Ann Intern Med 2003; 138(3):212–214.

93. Lebovitz HE, Austin MM, Blonde L, et al. ACE/AACE consensus conference on the implementation of outpatient management of diabetes mellitus: consensus conference recommendations. Endocr Pract 2006; 12(Suppl 1):6–12.

94. American Association of Clinical Endocrinologists. The American Association of Clinical Endocrinologists Medical Guidelines for the Management of Diabetes Mellitus: the AACE system of intensive diabetes self-management – 2000 update. Endocr Pract 2000; 6(1):43–84.

95. Stratton IM, Adler AI, Neil HA, et al. Association of glycaemia with macrovascular and microvascular complications of type 2 diabetes (UKPDS 35): prospective observational study. BMJ 2000; 321(7258):405–412.

96. Dixon JB, O'Brien PE, Playfair J, et al. Adjustable gastric banding and conventional therapy for type 2 diabetes: a randomized controlled trial. JAMA 2008; 299(3):316–323.

97. Type 2 diabetes. Ann Intern Med 2007; 146(1):ITC1–ITC15.

98. American Diabetes Association. Nutrition Recommendations and Interventions for Diabetes: a position statement of the American Diabetes Association. Diabetes Care 2007; 30(Suppl 1):S48–S65.

99. Brand-Miller J, Hayne S, Petocz P, Colagiuri S. Low-glycemic index diets in the management of diabetes: a meta-analysis of randomized controlled trials. Diabetes Care 2003; 26(8):2261–2267.

100. Boule NG, Haddad E, Kenny GP, Wells GA, Sigal RJ. Effects of exercise on glycemic control and body mass in type 2 diabetes mellitus: a meta-analysis of controlled clinical trials. JAMA 2001; 286(10):1218–1227.

101. Dunstan DW, Daly RM, Owen N, et al. High-intensity resistance training improves glycemic control in older patients with type 2 diabetes. Diabetes Care 2002; 25(10):1729–1736.

102. Castaneda C, Layne JE, Munoz-Orians L, et al. A randomized controlled trial of resistance exercise training to improve glycemic control in older adults with type 2 diabetes. Diabetes Care 2002; 25(12):2335–2341.

103. Dunstan DW, Daly RM, Owen N, et al. Home-based resistance training is not sufficient to maintain improved glycemic control following supervised training in older individuals with type 2 diabetes. Diabetes Care 2005; 28(1):3–9.

104. Nissen SE, Wolski K. Effect of rosiglitazone on the risk of myocardial infarction and death from cardiovascular causes. N Engl J Med 2007; 356(24):2457–2471.

105. Singh S, Loke YK, Furberg CD. Long-term risk of cardiovascular events with rosiglitazone: a meta-analysis. JAMA 2007; 298(10):1189–1195.

106. Lago RM, Singh PP, Nesto RW. Congestive heart failure and cardiovascular death in patients with prediabetes and type 2 diabetes given thiazolidinediones: a meta-analysis of randomised clinical trials. Lancet 2007; 370(9593):1129–1136.

107. Home PD, Pocock SJ, Beck-Nielsen H, et al. Rosiglitazone evaluated for cardiovascular outcomes - an interim analysis. N Engl J Med 2007; 357(1):28–38.

108. Lincoff AM, Wolski K, Nicholls SJ, Nissen SE. Pioglitazone and risk of cardiovascular events in patients with type 2 diabetes mellitus: a meta-analysis of randomized trials. JAMA 2007; 298(10):1180–1188.

109. Schwartz AV, Sellmeyer DE, Vittinghoff E, et al. Thiazolidinedione use and bone loss in older diabetic adults. J Clin Endocrinol Metab 2006; 91(9):3349–3354.

110. Aschner P, Kipnes MS, Lunceford JK, Sanchez M, Mickel C, Williams-Herman DE. Effect of the dipeptidyl peptidase-4 inhibitor sitagliptin as monotherapy on glycemic control in patients with type 2 diabetes. Diabetes Care 2006; 29(12):2632–2637.

111. Charbonnel B, Karasik A, Liu J, Wu M, Meininger G. Efficacy and safety of the dipeptidyl peptidase-4 inhibitor sitagliptin added to ongoing metformin therapy in patients with type 2 diabetes inadequately controlled with metformin alone. Diabetes Care 2006; 29(12):2638–2643.

112. Rosenstock J, Brazg R, Andryuk PJ, Lu K, Stein P. Efficacy and safety of the dipeptidyl peptidase-4 inhibitor sitagliptin added to ongoing pioglitazone therapy in patients with type 2 diabetes: a 24-week, multicenter, randomized, double-blind, placebo-controlled, parallel-group study. Clin Ther 2006; 28(10):1556–1568.

113. Heine RJ, Van Gaal LF, Johns D, Mihm MJ, Widel MH, Brodows RG. Exenatide versus insulin glargine in patients with suboptimally controlled type 2 diabetes: a randomized trial. Ann Intern Med 2005; 143(8):559–569.

114. Ratner RE, Want LL, Fineman MS, et al. Adjunctive therapy with the amylin analogue pramlintide leads to a combined improvement in glycemic and weight control in insulin-treated subjects with type 2 diabetes. Diabetes Technol Ther 2002; 4(1):51–61.

115. Hollander PA, Levy P, Fineman MS, et al. Pramlintide as an adjunct to insulin therapy improves long-term glycemic and weight control in patients with type 2 diabetes: a 1-year randomized controlled trial. Diabetes Care 2003; 26(3):784–790.

116. Nathan DM. Thiazolidinediones for initial treatment of type 2 diabetes? N Engl J Med 2006; 355(23):2477–2480.

117. Nathan DM, Buse JB, Davidson MB, et al. Management of hyperglycemia in type 2 diabetes: a consensus algorithm for the initiation and adjustment of therapy: a consensus statement from the American Diabetes Association and the European Association for the Study of Diabetes. Diabetes Care 2006; 29(8):1963–1972.

118. Nathan DM, Buse JB, Davidson MB, et al. Management of hyperglycaemia in type 2 diabetes mellitus: a consensus algorithm for the initiation and adjustment of therapy: update regarding the thiazolidinediones. Diabetologia 2008; 51(1):8–11.

119. Garber AJ, Larsen J, Schneider SH, Piper BA, Henry D. Simultaneous glyburide/metformin therapy is superior to component monotherapy as an initial pharmacological treatment for type 2 diabetes. Diabetes Obes Metab 2002; 4(3):201–208.

120. Dailey GE, III, Noor MA, Park JS, Bruce S, Fiedorek FT. Glycemic control with glyburide/metformin tablets in combination with rosiglitazone in patients with type 2 diabetes: a randomized, double-blind trial. Am J Med 2004; 116(4):223–229.
121. Schwartz S, Sievers R, Strange P, Lyness WH, Hollander P. Insulin 70/30 mix plus metformin versus triple oral therapy in the treatment of type 2 diabetes after failure of two oral drugs: efficacy, safety, and cost analysis. Diabetes Care 2003; 26(8):2238–2243.

17 Surgical Management of Obesity and Postoperative Care

George L. Blackburn, Torsten Olbers,
Benjamin E. Schneider, Vivian M. Sanchez,
Aoife Brennan, Christos S. Mantzoros,
and Daniel B. Jones

KEY POINTS

- An estimated 8–10 million people suffer from extreme obesity, defined as a body mass index (BMI) of greater than 40 kg/m^2.
- Bariatric surgery has advanced significantly over the years and can reverse or greatly ameliorate numerous life-threatening comorbidities associated with obesity.
- There are two main types of bariatric surgery: restrictive surgeries, such as gastric banding, and malabsorptive surgeries, which include Roux-en-Y gastric bypass (RYGB), biliopancreatic diversion (BPD), and sleeve gastrectomy.
- Because of the increasing number of surgeries performed worldwide each year, a working knowledge of the preoperative evaluation, surgeries performed, and the resulting changes in nutritional requirements, gut function, and physiology is recommended for all healthcare professionals.
- Through selection of appropriate surgical candidates and limiting surgery to regional centers with high-volume bariatric surgery, perioperative mortality can be minimized.
- Structured postoperative follow-up can improve effectiveness and long-term safety for patients.

Key Words: Gastric bypass, Gastric banding, Obesity, Bariatric surgery, Weight loss

1. INTRODUCTION

Worldwide an estimated 300 million individuals are obese and in the USA alone, an estimated 8–10 million people suffer from extreme obesity, defined as a body mass index (BMI) of greater than 40 kg/m^2. Weight-loss surgery (WLS) is the only effective treatment for severe, medically complicated, and refractory obesity. Bariatric surgery reverses, eliminates, or significantly ameliorates numerous life-threatening medical

From: *Nutrition and Health: Nutrition and Metabolism*
Edited by: C.S. Mantzoros, DOI: 10.1007/978-1-60327-453-1_17
© Humana Press, a part of Springer Science+Business Media, LLC 2009

comorbidities associated with obesity and recent advances have improved safety and patient acceptability; WLS has recently been shown to reduce long-term mortality in two large, long-term studies *(1,2)*. Because of the increasing number of surgeries performed worldwide each year, all healthcare professionals require a working knowledge of the preoperative evaluation, surgeries performed and the resulting changes in nutritional requirements, gut function, and physiology. Preoperative evaluation with multidisciplinary assessment, perioperative care, and careful postoperative follow-up are essential elements of therapy. Appropriate candidates for bariatric surgery include those who have severe obesity; typically identified with a BMI > 40 kg/m^2 or those with a BMI > 35 kg/m^2 and significant comorbidities. Individual patient selection and appropriate informed consent require a comprehensive, evidence-based protocol.

Three groups of indication for WLS have been defined: metabolic, quality of life, and difficulty weight bearing. In addition, an assessment of the severity of each comorbid condition can be stratified within three levels: (1) life threatening or life shortening, (2) leading to deterioration and loss of quality-adjusted life years, and (3) improvements desirable. Within these three basic priority levels, an integrated scoring system can be created, with higher score indicating greater potential benefit from surgery (*see* Table 1).

Table 1
Assessment of Obesity-Related Morbidity

Heart disease	No		
	Yes	Angina pectoris	2
		Heart failure, mild	2
		Heart failure, severe	3
		Obesity related cardiomyopathy	3
		Previous myocardial infarction	3
Pulmonary disease	No		
	Yes	Asthma bronchial	1
		Sleep apnea syndrome	2
		Sleep apnea syndrome – unstable on treatment	3
		Obesity hypoventilative syndrome	3
		Pulmonary hypertension	3
Diabetes	No		
	Yes	Impaired glucose tolerance and hyperinsulinemia	1
		Type 2 diabetes – stable on oral treatment	2
		Type 2 diabetes – with insulin treatment	3
		Type 2 diabetes – uncontrolled despite treatment	3
Cardiovascular risk (as assessed by Risk Score)	No		
	Yes	Low	1

(continued)

Table 1
(continued)

		Moderate	2
		High	3
Pseudotumor cerebri	No		
	Yes	Headache, dizziness, and visual symptoms	1
		Diagnose established, stable on diuretics	2
		Diagnose established, unstable on diuretics	2
Joint pain/arthritis	No		
	Yes	Intermittent medical treatment	1
		Constant need for pain medication	2
		Degenerative findings on X-rays	2
		Awaiting joint replacement	2
		Leading to work inability	2
Lower extremity edema	No		
	Yes	Need for compression stocking, etc	1
		History of deep venous thrombosis	2
		Venous stasis ulcers or pulmonary embolism	3
Back pain	No		
	Yes	Occasional pain medication	1
		Constant need for pain medication	2
		Leading to work inability	2
Gastroesophageal reflux	No		
	Yes	Occasional medical treatment	1
		Continuous medical treatment	2
		Volume reflux	2
Stress/urinary incontinence	No		
	Yes	Any degree	1

Assessment of obesity-related morbidity can be stratified as:
1: Life threatening or life shortening,
2: Leading to deterioration,
3: Improvements desirable

2. PREOPERATIVE EVALUATION

The number of bariatric surgeries performed is increasing each year. Unfortunately, some patients will suffer mortality and other serious complications of surgery, while others may have poor weight loss despite the risks and costs of surgery *(3)*. Thus, it remains a priority to examine the appropriateness of candidates for WLSs. Multidisciplinary preoperative assessment, through proper patient selection and treatment of coexistent medical and psychological factors, can greatly improve both safety and efficacy of bariatric surgery in patients with extreme obesity. The preoperative assessment team should include surgeon, physician, psychologist/psychiatrist, and nutritionist working in liaison with other specialists where appropriate *(4)*. The main aims of preoperative assessment are as follows:

Ensure that the patient meets recommended criteria for bariatric surgery.

- Suitable patients should have a BMI of >40 or >35 with comorbidities. They should have documented or high probability of failure of nonsurgical weight-loss treatments. In addition, they should have no medical or psychological contraindications and should be well-informed, compliant, and motivated.
- To identify and treat any causes of secondary obesity, such as hypothyroidism and Cushing's disease, and to identify medications that may contribute to weight gain which may be switched for alternatives.
- To identify factors which may increase the patients perioperative risk and to intervene preoperatively where possible. These factors include untreated nutritional deficiencies, coronary artery disease, untreated obstructive sleep apnea, smoking, and cirrhotic liver disease. These conditions should be screened using complete medical history, including detailed weight history, physical examination, and laboratory testing.
- To identify factors that may reduce the probability of long-term successful weight loss and put the patient at risk for long-term complications. A detailed nutritional history may identify factors that would limit the success of bariatric surgery such as high intake of sugary drinks. In addition, education regarding dietary expectations after surgery can identify individuals who will be unable to comply with the lifestyle restrictions imposed by the procedure. Psychological conditions such as untreated depression or a history of trauma or sexual abuse may be uncovered as part of the assessment and these patients may be referred for treatment preoperatively.

In addition to the above factors, and in order to maximize successful weight loss postoperatively, several programs mandate that patients achieve some weight loss before surgery. Preoperative weight loss is thought to predict motivation, adherence with postoperative dietary restriction, and surgical outcome. The evidence base for this approach is lacking, however, as the three studies performed to date have had differing results *(5–7)*. Similarly, exercise is also seen as an important element of preparation for surgery in several programs; however, screening for coronary artery disease is recommended prior to the initiation of exercise intervention program in individuals with multiple cardiovascular risk factors *(8)*.

Expert opinion suggests that registered dietitians are best qualified to provide nutritional care, including preoperative assessment and postoperative education, counseling, and follow-up. Bariatric surgery patients need to learn important new skills including self-monitoring and meal planning. Patients who undergo surgery need lifelong nutritional supplements and medical monitoring *(9)*. Dedicated dietitians can help them during their preoperative education on new dietary requirements and stipulations *(10)*, and their postsurgical adjustment to those requirements *(11)*.

3. CURRENTLY PERFORMED SURGERIES

3.1. Roux-en-Y Gastric Bypass

RYGB involves creation of a small gastric pouch that is then connected to a distal segment of small intestine (alimentary limb) *(see* Figs. 1 and 2). The remainder of the stomach is left in situ but is disconnected from the normal food stream. The bilopancreatic

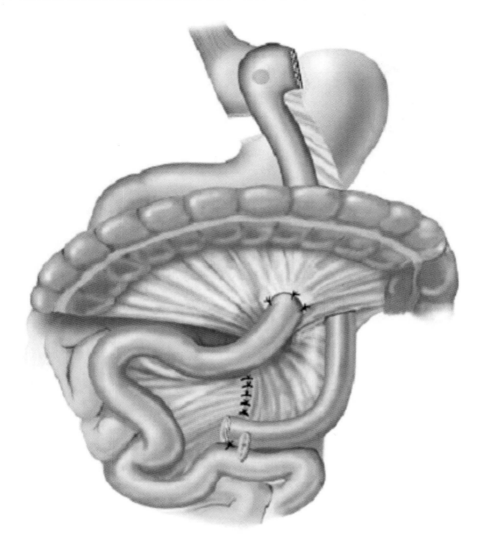

Fig. 1. Roux-en-y gastric bypass (with permission from Jones et al. Atlas of Minimally Invasive Surgery, CineMed, CT, 2007).

limb reconnects with the Roux limb at the jejunojejunostomy. The restrictive component is based on the small pouch as well as the narrow aperture connecting the gastric pouch to the jejunum. The malabsorptive component is marginal at best, as only 30–50 cm of small bowel is bypassed. The altered anatomic configuration leads to changes in gut hormones that may be associated with satiety, gastric emptying, and weight loss. Gastric bypass can be performed laparoscopically (LRYGB) or via the open approach with similar success rates *(12,13).* Thirty-day mortality rates associated with gastric bypass surgery are reported to be approximately 0.44% and 0.16% for open and laparoscopic procedures, respectively *(14).* Early complications associated with gastric bypass include leakage, bleeding, pulmonary embolus, gastrojejunal strictures, and death. Late complications include internal

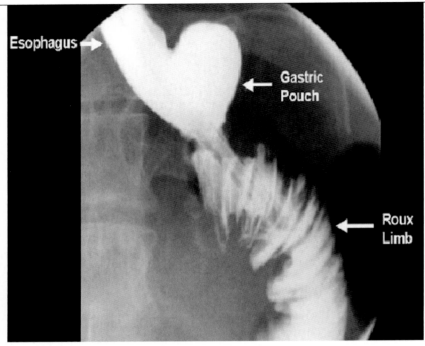

Fig. 2. Gastrograffin swallow demonstrates small pouch, patent anastomosis, and no leak prior to advancing diet.

hernias, bleeding, ulcers, vitamin deficiencies, and anemia. To prevent nutritional deficiencies, gastric bypass patients must take a daily multivitamin (with iron): B_{12}, folate, and calcium (*see* Sect. 6 below). Olbers et al. have reported an alteration in eating patterns, including a reduction in dietary fat intake important to long-term reduction in body fat and weight maintenance *(15)*.

3.2. Gastric Banding

The laparoscopic adjustable gastric band (LAGB) and the Swedish band are placed around the top portion of the stomach to reduce stomach size. They restrict the volume of ingested solid food. Both bands have been used widely throughout Europe, Australia, and South America for over a decade, but only the LAGB has been approved by the FDA for use in the USA since 2001. The band is wrapped around the cardia of the stomach, and a, gastrogastric imbrication anteriorly is performed to help prevent prolapse (*see* Fig. 3). The band itself is made of silicone and is connected via plastic tubing to a port implanted in the patient's abdominal wall (*see* Fig. 4). The quantity of fluid placed into the port gradually increases the restriction on the stomach and sense of satiety. Patients must have frequent follow-ups with their physicians to titrate the volume injected into the port. In contrast to gastric bypass operation, the gastrointestinal tract remains intact after the lap band and thus the procedure is completely reversible.

The mortality rate associated with the band is lower than it is with gastric bypass surgery. The difference might be due to the absence of leaks and shorter operating times *(16)*. While a mortality rate of 0.06% is relatively low *(14)*, patients must be

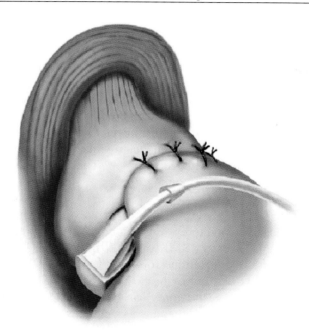

Fig. 3. Laparoscopic adjustable gastric band (with permission from Jones et al. Atlas of Minimally Invasive Surgery, CineMed, CT, 2007).

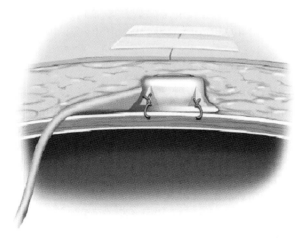

Fig. 4. Subcutaneous port of the laparoscopic adjustable gastric band (with permission from Jones et al. Atlas of Minimally Invasive Surgery, CineMed, CT, 2007).

counseled that there still is a real risk to an operation, and patients with multiple comorbid conditions are at higher risk. Postoperative complications associated with the band include erosions, slips, esophageal dilatation, infections, and port problems. In one study with 4-year follow-up, 22% of patients with gastric banding required some kind of reoperation *(17)*.

3.3. Biliopancreatic Diversion

BPD is a malabsorptive procedure in which a distal gastrectomy and Roux-en-Y configuration is created with a short common limb. The duodenal switch (DS) procedure is similar to BPD, but a duodenojejunostomy is performed to limit marginal ulceration. BPD is effective in inducing weight loss, particularly in "super-obese" patients (BMI > 50 kg/m^2) *(18)*, but is associated with significant complications *(19)*. It involves gastric resection and diversion of the biliopancreatic juices to the terminal ileum through an entero-entero anastomosis performed between the proximal limb of the transected jejunum and ileum, 50 cm proximal to the ileocecal valve. The distal end of the transected jejunum is anastomosed to the gastric pouch *(20)*.

3.4. Sleeve Gastrectomy

Still in its infancy, sleeve gastrectomy was first conceived as a bridge for surgery in patients with super extreme obesity (BMI > 50) *(20)*, though it is now being considered as a stand-alone restrictive technique for weight loss *(21)*. The procedure, which is exclusively restrictive, involves removing 80% of the stomach, leaving behind only a sleeve of the stomach. Sleeve gastrectomy can be performed laproscopically [called laparoscopic sleeve gastrectomy (LSG)] and is associated with lower surgical risk than more complex surgeries, such as BPD with DS or RYGB *(22,23)*. LSG may be particularly well-suited for the most surgically challenging high-risk patients, defined as those who are super-super obese (BMI > 60 kg/m^2) and those with severe comorbidities *(24)*. Such patients have higher perioperative morbidity and mortality with WLS. However, long-term data is still scarce, and sleeve gastrectomy does not appear to result in as profound a weight loss as RYGB or DS; in a series of 118 patients, sleeve gastrectomy only resulted in the loss of 47.3% of excess weight by 24 months *(25)*.

4. SURGICAL OUTCOMES

4.1. Weight Loss and Comorbidities

WLS is fundamentally different from dieting. Changes in physiology resulting from the operation can reset the energy equilibrium, affect the complex weight-regulatory system at multiple levels, inhibit environmental influences on weight regulation, and defeat powerful mechanisms that are inappropriately active in obesity. For example, the RYGB operation induces physiological and neuroendocrine changes that appear to affect the weight regulatory centers in the brain, suggesting alteration of the reward pathways in the central nervous system. Bariatric surgery is known to provide marked and lasting weight loss of 47.5–70.1% of excess body weight *(26)*. This is approximately 25–35% of baseline body weight. Such results have been obtained in relative safety, with operative mortality equal to or less than that for other major operative procedures (about 0.5%) *(26,27)*. RYGB and BPD induce an initial rapid weight loss, followed by a more gradual weight loss over the following year through both restrictive and malabsorptive mechanisms. The initial weight loss is not as marked after LAGB. On average, patients lose 0.25–0.5 kg/day for the initial 3 months, followed by an average weight reduction of 0.1–0.25 kg/day for the following year *(28)*. Approximately two-thirds of patients will succeed in maintaining a weight reduction of greater than 50% of preoperative excess weight after 7 years *(29)*.

Weight loss, possibly in association with changes in the gastrointestinal hormonal milieu, results in dramatic effects on the comorbid conditions of severe obesity *(30)*. A recent meta-analysis of 21 case series reported an improvement or resolution of diabetes in 64–100% of patients *(26)*. Defining the exact probability of resolution of diabetes is difficult, however, due to the heterogeneity in the reported series, particularly with regard to surgical techniques and definition as well as extent of improvement in diabetes.

Dixon et al. (2008) reported a randomized controlled trial of 60 patients (BMI > 30 and <40) with recently diagnosed (<2 years) type 2 diabetes comparing adjunctive gastric banding and conventional therapy for type 2 diabetes. A two-year follow-up revealed a remission of type 2 diabetes in 73% of the surgical patients and 13% remission in the conventional therapy group *(31)*.

Reversal or improvement has also been documented for the following comorbidities: dyslipidemia *(26)*, hypertension *(26)*, obstructive sleep apnea *(26)*, nonalcoholic fatty liver disease *(32)*, weight-bearing osteoarthritis *(33)*, gastroesophageal reflux disease *(34)*, polycystic ovarian syndrome *(35)*, and depression. Improvement is also reasonable and presumed for other comorbidities, including cardiac and peripheral vascular disease, and risk of carcinomas of the breast, uterus, ovary, prostate, colon, pancreas, and liver *(36)*. Furthermore, there are also improvements in quality of life factors related to body image, personal hygiene, sexual activity, employment opportunities, and socioeconomic status *(30)*. Finally, increasing epidemiological observational evidence suggests that WLS might increase longevity *(37)*. Long-term outcomes are discussed in more detail in Chap. 18.

4.2. Safety

Rapid advances in bariatric surgical technology, coupling with rapidly expanding numbers of operations performed, have made the development and implementation of performances standards and patient safeguards a national priority in the USA. Although a focus on surgical volume and the setting in which surgery is performed is a necessary step, it falls short of what is required to protect the well-being of patients and the best interests of physicians and facilities.

Standardization of presurgical education, patient selection, perioperative care, and postsurgical support is essential to minimize risk to patients and avoid confounding in studies of surgical effectiveness *(21,38)*. Compatibility of database technology and consistency in data collection are likewise essential in the analysis of morbidity and mortality rates. Current variability in coding, information systems infrastructure, and database analyses *(39,40)* highlights the need for a nationwide perspective in addressing broad-based standards and outcome reporting. Patient safety initiatives underscore the need for prospective, clinically derived outcome databases that will serve as a vehicle for quality improvement *(41)*, much like current systems for coronary artery bypass graft surgery established by the Society for Thoracic Surgeons *(42)*.

Efforts to address these shortfalls are part of a nationwide drive for quality control in the USA. Massachusetts was the first state to develop comprehensive evidence-based recommendations for best practices in WLS *(21,38)*. Many professional societies and other stakeholders have also moved forward with various patient protection and quality performance initiatives. The American College of Surgeons (ACS) program, for example, is in-depth and comprehensive. On the basis of the Massachusetts Lehman Center report

(38), it specifies the necessary physical and human resources, clinical and surgeon credentialing standards, data reporting standards, and verification/approvals processes required to receive designation as an ACS Bariatric Surgery Center. Such steps will serve as an impetus and a role model to others engaged in the practice of WLS globally and will ultimately lead to further improvements in safety for patients.

5. MECHANISMS OF SURGICALLY INDUCED WEIGHT LOSS

There are two major categories of WLS: gastric restriction and intestinal malabsorption. Restrictive operations create a small neogastric pouch and gastric outlet to decrease food intake. Malabsorptive procedures rearrange the small intestine in order to decrease the functional length or efficiency of the intestinal mucosa for nutrient absorption. Although the malabsorptive approach produces more rapid and profound weight loss than restrictive procedures, it also puts patients at risk of metabolic complications, such as vitamin deficiencies and protein-energy malnutrition *(36)*. Restrictive procedures are considered simpler and safer than their malabsorptive counterparts, but may result in a smaller amount of long-term weight loss *(43)*.

Bariatric surgery is also thought to produce weight loss through its effect on the entero-hypothalamic endocrine axis *(44)*. Dramatic improvements in glycemic control have been observed in subjects with type 2 diabetes following bariatric surgery, and specifically the RYGB procedure *(29,44–48)*. In many cases, normal fasting plasma glucose concentrations are achieved prior to substantial weight loss *(43,46,47)*. Emerging evidence suggests that changes in circulating gut hormones may promote improvements in glycemic control, reductions in appetite, and subsequent weight loss following bypass surgery *(15,46,49,50)*. A number of peptides released from the gastrointestinal tract have recently been shown to regulate appetite and food intake, effecting both orexigenic and anorexic outcomes through actions on the hypothalamic arcuate nucleus, but the entire spectrum of underlying mechanisms remains to be fully elucidated *(51,52)*. Peptides of interest include ghrelin, which increases expression of the orexigenic hypothalamic neuropeptide Y and stimulates food intake in rodents and humans *(44,53)*; peptide YY (PYY) and/or the presumably more active PYY3-36, which has been known to induce satiety and reduce food intake *(54)*; and glucagon-like peptide 1, which acts mainly as an incretin, promoting postprandial insulin release, improving pancreatic β-cell function, and inhibiting food intake in humans *(44)*. Pancreatic polypeptide and oxyntomodulin have also been shown to inhibit food intake and promote energy expenditure *(55)*, as discussed in detail in the relevant chapters.

le Roux et al. *(44)* have demonstrated a pleiotropic endocrine response to bariatric surgery, which might account for the appetite reduction that leads to long-term changes in body weight. Compared with lean and obese controls, postsurgical RYGB patients had increased postprandial plasma (PYY) and glucagon-like peptide 1, which favor enhanced satiety *(56)*. Furthermore, those patients had early and exaggerated insulin responses, potentially mediating improved glycemic control. None of these effects were observed in patients losing equivalent weight through gastric banding. Leptin, ghrelin, and pancreatic polypeptide were similar in both surgical groups *(44)*. In addition, it has recently been demonstrated that gastric bypass results in a more robust PYY response to caloric intake, which may contribute to the sustained efficacy of this procedure *(56)*.

6. POSTOPERATIVE CARE AND FOLLOW-UP

Patient commitment to long-term multidisciplinary care is central to ensuring long-term success and safety after bariatric surgery. Patients must be monitored for compliance with the lifestyle adjustments required to ensure long-term, sustained weight loss. In addition, prevention and monitoring for potential vitamin and mineral deficiencies, adjustment of the nutritional program as weight loss occurs, and monitoring changes in comorbid conditions and treatments are essential.

6.1. Fluid and Protein

In the early postoperative period, adequate oral intake of fluids and protein is a priority. A step-by-step approach is taken to gradually advance the composition and consistency of the diet and the patient's tolerance to each stage determines the rate of progression (see Table 2 for an example of postsurgical diet in use at our institution). Individuals vary in their readiness to move forward (57,58). Gastric bypass patients commonly experience intolerance to foods such as red meat, dry or tough poultry or pork, bread or doughy textured starches, celery, and coconut (59,60). The aim for patients is to achieve a daily intake of protein of approximately 1.0–1.5 g/kg of ideal body weight and a fluid intake of 35 ml/kg or 1 ml/kcal of estimated energy

Table 2
Diet Progression After Bariatric Surgery

Location and approximate schedule	Stage	General description	Length of stage
Starts after surgery with IV fluids continuing	1	Water (1 oz/h)	One day or less
Completed in the hospital	2	Low sugar, decaffeinated, noncarbonated clear liquids (2–4 oz/h)	One day or less
Getting ready for discharge, you will be introduced to stage 3 and evaluated for tolerance	3	Low sugar, high-protein modified full liquids (4–8 oz/h)	Three weeks
Home - follow-up in clinic (3 weeks postoperative)	4	Lean pureed/ground	Four to five weeks
Home - follow up in clinic (8 weeks postoperative)	5	Lean meat, fish and poultry, protein bars, fresh fruit, veggies, whole grains, legumes, healthy fat, low-fat dairy	Lifetime

In order to be successful losing weight and keeping it off, patients must learn how to modify eating behavior permanently. The primary objective is to maintain good nutrition, facilitate safe and sustained weight loss, and nurture independence toward a healthier lifestyle. The surgery is only part of the treatment. These diet stages progress through a series of five stages, the first four lasting a total of 8 weeks. The Bariatric Surgery Team has designed each diet stage to provide nutrition consistent with recovery, healing, and tolerance (progression may slightly vary with each individual and type of category). Provided by the Bariatric Surgery Team at the Beth Israel Deaconess Medical Center: Linda Veglia, MA RD, LDN, RN, Kelly Boyer, RD, LDN, and June Skoropowski, RD, LDN requirements *(61,62)*. Generally, patients should be able to tolerate foods of regular consistency with firmer texture 3 month postoperatively.

6.2. Postoperative Vomiting

Postoperative vomiting commonly leads to dehydration and can result in uncommon but potentially serious problems, for example, protein energy malnutrition and thiamine deficiency. Thiamine deficiency has occurred in patients without preoperative risk factors or concurrent alcohol abuse, and has developed as early as 1 week to 2 months postoperatively *(63–65)*. Both thiamine deficiency and PEM are most likely to occur with malabsorptive procedures, such as BPD and distal gastric bypass *(66–68)*.

6.3. Micronutrients

Energy intake during the first 3 months after bariatric surgery may be less than 1,000 kcal/day, and will not increase substantially *(62,69)*. In this setting, it is not surprising that nutritional deficiencies are a common complication, particularly in malabsorptive types of bariatric surgery (*see* Table 3 for evidence-based nutritional recommendations). Iron deficiency, in particular, can occur both early and late after surgery and frequent monitoring is required for life. In case series lasting 1–8 years, iron deficiency developed in 20–49% of gastric bypass patients and was most likely to occur in menstruating women; as a consequence, prophylactic iron supplementation has been recommended in this group *(70–72)*. Data has show that 640 mg/day of ferrous sulfate can prevent iron deficiency *(73)*, and that the addition of vitamin C to iron supplements can improve absorption in gastric bypass patients *(74)*. Gastric bypass surgery and other malabsorptive procedures have been associated with hypovitaminosis D, impaired calcium absorption, elevated markers of bone turnover, and osteopenia *(75–77)*. Patients may need supplementation with high-dose vitamin D in order to maintain serum 25-hydroxy vitamin D concentrations greater than 30 ng/ml and parathyroid hormone levels in the normal range. In addition, patients at risk for bone loss, such as postmenopausal women, should be screened for osteoporosis. Deficiencies of the other fat-soluble vitamins, A, E and K, can also occur after malabsorptive surgery, even in those taking daily multivitamins and monitoring of serum levels at 6 months and yearly postoperatively is generally recommended.

Because of limited body stores of water-soluble vitamins, both thiamine and vitamin B_1 deficiency can occur in the immediate postoperative period, and are generally associated with vomiting. Ingestion of daily multivitamins should prevent deficiency of these water-soluble vitamins in the long-term. Folic acid deficiency has also been reported in several case series, with reported rates of up to 38% of gastric bypass patients *(70,72,78,79)*; however, daily multivitamin intake is known to prevent folic acid deficiency postoperatively *(78)*. Vitamin B_{12} deficiency has been found in 25–75% of GBP patients postoperatively, due to lack of gastric acid and availability of intrinsic factor, which are both necessary for oral absorption. The majority of studies report rates of deficiency of approximately 35% *(70,80–82)*. As a consequence, parenteral, monthly vitamin B_{12} supplementation is required in patients who have had malabsorptive bariatric procedures. This supplementation has been found to prevent deficiency *(80)*.

Table 3
Nutrition Recommendations for Bariatric Surgery Patients (19)

Preoperative	• Preoperative education and counseling by a registered dietitian (category D) • Preoperative assessment for micronutrient deficiencies (category D)
Postoperative	• Early priority on adequate hydration and protein intake (category D) • A well-defined diet progression (category D) • Serum micronutrient assessment at 6 months postsurgery, and at least annually thereafter (category D) • Daily multivitamin (category A) and calcium supplement with added vitamin D (category D) • Consideration of thiamine supplementation for patients with persistent vomiting or inadequate nutrient intake (category C) • Regular use of iron supplements for patients at risk for iron and/or folic acid deficiency (with prenatal multivitamin option) (category A) • Periodic assessment for metabolic bone disease in patients who have had RYGB or other malabsorptive procedures, or who are at additional risk for metabolic bone disease (category A)
Levels of evidence	*Description*
Category A	Clear evidence obtained from at least one well-conducted randomized clinical trial or a systematic review of all relevant RCTs
Category B	Evidence from well-conducted prospective cohort studies, registry or meta-analysis of cohort studies, or population-based case-control studies
Category C	Supportive evidence obtained from uncontrolled or poorly controlled clinical trials, or retrospective case-control analyses, cross-sectional studies, case series, or case reports
Category D	Evidence consisting of opinion from expert consensus panels or the clinical experience of acknowledged experts

Evidence-Based Recommendations Grading System. Adapted from American Diabetes Association (Diabetes Care 2004;27:S1–S2) and Betsy Lehman Center for Patient Safety and Medical Error Reduction, Updated evidence-based recommendations for best practices in weight loss surgery (Obesity 2009, *in press*)

6.4. Other Long-Term Complications

Dumping syndrome can occur after RYGB due to the delivery of large volumes of simple carbohydrates into the intestine. Symptoms can be managed by avoidance of high-carbohydrate drinks and foods and the syndrome generally resolves after 1 year. A more recently recognized complication is postoperative hypoglycemia due to endogenous hyperinsulinemia. This uncommon complication can cause intractable hypoglycemia, requiring pancreatectomy *(83)*. Islet cell hypertrophy and nesidioblastosis are found on histological examination but the exact pathophysiology remains to be fully elucidated *(83,84)*. As a consequence, patients with symptoms consistent with postprandial hypoglycemia require thorough endocrine evaluation and work-up. An expected consequence of rapid weight loss is redundant skin which can result in recurrent skin infections, ulcerations, and back pain. Reconstructive plastic surgery may be needed and these procedures are usually deferred until 18–24 months after bariatric surgery, when weight loss has stabilized. Other possible long-term complications include gallstones, intestinal obstruction due to adhesions, internal herniation or stomal stricture, steatorrhea, and incisional herniation *(28)*.

7. CONCLUSION

WLS is the only effective treatment for severe, medically complicated, and refractory obesity as discussed in detail in Chap. 18. It reverses, eliminates, or significantly ameliorates numerous life-threatening medical comorbidities that occur as part of the pathophysiology of obesity. Rapid changes in surgical technology and in demand for WLS have made the field one of medicine's most dynamic. Ensuring short-term and long-term patient safety as well as sustained weight loss involves a multidisciplinary team-based approach, beginning with the preoperative assessment and continuing for life. Through selection of appropriate surgical candidates and limiting surgery to regional centers with high-volume bariatric surgery, perioperative mortality can be minimized. Structured postoperative follow-up can improve effectiveness and long-term safety for patients.

ACKNOWLEDGMENTS

The authors would like to acknowledge the support of the S. Daniel Abraham Teaching Fund, the Harvard Center for Healthy Living, the Center for Nutritional Research Charitable Trust, and the Boston Obesity Nutrition Research Center (BONRC) (Grant number P30DK46200).

REFERENCES

1. Adams TD, Gress RE, Smith SC et al. Long-term mortality after gastric bypass surgery. N Engl J Med 2007;357:753–761.
2. Sjostrom L, Narbro K, Sjostrom D, et al. Effects of bariatric surgery on mortality in Swedish obese subjects. N Engl J Med 2007;357:741–752.
3. Livingston EH, Langert J. The impact of age and Medicare status on bariatric surgical outcomes. Arch Surg 2006;141:1115–1120.
4. Collazo-Clavell ML, Clark MM, McAlpine DE, et al. Assessment and preparation of patients for bariatric surgery. Mayo Clin Proc 2006;81:S11–S17.
5. Liu RC, Sabnis AA, Forsyth C, et al. The effects of acute preoperative weight loss on laparoscopic Roux-en-Y gastric bypass. Obes Surg 2005;15:1396–1402.
6. Van de Weijgert EJ, Ruseler CH, Elte JW. Long-term follow-up after gastric surgery for morbid obesity: preoperative weight loss improves the long-term control of morbid obesity after vertical banded gastroplasty. Obes Surg 1999;9:426–432.
7. Still CD, Benotti P, Wood C, et al. Outcomes of preoperative weight loss in high-risk patients undergoing gastric bypass surgery. Arch Surg 2007;142:994–998.
8. Maron BJ, Araujo CG, Thompson PD, et al. Recommendations for preparticipation screening and the assessment of cardiovascular disease in masters athletes: an advisory for healthcare professionals from the working groups of the World Heart Federation, the International Federation of Sports Medicine, and the American Heart Association Committee on Exercise, Cardiac Rehabilitation, and Prevention. Circulation 2001;103:327–334.
9. Fobi MA. Surgical treatment of obesity: a review. J Natl Med Assoc 2004;96:61–75.

10. Bond DS, Evans RK, DeMaria EJ, et al. A conceptual application of health behavior theory in the design and implementation of a successful surgical weight loss program. Obes Surg 2004;14:849–856.

11. American College of Surgeons [ST-34] Recommendations for facilities performing bariatric surgery. http://www.facs.org/fellows_info/statements/st-34.html. Accessed October 5, 2004.

12. Smith SC, Edwards CB, Goodman GN, et al. Open vs laparoscopic Roux-en-Y gastric bypass: comparison of operative morbidity and mortality. Obes Surg 2004;14:73–76.

13. Nguyen NT, Ho HS, Palmer LS, et al. A comparison study of laparoscopic versus open gastric bypass for morbid obesity. J Am Coll Surg 2000;191:149–155; discussion 155–147.

14. Buchwald H, Estok R, Fahrbach K, et al. Trends in mortality in bariatric surgery: a systematic review and meta-analysis. Surgery 2007;142:621–635.

15. Olbers T, Bjorkman S, Lindroos A, et al. Body composition, dietary intake, and energy expenditure after laparoscopic Roux-en-Y gastric bypass and laparoscopic vertical banded gastroplasty: a randomized clinical trial. Ann Surg 2006;244:715–722.

16. Chapman AE, Kiroff G, Game P, et al. Laparoscopic adjustable gastric banding in the treatment of obesity: a systematic literature review. Surgery 2004;135:326–351.

17. Branson R, Potoczna N, Brunotte R, et al. Impact of age, sex and body mass index on outcomes at four years after gastric banding. Obes Surg 2005;15:834–842.

18. Gagner M, Matteotti R. Laparoscopic biliopancreatic diversion with duodenal switch. Surg Clin North Am 2005;85:141–149.

19. Blackburn GL, Hu FB, Hutter M. Updated evidence-based recommendations for best practices in weight loss surgery. Obesity 2009;17, in press.

20. Regan JP, Inabnet WB, Gagner M, et al. Early experience with two-stage laparoscopic Roux-en-Y gastric bypass as an alternative in the super-super obese patient. Obes Surg 2003;13:861–864.

21. Kelly J, Shikora SA, Jones DB, et al. Best practice updates for surgical care in weight loss surgery. Obesity 2009;17, in press.

22. Mognol P, Chosidow D, Marmuse JP. Laparoscopic sleeve gastrectomy (LSG): review of a new bariatric procedure and initial results. Surg Technol Int 2006;15:47–52.

23. Cottam D, Quresh FG, Mater SG, et al. Laparoscopic sleeve gastrectomy as an initial weight-loss procedure for high-risk patients with morbid obesity. Surg Endosc 2006;20:859–863.

24. Roa PE, Kaidar-Person O, Pinto D, et al. Laparoscopic sleeve gastrectomy as treatment for morbid obesity: technique and short-term outcome. Obes Surg 2006;16:1323–1326.

25. Hamoui N, Anthone GJ, Kaufman HS, et al. Sleeve gastrectomy in the high-risk patient. Obes Surg 2006;16:1445–1449.

26. Buchwald H, Braunwald E, Avidor Y, et al. Bariatric surgery: a systematic review and meta-analysis. JAMA 2004;292:1724–1737.

27. Nguyen NT, Root J, Zainabadi K, et al. Accelerated growth of bariatric surgery with the introduction of minimally invasive surgery. Arch Surg 2005;140:1198–1202.

28. McMahon MM, Sarr MG, Clark MM, et al. Clinical management after bariatric surgery: value of a multidisciplinary approach. Mayo Clin Proc 2006;81:S34–S45.

29. Pories WJ, Swanson MS, MacDonald KG, et al. Who would have thought it? An operation proves to be the most effective therapy for adult-onset diabetes mellitus. Ann Surg 1995;222:339–350.

30. Buchwald H. The future of bariatric surgery. Obes Surg 2005;15:598–605.

31. Dixon JB, O'Brien PE, Playfair J, et al. Adjustable gastric banding and conventional therapy for type 2 diabetes. JAMA 2008;299:316–323.

32. Klein S, Mittendorfer B, Eagon JC, et al. Gastric bypass surgery improves metabolic and hepatic abnormalities associated with nonalcoholic fatty liver disease. Gastroenterology 2006;130:1564–1572.

33. Abu-Abeid S, Wishnitzer N, Szold A, et al. The influence of surgically-induced weight loss on the knee joint. Obes Surg 2005;15:1437–1442.

34. Tolonen P, Victorzon M, Niemi R, et al. Does gastric banding for morbid obesity reduce or increase gastroesophageal reflux?. Obes Surg 2006;16:1469–1474.

35. Escobar-Morreale HF, Botella-Carretero JI, Alvarez-Blasco F, et al. The polycystic ovary syndrome associated with morbid obesity may resolve after weight loss induced by bariatric surgery. J Clin Endocrinol Metab 2005;90:6364–6369.

36. Blackburn GL, Mun EC. Weight loss surgery and major cardiovascular risk factors. Nat Clin Pract Cardiovasc Med 2005;2:585–591.

37. Christou NV, Sampalis JS, Liberman M, et al. Surgery decreases long-term mortality, morbidity, and health care use in morbidly obese patients. Ann Surg 2004;240:416–423.

38. Apovian CM, Cummings S, Anderson W. Best practice updates for multidisciplinary care in weight loss surgery. Obesity 2009;17, in press.

39. Zingmond DS, McGory ML, Ko CY. Hospitalization before and after gastric bypass surgery. JAMA 2005;294:1918–1924.

40. Santry HP, Gillen DL, Lauderdale DS. Trends in bariatric surgical procedures. JAMA 2005;294:1909–1917.

41. Wolfe BM, Morton JM. Weighing in on bariatric surgery: procedure use, readmission rates, and mortality. JAMA 2005;294:1960–1963.

42. Ferguson TBJr., Coombs LP, Peterson ED. Society of Thoracic Surgeons National Adult Cardiac Surgery Database. Related articles links preoperative beta-blocker use and mortality and morbidity following CABG surgery in North America. JAMA 2002;287:221–227.

43. Blackburn GL, Jones DB. Effective surgical treatment of diabetes for the obese patient. Current Diabetes Reports 2006;6:85–87.

44. le Roux CW, Aylwin SJ, Batterham RL, et al. Gut hormone profiles following bariatric surgery favor an anorectic state, facilitate weight loss, and improve metabolic parameters. Ann Surg 2006;243:108–114.

45. Pories WJ, MacDonald KG, Jr., Morgan EJ, et al. Surgical treatment of obesity and its effect on diabetes: 10-y follow-up. Am J Clin Nutr 1992;55:582S–585S.

46. Schauer PR, Burguera B, Ikramuddin S, et al. Effect of laparoscopic Roux-en Y gastric bypass on type 2 diabetes mellitus. Ann Surg 2003;238:467–484.

47. Clements RH, Gonzalez QH, Long CI, et al. Hormonal changes after Roux-en Y gastric bypass for morbid obesity and the control of type-II diabetes mellitus. Am Surg 2003;70:1–4.

48. Blackburn GL. Solutions in weight control: lessons from gastric surgery. Am J Clin Nutr 2005;82:248S–252S.

49. Cummings DE, Weigle DS, Frayo RS, et al. Plasma ghrelin levels after diet-induced weight loss or gastric bypass surgery. N Engl J Med 2002;346:1623–1630.

50. Rubino F, Marescaux J. Effect of duodenal-jejunal exclusion in a non-obese animal model of type 2 diabetes: a new perspective for an old disease. Ann Surg 2004;239:1–11.

51. Schwartz MW, Morton GJ. Obesity: keeping hunger at bay. Nature 2002;418:595–597.

52. Schwartz MW, Woods SC, Porte D, et al. Central nervous system control of food intake. Nature 2000;404:661–671.

53. Tschop M, Smiley DL, Heiman ML. Ghrelin induces adiposity in rodents. Nature 2000;407:908–913.

54. Batterham RL, Cohen MA, Ellis SM, et al. Inhibition of food intake in obese subjects by peptide YY3–36. N Engl J Med 2003;349:941–948.

55. Asakawa A, Inui A, Yuzuriha H, et al. Characterization of the effects of pancreatic polypeptide in the regulation of energy balance. Gastroenterology 2003;124:1325–1336.

56. Chan JL, Mun EC, Stoyneva V, et al. Peptide YY levels are elevated after gastric bypass surgery. Obesity (Silver Spring) 2006;14:194–198.

57. Flanagan L. Measurement of functional pouch volume following the gastric bypass procedure. Obes Surg 1996;6:38–43.

58. Stocker DJ. Management of the bariatric surgery patient. Endocrinol Metab Clin North Am 2003;32:437–457.

59. Elliot K. Nutritional considerations after bariatric surgery. Crit Care Nurs Q 2003;26:133–138.

60. Collene AL, Hertzler S. Metabolic outcomes of gastric bypass. Nutr Clin Pract 2003;18:136–140.

61. Marcason W. What are the dietary guidelines following bariatric surgery?. J Am Diet Assoc 2004;104:487–488.

62. Moize V, Geliebter A, Gluck ME, et al. Obese patients have inadequate protein intake related to protein intolerance up to 1 year following Roux-en-Y gastric bypass. Obes Surg 2003;13:23–28.

63. Salas-Salvado J, Garcia-Lorda P, Cuatrecasas G, et al. Wernicke's syndrome after bariatric surgery. Clin Nutr 2000;19:371–373.

64. Bozbora A, Coskun H, Ozarmagan S, et al. A rare complication of adjustable gastric banding: Wernicke's encephalopathy. Obes Surg 2000;10:274–275.
65. Toth C, Voll C. Wernicke's encephalopathy following gastroplasty for morbid obesity. Can J Neurol Sci 2001;28:89–92.
66. Bajardi G, Ricevuto G, Mastrandrea G, et al. Surgical treatment of morbid obesity with biliopancreatic diversion and gastric banding: report on an 8-year experience involving 235 cases. Ann Chir 2000;125:155–162.
67. Brolin RE, LaMarca LB, Kenler HA, et al. Malabsorptive gastric bypass in patients with superobesity. J Gastrointest Surg 2002;6:195–203.
68. Mason EE. Starvation injury after gastric reduction for obesity. World J Surg 1998;22:1002–1007.
69. Bobbioni-Harsch E, Huber O, Morel P, et al. Factors influencing energy intake and body weight loss after gastric bypass. Eur J Clin Nutr 2002;56:551–556.
70. Halverson JD. Micronutrient deficiencies after gastric bypass for morbid obesity. Am Surg 1986;52:594–598.
71. Avinoah E, Ovnat A, Charuzi I. Nutritional status seven years after Roux-en-Y gastric bypass surgery. Surgery 1992;111:137–142.
72. Brolin RE, Gorman RC, Milgrim LM, et al. Multivitamin prophylaxis in prevention of post-gastric bypass vitamin and mineral deficiencies. Int J Obes 1991;15:661–667.
73. Brolin RE, Gorman JH, Gorman RC, et al. Prophylactic iron supplementation after Roux-en-Y gastric bypass: a prospective, double-blind, randomized study. Arch Surg 1998;133:740–744.
74. Rhode BM, Shustik C, Christou NV, . Iron absorption and therapy after gastric bypass. Obes Surg 1999;9:17–21.
75. Goode LR, Brolin RE, Chowdhury HA, et al. Bone and gastric bypass surgery: effects of dietary calcium and vitamin D. Obes Res 2004;12:40–47.
76. Coates PS, Fernstrom JD, Fernstrom MH, et al. Gastric bypass surgery for morbid obesity leads to an increase in bone turnover and a decrease in bone mass. J Clin Endocrinol Metab 2004;89:1061–1065.
77. Shaker JL, Norton AJ, Woods MF, . Secondary hyperparathyroidism and osteopenia in women following gastric exclusion surgery for obesity. Osteoporosis Int 1991;1:177–181.
78. Brolin RE, Gorman JH, Gorman RC, et al. Are vitamin B12 and folate deficiency clinically important after roux-en-Y gastric bypass?. J Gastrointest Surg 1998;2:436–442.
79. Halverson JD. Metabolic risk of obesity surgery and long-term follow-up. Am J Clin Nutr 1992;55:602S–605S.
80. Rhode BM, Arseneau P, Cooper BA, et al. Vitamin B-12 deficiency after gastric surgery for obesity. Am J Clin Nutr 1996;63:103–109.
81. Schilling RF, Gohdes PN, Hardie GH. Vitamin B12 deficiency after gastric bypass surgery for obesity. Ann Int Med 1984;101:501–502.
82. Simon SR, Zemel R, Betancourt S, et al. Hematologic complications of gastric bypass for morbid obesity. South Med J 1989;82:1108–1110.
83. Patti ME, McMahon G, Mun EC, et al. Severe hypoglycaemia post-gastric bypass requiring partial pancreatectomy: evidence for inappropriate insulin secretion and pancreatic islet hyperplasia. Diabetologia 2005;48:2236–2240.
84. Service GJ, Thompson GB, Service FJ, et al. Hyperinsulinemic hypoglycemia with nesidioblastosis after gastric-bypass surgery. N Engl J Med 2005;353:249–254.

18 Long-Term Impact of Weight Loss on Obesity and Obesity-Associated Comorbidities

Janice Jin Hwang, George Blackburn, and Christos S. Mantzoros

KEY POINTS

- Obesity, a growing epidemic in the developing world, is associated with numerous comorbidities.
- This chapter reviews the current literature on the effects of weight loss on obesity and its comorbidities and focuses on the long-term efficacy of treatment modalities including behavioral modifications, pharmacotherapy, and bariatric surgery.
- Behavioral modifications including diet and exercise are first-line recommendations from the US Preventative Services Task Force and are associated with improvement in numerous comorbidities including body weight, lipid profile, blood pressure, and glycemic control; however, long-term compliance and sustainability has been an important issue.
- Currently, there are only two medications approved by the FDA for weight loss. While short-term data are promising, there is limited long-term data on weight loss and other comorbidities of obesity.
- For certain subgroups of obese patients, bariatric surgery yields dramatic and sustained effects on weight loss as well glycemic control and other comorbidities, and recent data suggests an improvement in long-term mortality associated with bariatric surgery; however, given the invasiveness and potential complications of bariatric surgery, more studies will be needed to clarify its future role in obesity treatment.

Key Words: Obesity, Diet, Exercise, Bariatic surgery

1. INTRODUCTION

Obesity, the prevalence of which is growing rapidly in affluent Western societies, is considered the epidemic of the twenty-first century. Prior to 1980, only 15% of US adults were overweight. Most recent estimates, however, suggest that currently 30% of Americans are obese with another 30% qualifying as overweight. Similar trends in

From: *Nutrition and Health: Nutrition and Metabolism*
Edited by: C.S. Mantzoros, DOI: 10.1007/978-1-60327-453-1_18,
© Humana Press, a part of Springer Science+Business Media, LLC 2009

the prevalence of obesity are being seen in developed countries around the world *(1)*. The etiology of this prevalent disorder is complex, multifactorial, and remains incompletely understood as the mechanisms of energy homeostasis are highly individualized and influenced by genetic, environmental, cultural, social, and psychological factors. Importantly, obesity is closely associated with significant comorbidities and leads to increased mortality, as outlined in previous chapters. A summary of the data establishing the relationship between obesity and its comorbidities is beyond the scope of this chapter, but has been extensively reviewed for all major comorbidities including type II diabetes *(2–7)*, dyslipidemia *(8)*, hypertension *(9,10)*, coronary artery disease *(11–13)*, biliary disease *(14)*, degenerative joint disease *(15–19)*, sleep apnea *(20)*, as well as some cancers *(21–23)*. As a consequence, both medical opinion and current diagnostic and therapeutic approaches have shifted toward considering obesity as a chronic disease requiring lifelong management.

The field of bariatrics, derived from the Greek words "baros" and "iatriki" for weight and medicine, respectively, has seen great changes in the last century. Essentially, all treatments for obesity either increase energy expenditure or decrease energy intake. However, this simple statement belies the incredibly complex homeostatic mechanisms, which make treatment notoriously difficult. For example, weight loss often induces a compensatory decrease in body energy expenditure, and all treatment modalities including behavioral modification such as exercise and dietary therapy, pharmacotherapy, and bariatric surgery are plagued by varying degrees of recidivism, or regaining of lost weight *(24)*.

This chapter examines the effects of weight loss on obesity and its comorbidities and focuses on the long-term efficacy of treatment modalities including behavioral modifications, pharmacotherapy, and bariatric surgery. Pertinent randomized control trial (RCT) and meta-analysis data will be summarized and discussed; however, when these are not available, case series data are reported.

2. BEHAVIORAL MODIFICATIONS: DIET AND EXERCISE

Achieving a negative energy balance through behavioral modifications such as increased exercise or dietary therapy is perhaps the most straightforward way to achieve weight loss, and thus represents the first-line recommendation of the US Preventive Services Task Force (USPSTF) (*see* Appendix). However, as most dieters can attest, even in the most successful cases, behavioral modifications achieve relatively small changes in weight lasting no longer than 4–6 months after which a plateau of weight loss usually occurs followed, ultimately, by return to baseline body weight. The lack of long-term success coupled with the rise in the prevalence of obesity has spurred numerous different weight loss diets and fads. A full discussion of different weight loss diets is beyond the scope of this chapter, but has been reviewed in previous chapters. For the purposes of this review, which focuses on long-term effects of weight loss, diets are grouped as either low-fat, low-carbohydrate, or moderate-monounsaturated fat/Mediterranean diet.

2.1. Long-Term Effects on Body Weight

The popular assumption that dietary fat intake is directly proportional to total body fat has generated great interest in low-fat diets, which have already been discussed in detail in previous chapters. The Women's Health Initiative Dietary Modification trial was a large, randomized intervention trial comparing an intervention group instructed to reduce total fat intake to 20% of total energy intake by increasing consumption of fruits, vegetables, etc. to a control group instructed to continue their usual diet. This trial found that compared to the control group, the intervention group had a 1.9 kg decrease in weight after 1 year and a 0.4 kg decrease in weight at 7.5 years. However, beyond 7.5 years, the weight differences became negligible *(25)*. Bray and Popkin reviewed 28 trials evaluating low-fat diets and found that decreases in daily fat intake reduce weight significantly in the short term (follow-up from 4 weeks to 18 months) *(26)*; however, again, longer-term trials do not support weight maintenance.

Another popular diet is the low-carbohydrate diet, with extreme forms of this diet associated with rapid short-term weight loss secondary to starvation ketosis and concomitant diuresis. A meta-analysis of five RCTs found that low carbohydrate diets result in greater weight loss than low-fat diets, but there is no difference after 12 months *(27)*. The high rates of recidivism for low-fat and low-carbohydrate diets are partially attributable to the poor palatability and lack of variety of foods. For this reason, the Mediterranean diets, which are characterized by moderate consumption of monounsaturated fatty acids, fruits, vegetables, nuts, and fish, have become increasingly popular. One RCT found that mean weight loss in a moderate-fat diet group was greater than in the low-fat group after 30 months *(28)*. Further research is needed to determine the long-term success of this diet.

The USPSTF reviewed the medical literature and summarized the results from 29 RCTs and concluded that with counseling for diet and exercise, average weight change was 3.3 kg weight loss (1.9 to −8.8 kg) corrected for change in controls after 12–60 months follow-up *(29)*. The Cochrane database analyzed 43 randomized controlled trials that examined weight change using physical activity interventions in adults with baseline obesity/overweight. The analysis found that exercise resulted in small but significant weight loss compared to no treatment, increasing intensity of exercise was associated with increased weight loss, and exercise plus diet resulted in more weight loss than diet alone *(30)*. However, in this analysis, the duration of the studies ranged from 3 to 12 months, including follow-up.

2.2. Effects on Cardiovascular Risk Factors Including Diabetes, Hypertension, and Dyslipidemia

In recent years, obesity has been grouped along with insulin resistance, hypertension, and dyslipidemia into the metabolic syndrome; however, thus far there has been no definitive long-term evidence establishing their interdependence or causality. Observational studies have found that weight loss improves glycemic control and delays and/ or prevents the onset of diabetes *(31)*, and weight gain is a known risk for developing hypertension *(32)*.

The Cochrane review reports that exercise and diet both reduce serum fasting glucose, and diet produces slightly greater reductions after 12 months *(30)*. A RCT comparing low-fat and low-carbohydrate diets concluded that low-carbohydrate diets produced slightly greater weight loss and improved glycemic control among obese diabetic subjects. The improvement in glycemic control was weight loss dependent, disappearing after adjustment for weight loss between the two study groups *(33)*. Beyond a few years, the effects of diet and exercise on diabetes appear negligible. The WHI Dietary

Modifications study recently found that low-fat diets had no significant long-term effects on markers for cardiovascular disease including glucose and insulin levels after a mean 8 years follow-up *(25,34)*.

In 2003, meta-analysis of 25 RCTs examining weight loss and hypertension with up to 60 months follow-up reported the weight loss of 5.1 kg by either energy restriction, increased physical activity, or both reduced systolic blood pressure by 4.44 mm Hg and diastolic blood pressure by 3.57 mm Hg *(35)*. Further studies have suggested that low-fat and low-carbohydrate diets are equally as effective in decreasing blood pressure *(33)*. Importantly, the benefits of exercise and diet on hypertension are also independent from weight loss. It has long been known that exercise alone can improve hypertension regardless of weight loss *(36–38)*. While this mechanism is incompletely understood, it may be related to falls in catecholamines such as norepinephrine *(37)*. Diet alone without weight change has also been associated with improvement in blood pressure. The TOMHS *(39)* and DASH *(40)* trials among numerous others have shown that dietary changes such as low sodium diet with fruits and vegetables is associated with decreases in blood pressure, as discussed in Chaps. 15 and 21.

There have been numerous studies in the literature comparing the effects of different diets on lipid profiles. One RCT comparing low-fat versus low-carbohydrate diets found that at 6 months, a low-carbohydrate diet was associated with decreased triglycerides, but no difference in total cholesterol, HDL, or LDL was observed between the two study groups *(33)*. The OmniHeart study examined carbohydrate-rich, protein-rich, and monounsaturated fat-rich diets on lipid profiles and cardiovascular risk. The study found that all interventions reduced blood pressure from baseline and all diets decreased total cholesterol and LDL levels *(41)*. While these studies are promising, it remains unclear if any diet can translate into true long-term changes in lipid profiles, and more importantly, decreased cardiovascular risk.

2.3. Effects on Risk for Malignancy

Previous observational studies have shown that excess body weight is associated with increased risk of cancers including endometrial, kidney, gallbladder, breast, colon, and esophagus, and a full discussion of the observational data has been reviewed in Chaps. 9. A prospective, cohort study of over 900,000 subjects by Calle et al. found that increased body weight was associated with increased death rates for all cancers. When compared to normal weight women, obese women had a significantly increased relative risk of death from uterine (RR 6.25), kidney (RR 4.75), and cervical (RR 3.2) cancers. Similarly, obese men also had significantly increased relative risk of death from liver (RR 4.52), pancreas (RR 2.61), and stomach (RR 1.94) cancers *(42)*. Postmenopausal breast cancer (RR 1.3 for overweight and 1.5 for obese women), esophageal adenocarcinoma (RR 2.0 and 3.0 for overweight and obese subjects, respectively), as well as colon cancer (RR 1.5 and 3.0 in men and 1.2 and 1.5 in women, respectively) and probably prostate cancer are also associated with obesity. Furthermore, reviews by Calle et al. have estimated that the population attributable fractions for cancers strongly associated with obesity such as endometrial and esophageal are close to 55% for USA and 45% for Europe. Finally, it has also been estimated that between 4.2% and 14.2% of all deaths in men and between 14.3% and 19.8% of all deaths in women from cancer in USA may be attributable to overweight or obesity *(42)*.

On the basis of observational data, the International Agency for Research on Cancer has concluded that there is sufficient evidence to support avoidance of weight gain to prevent colon, breast (in postmenopausal women), endometrium, renal cell carcinoma, and esophageal adenocarcinoma *(43)*. While early animal and human observational studies suggested a correlation between increased fat and increased cancer risk, several recent interventional trials have cast doubt on this relationship. One RCT on prostate cancer found that a low-fat/high-soy diet had no effect on prostate-specific antigen levels in asymptomatic, hormonally naive prostate cancer patients with rising prostate specific antigen (PSA) values after 10 months of follow-up *(44)*. The WHI Dietary Modification Trial found that after mean follow-up of 8.1 years, a low-fat dietary pattern resulted in mild but significant weight loss, but did not reduce the risk of invasive breast cancer *(45)* or colorectal cancer *(46)* in postmenopausal women. In women already diagnosed with breast cancer, there have been some studies suggesting improved survival and clinical outcomes associated with a low-fat diet. The Women's Intervention Nutrition Study is an interventional RCT which at interim analysis of 60 months found that reducing dietary fat intake resulted in a significant weight loss and improved relapse-free survival of breast cancer patients receiving conventional treatments *(47)*. Clearly, further long-term studies (>10 years) are needed to further delineate the relationship, if any, between diet and cancer risk.

2.4. Effects on Other Comorbidities

The long-term effects of diet and exercise on other comorbidities such as bone disease and biliary disease remain unclear. There is short-term evidence to suggest that bone loss accompanies weight loss induced by caloric restriction. One recent RCT compared the effects of bone loss between caloric restriction versus exercise and found that after one year, weight loss was similar between the two treatment groups, but caloric restriction was associated with decreased bone mineral density at important sites (hip, femoral neck, spine, and trochanter) whereas exercise did not induce any decreases in bone mineral density at any site *(48)*. Trials examining the long-term effects of diet and exercise on bone disease have demonstrated that the addition of exercise prevents the weight loss induced by changes in bone density. Similarly, the long-term effects of diet and weight loss on biliary disease are largely unknown. Gallstone formation is associated with very low-calorie diets and rapid weight loss *(49)*, but the association between long-term weight loss from dietary or exercise modifications and gallstone formation remains to be fully elucidated.

3. PHARMACOTHERAPY

The high degree of recidivism and difficulty in adhering to various diet and exercise regimens has resulted in great interest in pharmacotherapy for obesity. Most weight loss medications work either by decreasing nutrient absorption or by appetite suppression via increasing the availability of anorexigenic neurotransmitters such as norepinephrine and serotonin. However, early pharmaceutical treatments proved to be either nondurable and/or were associated with unacceptable cardiac side effects. As of 1997, five drugs had been removed from USA and international markets because of efficacy and safety concerns *(50)*. Since then, numerous new drugs have been studied and drug development is an area of great interest *(51,52)*, but there is a lack of long-term data on the efficacy of most currently available medications and there are even fewer data on their effects on comorbidities. The following sections will examine the literature to date focusing on effects on weight loss and cardiovascular comorbidities.

3.1. Long-Term Effects on Body Weight

Currently, the American College of Physicians recommends pharmacological therapy only to patients who are obese and who have failed to achieve weight loss through diet and exercise. Pharmacological therapy in combination with behavioral modifications has been shown to result in more weight loss than either modality alone *(53)*. The recommended drug options include sibutramine, orlistat, phentermine, diethylpropion, fluoxetine, and bupropion. Of these, orlistat and sibutramine are the only two drugs that FDA approved for long-term use *(50)*.

A meta-analysis of 79 studies, mostly randomized controlled trials, found that the placebo subtracted difference in weight loss for sibutramine was 3.4–6 kg at 6 months and 4.5 kg at 12 months; for orlistat, 2.59 kg at 6 months and 2.89 kg at 12 months; for phentermine, 3.6 kg at 6 months and no 12 month data; for diethylpropion, 3.0 kg at 6 months and no 12 month data; and for bupropion, 2.77 kg at 6–12 months. Data for fluoxetine was inconclusive *(54)*. A Cochrane review meta-analysis including RCTs with at least 12 months follow-up examining the efficacy of different medications found that among trials for eight antiobesity agents investigated, only 11 orlistat and 5 sibutramine trials met inclusion criteria. Compared to placebo, orlistat-treated patients lost 2.7 kg (95% CI: 2.3–3.1) more weight and patients on sibutramine experienced 4.3 kg (95% CI: 3.6–4.9) greater weight loss at 12 months (6-month data was not reported) *(55)*.

3.2. Effects on Cardiovascular Risk Factors

The effect of pharmacotherapy on other comorbidities associated with obesity has been poorly studied in part because no long-term data is available. One of the longest trials of orlistat with behavioral modifications is the XENDOS study, a 4-year RCT of Swedish obese patients, which showed that at 1 year, orlistat reduced weight by 10.6 kg compared to 6.2 kg in the placebo group. After 4 years, placebo-compared weight loss was 2.8 kg greater in the orlistat group (orlistat, 5.8 kg vs placebo, 3.0 kg). In this same study, cumulative incidence of type II diabetes was 9.0% in placebo group compared with 6.3% in the orlistat group *(56)*. A meta-analysis of 11 RCTs at 1-year follow-up found that, compared to placebo, orlistat reduced systolic blood pressure by 1.8 mmHg, decreased total cholesterol by 0.33 mmol/liter, decreased LDL by 0.27 mmol/liter, decreased HDL by 0.02 mmol/liter, and decreased triglycerides by 0.05 mmol/liter. Fasting glucose was 0.1–1.3 mmol/liter lower than controls. Sibutramine was associated with a 0.08 mmol/liter increase in HDL, 0.18 mmol/liter decrease in triglycerides, and no change in total cholesterol or LDL when compared to placebo *(55)*. No data was reported on long-term mortality and morbidity outcomes *(55)*. Sibutramine is currently being evaluated for long-term effects in the ongoing Sibutramine cardiovascular outcomes trial, which is scheduled for completion in 2008.

3.3. Effects on Other Comorbidities

Because the current available pharmacotherapies have only been studied for less than 5 years, there is no data available on long-term effects on other obesity comorbidities.

4. BARIATRIC SURGERY

With improvements in technique and approach, surgery has become an increasingly popular option in the field of bariatric medicine over the last few decades.

Bariatric surgery is generally reserved for the class II obesity or higher, although, recently there has been literature evaluating its effectiveness in lesser degrees of obesity. In 1991, the National Institutes of Health established guidelines approving bariatric surgery in patients with body mass index (BMI)$\geq$40 kg/m^2 or $\geq$35 kg/m^2 and two or more comorbidities. Even then, surgery should be approached only after less-invasive alternatives have failed (1).

The remainder of this chapter will summarize and evaluate the efficacy of bariatric surgery on obesity and its comorbidities including the cardiovascular risk factors mentioned above as well as obstructive sleep apnea (OSA), degenerative bone disease, cancer, biliary disease, and general well being.

4.1. Types of Bariatric Surgery

A full discussion of the techniques and different types of bariatric procedures is beyond the scope of this chapter and can be found in chapter 17. Briefly, current surgical options can be categorized as malabsorptive, restrictive, or both. Malabsorptive procedures such as biliopancreatic diversion consist of small bowel reconstruction to reduce the area of bowel available for nutrient resorption. While these techniques are effective at inducing weight loss, they are rarely performed in the USA due to numerous side effects including severe protein and vitamin deficiency, metabolic bone disease, hepatic cirrhosis, and foul-smelling diarrhea (57). Restrictive surgeries, such as vertical banded gastroplasty and adjustable gastric banding (AGB), cause weight loss directly by decreasing stomach capacity and the amount of food that the patient can ingest (57,58).

By far, the most common bariatric operation performed in the USA is the Roux-en-Y gastric bypass, which consists of elements of both restrictive and malabsorptive operations. The procedure, which can be performed either as open or laparoscopically, involves creation of a small proximal stomach pouch and a Roux-en-Y small bowel arrangement. In this configuration, ingested food bypasses 95% of the stomach, all of the duodenum, and a small portion of the jejunum; however, because most of the small bowel is intact, there are significantly fewer side effects such as dumping syndrome. The effects on weight loss and decreases in comorbidities are also significantly better than most other techniques (57,59–62).

4.2. Long-Term Effects on Body Weight

Bariatric surgery has been extremely successful in producing dramatic and long-term weight reductions. One recent RCT comparing AGB to intensive medical therapy in mild-to-moderate obesity showed that at 6 months, both surgical and medical therapy resulted in the same amount of weight loss from baseline (13.4 vs 13.2 kg, respectively). However, at 12 months, weight loss from baseline was 18.7 kg in the surgical group compared with 9.5 kg in the medical group, and the margins widened further at 24 months, with a 20.5 kg weight loss in the surgery group and 5.3 kg loss in the medical group (63).

Two large meta-analysis by Maggard et al. *(64)* and Buchwald et al. *(65)* have examined the effectiveness of surgical treatments for obesity. Maggard et al. report that pooled results from 89 studies revealed a 43.46 kg weight loss from baseline weight associated with Roux-en-Y gastric bypass at 12 months, and 41.46 kg loss at ≥36 months *(64)*. As seen in Fig. 1, the Swedish Obesity Subjects (SOS) study, the longest prospective, controlled study to date has shown that at 10 years of follow-up, gastric bypass patients maintained a 25% decrease in weight compared to matched controls (1.8 kg weight gain in controls vs 30.0 kg weight loss in gastric bypass) *(66)*. While the majority of the studies are case-control studies and there are only a few randomized trials *(67–71)*, the bulk of the literature demonstrates that bariatric surgery is an extremely effective option to reduce obesity, although weight loss to ideal body weight is not always achieved *(65,72)*.

Furthermore, bariatric surgery patients have also been found to have significantly decreased mean energy intake compared to controls *(66)*. They exhibit appetite suppression and typically eat fewer meals and voluntarily restrict calorie dense foods. Why this occurs is poorly understood, but may involve hormones secreted by the gastrointestinal tract such as ghrelin, an endogenous appetite stimulant secreted mainly in the stomach and duodenum *(73)*. Surgeries which preferentially affect these areas of the gastrointestinal tract, such as the Roux-en-Y gastric bypass, have been found in randomized trials to be more effective than other techniques which do not *(74)*, and the concept that postsurgical alterations in enteric hormone homeostasis result in sustainable weight loss has generated a great deal of promising research on ghrelin as well as other enteric

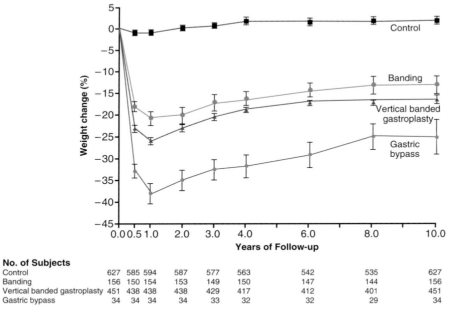

Fig. 1. Weight changes among subjects in the Swedish Obesity Subjects (SOS) study over a 10-year period. All data are for subjects who completed 10 years of the study. The average weight change in the entire group of surgically treated subjects was almost identical to that in the subgroup of subjects who underwent vertical banded gastroplasty. I bars represent the 95% confidence intervals. Permission granted from Sjostrom et al. NEJM. 2004. 351:2683.

hormones such as cholecystokinin, glucagon-like peptide-1 (GLP-1), oxyntomodulin, and peptide YY *(58,75–77)*. This area remains an active area of research.

4.3. Effects on Diabetes

There is a growing body of literature supporting bariatric surgery as a sustainable method to improve glycemic control and, at times, even to eliminate diabetes. In the meta-analysis by Buchwald et al. 1,417 of 1,846 (76.8%) patients had complete resolution of diabetes, defined as the ability to maintain blood glucose within the normal range and the cessation of all diabetes-related medications, and 414 of 485 (85.4%) had either resolved or improved diabetes; however, time points for these values were not specifically noted in the meta-analysis *(65)*. The SOS study reported that at 10 years of follow-up, the incidence of new onset diabetes in patients who underwent bariatric surgery was 7% compared to 24% in matched controls and surgical patients had significantly improved glycemic control compared to controls (Table 1) *(66)*.

Weight loss, decreased abdominal obesity, and subsequent improvement in insulin sensitivity have long been thought to be the major mechanisms behind the euglycemia observed in bariatric surgery. For example, muscle insulin receptor levels are increased postbariatric surgery, and levels of adiponectin, an endogenous insulin sensitizer, are increased both in response to long-term weight loss and in bariatric surgery patients *(78,79)*. However, there is also evidence to suggest that the surgery itself, independent of weight loss, may also play a role in diabetes control. For example, liposuction to reduce subcutaneous adipose tissue is not associated with any benefits toward diabetes or coronary risk factors *(80)*, and several reports have indicated that in many cases of post-Roux-en-Y bypass, glycemic normalization occurs before any significant weight loss. In fact, diabetic patients can become euglycemic and discontinue all diabetic medications by 1-week postsurgery *(81)*. While the beneficial glycemic effects are seen across the board with all bariatric procedures, the greatest effect is seen in biliopancreatic diversion or duodenal switch, followed by gastric bypass, gastroplasty, and gastric banding *(65,81–83)*.

The exact mechanisms underlying differences in efficacy and rapidity of effect observed between different surgical techniques remain unclear. A series of elegant experiments by Rubino and Marescaux studying Goto-Kakizaki type 2 diabetic rats has helped shed some light on this issue. Rats that underwent duodenal switch, a stomach-sparing, intestinal bypass operation, experienced resolution of diabetes compared to sham-operated animals with similar preoperative and postoperative features, suggesting that diabetes remission can be obtained by intestinal bypass without changes in food intake or weight loss *(84)*. In a follow-up experiment, rats that underwent duodenal-jejunal bypass, a stomach sparing, but duodenum bypassing operation, had significantly improved glycemic control compared to rats that underwent gastrojejunostomy, which maintained nutrient stimulation to the duodenum. Furthermore, the effects on glycemic control were reversible with revision surgery *(85)*. These studies strongly suggest that the duodenum plays an important, but yet to be fully elucidated, role in non-insulin-dependent diabetes mellitus (NIDDM). Several hormones secreted by the stomach and small bowel have been proposed as key mediators including ghrelin and GLP-1. Ghrelin is associated with increased feeding, weight gain, and has several diabetogenic effects such as stimulating insulin counter-regulatory hormones *(86)* and antagonizing insulin-mediated

Table 1

Percentage Changes in Weight, Anthropometric Variables, Risk Factors, and Energy Intake at 2 and 10 Years[a]

Variable	Changes at 2 years[b]			Changes at 10 years[b]			Changes at 10 years in surgery subgroups		
	Control Group (N=1,660)	Surgery Group (N=1,845)	Difference (95% CI)	Control Group (N=627)	Surgery Group (N=641)	Difference (95% CI)	Banding (N=156)	Vertical banded gastroplasty (N=451)	Gastric bypass (N=34)
	Percent			Percent			Percent		
Weight	0.1	−23.4	22.2 (21.6 to 22.8)*	1.6	−16.1	16.3 (14.9 to 17.6)*	−13.2	−16.5**	−25.0*
Height	−0.01	−0.06	0.06 (0.02 to 0.10)**	−0.3	−0.3	−0.01 (−0.12 to 0.10)	−0.2	−0.3	−0.8*
BMI	0.1	−23.3	22.1 (21.5 to 22.7)*	2.3	−15.7	16.5 (15.1 to 17.8)*	−12.8	−16.0**	−23.8*
Waist	0.2	−16.9	16.0 (15.4 to 16.5)*	2.8	−10.1	11.3 (10.3 to 12.4)*	−7.6	−10.2**	−19.3*
Systolic blood pressure	0.5	−4.4	2.8 (2.1 to 3.6)*	4.4	0.5	1.1 (−0.3 to 2.6)	2.1	0.4	−4.7
Diastolic blood pressure	0.3	−5.2	3.2 (2.4 to 3.9)*	−2.0	−2.6	−2.3 (−3.5 to −1.0)*	−1.4	−2.5	−10.4
Pulse pressure	3.2	0.6	−0.5 (−2.3 to 1.3)	18.0	10.8	3.5 (0.1 to 6.9)**	13.8	10.1	6.3
Glucose	5.1	−13.6	16.6 (15.0 to 18.3)*	18.7	−2.5	18.4 (14.7 to 22.1)*	−0.8	−2.5	−10.0
Insulin	10.3	−46.2	51.4 (48.0 to 54.8)*	12.3	−28.2	30.3 (23.9 to 36.6)*	−25.3	−27.2	−54.0*

Uric acid	−0.4	−14.9	13.5 (12.5 to 14.6)*	3.9	−6.2	8.8 (6.4 to 11.1)*	−5.2	−6.1	−12.3
Triglycerides	6.3	−27.2	29.9 (27.4 to 32.5)*	2.2	−16.3	14.8 (10.4 to 19.1)*	−18.0	−14.9	−28.0**
HDL cholesterol	3.5	22.0	−18.7 (−20.1 to −17.3)*	10.8	24.0	−13.6 (−16.5 to −10.6)*	20.4	23.5	47.5**
Total cholesterol	0.1	−2.9	1.0 (0.1 to 1.9)**	−6.0	−5.4	−2.0 (−0.2 to −3.8)**	−5.0	−5.0	−12.6*
Energy intake	−2.8	−28.6	19.1 (16.0 to 22.2)*	−1.0	−20.7	11.6 (8.1 to 15.0)*	−19.7	−21.6	−12.6

P values are for the comparison with the banding subgroup

*P<0.001.

**P<0.05.

[a]Data are for all subjects who completed 2 and 10 years of the study and are independent of diagnosis and medications at or after baseline. The changes within each treatment group are unadjusted, whereas the differences between the groups in the changes have been adjusted for sex, age, body-mass index (BMI), and the baseline level of the respective variable. CI confidence interval, HDL high-density lipoprotein.

[b]For values within each group, minus signs denote decreases; for differences between the groups, minus signs denote smaller reductions or (in the case of HDL cholesterol) larger increases in the surgical group than in the control group.

intracellular signaling pathways in vitro *(87)*. GLP-1, secreted mainly in the distal ileum, stimulates insulin secretion in response to food ingestion, and operations which bypass the proximal bowel and shunt food more readily to the distal bowel have been proposed to enhance GLP-1 and, hence, insulin secretion *(88–91)*. Other hormones such as peptide YY, neurotensin, oxyntomodulin, pancreatic polypeptide, and enteroglucagon have also been examined as possible mediators for the dramatic response in glycemic control seen after surgery *(58)*. Current studies are under way to further delineate the role of these hormones in glycemic control.

4.4. Effects on Mortality

Until recently, the long-term effects of bariatric surgery on mortality remained unclear. New evidence has emerged from the SOS study group *(92)* demonstrating that at 15 years postsurgery, the unadjusted hazard ratio was 0.76 (*P*=0.04) in the surgery group compared to controls (Fig. 2.) In another recently published restrospective cohort study of 7,925 subjects who had undergone gastric bypass and 7,925 matched controls, gastric bypass significantly reduced mortality associated with diabetes, heart disease, and cancer. However, rates of death associated with accidents and suicide were significantly higher in the surgery groups *(93)*. While these studies are promising, it is notable that the relative decrease in mortality associated with bariatric surgery is still significantly less than the potential benefits of other lifestyle modifications such as smoking cessation. Finally, further studies are needed to clarify which subgroups of individuals stand to benefit the most from these bariatric procedures.

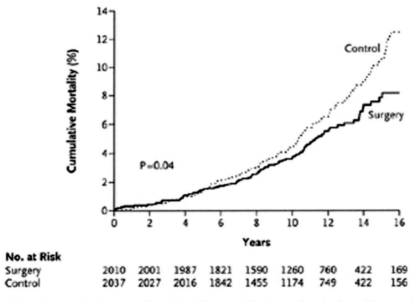

No. at Risk									
Surgery	2010	2001	1987	1821	1590	1260	760	422	169
Control	2037	2027	2016	1842	1455	1174	749	422	156

Fig. 2. Unadjusted cumulative mortality after 15 years. The hazard ratio for subjects who underwent bariatric surgery, as compared with control subjects, was 0.76 (95% confidence interval, 0.59–0.99; *P* = 0.04), with 129 deaths in the control group and 101 in the surgery group. Permission granted from Sjostrom et al. NEJM 2007. 357:741.

4.5. Effects on Hypertension

In a case series of 1,025 gastric bypass patients by Sugerman et al. at 2 years, 69% of preoperative hypertensive patients were no longer hypertensive after surgery, and at 10–12 years, 51% of these patients remained normotensive *(94)*. In the meta-analysis by Buchwald et al. improvement or complete resolution of hypertension was observed in 78.5% and 62% of patients, respectively, at two or less years of follow-up *(65)*. The SOS study found that at 2 years, the systolic blood pressure was increased by 0.5% (0.68 mmHg) in the control group compared to a 4.4% decrease (6.3 mmHg) in the surgical group; however, by 10 (and possibly as early as 3–4) years, systolic hypertension had recurred and there was no significant difference between control and surgical groups *(66)*. Thus, it remains unclear whether bariatric surgery has any significant long-term effects on blood pressure. The majority of studies in the literature are case series which extend to, on average, 2 years follow-up *(94–96)*. Beyond the SOS study, there are no other large, controlled studies with long-term data. The lack of controlled studies makes it difficult to determine whether the increase of blood pressure is weight related or secondary to other factors. Furthermore, changes in blood pressure appear to be more closely associated with the direction of ongoing weight change as opposed to the absolute weight lost. Whether there is a weight threshold for hypertension remains unclear, and this remains an active area of research.

4.6. Effects on Dyslipidemia

The direct relationship between lower cholesterol levels and increased coronary artery disease risk was partly established in the early 1990 s by the Program on the Surgical Control of the Hyperlipidemias, a multicenter, randomized, secondary intervention trial designed to assess whether cholesterol lowering induced by partial ileal bypass surgery would favorably effect morbidity and mortality associated with coronary artery disease. This study, which was not designed to study obesity per se, was one of the longest randomized studies of a surgical method to reduce hyperlipidemia. Mean follow-up was 9.7 years and revealed 23% lower total cholesterol, 38% lower LDL, and 4% higher HDL levels in patients after partial ileal bypass compared to controls *(97)*. A different study showed that, after more than 20 years postoperation, partial ileal bypass was able to sustain reduction of total cholesterol levels by 30% *(98)*.

In the obese population, the effects of bariatric procedures on lipid profiles have been positive in the short term *(99–102)*. The SOS study results reveal that at 2 years, the control group experienced a 0.1% increase in total cholesterol, 3.5% increase in HDL, and 6.3% increase in triglycerides compared to the surgical arm, which experienced a 2.9% decrease in total cholesterol, 22% increase in HDL, and 27.2% decrease in triglycerides. At 10 years follow-up, the control arm had a 6% decrease in total cholesterol, 11% increase in HDL, and 2.2 increase in triglycerides compared with surgical patients with 5.4% decrease in total cholesterol, 24% increase in HDL, and 16.3% decrease in triglycerides *(66)*. Notably, the SOS study found that at 10 years, there was no significant improvement in total cholesterol levels in gastric bypass patients in comparison to controls *(66)*. It is unclear why the initial benefits observed do not persist. Whether any of these changes translate into changes in coronary artery disease risk is completely unknown but is currently being evaluated by the SOS study group.

4.7. Effects on Bone Disease

4.7.1. Osteomalacia/Osteoporosis

Bone mineral density, the strongest predictor of future osteoporotic fracture, is directly related to body weight, and numerous interventional trials have shown that weight loss results in bone loss and bone resorption *(103–105)*. Not surprisingly, the dramatic weight loss seen in bariatric surgery patients is also associated with increased bone turnover and decreased bone mineral density. One recent study revealed that by 9 months post-Roux-en-Y gastric bypass, patients had dramatic weight loss, and bone mineral density decreased 7.8% at the hip, 9.3% at trochanter, and 1.6% at the total body *(106)*. However, very little is known about long-term effects, and the preliminary data is conflicting. It has been suggested that different surgical techniques and subgroups of patients are associated with different risks for developing osteoporosis. For example, one small, prospective study found that AGB had no significant effect on bone mineral content compared to a control group. However, Roux-en-Y was associated with significantly decreased bone mineral content *(107)*. Another study comparing pre- and postmenopausal women who received Roux-en-Y bypass with matched controls found that significant differences in bone mineral density between the surgical and nonsurgical patients did not appear until after menopause *(108)*. Further studies are needed to clarify these conflicting results.

The mechanisms underlying the bone loss seen in bariatric surgery patients remain unclear, but may involve decreased mechanical load on the skeleton, alterations in mineral absorption and calcium/vitamin D metabolism, as well as changes in other hormones such as insulin, leptin, or enteric hormones *(109–112)*. The exact impact of malabsorption is unclear as serum calcium and phosphate levels are most often normal in postgastrectomy states; however, calcium levels may be normal, secondary to mobilization of calcium from bone. Serum alkaline phosphatase, vitamin D metabolites, and PTH levels have been shown to be variable, however. One study examining the effects of calcium and vitamin D supplementation following bariatric surgery found that postmenopausal women after Roux-en-Y gastric bypass showed evidence of secondary hyperparathyroidism and elevated bone resorption that was not reversed with modest calcium and vitamin D supplementation *(108)*. The observation that osteoporotic bone is characterized by a higher percentage of adipocytes compared to normal bone has raised interest in the role of other factors such as leptin, an adipocyte-derived hormone associated with obesity *(113)*. Similarly, the interplays between bone density and insulin and enteric hormones are also being explored. At this time, there is not enough evidence (short-term or long-term) to make any conclusive opinions regarding risk of developing osteoporosis after bariatric surgery, although the general evidence seems to suggest that decreased bone mineral density is certainly a complication that should be monitored closely among patients.

4.7.2. Osteoarthritis

Obesity is perhaps the strongest modifiable risk factor for the development of osteoarthritis, a degenerative joint disease associated with significant morbidity *(114,115)*. There are numerous reports in the literature reviewing the relationship between obesity and osteoarthritis *(116,117)*. Notably, the association of obesity as a risk factor for osteoarthritis varies by joint and is more strongly associated with the knees and hands than the hips. One report of 64 patients with osteoarthritis from the Framingham knee osteoarthritis study noted that most cases of osteoarthritis occurred in women who had gained between 2 and 4 BMI units from their baseline weight 10 years ago *(114)*. While the study was limited by significant recall bias, it strongly implies that weight loss decreases osteoarthritis risk. The weight loss associated with bariatric procedures also results in significant improvement in osteoarthritis with one case series following 275 subjects up to 31 months reporting 47% improvement and 41% complete resolution of symptoms associated with degenerative joint disease *(118)*. Again, long-term data is needed to further evaluate the effects of bariatric surgery on this disease.

4.8. Effects on Obstructive Sleep Apnea

OSA is characterized by excessive daytime sleepiness, snoring, and hypertension and is classically observed in obese men with large neck circumferences. The prevalence of OSA is rising in parallel with the increase in obesity; one study estimated that the concomitant diagnosis of OSA doubles the costs of treatment for all other additional comorbidities *(119)*. Weight loss is the standard recommendation for these patients, and bariatric surgery has proven to be very effective means to treat OSA. Many studies on sleep apnea are confounded by poor long-term follow-up and difficulty obtaining subjects for repeat polysomnography postintervention. Two-year follow-up data indicate that there are beneficial effects of bariatric surgery for resolving OSA; however, more studies are needed to evaluate long-term effects *(120)*.

4.9. Effects on Risk of Malignancy

The effects of weight loss from bariatric surgery on cancer risk remain unclear. At 10 years of follow-up in the SOS study, analysis of incidence of cancer remained ongoing, presumably because of inadequate person-years of follow-up. The SOS study is marked for continuation until 2020 and 40,000 person-years of follow-up have been attained *(66,121)*.

4.10. Effects on Biliary Disease

Obesity is a very well established risk factor for the development of cholesterol gallstones *(14,122,123)*, and rapid weight loss is associated with additional risks of developing gallstones. Not surprisingly, bariatric surgeries are associated with high rates of gallstone formation as early as 3 months following surgery *(124,125)*. Two-year data from the SOS study revealed that 4% of postsurgical men had cholelithiasis, 2.5% had cholecystitis, and 3.4% required cholecystectomy compared to 1.2%, 0.7%, and 0.7%, respectively, in control men. In women, there was no statistically significant difference between surgical and control groups *(126)*. Another study by Shiffman et al. found that 38% of patients developed gallstones, and 15% of patients developed symptomatic gallstones requiring cholecystectomy within 3 years of gastric bypass *(127)*. Clearly, gallstone formation is an important complication of the rapid weight loss associated with bariatric surgery. Treatment methods and prophylaxis for this complication have been discussed in Chap. 17.

4.11. Effects on Quality of Life

Obesity has a tremendous impact on the psychosocial, physical, and economic health of those afflicted by it. Depression, anxiety, increased dissatisfaction with body image, unsatisfactory marital relationships, difficulties with sexual function, physical limitations, bodily pain, and fatigue are just a few of the factors impaired in obesity. Many of the psychosocial and behavioral aspects of bariatric surgery have been well summarized in a review by Sarwer et al. who note that between 20% and 60% of bariatric candidates suffer from an Axis I psychiatric disorder *(128)*.

The overwhelming majority of studies have found that bariatric surgery improves quality of life, and the specific details of quality of life measurements have been reviewed elsewhere *(129)*. The SOS study found that 1 year after bariatric surgery, patients reported significant reductions in depression and anxiety. Furthermore, peak improvements in health-related quality of life were seen at 6–12 months, with a slight decline at 2 years of follow-up *(130)*. In general, improvements in psychosocial markers directly correspond with the amount of retained weight loss. Unfortunately, the data is scarce beyond several years of follow-up. Furthermore, some studies have suggested that the socioeconomic impact of morbid obesity persists long after a reduction in weight and improvement in quality of life. For example, one study found that after 5 years post-Roux-en-Y gastric bypass, only 16% of subjects who had initially attributed their disability to morbid obesity were gainfully employed despite significant weight loss and improvement in quality of life *(131)*. In another study from the SOS study group, there was no difference between the number of hospitalization days and total hospitalization costs for surgically and conventionally treated obese patients followed for 7 years *(132)*. Thus, while early data appear very promising, these findings need to be replicated in larger cohorts of patients followed for longer time periods before definitive conclusions can be made regarding the psychosocial outcomes of bariatric surgery.

5. CONCLUSIONS

Obesity is the epidemic of our times and is associated with major morbidity and mortality. Despite its prevalence, relatively little is known about the pathogenesis of this complex disease, and even less is known about the long-term efficacy of the potential treatment methods. Diet and exercise, while first-line treatments for obesity, have proven to be inadequate in the face of the genetic, biochemical, environmental, and socioeconomic obstacles hindering maintenance of long-term weight loss. Current breakthroughs in pharmacotherapy and bariatric surgery are very promising and exciting, but these are essentially new areas of study limited by lack of long-term follow-up and/or adequate randomized, interventional trials. Virtually nothing is known about the effects of any of these treatment modalities on mortality, and the side effects associated with these treatments are not trivial. As such, current treatments for obesity should be utilized cautiously, and as further progress is made to clarify the long-term effects of behavioral modifications, pharmacotherapy, and surgery on obesity and its comorbidities, more light will be shed on the pathophysiology of this complicated disease. This will hopefully provide physicians new strategies for prevention and cure and will eventually provide tangible benefits to patients who are striving to decrease their excessive body weight.

REFERENCES

1. *The practical guide: identification, evaluation, and treatment of overweight and obesity in adults. (NIH publication no. 00-4048)*. 2000, National Heart, Lung, and Blood Institute. North American Association for the Study of Obesity: Bethesda, MD.

2. Ford, E.S., Body mass index, diabetes, and C-reactive protein among U.S. adults Diabetes Care 1999; 22, 1971–7.

3. Ford, E.S., Giles, W.H., and Mokdad, A.H., Increasing prevalence of the metabolic syndrome among U.S. adults Diabetes Care 2004; 27, 2444–9.

4. Mensah, G.A., Mokdad, A.H., Ford, E., et al. Obesity, metabolic syndrome, and type 2 diabetes: emerging epidemics and their cardiovascular implications. Cardiol Clin 2004; 22, 485–504.

5. Mokdad, A.H., Bowman, B.A., Ford, E.S., et al. The continuing epidemics of obesity and diabetes in the United States. JAMA 2001; 286, 1195–200.

6. Mokdad, A.H., Ford, E.S., Bowman, B.A., et al. Prevalence of obesity, diabetes, and obesity-related health risk factors, 2001. JAMA 2003; 289, 76–9.

7. Lipton, R.B., Liao, Y., Cao, G., et al. Determinants of incident non-insulin-dependent diabetes mellitus among blacks and whites in a national sample. The NHANES I Epidemiologic Follow-up Study. Am J Epidemiol 1993; 138, 826–39.

8. Tchernof, A., Lamarche, B., Prud'Homme, D., et al. The dense LDL phenotype. Association with plasma lipoprotein levels, visceral obesity, and hyperinsulinemia in men. Diabetes Care 1996; 19, 629–37.

9. Dyer, A.R., and Elliott, P., The INTERSALT study: relations of body mass index to blood pressure. INTERSALT Co-operative Research Group J Hum Hypertens 1989; 3, 299–308.

10. Dyer, A.R., Elliott, P., and Shipley, M., Body mass index versus height and weight in relation to blood pressure. Findings for the 10,079 persons in the INTERSALT Study. Am J Epidemiol 1990; 131, 589–96.

11. Havlik, R.J., Hubert, H.B., Fabsitz, R.R., et al. Weight and hypertension. Ann Intern Med 1983; 98, 855–9.

12. Hubert, H.B., The nature of the relationship between obesity and cardiovascular disease. Int J Cardiol 1984; 6, 268–74.

13. Hubert, H.B., Feinleib, M., McNamara, P.M., et al. Obesity as an independent risk factor for cardiovascular disease: a 26-year follow-up of participants in the Framingham Heart Study. Circulation 1983; 67, 968–77.

14. Stampfer, M.J., Maclure, K.M., Colditz, G.A., et al. Risk of symptomatic gallstones in women with severe obesity. Am J Clin Nutr 1992; 55, 652–8.

15. Gelber, A.C., Hochberg, M.C., Mead, L.A., et al. Body mass index in young men and the risk of subsequent knee and hip osteoarthritis. Am J Med 1999; 107, 542–8.

16. Hochberg, M.C., Risk factors for the development and progression of hip osteoarthritis. J Rheumatol 2005; 32, 1135–6.

17. Hochberg, M.C., Lethbridge-Cejku, M., Scott, W.W., Jr., et al. Obesity and osteoarthritis of the hands in women. Osteoarthritis Cartilage 1993; 1, 129–35.

18. Hochberg, M.C., Lethbridge-Cejku, M., Scott, W.W., Jr., et al. The association of body weight, body fatness and body fat distribution with osteoarthritis of the knee: data from the Baltimore Longitudinal Study of Aging. J Rheumatol 1995; 22, 488–93.

19. Tepper, S., and Hochberg, M.C., Factors associated with hip osteoarthritis: data from the First National Health and Nutrition Examination Survey (NHANES-I). Am J Epidemiol 1993; 137, 1081–8.

20. Young, T., Palta, M., Dempsey, J., , The occurrence of sleep-disordered breathing among middle-aged adults. N Engl J Med 1993; 328, 1230–5.

21. Chute, C.G., Willett, W.C., Colditz, G.A., et al. A prospective study of body mass, height, and smoking on the risk of colorectal cancer in women. Cancer Causes Control 1991; 2, 117–24.

22. Giovannucci, E., Ascherio, A., Rimm, E.B., et al. Physical activity, obesity, and risk for colon cancer and adenoma in men. Ann Intern Med 1995; 122, 327–34.

23. Giovannucci, E., Colditz, G.A., Stampfer, M.J., et al. Physical activity, obesity, and risk of colorectal adenoma in women (United States). Cancer Causes Control 1996; 7, 253–63.

24. Goldstein, D.J., and Potvin, J.H., Long-term weight loss: the effect of pharmacologic agents. Am J Clin Nutr 1994; 60, 647–57; discussion 658–9.

25. Howard, B.V., Manson, J.E., Stefanick, M.L., et al. Low-fat dietary pattern and weight change over 7 years: the Women's Health Initiative Dietary Modification Trial. JAMA 2006; 295, 39–49.

26. Bray, G.A., and Popkin, B.M., Dietary fat intake does affect obesity! Am J Clin Nutr 1998; 68, 1157–73.

27. Nordmann, A.J., Nordmann, A., Briel, M., et al. Effects of low-carbohydrate vs low-fat diets on weight loss and cardiovascular risk factors: a meta-analysis of randomized controlled trials. Arch Intern Med 2006; 166, 285–93.

28. McManus, K., Antinoro, L., and Sacks, F., A randomized controlled trial of a moderate-fat, low-energy diet compared with a low fat, low-energy diet for weight loss in overweight adults. Int J Obes Relat Metab Disord 2001; 25, 1503–11.

29. McTigue, K.M., Harris, R., Hemphill, B., et al. Screening and interventions for obesity in adults: summary of the evidence for the U.S. preventive services task force. Ann Intern Med 2003; 139, 933–949.

30. Shaw, K., Gennat, H., O'Rourke, P., et al. Exercise for overweight or obesity Cochrane Database Syst Rev 2006, CD003817.

31. Knowler, W.C., Barrett-Connor, E., Fowler, S.E., et al. Reduction in the incidence of type 2 diabetes with lifestyle intervention or metformin. N Engl J Med 2002; 346, 393–403.

32. Huang, Z., Willett, W.C., Manson, J.E., et al. Body weight, weight change, and risk for hypertension in women. Ann Intern Med 1998; 128, 81–8.

33. Samaha, F.F., Iqbal, N., Seshadri, P., et al. A low-carbohydrate as compared with a low-fat diet in severe obesity. N Engl J Med 2003; 348, 2074–81.

34. Howard, B.V., Van Horn, L., Hsia, J., et al. Low-fat dietary pattern and risk of cardiovascular disease: the Women's Health Initiative Randomized Controlled Dietary Modification Trial. JAMA 2006; 295, 655–66.

35. Neter, J.E., Stam, B.E., Kok, F.J., et al. Influence of weight reduction on blood pressure: a meta-analysis of randomized controlled trials. Hypertension 2003; 42, 878–84.

36. Kelemen, M.H., Effron, M.B., Valenti, S.A., et al. Exercise training combined with antihypertensive drug therapy. Effects on lipids, blood pressure, and left ventricular mass. JAMA 1990; 263, 2766–71.

37. Nelson, L., Jennings, G.L., Esler, M.D., et al. Effect of changing levels of physical activity on blood-pressure and haemodynamics in essential hypertension. Lancet 1986; 2, 473–6.

38. Whelton, S.P., Chin, A., Xin, X., et al. Effect of aerobic exercise on blood pressure: a meta-analysis of randomized, controlled trials. Ann Intern Med 2002; 136, 493–503.

39. Neaton, J.D., Grimm, R.H., Jr., Prineas, R.J., et al. Treatment of Mild Hypertension Study. Final results. Treatment of Mild Hypertension Study Research Group. JAMA 1993; 270, 713–24.

40. Sacks, F.M., Svetkey, L.P., Vollmer, W.M., et al. Effects on blood pressure of reduced dietary sodium and the Dietary Approaches to Stop Hypertension (DASH) diet. DASH-Sodium Collaborative Research Group. N Engl J Med 2001; 344, 3–10.

41. Appel, L.J., Sacks, F.M., Carey, V.J., et al. Effects of protein, monounsaturated fat, and carbohydrate intake on blood pressure and serum lipids: results of the OmniHeart randomized trial. JAMA 2005; 294, 2455–64.

42. Calle, E.E., Rodriguez, C., Walker-Thurmond, K., et al. Overweight, obesity, and mortality from cancer in a prospectively studied cohort of U.S. adults. N Engl J Med 2003; 348, 1625–38.

43. IARC Handbooks on Cancer Prevention: Weight Control and Physical Activity 2002; 6.

44. Spentzos, D., Mantzoros, C., Regan, M.M., et al. Minimal effect of a low-fat/high soy diet for asymptomatic, hormonally naive prostate cancer patients. Clin Cancer Res 2003; 9, 3282–7.

45. Prentice, R.L., Caan, B., Chlebowski, R.T., et al. Low-fat dietary pattern and risk of invasive breast cancer: the Women's Health Initiative Randomized Controlled Dietary Modification Trial. JAMA 2006; 295, 629–42.

46. Beresford, S.A., Johnson, K.C., Ritenbaugh, C., et al. Low-fat dietary pattern and risk of colorectal cancer: the Women's Health Initiative Randomized Controlled Dietary Modification Trial. JAMA 2006; 295, 643–54.

47. Chlebowski, R.T., Blackburn, G.L., Thomson, C.A., et al. Dietary fat reduction and breast cancer outcome: interim efficacy results from the Women's Intervention Nutrition Study. J Natl Cancer Inst 2006; 98, 1767–76.

48. Villareal, D.T., Fontana, L., Weiss, E.P., et al. Bone mineral density response to caloric restriction-induced weight loss or exercise-induced weight loss: a randomized controlled trial. Arch Intern Med 2006; 166, 2502–10.

49. Andersen, T., Liver and gallbladder disease before and after very-low-calorie diets. Am J Clin Nutr 1992; 56, 235S–9S.

50. Snow, V., Barry, P., Fitterman, N., et al. Pharmacologic and surgical management of obesity in primary care: A Clinical Practice Guideline from the American College of Physicians. Ann Intern Med 2005; 142, 525–31.

51. Cooke, D., and Bloom, S., The obesity pipeline: current strategies in the development of anti-obesity drugs. Nat Rev Drug Discov 2006; 5, 919–31.

52. Padwal, R.S., and Majumdar, S.R., Drug treatments for obesity: orlistat, sibutramine, and rimonabant. Lancet 2007; 369, 71–7.

53. Wadden, T.A., Berkowitz, R.I., Womble, L.G., et al. Randomized trial of lifestyle modification and pharmacotherapy for obesity. N Engl J Med 2005; 353, 2111–20.

54. Li, Z., Maglione, M., Tu, W., et al. Meta-analysis: pharmacologic treatment of obesity. Ann Intern Med 2005; 142, 532–46.

55. Padwal, R., Li, S.K., and Lau, D.C., Long-term pharmacotherapy for obesity and overweight Cochrane Database Syst Rev 2003, CD004094.

56. Torgerson, J.S., Hauptman, J., Boldrin, M.N., et al. XENical in the prevention of diabetes in obese subjects (XENDOS) study: a randomized study of orlistat as an adjunct to lifestyle changes for the prevention of type 2 diabetes in obese patients. Diabetes Care 2004; 27, 155–61.

57. Brolin, R.E., Bariatric surgery and long-term control of morbid obesity. JAMA 2002; 288, 2793–6.

58. Cummings, D.E., Overduin, J., and Foster-Schubert, K.E., Gastric bypass for obesity: mechanisms of weight loss and diabetes resolution. J Clin Endocrinol Metab 2004; 89, 2608–15.

59. Alvarado, R., Alami, R.S., Hsu, G., et al. The impact of preoperative weight loss in patients undergoing laparoscopic Roux-en-Y gastric bypass. Obes Surg 2005; 15, 1282–6.

60. Barrow, C.J., Roux-en-Y gastric bypass for morbid obesity. Aorn J 2002; 76, 590, 593–604; quiz 606–8.

61. Cottam, D.R., Atkinson, J., Anderson, A., et al. A case-controlled matched-pair cohort study of laparoscopic Roux-en-Y gastric bypass and Lap-Band patients in a single US center with three-year follow-up. Obes Surg 2006; 16, 534–40.

62. Crookes, P.F., Surgical treatment of morbid obesity. Annu Rev Med 2006; 57, 243–64.

63. O'Brien, P.E., Dixon, J.B., Laurie, C., et al. Treatment of mild to moderate obesity with laparoscopic adjustable gastric banding or an intensive medical program: a randomized trial. Ann Intern Med 2006; 144, 625–33.

64. Maggard, M.A., Shugarman, L.R., Suttorp, M., et al. Meta-analysis: surgical treatment of obesity. Ann Intern Med 2005; 142, 547–59.

65. Buchwald, H., Avidor, Y., Braunwald, E., et al. Bariatric surgery: a systematic review and meta-analysis. JAMA 2004; 292, 1724–37.

66. Sjostrom, L., Lindroos, A.K., Peltonen, M., et al. Lifestyle, diabetes, and cardiovascular risk factors 10 years after bariatric surgery. N Engl J Med 2004; 351, 2683–93.

67. Ashy, A.R., and Merdad, A.A., A prospective study comparing vertical banded gastroplasty versus laparoscopic adjustable gastric banding in the treatment of morbid and super-obesity. Int Surg 1998; 83, 108–10.

68. Hall, J.C., Watts, J.M., O'Brien, P.E., et al. Gastric surgery for morbid obesity. The Adelaide Study. Ann Surg 1990; 211, 419–27.

69. Mingrone, G., Greco, A.V., Giancaterini, A., et al. Sex hormone-binding globulin levels and cardiovascular risk factors in morbidly obese subjects before and after weight reduction induced by diet or malabsorptive surgery. Atherosclerosis 2002; 161, 455–62.

70. Nguyen, N.T., Goldman, C., Rosenquist, C.J., et al. Laparoscopic versus open gastric bypass: a randomized study of outcomes, quality of life, and costs. Ann Surg 2001; 234, 279–89; discussion 289–91.

71. Thorne, A., Lonnqvist, F., Apelman, J., et al. A pilot study of long-term effects of a novel obesity treatment: omentectomy in connection with adjustable gastric banding. Int J Obes Relat Metab Disord 2002; 26, 193–9.

72. Maggard, M.A., Shugarman, L.R., Suttorp, M., et al. Meta-analysis: surgical treatment of obesity. Ann Intern Med 2005; 142, 547–59.

73. Cummings, D.E., Weigle, D.S., Frayo, R.S., et al. Plasma ghrelin levels after diet-induced weight loss or gastric bypass surgery. N Engl J Med 2002; 346, 1623–30.

74. Sugerman, H.J., Starkey, J.V., and Birkenhauer, R., A randomized prospective trial of gastric bypass versus vertical banded gastroplasty for morbid obesity and their effects on sweets versus non-sweets eaters. Ann Surg 1987; 205, 613–24.

75. Cummings, D.E., Overduin, J., Shannon, M.H., et al. Hormonal mechanisms of weight loss and diabetes resolution after bariatric surgery. Surg Obes Relat Dis 2005; 1, 358–68.

76. Chan, J.L., Mun, E.C., Stoyneva, V., et al. Peptide YY levels are elevated after gastric bypass surgery. Obesity (Silver Spring) 2006; 14, 194–8.

77. le Roux, C.W., Aylwin, S.J., Batterham, R.L., et al. Gut hormone profiles following bariatric surgery favor an anorectic state, facilitate weight loss, and improve metabolic parameters. Ann Surg 2006; 243, 108–14.

78. Pender, C., Goldfine, I.D., Tanner, C.J., et al. Muscle insulin receptor concentrations in obese patients post bariatric surgery: relationship to hyperinsulinemia. Int J Obes Relat Metab Disord 2004; 28, 363–9.

79. Ronti, T., Lupattelli, G., and Mannarino, E., The endocrine function of adipose tissue: an update. Clin Endocrinol (Oxf) 2006; 64, 355–65.

80. Klein, S., Fontana, L., Young, V.L., et al. Absence of an effect of liposuction on insulin action and risk factors for coronary heart disease. N Engl J Med 2004; 350, 2549–57.

81. Schauer, P.R., Burguera, B., Ikramuddin, S., et al. Effect of laparoscopic Roux-en Y gastric bypass on type 2 diabetes mellitus. Ann Surg 2003; 238, 467–84; discussion 84–5.

82. Dixon, J.B., and O'Brien, P.E., Changes in comorbidities and improvements in quality of life after LAP-BAND placement. Am J Surg 2002; 184, 51S–4S.

83. Pontiroli, A.E., Pizzocri, P., Librenti, M.C., et al. Laparoscopic adjustable gastric banding for the treatment of morbid (grade 3) obesity and its metabolic complications: a three-year study. J Clin Endocrinol Metab 2002; 87, 3555–61.

84. Rubino, F., and Marescaux, J., Effect of duodenal-jejunal exclusion in a non-obese animal model of type 2 diabetes: a new perspective for an old disease. Ann Surg 2004; 239, 1–11.

85. Rubino, F., Forgione, A., Cummings, D.E., et al. The mechanism of diabetes control after gastrointestinal bypass surgery reveals a role of the proximal small intestine in the pathophysiology of type 2 diabetes. Ann Surg 2006; 244, 741–9.

86. Takaya, K., Ariyasu, H., Kanamoto, N., et al. Ghrelin strongly stimulates growth hormone release in humans. J Clin Endocrinol Metab 2000; 85, 4908–11.

87. Broglio, F., Arvat, E., Benso, A., , Ghrelin, a natural GH secretagogue produced by the stomach, induces hyperglycemia and reduces insulin secretion in humans. J Clin Endocrinol Metab 2001; 86, 5083–6.

88. Guidone, C., Manco, M., Valera-Mora, E., et al. Mechanisms of recovery from type 2 diabetes after malabsorptive bariatric surgery. Diabetes 2006; 55, 2025–31.

89. Naslund, E., Backman, L., Holst, J.J., et al. Importance of small bowel peptides for the improved glucose metabolism 20 years after jejunoileal bypass for obesity. Obes Surg 1998; 8, 253–60.

90. Naslund, E., Barkeling, B., King, N., et al. Energy intake and appetite are suppressed by glucagon-like peptide-1 (GLP-1) in obese men. Int J Obes Relat Metab Disord 1999; 23, 304–11.

91. Naslund, E., and Kral, J.G., Impact of gastric bypass surgery on gut hormones and glucose homeostasis in type 2 diabetes. Diabetes 2006; 55 (Suppl 2), S92–7.

92. Sjostrom, L., Narbro, K., Sjostrom, C.D., et al. Effects of bariatric surgery on mortality in Swedish obese subjects. N Engl J Med 2007; 357, 741–52.

93. Adams, T.D., Gress, R.E., Smith, S.C., et al. Long-term mortality after gastric bypass surgery. N Engl J Med 2007; 357, 753–61.

94. Sugerman, H.J., Wolfe, L.G., Sica, D.A., et al. Diabetes and hypertension in severe obesity and effects of gastric bypass-induced weight loss Ann Surg 2003; 237, 751–6; discussion 757–8.

95. Carson, J.L., Ruddy, M.E., Duff, A.E., et al. The effect of gastric bypass surgery on hypertension in morbidly obese patients. Arch Intern Med 1994; 154, 193–200.

96. Foley, E.F., Benotti, P.N., Borlase, B.C., et al. Impact of gastric restrictive surgery on hypertension in the morbidly obese. Am J Surg 1992; 163, 294–7.

97. Buchwald, H., Varco, R.L., Matts, J.P., et al. Effect of partial ileal bypass surgery on mortality and morbidity from coronary heart disease in patients with hypercholesterolemia. Report of the Program on the Surgical Control of the Hyperlipidemias (POSCH). N Engl J Med 1990; 323, 946–55.

98. Buchwald, H., Stoller, D.K., Campos, C.T., et al. Partial ileal bypass for hypercholesterolemia. 20- to 26-year follow-up of the first 57 consecutive cases. Ann Surg 1990; 212, 318–29; discussion 329–31.

99. Brizzi, P., Angius, M.F., Carboni, A., et al. Plasma lipids and lipoprotein changes after biliopancreatic diversion for morbid obesity. Dig Surg 2003; 20, 18–23.

100. Brolin, R.E., Bradley, L.J., Wilson, A.C., et al. Lipid risk profile and weight stability after gastric restrictive operations for morbid obesity. J Gastrointest Surg 2000; 4, 464–9.

101. Corradini, S.G., Eramo, A., Lubrano, C., et al. Comparison of changes in lipid profile after bilio-intestinal bypass and gastric banding in patients with morbid obesity. Obes Surg 2005; 15, 367–77.

102. Garcia-Diaz Jde, D., Lozano, O., Ramos, J.C., et al. Changes in lipid profile after biliopancreatic diversion. Obes Surg 2003; 13, 756–60.

103. Chao, D., Espeland, M.A., Farmer, D., et al. Effect of voluntary weight loss on bone mineral density in older overweight women. J Am Geriatr Soc 2000; 48, 753–9.

104. Fogelholm, G.M., Sievanen, H.T., Kukkonen-Harjula, T.K., et al. Bone mineral density during reduction, maintenance and regain of body weight in premenopausal, obese women. Osteoporos Int 2001; 12, 199–206.

105. Jensen, L.B., Quaade, F., and Sorensen, O.H., Bone loss accompanying voluntary weight loss in obese humans. J Bone Miner Res 1994; 9, 459–63.

106. Coates, P.S., Fernstrom, J.D., Fernstrom, M.H., et al. Gastric bypass surgery for morbid obesity leads to an increase in bone turnover and a decrease in bone mass. J Clin Endocrinol Metab 2004; 89, 1061–5.

107. von Mach, M.A., Stoeckli, R., Bilz, S., et al. Changes in bone mineral content after surgical treatment of morbid obesity. Metabolism 2004; 53, 918–21.

108. Goode, L.R., Brolin, R.E., Chowdhury, H.A., et al. Bone and gastric bypass surgery: effects of dietary calcium and vitamin D. Obes Res 2004; 12, 40–7.

109. Bisballe, S., Eriksen, E.F., Melsen, F., et al. Osteopenia and osteomalacia after gastrectomy: interrelations between biochemical markers of bone remodelling, vitamin D metabolites, and bone histomorphometry. Gut 1991; 32, 1303–7.

110. Glatzle, J., Piert, M., Meile, T., et al. Prevalence of vertebral alterations and the effects of calcium and vitamin D supplementation on calcium metabolism and bone mineral density after gastrectomy. Br J Surg 2005; 92, 579–85.

111. Klein, K.B., Orwoll, E.S., Lieberman, D.A., et al. Metabolic bone disease in asymptomatic men after partial gastrectomy with Billroth II anastomosis. Gastroenterology 1987; 92, 608–16.

112. Zittel, T.T., Zeeb, B., Maier, G.W., et al. High prevalence of bone disorders after gastrectomy. Am J Surg 1997; 174, 431–8.

113. Rosen, C.J., and Bouxsein, M.L., Mechanisms of disease: is osteoporosis the obesity of bone? Nat Clin Pract Rheumatol 2006; 2, 35–43.

114. Felson, D.T., Zhang, Y., Anthony, J.M., et al. Weight loss reduces the risk for symptomatic knee osteoarthritis in women. The Framingham Study. Ann Intern Med 1992; 116, 535–9.

115. Hartz, A.J., Fischer, M.E., Bril, G., , The association of obesity with joint pain and osteoarthritis in the HANES data. J Chronic Dis 1986; 39, 311–9.

116. Bliddal, H., and Christensen, R., The management of osteoarthritis in the obese patient: practical considerations and guidelines for therapy. Obes Rev 2006; 7, 323–31.

117. Burnett, B.P., Levy, R., and Cole, B.J., Metabolic mechanisms in the pathogenesis of osteoarthritis. A review. J Knee Surg 2006; 19, 191–7.

118. Schauer, P.R., Ikramuddin, S., Gourash, W., et al. Outcomes after laparoscopic Roux-en-Y gastric bypass for morbid obesity. Ann Surg 2000; 232, 515–29.

119. Ronald, J., Delaive, K., Roos, L., et al. Obstructive sleep apnea patients use more health care resources ten years prior to diagnosis. Sleep Res Online 1998; 1, 71–4.

120. Guardiano, S.A., Scott, J.A., Ware, J.C., et al. The long-term results of gastric bypass on indexes of sleep apnea. Chest 2003; 124, 1615–9.

121. Vlassov, V.V., Long-term outcome of bariatric surgery. N Engl J Med 2005; 352, 1495–6; author reply 1495–6.

122. Mabee, T.M., Meyer, P., DenBesten, L., et al. The mechanism of increased gallstone formation in obese human subjects. Surgery 1976; 79, 460–8.

123. Maclure, K.M., Hayes, K.C., Colditz, G.A., et al. Weight, diet, and the risk of symptomatic gallstones in middle-aged women. N Engl J Med 1989; 321, 563–9.
124. Liddle, R.A., Goldstein, R.B., and Saxton, J., Gallstone formation during weight-reduction dieting. Arch Intern Med 1989; 149, 1750–3.
125. Worobetz, L.J., Inglis, F.G., and Shaffer, E.A., The effect of ursodeoxycholic acid therapy on gallstone formation in the morbidly obese during rapid weight loss. Am J Gastroenterol 1993; 88, 1705–10.
126. Torgerson, J.S., Lindroos, A.K., Naslund, I., et al. Gallstones, gallbladder disease, and pancreatitis: cross-sectional and 2-year data from the Swedish Obese Subjects (SOS) and SOS reference studies. Am J Gastroenterol 2003; 98, 1032–41.
127. Shiffman, M.L., Sugerman, H.J., Kellum, J.M., et al. Changes in gallbladder bile composition following gallstone formation and weight reduction. Gastroenterology 1992; 103, 214–21.
128. Sarwer, D.B., Cohn, N.I., Gibbons, L.M., et al. Psychiatric diagnoses and psychiatric treatment among bariatric surgery candidates. Obes Surg 2004; 14, 1148–56.
129. Sarwer, D.B., Wadden, T.A., and Fabricatore, A.N., Psychosocial and behavioral aspects of bariatric surgery. Obes Res 2005; 13, 639–48.
130. Karlsson, J., Sjostrom, L., and Sullivan, M., Swedish obese subjects (SOS) - an intervention study of obesity. Two-year follow-up of health-related quality of life (HRQL) and eating behavior after gastric surgery for severe obesity. Int J Obes Relat Metab Disord 1998; 22, 113–26.
131. Velcu, L.M., Adolphine, R., Mourelo, R., et al. Weight loss, quality of life and employment status after Roux-en-Y gastric bypass: 5-year analysis. Surg Obes Relat Dis 2005; 1, 413–6; discussion 417.
132. Agren, G., Narbro, K., Jonsson, E., et al. Cost of in-patient care over 7 years among surgically and conventionally treated obese patients. Obes Res 2002; 10, 1276–83.

VI APPENDIX

19 Methods for Classifying, Diagnosing, and Monitoring Obesity

Christos S. Mantzoros

From: *Nutrition and Health: Nutrition and Metabolism*
Edited by: C.S. Mantzoros, DOI: 10.1007/978-1-60327-453-1_19,
© Humana Press, a part of Springer Science+Business Media, LLC 2009

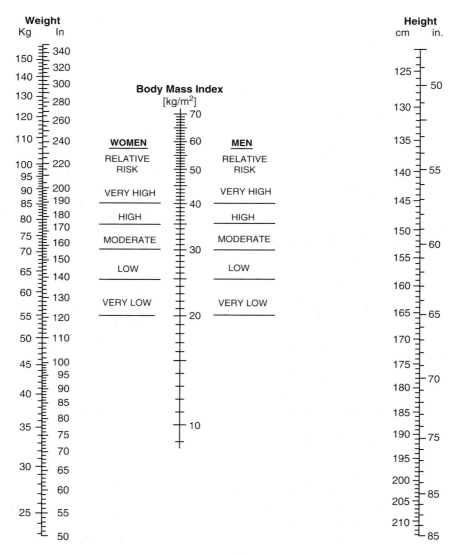

Fig. 1. Nomogram for determining body mass index.
To use this nomogram, place a ruler or other straight edge between the body weight (without clothes) in kilograms or pounds located on the left-hand line and the height (without shoes) in centimeters or in inches located on the right-hand line. The body mass index is read from the middle of the scale and is in metric units. (Copyright 1978, George A. Bray, MD. With permission.)

Your weight in kilograms

	52	54	57	59	61	63	66	68	70	72	75	77	79	82	84	
6'4"	14	15	15	16	16	17	18	18	19	19	20	21	21	22	23	190
6'3"	14	15	16	16	17	17	18	19	19	20	21	21	22	22	23	187.5
6'2"	15	15	16	17	17	18	19	19	20	21	21	22	22	23	24	185
6'1"	15	16	16	17	18	18	19	20	20	21	22	22	23	24	24	182.5
6'0"	16	16	17	18	18	19	20	20	21	22	22	23	24	24	25	180
5'11"	16	17	17	18	19	20	20	21	22	22	23	23	24	25	26	177.5
5'10"	17	17	18	19	19	20	21	22	22	23	23	24	25	26	27	175
5'9"	17	18	18	19	20	21	21	22	23	24	24	25	26	27	27	172.5
5'8"	17	18	19	20	21	21	22	23	24	24	25	26	27	27	28	170
5'7"	18	19	20	20	21	22	23	23	24	25	26	27	27	28	29	167.5
5'6"	19	19	20	21	22	23	23	24	25	26	27	27	28	29	30	165
5'5"	19	20	21	22	22	23	24	25	26	27	27	28	29	30	31	162.5
5'4"	20	21	21	22	23	24	25	26	27	27	28	29	30	31	32	160
5'3"	20	21	22	23	24	25	26	27	27	28	29	30	31	32	33	157.5
5'2"	21	22	23	24	25	26	27	27	28	29	30	31	32	33	34	155
5'1"	22	23	24	25	26	26	27	28	29	30	31	32	33	34	35	152.5
5'0"	22	23	24	25	26	27	28	29	30	31	32	33	34	35	36	150
	8,2	8,6	8,9	9,3	9,6	10	10,4	10,7	11,1	11,4	11,8	12,1	12,5	12,9	13,2	

Your height in feet and inches (left) — Your height in centimetres (right)

Your weight in stone and pounds

☐ BMI less than 18.5 (underweight)   ☐ BMI 25–29.9 (overweight)
☐ BMI 18.5–24.9 (normal weight)   ☐ BMI 30+ (obese)

Fig. 2. BMI chart:
To use the BMI chart, determine one's height (without shoes) in feet and inches or centimeters and locate the value on the left or right side. Determine one's weight (without clothes) in stone and pounds or kilograms located on the bottom or top. Find where one's height and weight intersect to determine one's BMI value. Use the legend to determine one's weight category. [From Cooke D. and Bloom S. The obesity pipeline: current strategies in the development of anti-obesity drugs. Nature 2006; 5: 919–930 (with permission).]

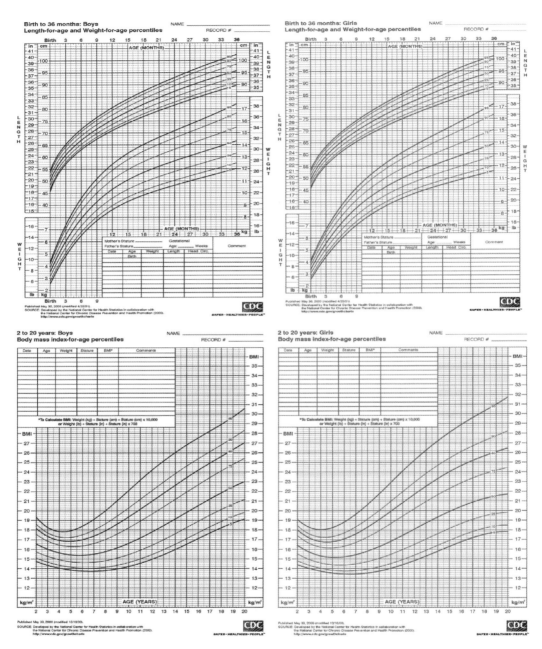

Fig. 3. Length-for-age and weight-for-age percentiles (top panels) and body mass index-for-age percentiles (lower panels).
CDC growth charts available at http://www.cdc.gov/nchs/about/major/nhanes/growthcharts/clinical_charts.htm

Table 1
Classification of Obesity Using Different Criteria

A. Obesity (BMI, kg/m^2)

BMI ranges	Classes	Health risk based on BMI	Health risk adjusted for presence of comorbid conditions
18–24.9	Normal	Minimal	Low
25.0–29.9	Overweight	Low	Moderate
30.0–34.9	Obesity class I	High	Very high
35.0–39.9	Obesity class II	Very high	Extremely high
40 or greater	Obesity class III	Extremely high	Extremely high

B. Central obesity (waist circumference)

Country/Ethnic group	Waist circumference[d] Male (cm)	Female (cm)
Europids[a]	≥94	≥80
South Asians[b]	≥90	≥80
Chinese	≥90	≥80
Japanese[c]	≥85	≥90
Ethnic South and Central Americans	Use South Asian recommendations until more specific data are available	
Sub-Saharan Africans	Use European data until more specific data are available	
Eastern Mediterranean and Middle[d] East (Arab) populations	Use European data until more specific data are available	

Although a higher cut-point is currently used for all ethnic groups in the USA for clinical diagnosis, it is strongly recommended that for epidemiological studies and, wherever possible, for case detections, ethnic group-specific cut-points should be used for people of the same ethnic group wherever they are found. Thus, the criteria recommended for Japan would also be used in expatriate Japanese communities, as would those for South Asian males and females regardless of place and country of residence

Data derived from: The IDF consensus definition of the metabolic syndrome page 2 of 7. http://idf.gov and Alberti KG, Zimmet P, Shaw J. Metabolic syndrome – a new worldwide definition. A Consensus Statement from the International Diabetes Federation. Diabete Med 2006; 23(5): 469–480
[a]In the USA, the ATP III values (102 cm male; 88 cm female) are likely to continue to be used for clinical purpose.
[b] on the basis of Chinese, Malay, and Asian-Indian population.
[c]Subsequent data analyses suggest that Asian values (male, 90 cm; female 80 cm) should be used for Japanese populations until more data are available.
[d]In the future epidemiological studies of populations of Europid origin, prevalence should be given using both European and North-American cut-points to allow better comparisons.

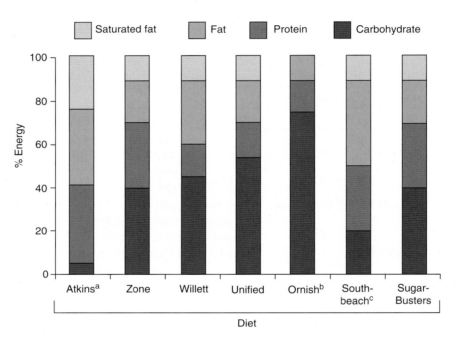

Fig. 4. Comparison of popular weight-loss diets. A comparison of popular weight-loss diets by percent macronutrient and saturated fat. [a]Composition represents the induction phase of the Atkins diet. [b]Recommendation for saturated fat is polyunsaturated:saturated fat ratio more than. [c]Composition represents the average for phase 1 of the South Beach Diet.

From Malik V.S. and Hu F.B. Popular weight-loss diets: from evidence to practice. Nat Clin Prac 2007; 4(1): 34–41 (with permission).

Table 2
Ideal Body Weight for Men and Women (According to Publications in Chronological Order)

Source	Equation
Broca (1871)/H-index	IBW (kg) = height (cm) − 100
Homwi (1964)	IBW (men) = 106 lb + 6 lb/in. over 5 ft
	IBW (women) = 100 lb + 5 lb/in. over 5 ft
Devine (1974)	IBW (men) = 50 kg + 2.3 kg/in. over 5 ft
	IBW (women) = 4.45 kg + 2.3 kg/in.
Robinson et al. (1983)	IBW (men) = 52 kg + 1.9 kg/in. over 5 ft
	IBW (women) = 49 kg + 1.7 kg/in. over 5 ft
Miller et al. (1983)	IBW (men) = 55.7 kg + 1.39 kg/in. over 5 ft
	IBW (women) = 53 kg + 1.33 kg/in. over 5 ft
Hammond (2000)	IBW (men) = 48 kg for 150 cm + 1.1 kg/cm
	IBW (women) = 45 kg for 150 cm + 0.9 kg/cm

Hamwi G.J. Therapy: changing dietary concepts. In: Danwoski TS, ed. Diabetes Mellitus: Diagnosis and Treatment. New York, NY; American Diabetes Association 1964: 75–78

For Hamwi and Hammond for a light frame, the calculated weight may be subtracted by 10%, and for a heavy frame, it may be added by 10%. Miller et al. formula is for a medium frame

Devine B.J. Gentamicin therapy. Drug Intell Clin Pharm 1974; 8: 650–655

Robinson J.D., Lupkiewicz S.M., Palenik L., et al. Determination of ideal body weight for drug dosage calculations. Am J Hosp Pharm 1983; 40: 1016–1018

Miller DR, Carlson JD, Lyod BJ, Day BJ. Determining body weight. Am J Hops Pharm. 1983; 40: 1622

Hammond KA. Dietary and clinical assessment. In: Mahan LK, Stump SE, eds. Krause's Food, Nutrition Therapy. 10th ed Philadelphia, PA: Saunders 2000: 358–379

Table 3
Height-Weight Tables

	Men				Women		
Height (cm)	Small frame (kg)	Medium frame (kg)	Large frame (kg)	Height (cm)	Small frame (kg)	Medium frame (kg)	Large frame (kg)
157.5	58.2–60.9	59.4–64.1	62.7–68.2	147.5	46.4–50.5	49.5–55.0	53.6–59.5
160	59.1–61.8	60.5–65.0	63.6–69.5	150	46.8–51.4	50.5–55.9	54.5–60.9
162.5	60.0–62.7	61.4–65.9	64.5–70.9	152.5	47.3–52.3	51.4–57.3	55.5–62.3
165	60.9–63.7	62.3–67.6	65.5–72.7	155	48.2–53.6	52.3–58.6	56.8–63.6
167.5	61.8–64.5	63.2–68.6	66.4–74.5	157.5	49.1–55.0	53.6–60.0	58.2–65.0
170	62.7–65.9	64.5–70.0	67.7–76.4	160	50.5–56.4	55.0–61.4	59.5–66.8
173	63.6–67.3	65.9–71.4	69.1–78.2	162.5	51.8–57.7	56.4–62.7	60.9–68.6
175	64.5–68.6	67.3–72.7	70.5–80.0	165	53.2–59.1	57.7–64.1	62.3–70.5
178	65.4–70.0	68.6–74.1	71.8–81.8	167.5	54.5–60.5	59.1–65.5	63.6–72.3
180	66.4–71.4	70.0–75.5	73.2–83.6	170	55.9–61.8	60.5–66.8	65.0–74.1
183	67.7–72.7	71.4–77.3	74.5–85.6	173	57.3–63.2	61.8–68.2	66.4–75.9
185.5	69.1–74.5	72.7–79.1	76.4–87.3	175	58.6–64.5	63.2–69.5	67.7–77.3
188	70.5–76.4	74.5–80.9	78.2–89.5	178	60.0–65.9	64.5–70.9	69.1–78.6
190.5	71.8–78.2	75.9–82.7	80.0–91.8	180	61.4–67.3	65.9–72.3	70.5–80.0
193	73.6–80.0	77.7–85.0	82.3–94.1	183	62.3–68.6	67.3–73.6	71.8–81.4

The 1983 Metropolitan Height-Weight Tables are based on the 1979 Build Study
The values are statistical computations from individuals ranging from 25 to 59 years of weights by height and body frame at which mortality has been found to be the lowest or longevity the highest. Metropolitan life does not advocate the use for the term "ideal," which has different meaning to various individuals, because the term was used originally in their 1942–1943 tables. If one wishes to use these tables in the sense that they are "ideal" in terms of lowest mortality, they are "appropriate" in that context. These tables do not provide weights related to minimizing illness, optimizing job performance, or creating the best appearance

Adapted from the Metropolitan Life Insurance Company, New York

Table 4
Fat Content, as Percentage of Body Weight, Estimated on the Basis of a Range of Values Calculated as the Sum of Four Skinfolds[a]

	Men (age in years)				Women (age in years)			
Skinfolds	17–29	30–39	40–49	50+	16–29	30–39	40–49	50+
15	4.8	–	–	–	10.5	–	–	–
20	8.1	12.2	12.2	12.6	14.1	17.0	19.8	21.4
25	10.5	14.2	15.0	15.6	16.8	19.4	22.2	24.0
30	12.9	16.2	17.7	18.6	19.5	21.8	24.5	26.6
35	14.7	17.7	19.6	20.8	21.5	23.7	26.4	28.5
40	16.4	19.2	21.4	22.9	23.4	25.5	28.2	30.3
45	17.7	20.4	23.0	24.7	25.0	26.9	29.6	31.9
50	19.0	21.5	24.6	26.5	26.5	28.2	31.0	33.4
55	20.1	22.5	25.9	27.9	27.8	29.4	32.1	34.6
60	21.2	23.5	27.1	29.2	29.1	30.6	33.2	35.7
65	22.2	24.3	28.2	30.4	30.2	31.6	34.1	36.7
70	23.1	25.1	29.3	31.6	31.2	32.5	35.0	37.7
75	24.0	25.9	30.3	32.7	32.2	33.4	35.9	38.7
80	24.8	26.6	31.2	33.8	33.1	34.3	36.7	39.6
85	25.5	27.2	32.1	34.8	34.0	35.1	37.5	40.4
90	26.2	27.8	33.0	35.8	34.8	35.8	38.3	41.2
95	26.9	28.4	33.7	36.6	35.6	36.5	39.0	41.9
100	27.6	29.0	34.4	37.4	36.4	37.2	39.7	42.6
105	28.2	29.6	35.1	38.2	37.1	37.9	40.4	43.3
110	28.8	30.1	35.8	39.0	37.8	38.6	41.0	43.9
115	29.4	30.6	36.4	39.7	38.4	39.1	41.5	44.5
120	30.3	31.1	37.0	40.4	39.0	39.6	42.0	45.1
125	31.0	31.5	37.6	41.1	39.6	40.1	42.5	45.7
130	31.5	31.9	38.2	41.8	40.2	40.6	43.0	46.2

(continued)

Table 4
(continued)

Skinfolds	Men (age in years)				Women (age in years)			
	17–29	30–39	40–49	50+	16–29	30–39	40–49	50+
135	32.0	32.3	38.7	42.4	40.8	41.1	43.5	46.7
140	32.5	32.7	39.2	43.0	41.3	41.6	44.0	47.2
145	32.9	33.1	39.7	43.6	41.8	42.1	44.5	47.7
150	33.3	33.5	40.2	44.1	42.3	42.6	45.0	48.2
155	33.7	33.9	40.7	44.6	42.8	43.1	45.4	48.7
160	34.1	34.3	41.2	45.1	43.3	43.6	45.8	49.2
165	34.5	34.6	41.6	45.6	43.7	44.0	46.2	49.6
170	34.9	34.8	42.0	46.1	44.1	44.4	46.6	50.0
175	35.3	–	–	–	–	44.8	47.0	50.4
180	35.6	–	–	–	–	45.2	47.4	50.8
185	35.9	–	–	–	–	45.6	47.8	51.2
190	–	–	–	–	–	45.9	48.2	51.6
195	–	–	–	–	–	46.2	48.5	52.0
200	–	–	–	–	–	46.5	48.8	52.4
205	–	–	–	–	–	–	49.1	52.7

Adapted from Durnin J.V. and Womersley J. Body fat assessed from total body density and its estimation from skinfold thickness measurements of 48 men and women aged 16 thru 72 years. Br J Nutr 1974; 32(1): 77–97

[a]Biceps, triceps, subscapular, and suprailiac of men and women of different ages.

Table 5
Basal Metabolic Rate in Adult Men and Women in Relation to Height and Median Acceptable Weight for Height
(Values Are Given in kcal with MJ in Parentheses)[a]

Height (m)	Weight[b] (kg)	18–30 years		30–60 years		>60 years	
		Per kg per day	Per day	Per kg per day	Per day	Per kg per day	Per day
Men							
1.5	49.5	29.0 (121)	1,440 (6.03)	29.4 (123)	450 (6.07)	23.2 (98)	1,150 (4.81)
1.6	56.5	27.4 (115)	1,540 (6.44)	27.2 (114)	1,530 (6.40)	22.2 (93)	1,250 (5.23)
1.7	63.5	26.0 (109)	1,650 (6.90)	25.4 (106)	1,620 (6.78)	21.2 (89)	1,350 (5.65)
1.8	71.5	24.8 (104)	1,770 (7.41)	23.9 (99)	1,710 (7.15)	20.3 (85)	1,450 (6.07)
1.9	79.5	23.9 (100)	1,890 (7.91)	22.7 (95)	1,800 (7.53)	19.6 (82)	1,560 (6.53)
2.0	88	23.0 (96)	2,030 (8.49)	21.6 (90)	1,900 (7.95)	19.0 (80)	1,670 (6.99)
Women							
1.4	41	26.7 (112)	1,100 (4.60)	28.8 (120)	1,240 (5.19)	25.0 (105)	1,090 (4.56)
1.5	47	25.2 (105)	1,190 (4.98)	26.3 (110)	1,300 (5.44)	23.1 (97)	1,160 (4.85)
1.6	54	23.9 (100)	1,290 (5.40)	24.1 (101)	1,360 (5.69)	21.6 (90)	1,230 (5.15)
1.7	61	22.9 (96)	1,390 (5.82)	22.4 (94)	1,420 (5.94)	20.3 (85)	1,310 (5.48)
1.8	68	22.0 (92)	1,500 (6.28)	20.9 (87)	1,190 (4.98)	19.3 (81)	1,030 (4.31)

Adapted from Energy and Protein Requirements: Report of a Joint FAO/WHO/UNU Expert Consultation. Technical Repost Series No. 724. Geneva, World Health Organization, 1985: 72

[a] BMR: Men = 17.5 + 651 kcal$_{th}$/day (2.72 MJ/day). Women = 12.2 W + 746 kcal$_{th}$/day (3.12 MJ/day).

[b] Weight taken as median acceptable weight for height: body mass index (wt/ht^2) = 22 in men and 21 in women.

Table 6
Average Daily Requirement of Adults Whose Occupational Work Is Classified as Light, Moderate, or Heavy, Expressed as a Multiple of Basal Metabolic Rate

	Light	*Moderate*	*Heavy*
Men	1.55	1.78	2.10
Women	1.56	1.64	1.82

Adapted from Energy Protein Requirements: Report of a Joint FAO/WHO/UNU Expert Consultation. Technical Report Series No. 274. Geneva, World Health Organization, 1985: 78

Table 7
Behavioral Therapy Techniques for Weight Loss

Weight loss technique	*Example*	*Suggestions for implementation*
Self-monitoring	Keep track of energy ingested	Consider handheld computer calorie-tracking programs; record food intake as consumed, not at the end of the day or week
Environmental modification	Keep track of exercise activity	Set realistic goals for time and distance walked
Physical environment	Goal: permanent change in eating habits, not short-term diets	Reduce energy intake and consumption of high-fat foods and increase consumption of fruits, vegetables, and fiber; keep fruit on the counter; avoid fruit juices and other sugary beverages; referral to a dietitian is recommended
	Be mindful of weight-loss goals while grocery shopping are tempting	Buy fruits and vegetables; avoid foods that result in weight gain
	Reduce consumption of food outside the home	Choose wisely in restaurants (share meals, skip dessert); bring food to work rather than eating at cafeterias and snacking; minimize fast foods
	Increase physical activity	Set aside time for walking every day; walk when talking on the phone at home and at work; park further away from entrances in parking lots (or walk or bike to your destination); find an exercise partner; use the stairs, not the elevator; understand that increased physical activity is the single most important predictor of maintaining weight loss; if feasible, assistance from trainers and exercise therapists is recommended

(continued)

Table 7
(continued)

Weight loss technique	Example	Suggestions for implementation
Thinking patterns	Create an environment in which self-control can succeed	Avoid temptation if possible rather than trying to resist; use distraction (e.g., go for a walk after dinner rather than snaking); reframe temptations (think less pleasant aspects of the temptation rather than focusing on the desirable aspects)
	Plan ahead for high-risk circumstances	Be aware that most people break their eating plan when they come home from work or before bedtime; plan ahead ("If faced with temptation x, I will do y instead")
Self-efficacy	Set clear and attainable short-term goals needed to reach the long-term goal	Set specific, reasonable, and proximate goals ("I will walk 20 min 5 days a week for the next 2 weeks") needed for long-term success; when goals are attained, set a new goal; if goals are not attained, determine what went wrong – if the strategy was correct but was not executed, try again; if the strategy was the problem, develop another one
Social supports	Do not dwell on guilt	Guilt is an ineffective modifier of long-term behavior; it is counterproductive
	Focus on success, not failure	Expect setbacks and do not let them destroy your belief in your ability to effect change; focus on learning and implementing new strategies rather than on blame and guilt; referral to a behavioral psychologist is recommended if feasible
	Family	Explain to your family that their help is needed and appreciated; enlist their help in avoiding temptation and increasing exercise (which often entails a change in other family members' eating and exercise habits)
	Physician	Continue to be optimistic; work with patients to view lack of success as a learning opportunity to refine strategies rather than as a failure; avoid excessive optimism regarding how much weight a patient will lose; facilitate frequent follow-up

From Thompson W.G., Cook D.A, Clark M.M, et al. Treatment of obesity. Mayo Clin Proc 2007; 82(1): 93–102

20

Methods for Classifying, Diagnosing, and Monitoring Type II Diabetes

Christos S. Mantzoros

From: *Nutrition and Health: Nutrition and Metabolism*
Edited by: C.S. Mantzoros, DOI: 10.1007/978-1-60327-453-1_20,
© Humana Press, a part of Springer Science + Business Media, LLC 2009

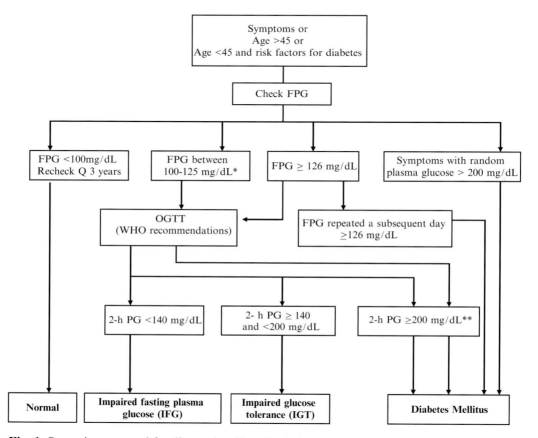

Fig. 1. Screening protocol for diagnosis of impaired glucose tolerance and type 2 diabetes.

*If the clinical suspicion is still very high, some authors recommend performing an OGTT (to be done after 8–14 h fast and at least 3 days of unrestricted diet, i.e., >150 g carbohydrates per day).

**Two values of 2-h PG need to be higher than 200 mg/dl for diabetes to be diagnosed in the normal and impaired fasting glucose groups.

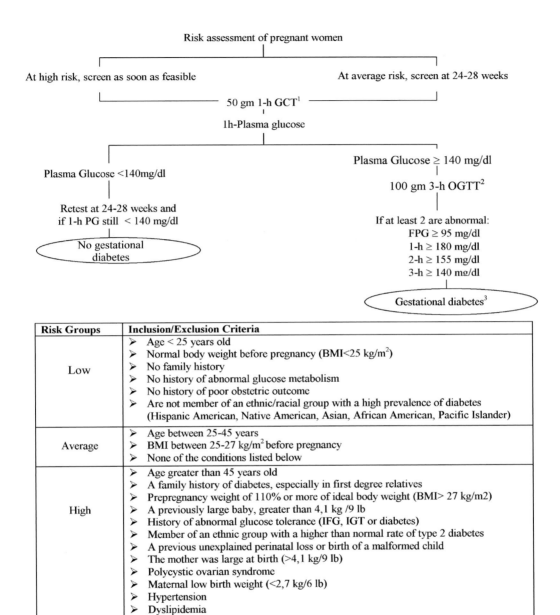

Fig. 2. Risk assessment and screening protocol for gestational diabetes:

1. GCT: oral glucose challenge test.
2. OGTT: Oral glucose tolerance test (to be done in the morning after 8–14 h fast and after at least 3 days of unrestricted diet, i.e., >150 g carbohydrate per day).
3. At least 6 weeks after pregnancy ends, the women should receive an OGTT and be reclassified as having diabetes, normal glucose tolerance, impaired glucose tolerance, or impaired fasting glucose on the basis of diagnostic criteria.

Table 1
Methods for Measuring Insulin Resistance

Indices	Formulas	Normal level
Insulin fasting level	N/A	<15 µUI/ml
Insulin peak level during OGTT	N/A	<150 µUI/ml
2-h Insulin level post-OGTT	N/A	<75 µUI/ml
HOMA-IR	Fasting glucose (mmol/liter) × fasting insulin (µUI/ml)/22,5	2.1–2.7
QUICKI	1/[log (Ins 0) + log (Glu 0)]	Mean value: 0.382 in lean subjects
Cederholm and Wibell (SI)	[75,000 + (Glu 0 − Glu 2 h) × 1.15 × 180 × 0.19 × BW]/ [120 × log (mean Ins) × mean Glu]	79 ± 14
Belfiore (ISI)	2/[(AUC insulin × AUC glucose) + 1]	Over or around 1.0
Gutt (ISI$_{0,120}$)	[75,000 + (Glu 0 − Glu 2 h) × 0.19 × BW]/[120 × log (insulin 0/2 + insulin 2 h/2) × (Glu 0/2 + Glu 2 h/2]	89 ± 39 lean controls 58 ± 23 obese controls
Matsuda (ISI composite)	10,000/ √(Ins 0 × Glu 0 × mean insulin × mean glucose during OGTT)	
Stumvoll (ISI)	0.22 − 0.0032 × BMI − 0.0000645 × Ins 2 h − 0.0037 × Glu 1.5 h	
Avignon (Si2h and SiM)	Si2h = 10^8/(Ins 2 h × Glu 2 h × 150)	1.79 ± 0.33
	SiM = [0.137 × 10^8/ (Ins 0 × Glu 0 × 150) + Si2h]/2	1.71 ± 0.24
Insulin tolerance test	K$_{ITT}$ = 0.693/plasma glucose half time × 100	>2%/min
FSIVGTT insulin sensitivity	Si = the glucose clearance rate per change in plasma insulin concentration	5–7 in nonobese; 2–3.5 min^{-1}/µU/ml in obese subjects
Euglycemic hyperinsulinemic clamp	M value = glucose infused per unit of time	4.7–8.7 mg/kg/min

Adapted from Barb D, Mantzoros CS. Diagnosing Obesity, Diabetes Mellitus, and the Insulin Resistance Syndrome. *In* Mantzoros CS, Obesity and Diabetes, Humana Press, 2006, p. 129–155

Abbreviations: *N/A* not applicable, *BW* body weight, *Ins 0 and 2 h* plasma insulin level at time 0 and 2 h after an oral glucose tolerance test, *Glu 0 and 2 h* plasma glucose level at time 0 and 2 h after an oral glucose tolerance test, *ISI/SiM* insulin sensitivity index, *Si* insulin sensitivity, *FSIVGTT* frequently sampled intravenous glucose tolerance test, *AUC* area under the curve, *ITT* insulin tolerance test, *K$_{ITT}$* percentage of decline in plasma glucose concentration

Table 2
Criteria for Testing for Diabetes in Asymptomatic Adult Individuals

1. Testing should be considered in all adults who are overweight (BMI $\geq$ 25 kg/m^{2a}) and have additional risk factors:
   - physical inactivity
   - first-degree relative with diabetes
   - members of a high-risk ethnic population (e.g., African-American, Latino, Native American, Asian-American, and Pacific Islander)
   - women who delivered a baby weighing >9 lb or were diagnosed with GDM
   - hypertension ($\geq$140/90 mmHg or on therapy for hypertension)
   - HDL cholesterol level < 35 mg/dl (0.90 mmol/liter) and/or triglyceride level > 250 mg/dl (2.82 mmol/liter)
   - women with PCOS
   - IGT or IFG on previous testing
   - other clinical conditions associated with insulin resistance (e.g., severe obesity and acanthosis nigricans)
   - history of CVD
2. In the absence of the above criteria, testing for prediabetes and diabetes should begin at age of 45 years
3. If results are normal, testing should be repeated at least at 3-year intervals, with consideration of more frequent testing depending on initial results and risk status

From American Diabetes Association. Standards of medical care in diabetes. Diabetes Care. 2008;31:S12–S54 (with permission)
GDM gestational diabetes mellitus, *IGT* impaired glucose tolerance, *IFG* impaired fasting glucose, *PCOS* polycystic ovarian syndrome
^{a}At-risk BMI may be lower in some ethnic groups.

Table 3
Etiological Classification of Diabetes Mellitus

I. Type 1 diabetes (β-cell destruction, usually leading to absolute insulin deficiency)
   A. Immune-mediated
   B. Idiopathic
II. Type 2 diabetes (may range from predominantly insulin resistance with relative insulin deficiency to a predominantly secretory defect with insulin resistance)
III. Other specific types
   A. Genetic defects to β-cell function
      1. Chromosome 12, HNF-1α (MODY3)
      2. Chromosome 7, glucokinase (MODY2)
      3. Chromosome 20, HNF-4α (MODY1)
      4. Chromosome 13, insulin promoter factor-1 (IPF-1; MODY4)
      5. Chromosome 17, HNF-1β (MODY5)
      6. Chromosome 2, *NeuroD1* (MODY6)
      7. Mitochondrial DNA
      8. Others
   B. Genetic defects in insulin action
      1. Type A insulin resistance
      2. Leprechaunism
      3. Rabson-Mendenhall syndrome
      4. Lipoatrophic diabetes
      5. Others
   C. Diseases of the exocrine pancreas
      1. Pancreatitis
      2. Trauma/pancreatectomy
      3. Neoplasia
      4. Cystic fibrosis
      5. Hemochromatosis
      6. Fibrocalculous pancreatopathy
      7. Others
   D. Endocrinopathies
      1. Acromegaly
      2. Cushing's syndrome
      3. Glucagonoma
      4. Pheochromocytoma
      5. Hyperthyroidism
      6. Somatostatinoma
      7. Aldosteronoma
      8. Others

(continued)

Table 3
(continued)

  E. Drug- or chemical-induced
    1. Vacor
    2. Pentamidine
    3. Nicotinic acid
    4. Glucocorticoids
    5. Thyroid hormone
    6. Diazoxoid
    7. β-Adrenergic agonists
    8. Thiazides
    9. Dilantin
    10. α-Interferon
    11. Others
  F. Infections
    1. Congenital rubella
    2. Cytomegalovirus
    3. Others
  G. Uncommon forms of immune-mediated diabetes
    1. "Stiff-man" syndrome
    2. Anti-insulin receptor antibodies
    3. Others
  H. Other genetic syndromes sometimes associated with diabetes
    1. Down's syndrome
    2. Klinefelter's syndrome
    3. Turner's syndrome
    4. Wolfram's syndrome
    5. Friedreich's ataxia
    6. Huntington's chorea
    7. Laurence-Moon-Biedl syndrome
    8. Myotonic dystrophy
    9. Porphyria
    10. Prader-Willi syndrome
    11. Others
IV. Gestational diabetes mellitus

Patients with any form of diabetes may require insulin treatment at some stage of their disease. Such use of insulin does not, by itself, classify a patient

From American Diabetes Association. Diagnosis and classification of diabetes mellitus. Diabetes Care. 2008;31S55–S60 (with permission)

21

Major Nutrition Recommendations and Interventions for Subjects with Hyperlipidemia, Hypertension, and/or Diabetes

Christos S. Mantzoros

From: *Nutrition and Health: Nutrition and Metabolism*
Edited by: C.S. Mantzoros, DOI: 10.1007/978-1-60327-453-1_21,
© Humana Press, a part of Springer Science+Business Media, LLC 2009

Table 1
Lifestyle Modifications for the Management and Prevention of Hypertension
A. Recommendations

- Discontinue smoking
- Maintain a healthy weight; if needed and if possible, lose weight
- Reduce sodium intake
- Increase physical activity
- Maintain adequate potassium, magnesium, and calcium by eating a diet rich in fruits, vegetables, and low-fat dairy foods
- Reduce intake of dietary saturated fat and cholesterol
- Limit alcohol intake

B. Expected efficacy of recommendations

Modification	Recommendation	Approximate range of systolic blood pressure reduction (mmHg)
Weight reduction (if overweight or obese)	Maintain normal body weight (as indicated by BMI 18.5–24.9 kg/m^2)	5–20 per 10 kg weight loss
Adopt DASH or Mediterranean diet	Consume a diet rich in fruits, vegetables, and low-fat dairy products with reduced content of saturated and total fat	5–8
Reduction in dietary sodium	Reduce intake to no more than 2.3 g (2,300 mg) sodium or 6 g sodium chloride	2–8
Increase physical activity level	Engage in regular aerobic physical activity such as brisk walking (at least 30 min/day, most days of the week)	4–9
Moderation in alcohol consumption	Limit consumption to no more than two drinks per day in adult men and to no more than one drink per day in adult women and lighter weight people (1 drink = 15 g alcohol, e.g., 12 oz of beer, 5 oz of wine, or 1.5 oz of 80-proof distilled spirits)	2–4
Comprehensive lifestyle modifications	Combination of lifestyle modifications: sodium reduction, weight loss, DASH diet, and regular aerobic exercise	9–11

Adapted from (1) Chobanian AV, Bakris GL, Cushman WC, Green LA, Izzo JL Jr, Jones DW, Maataerson BJ, Oparil S, Wright JT Jr, Roccella EJ; National Heart, Lung, and Blood institute; Joint National Committee on Prevention, Detection, Evaluation, and Treatment of Blood Pressure; National High Blood Pressure Education Program Coordinating Committee: The Seventh Report of the Joint Committee on Prevention, Detection, Evaluation, and Treatment of High Blood Pressure. JAMA 289:2560–2572,2003. (2) Whitworth JA, Chalmers J: World Health Organization-International Society of Hypertension (WHO/ISH) hypertension guidelines. Clin Exp Hypertens 26:747–752, 2004

Table 2
DASH Diet

A. Food groups, number of daily servings, and serving sizes according to the DASH diet

Food and servings per day	Sample serving sizes
Grains and grain products 7–8 daily	1 slice of bread, ¾ cup dry cereal, ½ cup cooked rice, pasta, or cereal
Vegetables 4–5 daily	1 cup raw leafy vegetables, ½ cup cooked vegetables, 6 oz vegetable juice
Fruits 4–5 daily	1 medium fruit, cup dried fruits, ½ cup fresh frozen or canned fruit, 6 oz fruit juice
Low-fat or nonfat dairy foods 2–3 daily	8 oz skim or 1% milk, 1 cup yogurt, 1½ oz low-fat cheese
Meat, poultry, fish ≤2 daily	3 oz cooked lean meat, poultry (skinless, white meat), or fish
Nuts, seeds, and legumes 4–5 per week	1½ oz or ⅓ cup nuts, ½ oz or 2 tsps seeds, ½ cup cooked legumes
Fats and oils 2–3 daily	1 tsp soft margarine or butter, 1 tbsp low-fat mayonnaise, 1 tbsp salad dressing or 2 tbsps light salad dressing, 1 tsp oil (olive, corn, canola, safflower, flaxseed, or other)
Sweets 5 per week	⅓ cup sherbet, 3 pieces of candy, small piece (2 oz) angel food cake

B. An example of a menu according to the DASH diet with <2,000 mg sodium and carbohydrate counting

DASH menu items (carbohydrate servings)
  Breakfast:
1 small banana (1), ¾ cup corn flakes (1), 1 cup nonfat or low-fat milk (1), 1 slice whole-wheat bread (1) with 1 tsp soft margarine
Total carbohydrate servings: 4
Lunch:
¾ cup chicken salad for sandwich, pita bread (2), raw vegetables: 3–4 carrot sticks, 3–4 celery sticks, 2 lettuce leaves, 1 cup nonfat or low-fat milk (1), small apple (1)
Total carbohydrate servings: 4
Dinner:
3 oz lean roast beef, ½ large baked potato (2), 1 tbsp reduced fat sour cream, ½ cup steamed broccoli, spinach salad: ½ cup raw spinach, 2 cherry tomatoes, ½ cup sliced cucumber, 1 tbsp light Italian dressing, 1 small whole-wheat dinner roll (1), 1 tsp soft margarine, 1 cup melon balls (1)
Total carbohydrate servings: 4
Snacks (morning, afternoon, evening, or added to meals):
¼ cup dried apricots (1), ½ cup orange juice or 1 orange (1), ¾ cup unsalted mini pretzels (1), 1 cup low-fat yogurt (1), 2 tbsps unsalted mixed nuts
Total carbohydrate servings: 4
Total carbohydrate servings for the day: 16

Adapted from the DASH website: http://dash.bwh.harvard.edu

Table 3
Summary of National Cholesterol Education Program (NCEP) Adult Treatment Panel III (ATP III) Recommendations for the Treatment of Hyperlipidemia

Step	Description
1. Obtain fasting plasma lipoprotein profile	Calculate LDL by formula: total cholesterol − HDL-C − TG/5, as long as TG < 4.52 mmol/liter (<400 mg/dL) Major goal is LDL-C levels: Optimal: <2.59 mmol/liter (<100 mg/dL), near/above optimal: 2.59–3.34 mmol/liter × (100–129 mg/dL), borderline high: 3.36–4.11 mmol/liter (130–159 mg/dL), high: 4.14–4.89 mmol/liter (160–189 mg/dL), very high: ≥4.91 mmol/liter (≥190 mg/dL)
2. Identify presence of CDA or risk equivalent	Presence of clinical atherosclerotic disease associated with high risk for CAD events (>20% over 10 years) Clinical CAD, symptomatic or significant carotid artery disease, peripheral arterial disease, abdominal aortic aneurysm, diabetes mellitus
3. Determine presence of major risk factors (other than elevated LDL)	Cigarette smoking, hypertension (BP ≥ 140/90 mmHg or taking antihypertensive medication), low HDL-C: <1.04 mmol/liter (<40 mg/dL), family history of premature CAD (CAD in male first-degree relative <55 years or female first-degree relative <65 years), age (men ≥ 45 years, women ≥ 55 years)
4. Assess 10-year CAD risk	Only necessary if ≥2 risk factors (other than elevated LDL) are present without CAD or CAD risk equivalent Levels of risk: >20% (CAD risk equivalent), 10–20%, <10%
5. Determine risk category to establish LDL-C goal of therapy	Determine need for TLC Determine LDL-C level for drug consideration
6. Initiate TLC if LDL-C is above goal	TLC includes diet (saturated fat < 7% of calories, cholesterol < 200 mg/day, increased viscous fiber 10–24 g/day, and plant stanols/sterols 2 g/day to enhance LDL lowering), weight management, increased physical activity
7. Consider adding drug therapy if LDL-C exceeds recommended levels	Consider drug simultaneously with TLC for patients at high risk For other risk categories, consider adding lipid-lowering drug to TLC after 3 months: statins, bile acid sequestrants, nicotinic acid, and fibrate
8. Identify the metabolic syndrome and treat if present after 3 months of TLC	Metabolic syndrome is identified by three of the following: abdominal obesity (increased waist circumference: men > 101.6 cm [>40 in.], women > 88.9 cm [>35 in.]), high TG ≥ 1.70 mmol/liter (≥150 mg/dL), low HDL (men, <1.04 mmol/liter [<40 mg/dL], women, <1.30 mmol/liter [<50 mg/dL]), high blood pressure (≥130/85 mmHg), high fasting plasma glucose ≥6.11 mmol/liter (≥110 mg/dL)[a]

(continued)

Table 3
(continued)

Step	Description
9. Treat elevated plasma TG ($\geq$1.70 mmol/liter [$\geq$150 mg/dL])	Primary aim is to reach LDL-C goal: if TG $\geq$2.26 mmol/liter ($\geq$200 mg/dL) after LDL goal is reached, set secondary goal for non-HDL at 0.78 mmol/liter (30 mg/dL) higher than LDL-D goal; if TG = 2.26–5.64 mmol/liter (200–499 mg/dL) after LDL-C goal is reached, consider adding drug to reach non-HDL-C goal; if TG > 5.56 mmol/liter (>500 mg/dL), first lower TG with very-low-fat diet to prevent pancreatitis
10. Consider treatment of low HDL-C (a component of step 9 in ATP III algorithm, but separated here for clarity)	First reach LDL goal, then: Intensity weight management and increase physical activity If TG = 2.26–5.64 mmol/liter (200–499 mg/dL), achieve non-HDL-C goal If TG < 2.26 mmol/liter (<200 mg/dL) in patients with CAD or CAD equivalent, consider nicotinic acid

Adapted from the National Cholesterol Education Program. ATP III Guidelines At-a-Glance Quick Desk Reference. Bethesda, MD: Department of Health and Human Services, Public Health Service; 2001. NIH Publication No. 01-3305. Available at: http://www.nhlbi.nih.gov/guidelines/cholesterol/atglance.pdf. Accessed January 1, 2005

BP blood pressure, *CAD* coronary artery disease, *HDL-C* high-density lipoprotein cholesterol, *LDL-C* Low-density lipoprotein cholesterol, *TG* triglycerides, *TLC* therapeutic lifestyle change

[a]The American Diabetes Association has suggested lowering this threshold to 5.5 mmol/liter (100 mg/dL).

Table 4
Major Nutrition Recommendations and Interventions for Diabetes

Effectiveness of medical nutrition therapy (MNT)
- Individuals who have prediabetes or diabetes should receive individualized MNT; such therapy is best provided by a registered dietitian familiar with the components of diabetes MNT.
- Nutrition counseling should be sensitive to the personal needs, willingness to change, and ability to make changes of the individual with prediabetes or diabetes.

Energy balance, overweight, and obesity
- In overweight and obese insulin-resistant individuals, modest weight loss has been shown to improve insulin resistance. Thus, weight loss is recommended for all individuals who have or are at risk for diabetes.
- For weight loss, either low-carbohydrate or low-fat calorie-restricted diets may be effective in the short term (up to 1 year).
- For patients on low-carbohydrate diets, monitor lipid profiles, renal function, and protein intake (in those with nephropathy), and adjust hypoglycemic therapy as needed.
- Physical activity and behavior modification are important components of weight loss programs and are most helpful in maintenance of weight loss.
- Weight loss medications may be considered in the treatment of overweight and obese individuals with type 2 diabetes and can help achieve a 5–10% weight loss when combined with lifestyle modification.
- Bariatric surgery may be considered for some individuals with type 2 diabetes and BMI ≥ 35 kg/m^2 and can result in marked improvements in glycemia. The long-term benefits and risks of bariatric surgery in individuals with prediabetes or diabetes continue to be studied.

Preventing diabetes (primary prevention)
- Among individuals at high risk for developing type 2 diabetes, structured programs that emphasize lifestyle changes that include moderate weight loss (7% body weight) and regular physical activity (150 min/week) with dietary strategies including reduced calories and reduced intake of dietary fat can reduce the risk for developing diabetes and are therefore recommended.
- Individuals at high risk for type 2 diabetes should be encouraged to achieve the USDA recommendation for dietary fiber (14 g fiber/100 kcal) and foods containing whole grains (one-half of grain intake).
- There is not sufficient, consistent information to conclude that low-glycemic load diets reduce the risk for diabetes. Nevertheless, low-glycemic index foods that are rich in fiber and other important nutrients are to be encouraged.
- Observational studies report that moderate alcohol intake may reduce the risk of diabetes, but the data did not support recommending alcohol consumption to individuals at risk for diabetes.
- No nutrition recommendation can be made for preventing type 1 diabetes.

Although there are insufficient data at present to warrant any specific recommendations for prevention of type 2 diabetes in youth, it is reasonable to apply approaches demonstrated to be effective in adults as long as nutritional needs for normal growth and development are maintained.

(continued)

Table 4
(continued)

Controlling diabetes (secondary prevention)

Carbohydrate in diabetes management

- A dietary pattern that includes carbohydrate from fruits, vegetables, whole grains, legumes, and low-fat milk is encouraged for good health.
- Monitoring carbohydrate, whether by carbohydrate counting, exchanges, or experienced-based estimation, remains a key strategy in achieving glycemic control.
- The use of glycemic index and load may provide a modest additional benefit over that observed when total carbohydrate is considered alone.
- Sucrose-containing foods may be substituted for other carbohydrates in the meal plan or, if added to the meal plan, covered with insulin or other glucose-lowering medications. Care should be taken to avoid excess energy intake.
- As for the general population, people with diabetes are encouraged to consume a variety of fiber-containing foods. However, evidence is lacking to recommend a higher fiber intake for people with diabetes than for the population as a whole.
- Sugar alcohols and nonnutritive sweeteners are safe when consumed within the daily intake levels established by the FDA.

Fat and cholesterol in diabetes management

- Limit saturated fat to <7% of total calories.
- Intake of *trans* fat should be minimized.
- In individuals with diabetes, lower dietary cholesterol to <200 mg/day.
- Two or more servings of fish per week (with the exception of commercially fried fish filets) provide *n*-3 polyunsaturated fatty acids and are recommended.

Protein in diabetes management

- For individuals with diabetes and normal renal function, there is insufficient evidence to suggest that usual protein intake (15–20% of energy) should be modified.
- In individuals with type 2 diabetes, ingested protein can increase insulin response without increasing plasma glucose concentrations. Therefore, protein should not be used to treat acute or prevent nighttime hypoglycemia.
- High-protein diets are not recommended as a method of weight loss at this time. The long-term effects of protein intake >20% of calories on diabetes management and its complications are unknown. Although such diets may produce short-term weight loss and improved glycemia, it has not been established that these benefits are maintained on long term, and long-term effects on kidney function for persons with diabetes are unknown.

Alcohol in diabetes management

- If adults with diabetes choose to use alcohol, daily intake should be limited to a moderate amount (one drink per day or less for women and two drinks per day or less for men).
- To reduce the risk of nocturnal hypoglycemia in individuals using insulin or insulin secretagogues, alcohol should be consumed with food.
- In individuals with diabetes, moderate alcohol consumption (when ingested alone) has no acute effect on glucose and insulin concentrations but carbohydrate coingested with alcohol (as in a mixed drink) may raise blood glucose.

Micronutrients in diabetes management

- There is no clear evidence of benefit for vitamin or mineral supplementation in people with diabetes (compared with general population) who do not have underlying deficiencies.

(continued)

Table 4
(continued)

- Routine supplementation with antioxidants, such as vitamin E and C and carotene, is not advised because of lack of evidence of efficacy and concern related to long-term safety.
- Benefit from chromium supplementation in individuals with diabetes or obesity has not been clearly demonstrated and therefore cannot be recommended.

Nutrition interventions for type 1 diabetes
- For individuals with type 1 diabetes, insulin therapy should be integrated into an individual's dietary and physical activity pattern.
- Individuals using rapid-acting insulin by injection or an insulin pump should adjust the meal and snack insulin doses based on the carbohydrate content of the meals and snacks.
- For individuals using fixed daily insulin doses, carbohydrate intake on a day-to-day basis should be kept consistent with respect to time and amount.
- For planned exercise, insulin doses can be adjusted. For unplanned exercise, extra carbohydrates may be needed.

Nutrition interventions for type 2 diabetes
- Individuals with type 2 diabetes are encouraged to implement lifestyle modifications that reduce intakes of energy, saturated and *trans* fatty acids, cholesterol, and sodium and to increase physical activity in an effort to improve glycemia, dyslipidemia, and blood pressure.
- Plasma glucose monitoring can be used to determine whether adjustments in foods and meals will be sufficient to achieve blood glucose goals or if medications(s) needs to be combined with MNT.

Nutrition interventions for pregnancy and lactation with diabetes
- Adequate energy intake that provides appropriate weight gain is recommended during pregnancy. Weight loss is not recommended, however, for overweight and obese women with gestational diabetes mellitus (GDM); modest energy and carbohydrate restriction may be appropriate.
- Ketonemia from ketoacidosis or starvation ketosis should be avoided.
- MNT for GDM focuses on food choices for appropriate weight gain, normoglycemia, and absence of ketones.
- Because GDM is a risk factor for type 2 diabetes after delivery, lifestyle modifications aimed at reducing weight and increasing physical activity are recommended.

Nutrition interventions for older adults with diabetes
- Obese older adults with diabetes may benefit from modest energy restriction and an increase in physical activity; energy requirements may be less than for a younger individual of a similar weight.
- A daily multivitamin supplement may be appropriate, especially for older adults with restricted energy intake.

Treating and controlling diabetes complications (tertiary prevention)
Microvascular complications
- Reduction of protein intake to 0.8–1.0 g kg body wt^{-1} day^{-1} in individuals with diabetes and the earlier stages of chronic kidney disease (CKD) and to 0.8 g kg body wt^{-1} day^{-1} in the later stages of CKD may improve measures of renal function (urine albumin excretion rate, glomerular filtration rate) and is recommended.

(continued)

Table 4
(continued)

- MNT that favorably affects cardiovascular risk factors may also have a favorable effect on microvascular complications such as retinopathy and nephropathy.

Treatment and management of CVD risk
- Target A1C is as close to normal as possible without significant hypoglycemia.
- For patients with diabetes at risk for CVD, diets high in fruits, vegetables, whole grains, and nuts may reduce the risk.
- For patients with diabetes and symptomatic heart failure, dietary sodium intake of <2,000 mg/day may reduce symptoms.
- In normotensive and hypertensive individuals, a reduced sodium intake (e.g. 2,300 mg/day) with a diet high in fruits, vegetables, and low-fat dairy products lowers blood pressure.
- In most individuals, a modest amount of weight loss beneficially affects blood pressure.

Hypoglycemia
- Ingestion of 15–20 g glucose is the preferred treatment for hypoglycemia, although any form of carbohydrate that contains glucose may be used.
- The response treatment of hypoglycemia should be apparent in 10–20 min; however, plasma glucose should be tested again in ~60 min, as additional treatment may be necessary.

Acute illness
- During acute illnesses, insulin and oral glucose-lowering medications should be continued.
- During acute illnesses, testing of plasma glucose and ketones, drinking adequate amounts of fluids, and ingesting carbohydrates are all important.

Acute care facilities
- Establishing an interdisciplinary team, implementation of MNT, and timely diabetes-specific discharge planning improves the care of patients with diabetes during and after hospitalizations.
- Hospitals should consider implementing a diabetes meal-planning system that provides consistency in the carbohydrate content of specific meals.

Long-term care facilities
- The imposition of dietary restrictions on elderly patients with diabetes in long-term care facilities is not warranted. Residents with diabetes should be served a regular menu, with consistency in the amount and timing of carbohydrates.
- An interdisciplinary team approach is necessary to integrate MNT for patients with diabetes into overall management.
- There is no evidence to support prescribing diets such as "no concentrated sweets" or "no sugar added."
- In the institutionalized elderly, undernutrition is likely and caution should be exercised when prescribing weight loss diets.

From American Diabetes Association, Nutrition Recommendations and Interventions for Diabetes: A position statement of the American Diabetes Association. *Diabetes Care.* 2008;31:S61–S78 (with permission)

Table 5
Glycemic Index Values of Certain Foods Adjusted in Relation to the Glycemic
Index of White Bread Considered as 100[a]

Food	Mean	Food	Mean
Breads		**Legumes**	
Rye (crispbread)	95	Baked beans (canned)	70
Rye (wholemeal)	89	Bengal gram dal	12
Rye (whole grain, e.g.. pumpernickel)	68	Butter beans	46
Wheat (white)	100	Chick peas (dried)	47
Wheat (wholemeal)	100	Chick (peas (canned)	60
Pasta		Green peas (canned)	50
Macaroni (white, boiled 5 min)	64	Green peas (dried)	65
Spaghetti (brown, boiled 15 min)	61	Garden peas (frozen)	65
Spaghetti (white, boiled 5 min)	67	Haricot beans (white, dried)	54
Star pasta (white, boiled 5 min)	54	Kidney beans (dried)	43
Cereal grains		Kidney beans (canned)	74
Barley (pearled)	36	Lentils (green, dried)	36
Buckwheat	78	Lentils (green, canned)	74
Bulgur	65	Lentils (red, dried)	38
Millet	103	Pinto beans (dried)	60
Rice (brown)	81	Pinto beans (canned)	64
Rice (instant, boiled 1 min)	65	Peanuts	15
Rice (polished, boiled 5 min)	58	Soya beans (dried)	20
Rice (polished, boiled 10–25 min)	81	Soya beans (canned)	22
Rice (parboiled, boiled 5 min)	54	**Fruit**	
Rice (parboiled, boiled 15 min)	68	Apple	52
Rye kernels	47	Apple juice	45
Sweet corn	80	Banana	84
Wheat kernels	63	Orange	59
Breakfast cereals		Orange juice	71
"All Bran"	74	Raisins	93
Cornflakes	121	**Sugars**	
Muesli	96	Fructose	26
Porridge oats	89	Glucose	138
Puffed rice	132	Honey	126
Puffed wheat	110	Lactose	57
Shredded wheat	97	Maltose	152
"Weetabix"	109	Sucrose	83
Cookies		**Dairy products**	
Digestive	82	Custard	59
Oatmeal	78	Ice cream	69
"Rich tea"	80	Skim milk	46
Plain crackers (water biscuits)	100	Whole milk	44
Shortbread cookies	88	Yogurt	52
Root vegetables		**Snack foods**	
Potato (instant)	120	Corn chips	99

(continued)

Table 5
(continued)

Food	Mean	Food	Mean
Potato (mashed)	98	Potato chips	77
Potato (new/white boiled)	80		
Potato (russet, baked)	116		
Potato (sweet)	70		
Yam	74		

[a]Glycemic index is defined as the blood glucose response to a 50-g available carbohydrate portion of a food expressed as a percentage of the response to the same amount of carbohydrate from a standard food, in this case white bread.

Table 6
Common Nutrition Issues in Hospitalized Patients with Diabetes: Considerations for Healthcare Professionals

Decreased appetite with poor oral intake

- Consistent carbohydrate intake is the goal whether the individual with diabetes is eating regular food or on a progression diet (e.g., clear liquid or full liquid).
- Amount of carbohydrate is more important than source. Allow individuals with diabetes to make substitutions of carbohydrate-containing foods with similar carbohydrate content to maintain consistent intake.
- Snacks and/or supplements may need to be included for individuals with diabetes to ensure adequate calorie and protein intake. The need for snacks should be individualized.
- Insulin dose requirements should be based on "basal" and "nutritional" needs. The "nutritional insulin requirement" includes the amount of insulin necessary to cover enteral or parenteral nutrition, intravenous dextrose, meals, snacks, and/or supplements - not just discrete meals. Combination insulin therapy may be appropriate to cover basal needs and match intermittent nutritional intake.
- For individuals on insulin, it may be appropriate to inject rapid-acting insulin immediately after a meal so that the insulin dose can be more accurately matched to actual carbohydrate intake.

Delayed meals or inconsistent meal timing

- If meals will be delayed or missed due to tests or procedures, nutritional insulin may need to be withheld; however, basal insulin is typically still required.
- For individuals taking oral diabetes medications that may cause hypoglycemia, it may be appropriate to provide a snack if a meal delay is anticipated.

Inconsistent carbohydrate intake

- Inconsistent carbohydrate intake can contribute to either hypo- or hyperglycemia. Individuals who are eating may or may not need snacks, depending on their medication therapy. Individuals with poor nutritional intake may need medication adjustments (i.e., decrease in medications) based upon amount of carbohydrate intake.
- Individuals with diabetes, along with family and hospital volunteers, may need to be educated on the carbohydrate content of foods and to notify hospital staff when the patient is brought food in addition to that of the hospital diet.

(continued)

Table 6
(continued)

- Meal-coverage insulin should not be withheld for "normal" blood glucose levels. It is necessary to cover the carbohydrate content of the meal.

Decreased activity level

- Glucose-lowering medications may need to be adjusted as activity level increases or decreases.

Inconsistent blood glucose monitoring

- When individuals are eating, check blood glucose level before each meal and at bedtime.
- For individuals receiving nothing by mouth, check blood glucose every 4–6 h.

Timing of blood glucose monitoring to meal and insulin/medication delivery

- If the patient is on premeal rapid-acting insulin, wait until the meal tray arrives to give insulin. If the patient is on premeal regular insulin, it can be provided 30 min before the meal, depending on premeal blood glucose results.
- Premeal blood glucose monitoring and insulin injections should be timed in relation to the delivery of the meal, not a predetermined time of day.

Adapted from Swift C.S. and Boucher J.L. Nutrition therapy for the hospitalized patient with diabetes. Endocrine Practice 2006;12(3):61–67vv

VII   RESOURCES

Resources

1. INTRODUCTION

Inappropriate nutrition, increased calorie intake, and lack of exercise usually lead to obesity and the metabolic syndrome, which, in turn, are responsible for several chronic diseases that affect every aspect of a person s life. In addition to prevention and medical treatment, education is the single most important tool for their management. Education is also of major importance in raising public health awareness since it can hopefully help curb the global epidemic of obesity, diabetes, and other disease states associated with the metabolic syndrome.

Following is a list of government agencies and nongovernmental organizations that provide information and resources related to nutrition, obesity, and diabetes.

2. DIABETES ORGANIZATIONS

American Association of Diabetes Educators (AADE)

100 West Monroe, Suite 400
Chicago, IL 60603
Tel: 800-338-3633 or 312-424-2426
Fax: 312-424-2427
Diabetes Educator Access Line: 800-TEAMUP4 (800-832-6874)
Email: aade@aadenet.org
Internet: http://www.diabeteseducator.org

American Diabetes Association (ADA)

1701 North Beauregard Street
Alexandria, VA 22311
Tel: 800-DIABETES (800-342-2383)
Fax: 703-549-6995
Email: askada@diabetes.org
Internet: http://www.diabetes.org

American Podiatric Medical Association (APMA)

9312 Old Georgetown Road
Bethesda, MD 20814-1621
Foot Care Information Center: 800-FOOT-CARE (800-366-8227)
Tel: 301-581-9200
Fax: 301-530-2752
Email: askapma@apma.org
Internet: http://www.apma.org

Diabetes Exercise and Sports Association (DESA)

8001 Montcastle Drive
Nashville, TN 37221
Tel: 800-898-4322
Fax: 602-433-9331
Email: desa@diabetes-exercise.org
Internet: http://www.diabetes-exercise.org

Joslin Diabetes Center

One Joslin Place
Boston, MA 02215
Tel: 800-JOSLIN-1 or 617-732-2400
Internet: http://www.joslin.org

Juvenile Diabetes Research Foundation International (JDRF)

120 Wall Street
New York, NY 10005-4001
Tel: 800-533-CURE (2873)
Fax: 212-785-9595
Email: info@jdrf.org
Internet: http://www.jdf.org

International Diabetic Federation (IDF)

Avenue Emile De Mot 19 – B-1000
Brussels, Belgium
Tel: +32-2-538-55-11
Fax: +32-2-538-51-14
Email: info@idf.org
Internet: http://www.idf.org

Centers for Disease Control and Prevention (CDC)

National Center for Chronic Disease Prevention and Health Promotion
Division of Diabetes Translation
P.O. Box 8728
Silver Spring, MD 20910
Tel: 877-CDC-DIAB (877-232-3422)

Fax: 301-562-1050
Email: diabetes@cdc.gov
Internet: http://www.cdc.gov/diabetes

3. OBESITY ORGANIZATIONS

Academy for Eating Disorders (AED)

60 Revere Drive, Suite 500
Northbrook, IL 60062
Tel: 847-498-4274
Fax: 847-480-9282
Email: aed@aedweb.org
Internet: http://www.aedweb.org

American Obesity Association (AOA)

1250 24th Street, NW
Suite 300
Washington, DC 20037
Tel: 202-776-7711
Fax: 202-776-7712
Internet: http://www.obesity.org

American Society for Bariatric Surgery (ASBS)

100 SW 75th Street
Suite 201
Gainesville, FL 32607
Tel: 352-331-4900
Fax: 352-331-4975
Email: info@asbs.org
Internet: http://www.asbs.org

American Society of Bariatric Physicians (ASBP)

2821 S. Parker Rd., Ste. 625
Aurora, CO 80014
Tel: 303-770-2526
Fax: 303-779-4834
Email: info@asbp.org
Internet: http://www.asbp.org

International Association for the Study of Obesity (IASO)

231 North Gower Street, London NW1 2NS, UK
Tel: +44-20-7691-1900
Fax: +44-20-7387-6033
Email: inquiries@iaso.org/obesity@iotf.org
Internet: http://www.iaso.org/http://www.iotf.org

North American Association for the Study of Obesity (NAASO)

8630 Fenton Street, Suite 918
Silver Spring, MD 20910
Tel: 301-563-6526
Fax: 301-563-6595
Internet: http://www.naaso.org

4. NUTRITION

American Society for Nutrition (ASN)

9650 Rockville Pike
Suite L-5500
Bethesda, MD 20814
Tel: 301-634-7050
Fax: 301-634-7892
Email: sec@nutrition.org
Internet: http://www.nutrition.org

United States Department of Agriculture (USDA) Center for Nutrition Policy and Promotion

3101 Park Center Drive
Room 1034
Alexandria, VA 22302-1594
Tel: 1-888-7pyramid
Email: support@cnpp.usda.gov
Internet: http://www.mypyramid.gov

Harvard School of Public Health (HSPH) Department of Nutrition

665 Huntington Avenue
Boston, MA 02115
Tel: 617-432-1851
Fax: 617-432-2435
Email: cstover@hsph.harvard.edu
Internet: http://www.hsph.harvard.edu/academics/nutr

World Health Organization (WHO) Department of Nutrition for Health and Development

Avenue Appia 20
1211 Geneva 27
Switzerland
Fax: +41-22-791-41-56
Email: nutrition@who.int
Internet: http://www.who.int/nutrition

National Health Information Center

P.O. Box 1133
Washington, DC 20013-1133

Tel: 800-336-4797
Email: info@nhic.org
Internet: http://www.healthierus.gov

Aristides Daskalopoulos Foundation (IAD)

10, Ziridi str
Maroussi 15123, Greece
Tel: +30-211-3494101
Fax: +30-211-3494128
Email: infor@iad.gr
Internet: http://www.iad.gr

American Society for Parenteral and Enteral Nutrition (ASPEN)

8630 Fenton Street, Suite 412
Silver Spring, MD 20910
Tel: 800-727-4567 or 301-587-6315
Fax: 301-587-2365
Email: aspen@nutr.org
Internet: http://www.nutritioncare.org

Dietary Guidelines for Americans

U.S. Department of Agriculture and U.S. Department of Health and Human Services
Internet: http://www.health.gov/dietaryguidelines

U.S. Food and Drug Administration (FDA)

Office of Consumer Affairs
5600 Fishers Lane
Rockville, MD 20857
Tel: 888-INFO-FDA (463-6332) and 888-SAFE FOOD (888-723-3366) (Food Information Line)
Fax: 301-443-9767
Internet: http://www.fda.gov

Food and Nutrition Information Center (FNIC)

USDA/ARS/National Agricultural Library
10301 Baltimore Avenue, Room 105
Beltsville, MD 20705-2351
Tel: 301-504-5719; TTY: 301-504-6856
Fax: 301-504-6409
Email: fnic@nal.usda.gov
Internet: http://www.nal.usda.gov/fnic

U.S. Department of Agriculture (USDA)

1400 Independence Ave., SW
Washington, DC 20250

Tel: 800-727-9540 and 202-720-2791
Internet: http://www.usda.gov

U.S. Government's Food Safety Web Site

http://www.foodsafety.gov

5. ORGANIZATIONS OF COMMON INTEREST

American Academy of Pediatrics (AAP)

141 Northwest Point Boulevard
Elk Grove Village, IL 60007-1098
Tel: 847-434-4000 or 888-227-1770
Email: csc@aap.org
Internet: http://www.aap.org

American Association of Clinical Endocrinologists (AACE)

1000 Riverside Avenue
Suite 205, Jacksonville, FL 32204
Tel: 904-353-7878
Fax: 904-353-8185
Email: info@aace.com
Internet: http://www.aace.com

American Dietetic Association (ADA)

120 South Riverside Plaza, Suite 2000
Chicago, IL 60606-6995
Tel: 800-366-1655
Fax: 312-899-4739
Email: hotline@eatright.org
Internet: http://www.eatright.org

American Heart Association

7272 Greenville Avenue
Dallas, TX 75231-4596
Tel: 800-AHA-USA1 (800-242-8721) or 214-706-1220
Fax: 214-706-1341
Internet: http://www.americanheart.org

Endocrine Society

4350 East West Highway, Suite 500
Bethesda, MD 20814-4426
Tel: 301-941-0200
Fax: 301-941-0259
Email: societyservices@endo-society.org
Internet: http://www.endo-society.org

National Cancer Institute (NCI)

Public Inquiries Office
6116 Executive Boulevard
Room 3036A
Bethesda, MD 20892-8322
Tel: 800-4-CANCER (800-422-6237); TTY: 800-332-8615
Email: cancergovstaff@mail.nih.gov
Internet: http://www.cancer.gov

National Center on Sleep Disorders Research

National Heart, Lung, and Blood Institute
6705 Rockledge Drive
Suite 6022
Bethesda, MD 20892-7993
Tel: 301-435-0199
Fax: 301-480-3451
Email: ncsdr@nih.gov
Internet: http://www.nhlbi.nih.gov/sleep

National Heart, Lung, and Blood Institute (NHLBI) Information Center

Education Programs Information Center
P.O. Box 30105
Bethesda, MD 20824-0105
Tel: 301-592-8573; TTY: 240-629-3255
Fax: 240-629-3246
Email: nhlbiinfo@nhlbi.nih.gov
Internet: http://www.nhlbi.nih.gov

National Institute on Aging (NIA)

Information Center
P.O. Box 8057
Gaithersburg, MD 20898
Tel: 800-222-2225; TTY: 800-222-4225
Email: niaic@jbs1.com
Internet: http://www.nia.nih.gov

North American Society for Pediatric Gastroenterology, Hepatology, and Nutrition (NASPGHAN)

P.O. Box 6
Flourtown, PA 19031
Tel: 215-233-0808
Fax: 215-233-3918
Email: naspghan@naspghan.org
Internet: http://www.naspghan.org

Index

About the Editor

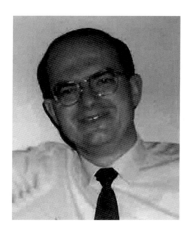

Christos Mantzoros is an Associate Professor of Medicine at Harvard Medical School and an Associate Professor in Environmental Health at the Harvard School of Public Health. He serves as the Clinical Research Overseer of the Division of Endocrinology Diabetes and Metabolism at Beth Israel Deaconess Medical Center and the Joslin Diabetes Center and he is a member of the Executive Committee of the Scholars in Clinical Science Program, a postgraduate clinical investigators training program at Harvard Medical School.

Dr. Mantzoros obtained an MD and DSc from the University of Athens Medical School, a Master's in Clinical Epidemiology from Harvard School of Public Health and a Master's in Medical Sciences (Clinical Investigation) from Harvard Medical School. He has received Board certification in Internal Medicine, Endocrinology, Diabetes and Metabolism and in Clinical Nutrition.

At the Harvard Medical School, he sees patients, teaches and conducts research on obesity and diabetes/metabolic diseases. His main research focus is the physiology, pathophysiology and potential therapeutic significance of adipokines, including leptin and adiponectin. Towards this goal, his lab utilizes a range of basic, translational and clinical research tools.

Dr. Mantzoros is an internationally recognized expert on obesity and diabetes and has published two books (one on *Diabetes and Obesity* and one on *Nutrition and Metabolism*), more than 200 original papers, more than 90 chapters and reviews and has received more than 10,000 citations. He serves on the Editorial Board of several journals including the *Journal of Clinical Endocrinology and Metabolism* and has been elected a member of ASCI. He has served as an advisor to Pharmaceutical and Diagnostics companies and is the scientific co-founder and Chair of the Scientific Advisory Board of InteKrin Metabolic Therapeutics. He has been given several awards including the prestigious American Association of Clinical Endocrinology Frontiers in Science Award, the Novartis Award in Diabetes and Metabolic Diseases, the Lilly Award by the North American Association for the Study of Obesity, the American Society for Nutrition Mead Johnson Award, the HypoCCS award in Paris, France, the Wilhelm Friedrich Bessel Award by the Humboldt Foundation of Germany, The Hygeia Award of the New England Hellenic Medical and Dental Society and the Outstanding Investigator Award by the American Federation of Medical Research. He is also the recipient of the BIDMC and Harvard Medical School award for excellence in Mentoring. Dr. Mantzoros is listed in Who's Who in America.

About the Series Editor

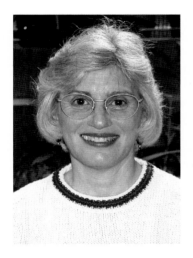

Dr. Adrianne Bendich is Clinical Director, Medical Affairs at GlaxoSmithKline (GSK) Consumer Healthcare, where she is responsible for leading the innovation and medical programs in support of many well-known brands including TUMS and Os-Cal. Dr. Bendich had primary responsibility for GSK's support for the Women's Health Initiative (WHI) intervention study. Prior to joining GSK, Dr. Bendich was at Roche Vitamins Inc. and was involved with the groundbreaking clinical studies showing that folic acid-containing multivitamins significantly reduced major classes of birth defects. Dr. Bendich has coauthored over 100 major clinical research studies in the area of preventive nutrition. Dr. Bendich is recognized as a leading authority on antioxidants, nutrition and immunity and pregnancy outcomes, vitamin safety, and the cost-effectiveness of vitamin/mineral supplementation.

Dr. Bendich is the editor of nine books including *Preventive Nutrition: The Comprehensive Guide for Health Professionals* coedited with Dr. Richard Deckelbaum, and is Series Editor of *Nutrition and Health* for Humana Press with 29 published volumes including *Probiotics in Pediatric Medicine* edited by Dr. Sonia Michail and Dr. Philip Sherman; *Handbook of Nutrition and Pregnancy* edited by Dr. Carol Lammi-Keefe, Dr. Sarah Couch and Dr. Elliot Philipson; *Nutrition and Rheumatic Disease* edited by Dr. Laura Coleman; *Nutrition and Kidney Disease* edited by Dr. Laura Byham-Grey, Dr. Jerrilynn Burrowes, and Dr. Glenn Chertow; *Nutrition and Health in Developing Countries* edited by Dr. Richard Semba and Dr. Martin Bloem; *Calcium in Human Health* edited by Dr. Robert Heaney and Dr. Connie Weaver; and *Nutrition and Bone Health* edited by Dr. Michael Holick and Dr. Bess Dawson-Hughes.

Dr. Bendich served as Associate Editor for *Nutrition* (the international journal), served on the Editorial Board of the *Journal of Women's Health and Gender-Based Medicine,* and was a member of the Board of Directors of the American College of Nutrition.

Dr. Bendich was the recipient of the Roche Research Award, was a *Tribute to Women and Industry* Awardee, and was a recipient of the Burroughs Wellcome Visiting Professorship in Basic Medical Sciences, 2000–2001. In 2008, Dr. Bendich was given the Council for Responsible Nutrition (CRN) Apple Award in recognition of her many contributions to the scientific understanding of dietary supplements. Dr. Bendich holds academic appointments as Adjunct Professor in the Department of Preventive Medicine and Community Health at UMDNJ and has an adjunct appointment at the Institute of Nutrition, Columbia University P&S, and is an Adjunct Research Professor, Rutgers University, Newark Campus. She is listed in Who's Who in American Women.